TEN THOUSAND CROSSROADS

Ten Thousand Crossroads

The Path as I Remember It

BALFOUR MOUNT

McGill-Queen's University Press
Montreal & Kingston • London • Chicago

© McGill-Queen's University Press 2020

ISBN 978-0-2280-0354-0 (cloth)
ISBN 978-0-2280-0490-5 (ePDF)
ISBN 978-0-2280-0491-2 (ePUB)

Legal deposit fourth quarter 2020
Bibliothèque nationale du Québec

Printed in Canada on acid-free paper that is 100% ancient forest free
(100% post-consumer recycled), processed chlorine free

Funded by the   Financé par le
Government   gouvernement   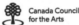   Canada Council   Conseil des arts
of Canada   du Canada   for the Arts   du Canada

We acknowledge the support of the Canada Council for the Arts.
Nous remercions le Conseil des arts du Canada de son soutien.

Library and Archives Canada Cataloguing in Publication

Title: Ten thousand crossroads : the path as I remember it / Balfour Mount.
Other titles: 10,000 crossroads
Names: Mount, Balfour M., author.
Description: Includes bibliographical references and index.
Identifiers: Canadiana (print) 20200229478 | Canadiana (ebook) 20200229516
 | ISBN 9780228003540 (cloth) | ISBN 9780228004905 (ePDF) | ISBN
 9780228004912 (ePUB)
Subjects: LCSH: Mount, Balfour M. | LCSH: Royal Victoria Hospital (Montréal,
 Québec)—Employees—Biography. | LCSH: Physicians—Canada—Biography.
 | LCSH: Surgeons—Canada—Biography. | LCSH: Palliative treatment—Canada—History.
 | LCSH: Hospice care—Canada—History. | LCSH: Terminal care—Canada—History.
 | LCGFT: Autobiographies.
Classification: LCC R464.M68 A3 2020 | DDC 610.92—dc23

This book was typeset in 10.5/13 Sabon.

For the patients, family members, and caregivers
who have been my teachers,
and
for Linda,
my partner and collaborator

Contents

Foreword

The current literature is replete with books on death and dying, suffering and its amelioration, and the spiritual component of our lives. They are penned by the dying, their caregivers, and professionals with varied backgrounds. There are also biographies of eminent people who have influenced our views and responses to these elements of the human condition.

Ten Thousand Crossroads: The Path As I Remember It is, I believe, the first autobiography of a seminal leader in the development of palliative care, a term encompassing the issues outlined above and indeed coined by the author, Dr Balfour Mount.

Dr Mount was a urologic oncology surgeon, and a good one. In the early 1970s he attended a talk by Elisabeth Kubler Ross at McGill University. It opened new circuits in an already fertile mind. The speaker brought the hospice work of Dr Cicely Saunders in England to his attention. Dr Mount contacted Dr Saunders, who invited him to spend a week with her at London's St Christopher's Hospice. The rest is history. He returned to McGill where, in a time of financial restraint, he convinced government, faculty, and hospital leaders to support a palliative-care program at Montreal's Royal Victoria Hospital. This program stands as the world's first fully articulated palliative-care initiative. Its components included a dedicated ward in a major teaching hospital, a home-care program, a consultation service for the active-treatment wards of the hospital, a unique volunteer section, music therapy, and a bereavement-support program for family members and caregivers. All of the above was built upon a scholarly research and education foundation endorsed by the McGill Faculty of Medicine.

While the call to develop "patient-centred care" is now universally accepted and gradually influencing practice, the Royal Victoria's Palliative Care Service was a groundbreaking initiative. It is also a model that remains valid today. As decades pass, this program, married with Dr Mount's research, writing, and powerful lectures, has had a significant impact on the adoption of the principles of palliative care in Canada, the United States, and across the international community.

The story of Dr Mount's life and the influences that caused a boy from Ottawa to become a leader of singular import is extraordinarily interesting. His is a tale of adventure, challenges (he personally encountered a variety of life-threatening events and, as a pioneer with insights far ahead of his time, many obstacles set up by "in the box" colleagues), and encounters with engaging and influential men and women.

William Osler said that "it helps a man immensely to be a bit of a hero worshipper" and Dr Mount illustrates the wisdom of this aphorism. He learned from many people and holds them as heroes even as he is held as a hero by those he has influenced. I must acknowledge my membership in this coterie. His discussion on the importance of spirituality and the imperative to include it in our lives and practice is essential reading. You may share my experience; while spirituality is often talked about in a somewhat mystical fashion, after reading this book I think I finally "get it." After all, Dr Mount is a surgeon, skilled at grasping the core of matters and describing them in lucid terms.

Above all, readers may look forward to an engrossing and witty read. Dr Mount's style is engaging; he is a man who loves all avenues of cultural expression – music, art, photography (he is a skilled artist and photographer himself), movies, theatre, and literature captivate him. He is an optimist and enthusiast about people and cultural events. How many times have I heard him say, "Neil, you MUST read this – or see that, it's FABULOUS!"

The product of a man of intellect combined with passion and broad interests and experiences, *Ten Thousand Crossroads* is a book delightful to read and to reflect upon. It will be welcomed by health-care professionals, but it will also be warmly received by a general audience. After all, Dr Mount's experience and insights touch on issues important to all of us. Enjoy.

Neil MacDonald
Emeritus Professor of Medicine and Oncology
McGill University and the University of Alberta

Acknowledgments

Considerable credit for this narrative goes to my wife, Linda, my mentor Ken MacKinnon, and indeed to all the teachers, both professional and non-professional, who have helped me to appreciate how difficult it is for me to be *radically present* and to *really listen.* In particular, I acknowledge my profound debt to my patients, their families, and my remarkably gifted and infinitely patient Royal Victoria Hospital and McGill-Queen's University Press colleagues.

Photographs of patients included here were always taken with the subject's permission and have been used over the decades in countless lectures relating to care of the dying. On such occasions they have been my valued colleagues in spreading the palliative-care message, as promised to each of them when I took the photograph.

Most photographs were taken by the author or received as a gift from the subject. In the case of professional portraits, acknowledgment is provided in the captions. The 1945 sketch of the author is by Winston Elliott. All other drawings and paintings are by the author.

In citing credit due, one must not omit existential and spiritual considerations, which are so essential to us all if there is to be light and meaning for our journey. The journey from self to Self, from ego to union, moves ever forward, but toward what end? Ah, there's the rub, as we each negotiate our ten thousand crossroads. In this sacred domain I gratefully acknowledge the lengthy and unexpectedly diverse assembly whom you will encounter in these pages.

Balfour Mount
Montreal
March 2020

TEN THOUSAND CROSSROADS

Beginning at 37

Home is where one starts from.

T.S. Eliot

A toddler, I was sitting on the kitchen floor clanging the lid clutched in my left hand against an array of cooking pots that I had laboriously pulled from the cupboard beside me in an effort to find the best fit. Mother was working quietly two or three feet away, near the window overlooking the back garden. Although I could see little of the sky from my vantage point, it felt like a sunny day. The counters and the cupboard doors were a cool, pale yellow. I don't recall any conversation between Mother and me. Perhaps she was humming. It was a safe, warm, expansive place to explore the world. It is, I believe, my earliest memory.

When I attempt to recapture similar early moments, I generally find myself at "37," the family enclave that would, over the ensuing eight decades, gain archetypal significance for three generations of Mounts. Other vignettes related to those years find me in various rooms of our Opeongo Road, Ottawa, home: waking from the quiet of an afternoon nap, riding perched on Dad's arms as he moved from room to room pointing out details in the paintings, enjoying the dazzling sun glinting off Dow's Lake sailboats just across the road, and playing games with my older sister, Alice, who was my constant companion in concocting adventures.

In the earliest recollection to which a date can be affixed, I am in the front hall, watching longingly as Dad and my brother, Jim, seven years my senior, were leaving to attend the 25 July 1941 memorial service in St Anthony, Newfoundland, honouring Sir Wilfred Grenfell who had died nine months earlier. How desperately I wanted to go with them! "He was a great man; he meant a lot to Mommy and Daddy, but no, Balfour, you won't be able to go with us this time." I was two years old.

Another, much later, moment comes to mind. It was Saturday and as I wakened that morning I was greeted by the sun pouring in through the window at the foot of my bed. The rays that bathed the room illuminated thousands of dancing, vibrating particles in the still air. I was transfixed, my attention held, as if suspended out of time. I can't estimate how long I lay there mesmerized, but the memory remains wrapped in a sense of wonder, this lifetime later.

Those early years were shaped by an experience of unconditional love coupled with clearly defined limits and expectations. "No, we don't think that an allowance is a good idea. If you need money for something, come and tell us and we will discuss it." Family prayers at meals and bedtime were the norm. Holy days, holidays, and Sunday services in the United Church were all celebrated as part of a taken-for-granted cultural reality, rather like the sable and white collies that sequentially lived in our backyard. "The proper place for a dog is outside in a kennel, not in the house. That's the way it was on the farm." Love and limits fostered enthusiasm. Central to it all, Mother was the glue. She was our compass, our centre of gravity, the wind in our sails.

SETTING AND CAST: AN OVERVIEW

37 Opeongo Road, or simply 37, was the family cornerstone. More than a house, more than a home, it was a responsive, welcoming catalyst for our lives, an active player weaving the fabric of each day as it accumulated layer upon layer of family lore, meaning, and the sense of community that marked our comings and goings. Its stately white clapboard elegance overlooked Dow's Lake across the road from a vantage point atop the steeply sloped property. Each detail of home and surroundings had been meticulously designed and planned by my mother, Maude Adeline Henry Mount. She led from the middle of the pack. She was best friend, confidante, and caregiver to each of us. Her shrewd insight, intuitive grasp of current circumstances, organizational skills, and fierce loyalty to each family member was shot through with humour. She planned the daily agenda and saw it through without fuss. She was where everything started and ended.

With auburn hair, brown eyes, and medium height, Mother radiated a dynamic energy that was other-person oriented, always directing attention and conversation away from herself toward others. Quietly ambitious yet self-effacing, she had little interest in politics, social status, theatre, classical music, philosophy, or literature. She enjoyed gardening. While radiating quiet confidence and determination in public, privately she was reflective and self-questioning. She was an admirer of strong Christian faith but often questioned her own. Though she actively attempted to live out the Gospel message as she understood it, she firmly believed that such troublesome legal details as speed limits, parking meters, and international customs regulations were meant for others and had little relevance to her.

Maudie was the third daughter of Addie and D.W. Henry, owner of the department store that dominated the crossroad community of Springfield, Ontario. In her late teens she qualified as a teacher at the Toronto Normal School, and then, following a brief pedagogical career that failed to fulfill her aspirations, she turned to a career in nursing training at St Luke's Hospital in New York City.

There was a part of Maude that was uneasy in some social circumstances, as seen in her agitation when asked to host a tea in our home for Norman Vincent Peale, the American minister, author, professional speaker, and popularizer of the power of positive thinking. That rather stilted event took place accompanied by my delight in whispered teasing: "A little over-impressed with celebrity status aren't we?" To which came her quick retort, "I've never heard of such stuff and nonsense!"

She added spice, flair, and a dash of innocent irreverence to all she touched. Her introductions at one particularly stiff Sunday dinner for ten illustrate the point. Her guests included a starchy visiting minister and his ever-so-prim wife, an elderly bachelor senator, and a couple who were neighbourhood friends – Harold Grey, a soft-spoken, internationally known entomologist, and his diminutive wife, Billie. When mother introduced Dr Grey to the good reverend's wife, the woman's response was decidedly cool, causing Mother to add enthusiastically, "Oh, you don't know Harold? Why he's one of the best-known buggers in Canada!" With that, as I recall, I coughed up my last spoonful of soup, while Dad, whose reserve was usually the real target of such zingers, managed a deadpan expression. From my earliest years, I sensed that he secretly cherished her flair. She was fun to be with.

Dad, Harry Telford Roy Mount, with his 6'2" stature, radiated an arresting aura of quiet presence. His hazel eyes, bushy black eyebrows, and evident interest in all around him gave him an attentive, evaluative air. He was, in a word, earnest. Though he was an Ontario farm boy at heart, his improbable journey from rural Ontario to the battles of Vimy Ridge and Passchendaele and then on to university (a first for his family) had resulted in him becoming a gifted neurosurgeon, Ottawa's first. His "back forty" and Mayo Clinic-honed abilities enabled him to be equally at home when wielding an axe to split firewood, resecting a brain tumour, or removing an advanced abdominal malignancy, each pursuit benefiting from his unwavering focused attention. His posture was always militarily erect, his dress immaculate, his gait brisk, measured, and always in exact step with his generally unaware partner.

He was a tireless advocate for his patients, and his medical/surgical practice was his constant preoccupation during the years he was "active in the profession." He was particularly seduced by diagnostic mysteries and surgical challenges and was at his best when solving a convoluted maze of clinical problems: the more complex, the more he was intrigued.

Following their June 1925 wedding and surgical training in Minnesota under the Brothers Mayo and their Canadian expatriate colleague, Dr Donald Balfour (my namesake), Harry and Maude made their way to St Anthony, Newfoundland, and the outports that dotted the Labrador coast. They spent three years working at the Grenfell Mission, my father as doctor and my mother as nurse and elementary school teacher. Their days were busy – driving dog teams and travelling by schooner; holding clinics in the tiny communities that dotted the barren coast; doing surgery, both in the operating room of the compact wood-frame St Anthony hospital with its sign boldly proclaiming "FAITH HOPE AND LOVE ABIDE BUT THE GREATEST OF THESE IS LOVE" and, as circumstances dictated, on the kitchen tables of humble family dwellings in the outports – and all the while they took great pleasure in the no-frills, bare-bones, adventure-filled world of the deep-sea fishers, hunters, and trappers who welcomed them to those rocky shores.

At home, Dad was the instigator of dinner discussions on topics ranging from current affairs to ethics, politics, and theology. On the infrequent evenings during my early years when he returned from the office before I was in bed, he would invite me to sit on his lap on the green-leather couch in the library while he read the comics to me from the evening newspaper. He was devoted to family but deferred to Mother in all decisions regarding family affairs and the day-to-day management of their alcohol-free home. Mysteriously, their alcohol prohibition did not extend to ultra-sweet, kosher Manischewitz wine in spite of its 11 per cent alcohol content. "Medicinal, you know."

Jim was the eldest of Mother and Dad's three children. He and I couldn't have differed more strikingly. He was blond, an introvert who read constantly (*War and Peace* and *Les Misérables* when he was fifteen) and often was retiring in relationships. From an early age, he loved philosophical discourse and classical music. He played the E-flat alto horn. Our seven-year age difference meant that he was a larger-than-life role model in my eyes. In response to my "damning" someone when I was perhaps eight, he cited biblical authority to advise me that my pronouncement placed me at risk of "eternal damnation." Though I wasn't sure what that meant, it didn't sound good.

Jim was responsible for introducing me to many of the finer things in life: making model airplanes from balsa wood, our endless succession of collies, a quality high-fidelity sound system equipped with a three-speed turntable, music from Beethoven to Swing (Benny Goodman, Glenn Miller, the Dorsey Brothers, and the incomparable Sinatra), a sporty metallic-blue convertible Singer car which somehow he persuaded Mother that she needed, alpine skiing, and the mysteries of the teen years, including breakneck, high-octane slaloming on the hills at Camp Fortune while lustily singing, "Cigareets, corn-whisky and Maybelline Linsky, they'll drive you crazy, they'll drive you insane!" – a ditty rendered at top volume by the members of his pick-up band that included his friends Russell Nixon ("Nix"), Al Carlyle ("Al Co-Hall"), and Al Hodgins ("Hadge"). I recall being included in Jim's activities only once during my formative years. When I was about ten, he took me with him to the Rockcliffe Air Show. What a thrill to accompany my big brother!

Our sister, Alice, sandwiched in age between her two brothers, was three years younger than Jim. Tall, brunette, and gangly as she negotiated the shoals of adolescence, she had the added burden of too many well-meaning advisers.

"Stand up straight."

"Use your napkin!"

"Always do this!"

"Never do that!"

"Al" found school less than captivating and considered academic prowess a poor yardstick of human worth. Taking her leave from the hurly-burly of home life, she spent her high school years at Ontario Ladies' College in Whitby and then returned home for secretarial courses prior to studying at Western University in London, Ontario. In her late teens, she developed singing skills, learned to play the cello, and, under the tutelage of Aunt Marian, became proficient in elocution, giving dramatic readings such as "The Moo Cow Moo" and "Seein' Things at Night" with considerable polish. She went on to develop a small group of close friends who remained loyal through life.

Al was more than a sister. She was my soulmate, friend, and the person with whom I shared childhood. We dressed up as pirates, royalty, courtiers, and any number of heroic folk immersed in high drama. Family car trips found us spending hours playing cards and pick-up-sticks on the back seat. I could always count on her openness and readiness to take her little brother seriously. She became my lifelong confidante and a source of unswerving support.

Our closeness in childhood was to lead to a connection that deepened over subsequent decades through letters, telephone calls, and visits to each other's home in Montreal and Cambridge, England. On hearing my voice on the line, whether from across the city or the Atlantic, her response was always the same – "Bal!!" – delivered in a half-shout that was tinged with overtones of seriousness and anticipated importance, respect, joy, and total presence. I always felt deeply blessed to have such a caring sister.

It was in the mid-1940s that Mother and Dad sought to recruit a live-in housekeeper. Helen appeared to meet the requirements and was hired for a three-month trial period. Within a couple of weeks, her true ambitions were clarified when, at the first empty-house opportunity, she cleaned out all cash, silverware, and moveable valuables before disappearing along with her pseudonym into the shifting crowds celebrating the end of the war.

Enter Corporal Nettie Dufour. Among Nettie's first day duties was the supervision of my evening bath, a level of personal exposure that I found frankly embarrassing until it became evident that, for Nettie, the task ranked with feeding the chickens back on the farm. A no-nonsense, down-to-earth gal had just joined the family.

Nettie, of Icelandic stock from Foam Lake, Saskatchewan, completed the family when she joined us in 1946 at the age of thirty-eight. She had been a cook (for several hundred at a sitting) in the Canadian Army during the war. Though she was self-effacing and quiet, her weathered face and diminutive, wiry frame were accompanied by surprising strength and prairie practicality. She wore her greying hair pulled tightly back. Ever-vigilant, Nettie kept an eagle eye on her particular kingdom – the family kitchen, the laundry, and the assorted artillery pieces related to household cleanliness.

While Nettie was considered an indispensable family member, she preferred to eat on her own, perched on her special four-legged stool in the kitchen where she could "keep an eye on things." For Nettie, the kettle always boiled more quickly if she stood over it, pressing down on the lid with both hands. Tea was sipped around a sugar cube held firmly between her front teeth and chores were, by definition, a dawn-to-dusk affair, as they had been on the farm. She and Mother were congenial semi-independent teammates, with Mother the token commandant. Mother's perennial good nature could, however, be seriously ruffled when, on occasion, Nettie would make an 11 p.m. unexpected visit to

Mother and Dad's bedroom, her arms loaded with freshly laundered, neatly folded clothes, commenting as she kicked their bedroom door open with her foot, "Don't let me interrupt. I just thought I'd put these things away."

Nettie had an enquiring mind. She read the daily newspaper intently and tracked all household activities and conversations with interest and attention to detail. During one of my parents' infrequent Sunday dinner parties, Dad was holding forth with a detailed description of the surgery he had recently performed on a head-injury patient, much to the chagrin of his blanching non-medical guests. "It became clear that the lad was bleeding heavily into his brain, and things were getting worse instead of settling down," he enthused.

Nettie was at the far end of the dining room, halfway through the door to the kitchen, having just delivered to Mother a tureen of piping hot soup. With Dad's description she froze in mid-stride and spun around, intrigued by his therapeutic dilemma. "What did you do, turn a bone flap?" she queried. "Exactly!" he roared back enthusiastically from his end of the astonished assembly. For twenty years, Nettie was a much loved and respected member of the family.

This family census must, of course, include Pal, Beau, Big Mike, and the other ever-alert collies that over the years faithfully patrolled our yard and the adjacent street. Jim's dog, Pal, the first in our long line of Lassie variants, served sentry duty during the early years and was the main catalyst for the intermittent Hatfield-McCoy tensions between the Mount clan and our neighbours, the Puddicombes.

It was obstetrician Dr John F. Puddicombe who, on 18 January 1943, attended Holland's Princess Juliana during the delivery of her baby girl at the Ottawa Civic Hospital (OCH). The thirty-three-year-old princess had been living in Ottawa since the German invasion of the Low Countries in the spring of 1940. While the birth elevated Dr Puddicombe to semi-regal status in some eyes, that perception escaped Pal, and the best our two families could manage was an uneasy truce, given Pal's incessant barking (a potential at all hours of the day and night) and her determined attempts to herd the Puddicombe's car.

Pal made a habit of concealing herself in the long grass on the strategic high bluff of the corner vacant lot adjacent to our home. It was an ideal spot from which to keep an eye on the Puddicombe garage, just up the hill on Crescent Heights. She could lie in wait unseen for hours watching for the emergence of the hated "four-wheeled creature" that lived there. Then, as the elegant vehicle floated past, Dr Puddicombe enthroned on the buffalo-skin robe that graced the driver's seat, she would suddenly materialize and rocket down the several yards of embankment to the road, all snarls and teeth. Undoubtedly, she was a formidable terrorist for both car and driver! When, in due course, Pal finally ended up under the wheels, she suffered a broken back. Since this distressing event occurred only days before Jim's year-end examinations, all steps were taken to save her. She was operated on, placed in a cast, and eventually made a remarkable recovery. But things had changed. Pal no longer chased the Puddicombe car. It was Mother's sharp eye and appreciation for irony that first led to our being aware of her new strategy. With intentionality that was hard to miss, Pal befriended the border collie pup recently acquired by the Puddicombes, taught it to join her at the vacant lot hideaway, and then trained it to deliver terrorist attacks on the Puddicombe family car. Pal watched with satisfaction as her pupil undertook the attacks alone while Pal supervised approvingly from the bluff above. The Puddicombes sold the dog in short order.

One additional person integral to family functioning must be mentioned. Andrew Hutchins served as an intermittent, but crucial, mainstay at 37, our carpenter, painter, plumber, repair man, and all-round building consultant. He was taciturn and spare in build and actions.

The diminutive Mr Hutchins had thinning, sandy-grey hair that peeked out from under a faded cloth cap. A pencil stub invariably protruded from behind his ear. He carried a small coil-bound, dog-eared pad of paper in his shirt pocket, along with the "fixings" for his anemic "roll-yer-owns." His overalls and work shoes had seen a lot of mileage and his pockets were home to an intriguing array of tools, most prominently an old penknife and a massive cloth appendage that served as a handkerchief, oil cloth, paint rag, and mop. I never learned when Hutchins first reached our shores from the old country, but he was living proof of the adage suggesting that while you can take the boy from the homeland, you can't take the homeland from the boy. On first meeting, he was asked to clarify his muttered name and replied with greater emphasis, "M'name is Handrew Utchins ... but you can call me Handy." And "Handy" he remained over all the years we were privileged to know him.

THE SECOND WORLD WAR, 1939–45

As I joined the family in 1939, the planet was being dragged into the Second World War. It was to be the deadliest military conflict in history, a global conflagration that spawned both unimaginable brutality and diabolic refinement in the capacity to kill. One hundred million military personnel were mobilized. There were more than sixty million fatalities, including civilian deaths by the millions through such horrors as the Holocaust, the fire bombings of Hamburg, Dresden, and Tokyo, and the first military use of atomic weapons at Hiroshima and Nagasaki. There were more than forty-four thousand Canadian military deaths.[1] I was six when the war ended.

Thanks to parental shielding, my memories of those years involve few war-related moments. These scattered recollections include the sun-drenched Sunday afternoon when the family rushed from the dinner table to the front lawn to shout our "Hurrahs" enthusiastically and wave our dinner napkins to cousin Bob Rogers as he and his crew roared over our home prior to heading their aircraft toward Europe. To me, it seemed *such* a celebration! Dad's stony silence, rigid posture, and stiffened expression left me puzzled.

There were few other reminders of war, but one evening I was tottering off to bed fuzzy-headed when the doorbell rang. It was Mr Mitchell, the august neighbour directly behind 37 on Crescent Heights. As he stood there framed in our doorway, the aura of formality that generally surrounded him in my young eyes was endlessly enhanced by the impressive tin hat that he wore. It featured an imposing "W" emblazoned across the front.

Dad's welcoming, "Why, hello Wellington. You and Mildred and the children are well, I trust?" was aborted by a prepared opening volley. "Evening, Doctor." (Perhaps he said "Harry" but the memorable formality of the visit brings to mind that more official salutation.) "As the designated air-raid warden for our community, I am calling at each home in the neighbourhood." Dad's expression was quizzical yet suitably sober. The notion of an air raid occurring in our tranquil surroundings seemed the height of incongruity, but the underlying principle of preparedness needed no explanation. We were, after all, at war. "Won't you come in?" At first, I thought Mr Mitchell was angry as he stepped into the foyer. "I want to ensure that you understand that *all* lights must be turned out when the air raid siren is sounded." His tone seemed threatening. "You may use a candle, but it must not be visible from outside. Finally, you must at all times have a pail of sand and a shovel at the ready in the attic." Dad nodded gravely as I tried to picture how that would protect us, but I found assurance in the certainty that my father would take care of everything. Meanwhile, Jim spent hours in our bedroom making his balsa-wood models of the legendary airplanes defending us, most memorably the de Havilland Mosquito, which, once completed, was suspended from the ceiling above the card table where he worked. I was strictly ordered *never* to touch these monumental, if frail, objects of reverence.

A further war-related memory has remained with me. I was perhaps five and the global conflict was at its height when I accompanied my parents to Uplands Airport. We were dressed in our Sunday attire to attend the graduation ceremony honouring a class of young pilot officers bound for active combat. It was a cold late-November day. The ceremony was held in a cavernous hangar that had been gussied up for the occasion with red, white, and blue bunting and the Royal Canadian Air Force ensign. Temporary bleachers were filled with family members, friends, the press, and the staff and officers of the Number 2 Service Flying Training School. The young men marched in as the Air Force band played glorious martial music. It seemed both grand and solemn.

At an appointed time in the proceedings, Dad was called to join the presiding officers, and I watched with pride as he pinned the graduation wings on the chest of a slim young officer standing stiffly at attention, the trace of a faint smile on his face. Shaking hands, they held each other in a meaning-filled gaze for what seemed a long time. While the full implications of all this were not clear to me, my father's respect and affection for this fine young pilot were evident. I felt proud of them both. The newspaper report of the ceremony read, in part:

> Having graduated with distinction, three Ottawa boys who yesterday afternoon received their wings at No. 2 S.F.T.S., Uplands, have been granted commissions in the R.C.A.F. ... P.O. C.O. Lyons, 408 Riverdale Avenue [sic] attained the standard which merited a commission but not without one serious setback. Some months ago, he was severely injured in a plane crash at Uplands, and it was thought that he might never recover, let alone fly again. However, he did recover under the care of Dr H.T.R. Mount. Evidence of his gratefulness to Dr. Mount was given in the fact that at his special request Dr. Mount yesterday afternoon pinned his wings on him.

Dad's personal account of Pilot Officer Lyons read:

> Having been active in the previous war, I felt it my duty to volunteer for service. I was not accepted in the armed forces but was appointed to take care of neurosurgical cases. My first patient in that field was a young fighter pilot trainee. In an accident, he had fractured the frontal bone on both sides of his head. Lying with his eyes swollen shut and forehead protruding, he appeared to be either fatally injured or unconscious. As I felt for his pulse, he whispered, "Am I going to be able to fly again?" He required two operative procedures.

On the first, it was found that a small portion of each frontal lobe had been destroyed and had to be removed by suction. During his convalescence from his first surgery, suitable artificial bone replacement was prepared. As soon as possible, he was again anesthetized and the frontal brain covered by an artificial plate. He made a rapid recovery and after some time he resumed his training. When he finally graduated as a flying officer, I had the extreme pleasure of pinning on his wings. I wrote to him during the nine months he was on active service – until the end of the war. I was anxious to know how he reacted under stress. He told me that when he had a "close one" his forehead would be dry and the remainder of his body wet, or vice versa. On his return to Canada, I believe he entered university but I have had no further contact with him. He was a brave lad.[2]

Other memories of those years involve music, and they have lasted a lifetime: music to power the assembly lines, factories, offices, and homes in support of the massive war effort, and music to buoy the spirits. There was the chocolate-syrup-and-testosterone voice of Vaughan Monroe, and the plaintive yet uplifting, strains of Vera Lynn as she called us through the glossy panelling of the upright radio in our den: *There'll be bluebirds over the white cliffs of Dover, tomorrow, just you wait and see. There'll be love and laughter, and peace ever after, tomorrow, when the world is free.* There was also music that made the adults smile, such as the tongue-in-cheek, ever-so precise diction of Noel Coward, presumably sporting a condescending monocle, as he intoned the lyrics of "Could You Please Oblige Us with a Bren Gun" or "Mad Dogs and Englishmen." And somehow, along with the dry wit, there came the message that there was a ramrod up the British spine and a fixed set to the jaw above it.

One knew that was true for their Allies as well, the fighting men and women who somehow seemed closer to us because of the songs: "Over the Rainbow," "Bewitched, Bothered and Bewildered," "Chattanoga Choo-Choo," "White Christmas," "Mairzy Doats," "Oh What a Beautiful Morning," "People Will Say We're in Love," "Don't Fence Me In" (I would happily render all verses at the slightest provocation), "Swinging on a Star," and "Sentimental Journey." These became the hymns of my childhood.

Then came the night when I was wakened by Mother. She informed me, as she helped me into my bathrobe, that I was to get up right away. Her excitement and wide grin confused me. "Alice and Jimmie are already awake and dressed," she blurted. There was an air of giddiness as my parents babbled on about some wondrous event we were about to attend. Everyone seemed excited, even Dad. Apparently, we were headed downtown. "Don't I need to get dressed!" Nothing made sense! "How can I go to a party in my pajamas?"

We bundled into the car and headed up Bank Street toward the Parliament Buildings. Soon we were in the midst of a great dancing crowd that thronged the streets. The world was laughing, shouting, singing! To my amazement, there seemed to be a lot of kissing. I felt very embarrassed to be in my pajamas.

Dad left the car at the side of the street and swung me onto his shoulders as we joined the crazy, joyous mass that swept us up Sparks Street. We came to a stop at the corner of O'Connor and Sparks. We were pinned on all sides by the huge, tumultuous, pulsating, delirious throng. The Parliament Buildings were just beyond my left shoulder. I caught Mother's attention in a vain attempt to explain how mortified I was to be there in my pajamas. She explained that no one would notice me; they were having too much fun, and furthermore, that she and Dad wanted me to be part of all this. "You will," she told me, "remember it for the rest of your life." It was 7 May 1945. The war in Europe had just ended.

WINSTON ELLIOTT

Not long after that, my most indelible reminder of those years found its way into our home. Harold Elliott, an old acquaintance of Dad's, called to say that his son, Winston, was, with the war's end, a newly minted veteran. Winston's career in the Royal Canadian Navy had been unusual. Remarkable, in fact. Soon after he enlisted, his spare-time sketches of shipmates came to the attention of the Navy's top brass. No snapshot images these! They were special. In Leonardo-fashion, these pencil, charcoal, and Conté portraits drew the viewer's attention from a head-and-shoulders overview to an in-depth exploration of face, eyes, and soul. The viewer experienced each of Elliott's comrades-in-arms as a distinct, wonderfully rugged, potentially vulnerable, unique individual. Young Winston Elliott's genius having been recognized, he was taken out of active service and commissioned to do portraits of the Canadian Navy servicemen who had been decorated more than twice. He did this for the remainder of the war.

Now, with VE Day, Winston was looking for work prior to his impending studies at the Ontario College of Art. Might Harry, Harold asked, know of any potential portrait work in these cash-strapped months? Indeed, he did! I was seven.

Winston (as my parents called him) positioned me leaning against the arm of the living-room couch. He suggested I examine the Venice scene oil painting on the wall directly in front of me. His vantage point was to my right, just out of my line of vision. As he worked, this gently smiling young man became absorbed in his private universe. I don't recall how often we met, but each session seemed to take forever. We both were undoubtedly convinced that I was about to perish with terminal wiggling. These were focused hours for both artist and subject.

I don't wish to romanticize those seemingly endless sittings, but a question comes to mind. Drawing was to become my passion and my first drawings were from about that period. Was it during those hours with Winston Elliott that I was seduced by the creative potential of art and the magic of capturing on paper something beyond the mechanical image? Could one suggest reality at a deeper level, something related to the *meaning* of the moment? It would begin with line, form, composition, colour, and play of light, to be sure, but was there something *more* than that? In the Venice painting, did the artist reveal something of the sound of the breeze in the trees in the foreground, the faint call of an unseen bird, the continual hypnotic lapping of the water as the gondola came toward the viewer? Perhaps great art can drop into the mysterious silence of a deeper way of knowing that transcends time. It seems to me that some of those ideas may have started to form in my mind through the gracious presence of that talented young veteran. If so, it was, for me, the genesis of a lifelong love affair.

During the years that followed, the Venice painting remained in its corner of the living room, and the completed Winston Elliott portrait found a home in the vestibule of 37, near the front door. They both spoke to me of the meaning of home. Finally, as life moved on and I had my own home, that early portrait, signed w.H. ELLIOTT 45 in the bottom-right corner, accompanied me.

The story ended there until sixty-four years later, when I got to wondering what had happened to that gifted young artist. Following several Canada 411 dead ends, there was one more call to a Vancouver listing.

"Hello, might this be the home of the portrait artist Winston Elliott?"

A welcoming woman's voice responded, "Why, yes, it is."

"May I speak to him, please."

"Just one moment ... Win, it's for you."

The man's voice was warm and strong.

"This is amazing. You won't remember me, but sixty-four years ago – the war had just ended and you did my portrait. Balfour Mount."

"Not only do I remember you, but stranger still, I am looking at you as we speak. You see, some time ago, I made a collage of some of my early works. You're among them, and you are across from where I am sitting right now."

A most improbable reunion. Addresses were exchanged. A DVD of a 2007 *Winston Elliott Vancouver Retrospective* was promised and plans to keep in touch by email were established.

A few days later the phone rang again.

"Balfour, this is Phyl Elliott. I'm calling for Win. After you phoned, he went through his archives and discovered a copy of your portrait. The thing is, it is *not* a copy, it's the original! Win can't recall how it happened. He must have exhibited it in a show. They require the original for that, you know. In any event, the portrait your parents and you have had all these years is a copy! We have the original here and we'll send it to you."

The carefully wrapped couriered parcel was unpacked along with countless memories of Mom and Dad and their deep interest in both model and artist. The original is signed in cursive script at the bottom left, Elliott 1946.

Set side by side, the original and the long-cherished copy are indistinguishable. In the smallest details, the texture of paper and image, subtleties of shading – in *every* aspect, they are identical. Strangely, however, when the original replaced the impostor on the wall, it leapt out of the frame with a new-found freshness and vibrancy that was startling.

The long-lost original *Elliott 1946* now hangs in our living room; W.H. ELLIOTT 45 is in my basement office, across from my desk as I write this and calls to mind our first meeting a lifetime ago.

TRANSITIONS AND GROWING PAINS

During the summer I was six, I was sent off to Camp Kagawong on Balsam Lake in the Kawartha chain, northwest of Peterborough, Ontario. I was, in the prevailing camp lingo, an "Inkie," that is, a member of the Incubator Section, a moniker designed to amuse God-knows whom. It was a nightmare. Each morning, I was afraid to open my eyes lest I find myself still at camp. After a week or so it became evident to all that I needed to return home and Mother and Dad came to pick me up, much to the relief of thirteen-year-old Jim, a mortified member of the lofty Junior Camp.

I would later spend several happy summers at Kagawong where its plethora of programs fostered my love of horses, canoe trips, camp fires, crafts, and the essences that for me define Canada. One abiding image of those summers involves early-morning sightings of the then elderly camp founder, Ernest Chapman, as he set out alone in one of the large camp sailboats, a craft that generally demanded a crew of three – the perfect image of a master mariner in complete harmony with wind and water, a vision of aging with grace and presence.

Not all transitions were as difficult as my early Kagawong experience. Pre-kindergarten years presented a number of more easily negotiated challenges: for example, foregoing an afternoon nap. The loss there was Mother's. I was ready to move on long before she was, though she encouraged me not to rush into it, warning that once I had given up napping during the day, it would likely disappear until I was very old – perhaps forty.

In general, the carefully structured life of kindergarten and grade one was comforting in its predictability: lining up in pairs to navigate the vast hallways outside the classroom, first holding hands with your partner, then without hands; sitting in a circle on the floor to listen to stories; taking part in singsongs; and downing milk and cookies on cue. Yet confusing transitions kept cropping up. There was the day in the driveway at 37 when Dad and Jim informed me, as they hurried off in the car on an errand, that they would be back "in the shake of a dead lamb's tail." What did that mean? Where would they find a lamb, let alone a dead one? And what incantations could be involved to assure the efficacy of shaking its tail? Similarly, there was the cloudy day when my enchantingly mysterious Aunt Marian assured me as we looked at the rain-soaked world beyond the dripping window pane that, if I could find enough blue up there to make a Dutchman's britches, it would be a fine day tomorrow. I wondered how small my Dutchman could be yet still meet the requisite demands?

Even more daunting conundrums were on the horizon. Rumour had it that girls were born *without* a penis! Now, I knew that was completely preposterous, and thus I concluded, in a process of deductive inference, that girls must be born *with* one, only to later lose it. But at what age did this tragic event occur? I decided, in a stroke of logic which decades later would have pleased my surgical chief-of-service, Lloyd ("When all else fails, examine the patient!") MacLean, that I should carry out an observational study. Watchful parents intervened, however, thereby nipping in the bud my promising career as a researcher.

But the most mind-stretching challenge lay ahead. It centred around where babies come from. As a young city dweller, I had missed the practicums that my rural cousins encountered on a regular basis. Such issues were treated with far more modesty and decorum back then. So, when informed by a fellow Kagawong camper concerning the facts as he understood them, I resorted to Socratic questioning to point out the embarrassing indelicacy of his hypothesis.

"Do you mean this applies to *your* parents, your *parents*?!" But he did not buckle under the weight of such towering incredulity. Stunned by his callousness, I pressed on, "And even *the King and Queen*?!" Surely I had him there! Several lifetimes later, all this came flooding back when my daughter announced on coming home from school that she knew "all about" where babies come from. "And?" I queried, my eyebrows arching toward the ceiling. "You don't want to know," she retorted, with evident disgust.

A year later, I was in grade two at Ottawa's Mutchmor Public School. It was the early fall, the dawn of a new school year. The smell of Dustbane and varnish permeated the sparkling classroom. Everything was arranged in its appropriate, sunny place. Dick and Jane books stood in neat lines on the shelves. The alphabet, displayed in large block letters on carefully spaced rows of white cards, circled us on the classroom walls high above our heads. Our motherly teacher, Miss Wilson, smiled and clucked encouragingly.

My problem was that everything seemed different. The comfortable familiarity of grade one was gone. My desk wasn't in the right place. There were too many girls and everyone seemed happier, more excited, and brighter than I was.

I walked the half-mile down familiar tree-lined neighbourhood streets for lunch with Mother and Dad (his being home at noon made it a *very* unusual occasion). Before heading back to school, I wandered into his book-lined study to say goodbye. He was sitting at his massive desk, ringed with textbooks, medical journals, and the business of current deadlines. A photo of his mentor, Sir Wilfred Grenfell, standing with Albert Schweitzer hung on the wall by the door. Mother's hand was resting on Dad's shoulder; they were gazing at the new passport on his desk. He had just turned fifty.

"My, Harry, how much older you look!" was all she said, but to my ears it was a death sentence. I felt a vice tighten around my chest.

At school, that afternoon, I could hold back the tears no longer. I buried my head in my arms and sobbed. Alarmed, Miss Wilson hovered. "What is it, Balfour?" I couldn't speak. How could I find words to admit that my Daddy was dying?

"Do you feel sick?" I shook my head.

"Are you worried about something?" I didn't respond.

"Is there trouble at home?" I nodded, feeling guilty in realizing that she was imagining marital strife or some other family problem. But I had hit a brick wall and could say no more. Awareness of transience and the death anxiety that is our constant shadowy companion had struck home for the first time.

The opening lines of J.M. Barrie's multilayered masterpiece *Peter Pan* are: "All children except one, grow up. They soon know that they will grow up, and the way Wendy knew was this. One day when she was two years old she was playing in a garden and she plucked another flower and ran with it to her mother. I suppose she must have looked rather delightful, for Mrs. Darling put her hand to her heart and cried, 'Oh, why can't you remain like this forever!' This was all that passed between them on the subject, but henceforth Wendy knew that she must grow up. You always know after you are two. Two is the beginning of the end."[3] Wendy was two; I had perhaps managed to repress the full weight of it a little longer.

Four years were to pass before I encountered the reality of death first-hand. Miss Stacey, an elderly family friend, had been a patient of Dad's for some time. Now she was dying. I accompanied him on the house call to the dimly lit home where she had lived alone for many years. The door was unlocked. In silence, we made our way to her second-floor bedroom and, with a pat on the shoulder, Dad told me to wait in the hall. Minutes passed, and then I was ushered in. Her complexion was pasty; she was faintly jaundiced, wasted, and drowsy. She smiled weakly as she took my hand and thanked me for coming. It was a gentle scene. There was no fear evident on the part of either Dad or Miss Stacey and because of that, I was not afraid. There was a sense of calm. It was clear to me that he understood what was needed and that everything was under control. Miss Stacey was comfortable and at peace. She died, I believe, later that day.

PRE-TEEN YEARS

Meeting Robert Ashley Cooper Benson early in our Mutchmor School years was to be a life changer. We quickly became brothers-in-arms as we engaged the mysteries encountered in growing through ages eight to eighteen. The Bensons lived on Kippewa Drive, a five-minute bike ride if you took the Madawaska shortcut.

While the details of our first encounter have faded from memory, Bob assures me that I confronted him from atop my trusty CCM steed with its flashy plastic pom-poms dangling from the handlebars. My challenging opening gambit caught him by surprise. I was, so I claimed, a member of the White Ship Gang. As we sized each other up, I graciously added that, if he liked, I would see if I could get him into the club. He never did comment on his reaction when he found out that he was the *only* other member of this elite group. It was to be a friendship that shaped my life on a daily basis until our parting of ways as we headed off to university.

We were inseparable, our friendship marked by the journey to school by foot or bike, Cubs and Scouts, summer cottage visits with forays picking raspberries for Mrs Benson's mouth-watering pies, camping, swimming, "throwing the old ball around," mastering croquet according to the idiosyncrasies of the Mounts' lawn as well as ping pong on our cobbled-together wartime table, cycling adventures, snowballs and building forts and tobogganing in the winter, devouring comic books, and hours spent listening to music and going to movies. "But Bal, you said the *last* film we saw was '*the best*' you'd ever seen! You're driving me crazy! They can't *all* be the best!"

"Well, actually, it *is* possible for each one to be better than all the others."

"You're driving me nuts!"

The Bensons welcomed me into their family – Bob's father, Ash, the trumpet-playing medical director of the Metropolitan Life Assurance Company, his mother, Alice, outgoing and welcoming, and Bob's two younger brothers: Ted, two years our junior, and Johnny, six years younger than Ted.

One sun-drenched early afternoon in the fall, Dad unexpectedly returned home as Mother and I sat at the piano in the living room, struggling through my obligatory daily practice session. My friends were manning our fort in the vacant lot just outside the window and Mother had a bolo-ball bat in her hand, an ever-ready sword of Damocles should my wandering attention not find instant renewed focus.

Instead of stopping, Dad swept busily along the hall, bound for a brief visit to the kitchen and his study prior to returning to the office with its meaning-charged appointments. Strange how apparently trivial moments can, over time, take on archetypal significance. Though a moment of no apparent import, for all three of us, it remained etched in his memory for life. Decades later, Dad wrote:

When Maude heard the door open, she turned, looked at me and smiled her beautiful smile, creating a picture I shall never forget. I have never been able to forgive myself for wordlessly passing by instead of entering the room to embrace them both and tell them of my love for them. Maude and I were both concerned that we should create the best possible environment for our children. I fear I left the major part of that responsibility to the mother. I loved my work and was determined to do everything possible for the welfare of my patients. As a result, almost every evening I felt it necessary to visit someone either pre or post–operative or to see in consultation a very troubled person. That left little time for family life.[4]

Life with Mother was never dull. Her free-spirit zest for life surfaced regularly. Take, for example, the day the jade plant, given to me several years earlier by Mother's florist, burst into bloom precisely *on* my birth-day. Miraculously, each separate bulbous leaf now sported a small red bloom at its tip. My friends, present for the party, were appropriately awestruck. None of us guessed that Mother had been up much of the night fastening the tiny cardboard blooms in place.

One day, Mother took me out of school to attend a Grenfell Tea hosted at Laurier House. "Well, after all, it *is* a National Historic Site! William Lyon Mackenzie King and Sir Wilfrid Laurier *both* lived there. Why, it's a chance to experience history first-hand!" The need to have someone take a head count at the fundraiser was passed over without acknowledgment.

Another day, she asked me over lunch whether I would like to go to a movie:

"But what about school?!"

"Oh, I think it will be alright," she reassured, adding something about dog teams and being like the Grenfell Mission. She took me to the film version of the novel *Mrs. Mike* that advertisements boasted "masterfully evokes the tender, touching moments that bring a man and a woman together forever." In its wake, my image of the Grenfell Mission needed sorting out for some time to come.

Memories of that period include the morning in the spring of 1947 when Alice and I were playing a game of tag on the ground floor. The only other person home at the time was my nineteen-year-old cousin, Don Connor, who was upstairs having a shower. There was a great deal of running and peals of laughter as I tagged Al and dashed off, declaring that she was "It." Tearing out of the living room and across the hall, I sped into the dining room, convulsing with laughter and totally preoccupied with how far behind me Al might be. On looking up, I ran headlong into the multi-paned glass door leading from dining room to side verandah. Instinctively, I attempted to grasp the door handle but my right hand and arm up to the elbow crashed through the pane of glass. I was amazed. Splinters of glass flew everywhere. My extended forearm was palm down through the broken window. In a reflex attempt to remove it, I jerked it back across the remaining shards, slicing open my forearm, which now resembled a filleted fish. There was blood everywhere. Responding to Al's screams, Don appeared from upstairs wrapped in a towel and grabbed my arm to stem the flow. "Am I going to die, Donnie?" His calm, soothing words were reassuring.

On arrival, Dad took over and confirmed that the radial artery had been spared by millimetres, and then asked me to open and close my fist. That too was intact, as was my response to light touch. The forearm was closed later that day in the Civic Hospital outpatient operating room.

The daily norm was for Dad to leave for the hospital before we children were awake and to return home after we were asleep. After a solitary supper, he would attack the lengthy list of telephone calls from patients, calls that were encouraged by his fatherly reassurance, "Don't hesitate to contact me if you are concerned about anything. Here, let me give you my home phone number."

Days, even weeks, would pass, affording us little more than a passing glimpse of him. He was driven, focused, caring, and determined in the face of high ideals and an unreachable goal – to be, perhaps, the Christian physician that he perceived in both Grenfell and Albert Schweitzer.

FAMILY ODYSSEY, 1947

The summer of 1947 was to be special. We were to have Dad completely to ourselves for six weeks owing to a carefully planned transcontinental family adventure in our trusty Hudson.5 A small house trailer was purchased for this landmark event. Complete with bunk beds, kitchenette, and a bathroom with a pocket-sized toilet and a sink, it offered just enough room for each of us to sleep, that is, as long as one of us slept on the back seat of the locked car (not always reassuring in campgrounds frequented by inquisitive bears). Since Jim was only fifteen, a year too young to have a learner's driving permit, he required special written clearance from the authorities to help out with the driving. This was duly obtained. The plan was to head west to Vancouver where Dad would leave us to fly home to his waiting patients, while we four undaunted pioneers undertook the long dusty drive home without him, Mother and Jim at the wheel. The scheme was all the more memorable since it was necessary for Jim to master the counter-intuitive task of backing a car into a parking spot with a trailer attached. "Remember, in backing up, you are *pushing*, not pulling. To back the trailer into a spot to your right, you have to move the car's hind quarters to the left," explained Dad in his usual earnest tone.

These decades hence, my first images of our vast, magnificent homeland remain crystal clear. We skirted south of lakes Huron, Michigan, and Superior to head north through Minnesota and nip the nose of Lake Superior at Duluth prior to re-entering Canada. Then it was on to Manitoba and Saskatchewan where we noted in passing the location of Foam Lake where Nettie grew up. We relished the romance of passing landmarks such as Moose Jaw, Swift Current, and Medicine Hat and were hypnotized by the endless sea of incandescent yellow-green around us. The prairies: fields of grain as far as the eye could see; an ocean of wheat swaying and shimmering under a brilliant blue sky with its marshmallow, grey-bottomed, cumulus clouds neatly lined up, away and away to the distant horizon. The arrow-straight railway line cut a path beside us as we journeyed west trailing clouds of dust from the unpaved roads, under the sentinel presence of the grain elevators that marked the passing miles. There were few cars, and anyway, you could see them coming for a hundred miles down that bowling- alley highway.

Somewhere on that leg of the trip, famished, and with the welcoming permission of the roadside farmer, we stopped for the night, pulling into his yard near the weathered farmhouse. Our sun-burnt, open-faced host was leaning against his fence as both families gathered and Dad asked how long they had lived here.

"Oh, we've been in these parts for a while. My granddad homesteaded here from out east in the seventies. Land's been good to us though we lost much of our topsoil in the drought ten years ago. But we should be up for another good harvest this year. Now, where did you say you folks are from?"

The high-domed prairie sky darkened and the clouds, now purple, accentuated the orange and reds of the blazing prairie sunset. We chatted, watched the foraging chickens, and smiled at the determination of the baby calf eagerly suckling in the field beside us.

A mumbled grace, a light supper, and then sleep followed in quick succession. We were exhausted by the newness of it all, the sense of having acquired new friends, and the grandeur of this boundless, bountiful land.

Approaching Calgary! All thoughts turned to the Stampede that awaited us. But what was that on the horizon? Ahead, where earth meets sky, there was a lumpy broken line that appeared and disappeared from view. The knotted image gradually came into focus and suddenly became clear. The foothills of the Rocky Mountains. Their mystical presence seemed to beckon, even at that first childhood acquaintance.

The Stampede parade inched along the crowded street as the attentive six-deep, neck-craning throng lined the frontier storefronts, all abuzz with excitement. It was a fantasy land, churned up before our eyes by the dizzying dancing mix of sun and sweat, the pungent scent of horses and waxed leather, fried potatoes, bacon, flapjacks, and maple syrup. All of it we experienced through intermittent wisps of wood smoke, peals of laughter, and the clouds of dust that filled the air, kicked up by a thousand hooves. The cowboys rode past in waves, their horses' heads and manes tossing proudly as their tails flicked at troublesome flies.

First Nations women, braided, beaded, buckskinned, and talisman-bedecked, were now upon us. Their impassive, weathered faces peered wisely down at me through thousand-year-old eyes. And instantly I knew that they could read the deepest secrets of my soul: knew beyond words, beyond endless white-man explanations. They were followed by twenty or thirty warriors on blanketed ponies, and, like the women, their expressionless countenances suggested a millennial wisdom that was theirs alone.

A regimental line of tanned and self-assured "community leaders" then appeared on their prancing, barely contained, steeds – skittish and with much snorting and pawing. These *men of substance* passed with practised indifference, Stetsons carefully positioned over bandana-wiped brows. Their embroidered shirts mirrored the opulence of their glittering tack with its hand-engraved silver conchos, buckles, tips, and hand-tooled leather while music poured from the streamer-decorated floats that followed.

Then, suddenly, I came upon her, or rather, she me: tall, gracious, straight, a slender poplar in full leaf, wise beyond the need for words but much younger than the others – in her late twenties perhaps, beautiful and adorned with a chief's splendid eagle-feather headdress. She stopped. The dusty street transformed itself into a timeless meadow. She smiled down at me and I experienced in her quiet grace a sense of shamanic mystery and a silent welcome to her world. A Brownie camera clicked; a float passed by the two of us, then a line of scarlet Mounties, and suddenly our private meadow once again had become the dust-blown, sunbaked street. With a smile and knowing nod, she bid me goodbye and moved on. The tumbling sights and sounds passed, as did the applause and chatter of the crowd. At least, that is how I now remember it. Did her near-mystical impact suggest greatness lived simply, or simplicity lived greatly, or both?

The Stampede, 7–12 July: a whirling world of risk and derring-do. Wild steers were wrestled, their horns tagged by buckaroos diving headlong off galloping steeds; convulsing bug-eyed stallions ejected all would-be riders; an endless succession of calves were roped, slammed to the ground, and tied as the cowpoke waved high to stop the timer that charted his prowess. An enraged Brahman bull catapulted from the chute, the rider's left hand fused to the cinch in a death grip, his right arm flailing the air as the massive humped beast contrived to move toward all four compass quadrants at the same moment as clouds of dust billowed and ominous horns flailed, the clock ticking. One sudden fearsome thrust and the cowboy's blanched face was driven into the dirt with terrible force, his body now limp. With bloodshot eyes and lowered horns, the bull twisted down and in, but in that same microsecond a clown arrived, artfully distracted the bull, and then danced free into the arms of a watchful rescuer who, with split-second timing, had arrived on his big pinto. A second rescuer retrieved the fallen cowboy; the furious bull snorted.

Finally, there was the chuckwagon race. Pandemonium erupted as the horn sounded, the screaming crowd competing with the bellowing PA system. The wagons careened around the first bend. Apparently out of control, they jostled for position. A collision seemed inevitable. They were moving at great speed heading into the next turn, the wagons rocking dangerously. We collectively held our breath as they thundered past, roaring toward the finish line. The drivers were standing, frantically slapping their reins and calling to their teams. A flag signalled victory and the crowd erupted with an enthusiastic roar for Johnny Phelan's team from Red Deer, and for Ronnie Glass, his driver. They had been the winners, the previous year, as well.

The other Stampede winners were announced, to further cheers. "All-round champion, Bill Linderman! Friends, a newcomer, Jim Like of Kim, Colorado, is our Champion bronc rider! And folks, one further piece of news you'll be interested in. Friday's attendance was 71,954, the largest single-day attendance in the history of the Stampede!"

Jim's new Stetson was midnight black. It came with a subtly elegant, twisted gold cord around the base of the crown. On each side, the brim was discretely curled upward, just so. He wore it with a casual off-hand air that filled me with envy. It added years to his already unfair advantage. I believe that his eyes narrowed into a thoughtful squint every time he put it on and I was certain that a passing cowpoke might easily mistake him for a local wrangler. He could even drive a car! Undoubtedly, *someone* was bound to ask him to mind their horse for a moment. Clearly, *I* would never be asked! Somehow, my *brown* cowboy hat always ended up on the back of my head, framing my face like a vast chocolate full moon. Instead of a gold cord, its crown was encircled by a brown shoelace derivative. Worst of all, whenever I adopted Jim's squint, Mother asked if I had something in my eye. And yet, in spite of all that, we were inseparable – my cowboy hat and me. I never did name it, the way my summer camp tent-mate Chucker Belford named his sailor's hat a few years later, but it remained my very closest friend – apart from Bob Benson.

Leaving Calgary, we headed south through Fort MacLeod to Pincher Creek, where Buckhorn Ranch, owned by Calgary oil baron Clifton C. Cross, sprawled in the shadow of the local landmark, Table Mountain. It had everything an eight-year-old could want: horses (mine, a fifteen-hand-old grey named CheeWee), cattle, real cowboys, trail-riding, branding, and bronco busting.[6]

It was on a Buckhorn Ranch trail ride that I had my first cup of coffee. Twenty of us had set out after an early breakfast on a cool but sunny day. Part way up a winding path leading to Table Mountain summit, we stopped at a clearing for sandwiches and fruit. We were still well below the tree line. Coffee was brewed by the cowboys over an open fire in a large cauldron, and, to my delight, it was being flavoured with pine cones thrown by all-comers from the perimeter of the camp site. My first attempt missed, but from then on they hit the bull's eye. The coffee was delicious. None has quite equalled it since.

Among the memories of our two weeks at Buckhorn, the most searing was the branding of the cattle with the tell-tale Buckhorn BU over a V (referred to as "BU hanging V"). The bellowing protests of the struggling steers, the smoke and pungent smell of burning flesh, and the perspiration of the straining cowboys led to long faces among us tenderfoot observers and reassurance from Stan, the Buckhorn wrangler: "There's an old saying, 'Trust your neighbour, but brand your stock.' You can't get tender-hearted. To get a good brand, you have to burn both hair and the outer layer of the skin. The brands got to last its whole life you know. You want it to always bring the animal home."

Always vigilant when monitoring my big brother, I was filled with awe by Jim's worldly sense of self. It was evident at every turn. *His* horse was particularly distinguished since *he* was *a pacer*! (a long explanation invariably followed). How embarrassing he found it to be a man of fifteen attending a *dude* ranch with his *family*; how great his disdain was as he informed me that ranchhand Sandy, who, at seventeen, was only two years older than Jim, was not a *real* cowboy since he was actually from Vancouver.

Many Buckhorn mental-snapshot moments remain with graphic clarity: Dad tending to a cowhand post-concussion after he was thrown from a bucking steer; the tranquility of the beaver pond I discovered in the forest and the beaver-crafted three-foot log that became my souvenir; CheeWee high-tailing it for the stable and coming close to clearing me off his back with the help of the low overhang on the barn door;

watching the surprising gentleness of the old cowpoke breaking in a wild mustang; the staff's high esteem for the Cross family; the addictive creak of leather and smell of horse on saddling up; and the inevitable magic of each evening campfire.

As we approached the Rocky Mountains on leaving Buckhorn, I became aware of a slight uneasiness. It wasn't fear, but it felt like fear. Then, without warning, we were in a small town, surrounded by pine forests. Extending high above the trees on all sides, in the rapidly falling evening light, there were great brooding walls of stone. They seemed overwhelmingly close yet completely remote. Each, I was informed, had a name: Mount Rundle, Sulphur Mountain, Mount Norquay, Cascade Mountain, and so on. As night was enveloping us, we drove down the deserted Banff Street and were suddenly confronted by a massive blackness directly ahead, towering over us to unimaginable heights. Majestic. Uncompromising. Overpowering. A final flash of sunlight caught a blazing band of snow at its towering western slope and it was then that a large bull elk meandered across the street, just fifty feet ahead of us.

The trip north from Banff to Jasper brought further wonders: Moraine Lake, Lake Louise, Bow Lake, the Columbia Icefield, the Athabaska Glacier, and Mount Edith Cavell. Bow Lake's Crowfoot Glacier prompted an impersonation from Mom that made Dad chuckle, as she mumbled in a gruff, gravely Churchillian voice, "Some chicken ... some neck!" (I had no idea what that was all about, no memory of Churchill's words when I was two, and so I simply concluded that I should chuckle too.) The Columbia Icefield, vast beyond visible limits, was silent at its timeless icy crest, yet at its melting leading edge in the valley it churned and roared as the turquoise and milk-white glacial runoff demanded full attention if we were to avoid slipping into the freezing maelstrom below the wet crossing plank we were negotiating.

Mount Edith Cavell, in the ever-changing afternoon light, represented sheer magnificence on a grand scale, while the mirror stillness of turquoise-blue glacier-fed Moraine Lake with the nearby grazing deer was like nothing I had ever seen. My unbridled wonderment as the day unfolded made me think of Bob. He would surely groan and say, "There you go again, Bal!" But sometimes, when you find yourself a smaller part of things in facing an overwhelmingly larger-than-life reality, that's simply the way it is! Right?

Dad was about to leave us. We continued west through the rugged terrain of the British Columbia interior, heading for Vancouver via the winding, unpaved road that followed the Fraser River Canyon. It twisted and turned, hugging the cliff face hundreds of feet above the turbulent

rapids far below. There were no guard rails. It was teeming rain. Passing
the occasional oncoming car or truck was accomplished with caution as
we negotiated the cliff face, the precipitous drop-off to one side and the
irregular rocky outcroppings above us on the other. It was then that a
cow moose rushed from the bluff above to cross the road directly ahead
of us, as Dad braked to a skidding stop. She plunged over the cliff face
on our left, to her apparent certain death in the Fraser River far, far
below. Jim asked Dad if he could get out to have a look. I followed. He
was almost at the cliff edge when he dashed back. The skittish moose
had simply chosen to retreat onto a favourite ledge ten or fifteen feet
below the brim and now was charging back up at us.

The long drive home without Dad included an encounter with a pudgy
rock-throwing youth who managed to crack our windshield one late
evening in the South Dakota Badlands. His unimpressed, unshaven, lean
and mean, flint-eyed family denied all responsibility as they stood in
their isolated roadside camp site cleaning their hunting rifles. Mother
drove on. There followed a fruitless search for a Badlands place to sleep.
"No Ma'am, there's no places to stay 'round here."

Mother vowed with vehemence, "This is the *last time* I will let Harry
return home before the rest of us!" That wasn't to be.

THE PATIENTS, THE PRACTICE, THE FAMILY

Throughout those years of personal change for Jim, Alice, and me,
Mother coordinated and supervised home and family with an enthusiasm that lent meaning to the crusade-like sacred trust Dad experienced
on a daily basis as he addressed his patients' problems. His medical
practice and Mother's guiding support determined how we came to
understand family life, community, caring, communication, and the
needs of others. The foundational cornerstone supporting all else was
the Practice of Medicine according to H.T.R. Mount, facilitated by
Maude. That is not to imply that this was a conscious dynamic for
us as children, but, like gravity, it was always part of the background
reality that shaped our perspective.

Having been trained in the pre-specialization days of the surgical generalist, Dad was adept at handling neurosurgical, abdominal, gynecological,
and, early on, orthopaedic challenges. A respectful formality characterized his professional relationships both with colleagues and with patients
and their families. He brought to everything he did a careful, systematic
approach that seemed to spring from the quietly gallant norms of an earlier age. His natural curiosity, diagnostic acumen, and thoughtfulness as a

tactician had been well honed during his Grenfell Mission and Mayo Clinic years. As a surgical craftsman and teacher, he ranked with the very best.

As I would later have the privilege of observing first-hand on a daily basis, he possessed a natural sure-handed grace that fostered a sense of calm in the operating theatre. His high standards of professional conduct and service were combined with a sense of surgical self confidence that left no question as to who was leading the team.

For example, there was the day he was doing battle with an upper-abdominal, locally advanced, cancer. Devilish distortion of the normal anatomy, matted adhesions, and troublesome bleeding marked each step of the resection, and, in a moment of uncertainty regarding how well his patient was tolerating the continuing blood loss, he asked the anesthetist to report on the blood pressure. There was no response. He turned his head to ask his colleague one more time, only to find that the anesthetist had left the room. He was managing, Dad was informed, synchronous cases in two adjacent theatres and had returned to the other room. With eyes blazing, H.T.R. roared for the anesthetist to report to him immediately. No one present soon forgot the scene that followed. With jaw set and eyes still glaring he barked, "I will *not* tolerate anesthesia in absentia! Ever! Don't *ever* do that again!" It never happened again.

An evident passion for his craft marked each hour of his long days which often commenced at 7:00 A.M., or earlier, as needed, to complete ward rounds prior to the day's operating-room (OR) list. His first surgical procedure was generally booked for 8:00 A.M. At the conclusion of his last case, he generally returned to the wards to review clinical problems with the residents and to meet with patients and their families for discussion of progress to date and upcoming potential issues.

His afternoon-office waiting room was generally filled to the doors prior to his unpredictable arrival, but he always conveyed focused, unhurried presence and deep interest in the person at hand. With four examining rooms running, he and his nurse would rarely leave for home before seven to nine o'clock each evening.

Decades later, Donna Munro, who, as a young nurse, ran Dad's office for six months, recounted the norms that shaped his practice:

One particular evening, my fiancée and I had plans for a special celebration and I wondered how I would ever get out of the office on time. At six o'clock, the waiting room was still completely full. What could I do? Assigning each of the next four patients to an examining room, I did their routine baselines – age, weight, pulse, blood pressure, temperature, urinalysis, blood work, and basal metabolic rate.

With these parameters charted and the four examining room patients undressed and ready to be examined, I turned to the crowded waiting room, completed the same assessments on each patient and lined up their charts in the proper order. But how was I going to tell him that I needed to leave? I knew that he didn't have a clue that I was there until nine o'clock many nights. It had never occurred to him.

Given the urgency of that particular evening, I said, "Dr. Mount, I have to tell you something. I hope you won't be annoyed. I have very important plans for tonight and I have to leave at seven o'clock." And he said, "Miss Munro, you get out of here as fast as you can and have a wonderful time!" I explained that I had all the patients ready for him and the charts arranged in order. "Thank you so much," he said. "I appreciate that, and I'll see you tomorrow." So I left. It was amazing. From then on, he would always say to me, "Now Miss Munro, it's seven o'clock, shouldn't you be out of here now?" It changed him completely. It was just that nobody had ever told him before. From then on he would be watching the clock to get me out on time.[7]

Following a rushed meal, Dad's evenings were taken up with the daily list of telephone calls. In answering an incoming call, we family members adhered to clear, time-honoured standards that were the result of training regarding the proper answering of the telephone: "Hello, Dr Mount's residence. No, I'm sorry, he is not in. May I take a message?" A pencil and pad lay by each telephone, awaiting collation at his arrival home. The number of calls – twenty or more was not unusual – was fanned by his legendary reassurance, "Call me if there is a problem."

Surgery is at its most efficient when the surgeon works with a consistent scrub-nurse assistant who, through long experience, is able to anticipate every move the surgeon makes and each instrument he will require. His hand extends without comment. His need for a second hemostat, or his favourite tie, then scissors, has been recognized and they are in his hand without a comment. "Cut." ... "Sponge." ... "Suction." ... "Cautery." ... "Retractor." The language is precise and sparse. Surgeon and nurse are in a near-wordless flow that seems little short of miraculous to the uninitiated. Each busy surgeon is on the lookout for just such a scrub-nurse partner when chaotic operating-room scheduling pressures permit that luxury. In the late 1950s, Dad enjoyed just such a partnership at the Ottawa Civic Hospital.

Lois Hollingsworth was good. A recent graduate, she had the right mix of focused attention, dynamic twinkle, and edgy, yet respectful, confidence. Holly, as she was known, was skilled, highly professional, well liked, and enjoyable to be with. She had assisted Dad several times when he approached Mary Armstrong, the Civic's OR director of nursing, to ask if Hollingsworth could be assigned to him whenever possible. Yes, Armstrong affirmed, in fact, it could start the next day when he had a major abdominal case booked. Holly was delighted.

"Would you like to make rounds with me and meet the patient before they bring her to the OR, Miss Hollingsworth?" Dad asked.

"Why, yes," replied the somewhat startled Holly. She had never heard of such a thing, but it sounded progressive, even cutting-edge.

"Fine, I'll meet you on the ward at seven," he replied.

They walked into the patient's room next morning at precisely 7:01. She was in her early sixties. Her condition was serious, perhaps grave, and the surgical outcome was far from certain. Approaching the bed, he pulled up a chair and sat down, gently taking her hand.

Decades later, Holly, who had, over the ensuing years, become my friend and Royal Victoria Hospital colleague in Montreal, described what followed:

We walked into her room. You know, he was always gentle with them and explained to them what was going to happen. He was very open in talking about the prognosis. If things looked serious, he would talk to them about it, which certainly wasn't the norm in the 1950s – but he was an up-front man! He didn't hide things. Well, she asked him questions and it was evident to me that they had talked like this before. A sense of trust had already been established. He was holding her hand when he mentioned again that things looked serious, but that he was going to do everything he could. Then, he gently asked her if she would like to have a word of prayer together. She nodded and he pushed the chair back and knelt at the bedside, head bowed. Well, I thought to myself, "This man is nuts! What are we doing here?!" Just then he looked over at me at the end of the bed; his eyebrow arched expectantly, as if to say, "Kneel!" I did!

It was a brief prayer. We prayed that the operation would go smoothly and that the outcome would be satisfactory. Nothing fancy. And I thought, "He's going to scare the hell out of her!" But the impact of all this on her was incredible. It was his approach, his honesty. He wasn't going to give her any garbage. You know, like, "everything will be just fine; I'm going to cure you." He sort of took it step by step. "This is the way it is going to happen, and hopefully things are going to work out." She became completely relaxed. It was as if she simply placed herself in his hands."

Then, after a pause, Holly added:

Everybody admired him. He was the kingpin, you know. They just
had such faith in him. It was really very stimulating. I've never experienced anything like that, before or since. A lot of nurses were afraid
of him, and I was as well, to a point, when I first started scrubbing
with him. He could be quite scary at times. I was an experienced
scrub nurse, but you know, scrubbing with him was like scrubbing
with the pope! You know, that's the way everybody felt. He was tall,
erect and severe looking. When he smiled he had a beautiful smile,
but he seldom smiled. I used to try to get him to laugh when I got
closer to him and every now and then he'd sort of let out a little
chuckle. He was very quiet. I never heard him blast anybody. He was
just a very well-respected man.
     When I became his regular scrub nurse I got to know him a little
better than the other girls. You didn't dare make a mistake. You
didn't hand him the wrong instrument. Not that he would ever comment on it, but he would look at you with a look that said, "What's
going on here?" You felt you wanted to work hard to get his respect.
But he also gave the impression that he respected *all* nurses.[8]

Holly's remarks were substantiated by OR Supervisor Armstrong.
"My first exposure to him was through his neurology lectures when I
was a student. I recall being fascinated by the brain and he was sincere,
serious, yet down to earth. We always understood him. He was very
earnest and clear. Later, on the wards, I remember him making rounds
and being very concerned and kind to the patients. Diane Boyle worked
in the Recovery Room. She recalls that he always had a prayer with
the patients before surgery. I can't confirm that, but I know that he did
always stop if the patient was on the OR table and he would have a quiet
moment with them and I suppose that was what was going on."[9]
Dad was the only neurosurgeon in Ottawa for approximately twenty
years until the mid-1950s. Initially, there were six operating rooms at the
Civic and the one or two neurosurgical cases each week were booked
in the two largest theatres. Later, the Civic operating-room suite was
enlarged to twelve general-surgery rooms, one x-ray room, and one room
reserved for neurosurgery procedures. At that time Dad did four or five
neurosurgery procedures each week in addition to three or four general-surgery cases. He admitted patients to the Ottawa General Hospital
and, after its founding in 1953, the Saint-Louis-Marie-de-Montfort
Hospital. As the years passed, the trend toward specialization increased

and, not surprisingly, less busy surgical colleagues became resentful of both the volume and diversity of his activities.

His gifts as a neurology and neurosurgery lecturer were appreciated by both nursing and medical students, who described him as sincere, earnest, and notable for the respect he showed each student. Armstrong commented: "If something wasn't going right he would explain it to us, but he was calm about it and he was friendly. He always knew us. Even as students, he spoke to us, and as graduate nurses he always called us by name. He knew who we were. That was not the norm at the time. Indeed, doctors in that era expected nurses to stand and offer up their seat if a doctor approached the nursing station. Similarly, the nurse was expected to step back at an elevator door to let the doctor enter first."

Holly recalled with amusement her first encounter with Dad. She was a first-year student-nurse probationer and was "scared to death" when a tall lab coat-clad surgeon encountered her struggling to manoeuvre a bed down the hospital corridor. "Now nurse, would you like a little help with that bed?" She responded that she would be delighted and they proceeded together with the patient in tow. She spent the rest of the day telling her astonished classmates the tale.

And so, the 1950s unfolded, with Dad manning the surgical battlements and Mother tending to the home front with consistent patience and infectious goodwill.

BOTTLE TOPS

The threat of change loomed large in June 1950 as the end of grade six approached. I had just been informed that at Glashan, the junior high school that I would attend in September for grades seven and eight, the students did *not* indulge in my favourite pastimes: marbles and bottle tops. While my skill at marbles was modest at best, I delighted in bottle tops. As the reader undoubtedly knows, bottle tops is a war game that involves the rocket-swift delivery of a cardboard milk-bottle top to knock down your opponent's as it leans against the schoolyard wall. The bottle top needs to be a "stiffy" (new, and not soaked with milk during its earlier lifetime atop the glass milk bottle delivered to your home that morning). This missile is released from its resting place between index and middle finger, with a well-aimed flick of the wrist. With practice, it can be delivered with deadly accuracy and surprising force.

My first solution to the looming catastrophe of a bottle-top-free life was the decision that I would introduce marbles and bottle tops at Glashan. I was certain I could get my peers to see the light. But that summer, in the course of many sleepless hours of sales-pitch plotting, it occurred to me that if they *didn't* indulge in these life-affirming endeavours at the new school, the chances were that they had discovered *other* diversions. I concluded that I would put my plans to proselytize on hold until I had done some research into those alternative activities.

The plan proved prudent. That September, I discovered girls, and found that they were at least as interesting as bottle tops. I recognized two life-shaping truths through that experience. First, life demands continual adaptation to change. Second, if we make age-appropriate choices and are successful in letting go of past preoccupations, life keeps getting better. It isn't that loss and suffering are eliminated, but coping skills are given a chance to come into play and as a result we may find ourselves opening to new, unimagined potentials. While at the time I might not have described these insights in exactly those terms, oddly enough, the lessons learned were *just* that clear in my mind. This was, for me, an epiphany.

It was September 1950. I was eleven and off to Glashan, my new centre-town school, four or five bicycled (trudged in winter) urban miles east of home. Coming and going to my new school, I passed a rambling bakery with delivery wagons (both motorized and horse-drawn) assembled in the adjacent yard, leaving their magic aroma of fresh bread a lasting reminder of those formative days.

My critical scan of the strangers clustered with me in that fenced-in schoolyard on my first morning at Glashan focused on one young fellow. He was the only student still sporting short pants and long wool socks. Harley Smyth was to achieve additional distinctions as time passed – gold medalist as a member of my medical-school class at Queen's, Rhodes scholar, monarchist, neurosurgeon, lay theologian, sailor, actor, and exceptionally gifted impersonator.

Other than my tall, dark-haired classmate Patsy, I recall few details of those Glashan years. Three come to mind: two of them wounding, one healing.

During our first weeks, the class was separated into two groups. Those who were identified as the more "promising" students were allocated seats in the main body of the class; those requiring "extra attention" were seated in the two rows nearest the door. I was assigned the latter. My sense of shame and self-doubt lingered as a result.

My second wound occurred shortly thereafter. The teacher had asked how many of us had a job after school. A good number put up their hands – delivering groceries on their bikes, stocking their father's corner store, a paper route. With an ill-considered urge to be part of the group, my hand shot up. The silence was deafening.

"Well, Balfour, *you* have a job?" the teacher asked with an incredulous emphasis that acknowledged by inference the general recognition of my father as a prominent neurosurgeon.

"What is *your* job?" I felt the ground slipping out from under me.

"Well," I stammered, flushing. "I help Mother with various jobs around the house." There was a roar of laughter. My humiliation was total. I had acquired a double shame – both a slow learner *and* a rich kid!

What of the healing experience? It remains my only memory of grade eight. Many years earlier, our perennially relaxed and somewhat ruffled teacher, Mr Shaver, had personally purchased a sufficient number of copies of Sir Walter Scott's historical novel *Ivanhoe* for there to be one for each student in his class. Since then, year after year, when his students had finished their daily work with time to spare, those well-worn, red- covered, slightly musty volumes would be extracted from their cardboard box near his desk and handed out as a priceless reward for a job well done. Then, each of us would sit glued to our seats as medieval magic transported us back to 1194 Norman England and the escapades of Sir Wilfred of Ivanhoe (a member of one of the remaining Saxon noble families), Locksley (to be known as Robin Hood), and their mesmerizing post-Crusade countrymen. This annual tradition had gone on sufficiently long that Shaver had memorized the book. We never tired of his theatrical flourish as he flawlessly read on after reaching the bottom of a page, his mist-covered eyes fixed in mid-air, his head tilted back as he continued the story, the page unturned. Mysteriously, the number of readings managed to be just enough to finish the glorious yarn by year's end, and so, as with many classes before us, we experienced our losses in parting multiplied as school closed for the summer – Ivanhoe, Locksley, the host of medieval friends that each of us had claimed as our own, *and* Mr Shaver.

GLEBE COLLEGIATE INSTITUTE, 1952–57

Glebe! Even as a child the word awakened in me a rich, earthy sense of the land. Perhaps I had heard someone refer to the word's origin as indicating the local territory assigned to a clergyman as part of his "benefice," or heard of our home district's history of the name as the hunting territory for local Algonquin tribes. While to this day, the Ottawa district surrounding 37 Opeongo remains "the Glebe," the high school of that name had more recent roots. In 1919 the Adolescent School Attendance Act decreed schooling compulsory until the age of sixteen. This necessitated expansion beyond the existing Ottawa Collegiate

Institute (later, Lisgar Collegiate) and a new four-storey brick facility, known as the Ottawa Collegiate Institute, Glebe Building, was constructed at the corner of Bronson and Carling avenues, the city outskirts at that time. It held its first classes in 1922.

From September 1952 to June 1957, Glebe provided the nutrient medium for our rapidly changing world as Bob and I morphed from oval to angular, soft to muscular, tweeter-voiced to unreliably rumbling, peach-faced to grittily stubbled, and watched in awe as our previously taken-for-granted companions of the opposite gender seamlessly evolved from angular to oval, board-like to soft, squeaking to lilting, and stupid to intellectually beyond us, all to the distracting background strains of "Jambalaya," "Your Cheatin' Heart," "Doggie in the Window," "I Believe," "Ebb Tide," and the like at regular weekend parties during that opening year of this process. Although the number in our year varied as the years passed, 181 graduated together at the end of grade thirteen, our fifth and final year at Glebe.

Grade nine, September '52: English, history, geography, mathematics, science, French, health and physical education, and art. I was perennially dizzy in an overwhelming new world. Suddenly we were part of a student body that varied from us uncertain neophytes to mature, confident men and women five years our senior. We were engulfed in a maze of corridors featuring an array of display-case trophies. The awe-inspiring school auditorium left us feeling very small. The generously windowed, book-lined classrooms had a similar impact.

All of this competed daily with the quicksand of my ever-shifting mental focus, a confusing array of dress codes, new social norms and expectations, endless distractions and anxieties, three-ring binders, pencil cases, countless lost pens, doodles and sketches entered on page margins, floating from class to class through random self-conscious crowds, crammed timetables, a forest of chalk-filled blackboards and the brushes that erase too soon what went before, not to mention our more pressing and omnipresent concerns: the uncertain cause of pimples, fascination with word play, the newest riddle making the rounds, and all things ribald.

Overlooking all of this was the host of otherworldly teachers: Taylor, Sonly, McClosky, Hewitt, Annable, Rorke, Thornton, O'Donnell, Berry, Thoms, Glibly, Waddell, Westington, Bullock – an apparently endless flow of pedagogic legends. There were landslides of homework, illegible notes, laid-back jocks on senior inter-collegiate athletic teams, the gym, pool, and associated dressing rooms with their uncomfortable risk of unaccustomed nudity, and, to further underscore our sense of inadequacy, the awe- inspiring maturity (physical, social, musical, academic, artistic, athletic, and theatrical) of our grade thirteen elders whose prowess was beyond our dazzled freshmen imaginings.

The weeks crept past or, alternatively, seemed to evaporate and suddenly our first year was almost over. While my academic performance had been marginal (to be charitable), my scrapbook documentation was far more upbeat. The weekly parties held in rotation at our various homes were a significant factor. What was more, I had been sketching more, egged on by endless hours spent over Mother's library of reference books on drawing and painting. In addition, during that year, I had linked up with my badminton-playing and accomplished pianist friend, Anne Caswell.

CF-EQL

Following lunch on Sunday, 3 May 1953, Dad invited Nettie and me to join him on a flying jaunt to Kingston where Jim was completing his second pre-medical year at Queen's University. It was to be a quick trip. Jim would meet us at the airport on his trusty motorcycle, a second-hand 650 cc BSA Golden Flash with a dented fuel tank (the latter due to a mishap that resulted in the death of its first owner). We were to return to Ottawa later that afternoon.

Dad acquired his pilot's licence late in life. Flying was to be his only diversion from surgery and patient-centred issues while "active in the profession." It was his holy grail, a passion born out of his childhood fascination with flight. Whatever its attractions, however, flying was definitely *not* a form of relaxation for him. Qualifying for his licence had been an epic challenge that resulted in many long nights that featured maps, charts, and teaching manuals spread over the dining-room table and Mother's unwavering encouragement. His Achilles heel in this process was the prerequisite that the student pilot must successfully put a plane into an intentional spin while diving toward the earth, for Dad an unimaginable request. Bravery was not the issue. He had settled the bravery question on Flanders Fields. His spin-anxiety was far more primal, like his fear of snakes or the response of many to spiders. It was a major hurdle, an obstacle of Everest proportions. It was therefore a source of great personal satisfaction when, in due course, he successfully soloed, completed the required spin, passed his licensing exams, and purchased a plane that we generally referred to by its aviation call signs – CF-EQL.

At Uplands Airport, we rolled Dad's single-engine Bellanca out of the hangar, filled her wing tanks with fuel and polished her with old rags until her scarlet skin shined, and then climbed in and buckled up as Dad went through the meticulous instrument check list. CF-EQL had dual controls. Dad was sitting on the left; I was on his right. Nettie sat behind us, on the roomy backseat.

We taxied onto the runway. Dad was all business, totally focused on becoming airborne. Noting that Nettie's seatbelt was a little loose, I suggested she tighten it. "If we're going to crash, I want to be able to jump out," she quipped in a characteristic Nettie mutter, and we were off.

We had just cleared the runway when we were suddenly jarred by violent shaking. Black clouds of oil began pouring back over the windscreen and fuselage. Dad asked me to take over as he reached over his left shoulder for the headphones to radio the tower that we were in trouble. Normally, this would be no problem. I had frequently handled the controls for brief periods once in flight.

But that day I was astonished at the task he had given me. Attempting to hold the plane steady required all my strength as CF-EQL bucked and reared with unimaginable force. What altitude we had gained in the few minutes we were airborne – a few hundred feet perhaps – we were now quickly losing. We passed over the pines at the nearby sandpits, then the river just beyond, with the more welcome prospect of landing on tilled Ottawa valley farmland within reach.

Time slowed, each second seemed a century, but gripped by the unfolding drama, each of us encountered these moments in isolation and in silence – alone. We were now only ten or fifteen feet above the ground, just above the farm fences that were rushing toward us, marking the border of each barren spring field. One after another, after another, they flashed under our feet. Our speed was approximately 90 mph. The clouds of oil were increasing. The associated overwhelming thunderous clatter was caused, we later learned, by a broken connecting rod repeatedly jamming into the engine block. The possibility of the engine dropping out of the plane, thus rendering us a tail-heavy projectile plummeting to earth, seemed great. I watched mesmerized as a hay stack approached before sliding past the right-wing tip beside me. Then, in an instant, the engine caught. Suddenly, it was firing smoothly again! *Have we been snatched from disaster?* We gained power and, with it, altitude. Our options began to multiply. *Should Dad attempt to return to the Uplands runway?* A split-second decision was required.

The teaching manuals all agree: "If you are disabled, pick the best spot to land and stick to your plan. We repeat. Do not change your plan of action. The risks increase greatly if you do." *But hitting one of those fields would be no picnic.*

Dad spoke once more to the tower. "Tower, CF-EQL. The engine is firing more smoothly. We will try to get back to you."

"We read you EQL and shall clear the runways. Emergency equipment is ready. Incidentally, the plane that followed you in takeoff is just above you, monitoring your progress. Good luck."

Pulling back on the controls, we climbed – 50 ft, 150 ft, 200 ft. We were accelerating as we climbed. Then, without warning, the pounding vibrations returned, more violent than ever. The billowing oil was back. Checkmate! The hard truth was clear to Dad and guessed by me. We couldn't get back and we were now too high to attempt a landing. Moreover, we were going too fast and were running out of space. One hundred yards away, directly ahead of us and rushing toward us at an alarming rate, was a row of stately mature elm trees. They stood directly across our flight path. They were about fifteen feet apart – too close to fly between, and too tall to get over. Moreover, a country road ran parallel to the elm trees. We would cross over the road, then hit the trees. Worse still, a formidable procession of Ontario Hydro power-line towers, running parallel to both trees and road, extended as far as the eye could see, to left and right. Finally, off to our right at 2 o'clock, on the far side of the country road and just beyond the last elm tree, there was a large stone farmhouse.

We would have to pass *under* the power line – and then what? Throw it to the right as we shot across the road. There was no other option.

The odds were obvious to both of us. Dad's hand settled on my knee and looking over he said in a controlled voice, "Well son, I'm sorry, I guess this is it." My foundational confidence as a son melted into the shared agony of a fellow victim.

I recalled that I had heard somewhere that there may be a second or two after impact prior to fuel-tank explosion. I reached for the twin door latches beside me and grasped them firmly with both hands as I closed my eyes. At that moment, we roared and belched under the hydro lines.

I felt the impact as the plane cartwheeled. A series of bumps and a chaotic spinning followed, then everything stopped. I remember realizing that our world was suddenly still; that I was alive. In attempting to escape before the plane exploded, I threw open the door and lurched up and out, onto what should have been the wing, but I found myself standing unsteadily on grass. The right wing had been torn off, only a few inches beyond my seat. It was disorienting. It seemed surreal.

"Dad, get out! Hurry!" But there was no answer. He was sitting, still buckled in, his tam clutched in his right hand, staring blankly straight ahead. He hadn't heard me. I called again, but he continued to stare

straight ahead, oblivious. I heard a noise from the back seat and turned
to help Nettie. She was bleeding from her chin but otherwise seemed
unhurt. I helped her out. Dad finally followed. I stared. The plane had
turned 180 degrees and was pointed back toward the airport. In crossing
the country road, it had lost its right wing and come to rest against a
tiny sapling, perhaps three inches in diameter. A metaphor came to mind
– a raging bull stopped by a school crossing guard's small sign. Massive
farm machinery lay feet from us along the direct path we had been hur-
tling along moments earlier. We were only feet from the farmhouse and
feet from having been impaled by massive manure-encrusted fangs of
the farm equipment. Silent thanks were given for the wrenching spin
initiated as our right wing hit the road.

Remarkably there was no fire, though both wing tanks of high-octane
gasoline had been emptied at our feet and the gathering crowd of folks
out for a Sunday drive on the country road insisted on throwing cigarettes into the fuel-soaked ground. Unnerved, I screamed a warning.

Where were we? It turned out that the farm was part of the tiny community of Merivale. The soft-spoken farmer shook Dad's hand, "Hello
there – Earl Mulligan. We watched you coming. We were sitting on the
porch. Can't believe we're all in one piece."

THE SUMMER OF 1953

Three weeks after our airborne brush with transience, the family headed
for London and the coronation of Queen Elizabeth II, and then on to
Vimy, Passchendaele, and other selected destinations. With Jim then twenty-one, Alice eighteen, and me fourteen, the timing of the trip had more to
do with the vanishing potential for such collective family adventures than
with any monarchist leanings. Indeed, as a First World War Canadian soldier, Dad had once been ordered to take part in building a raised walkway
for royalty to visit recent battle sites without getting their boots muddy;
"Sapper Mount-503173" emerged anything but a monarchist!

Not inclined to leave girlfriend Betty behind, Jim chose to remain in
Ottawa. Thus, boarding RMS *Franconia* in Quebec City, the remaining
four of us headed for centuries-old "Timber Cottage," in Croydon, home
of our cousins the Finches.

A coronation? In the mid-twentieth century? Was this an embarrassing
anachronism imposed on a struggling post-war people? Not at all! Indeed,
the 1950s promised to be a decade of rebuilding and increasing affluence in
England, a time of thanksgiving, confidence, and hope.[10] The country was
ready to honour anew the ancient traditions that had brought it thus far.

Reminders of the Second World War lingered. To be sure, London had been lovingly scrubbed and garbed for the splendid 2 June celebration, but the ordered rows of iconic buildings bore evidence of the devastation wrought by the Luftwaffe, places where the serene symmetry of the urban landscape lay ruptured with gaping holes. Now, eight years and longer after the fact, these painful souvenirs of suffering were carefully hidden away behind sheets of white plywood. To my mind, they resembled bandages lovingly placed over old wounds, carrying the message that the current collective joy was the product of *all* that had gone before.

Having given no previous thought to the monarchy, I was moved by the depth of personal meaning suggested by the words of the young princess.[11] It sounded more like a statement of deep religious commitment than a pledge to pageantry. At fourteen, I was surprised and impressed. The coronation of Her Most Gracious Majesty Elizabeth the Second, at age twenty-seven, promised to offer an evocation of both the secular and sacred values of her people.

My £4 coronation bleacher seat at Hyde Park near the Marble Arch came furnished with a cushion. With orders to be seated by 7:00 A.M., we left Croydon at 5. En route, the shout of newspaper hawkers told us of another celebratory event. Mount Everest had been conquered by the British Everest Expedition. New Zealander Edmund Hillary and Nepalese Sherpa Tenzing Norgay had scaled the 29,002-foot peak. The first to do so.

The driving wind and rain that began mid-morning notwithstanding, the festive spirit abroad in the sea of humanity lining the parade route was unquenchable.[12] Pomp and circumstance reigned. The Life Guards, the Blues, the Grenadiers and Coldstream, the Scots, the Irish, and the Welsh became outward expressions of a lineage woven with pride these centuries on. Ruler-straight rows of scarlet and blue, shining plumed helmets and bearskin hats, kilted pipers, prancing horses, marching bands – ramrod straight they came, eyes fixed. Each man marched in precise step with his neighbour, the lines stretching to the horizon and to memories far beyond. The steel-bound traditions of dress and deportment breathed excellence valued and camaraderie prized, honouring both the present and all that had been. Their very presence proclaimed, "In parade and in battle, on *my* watch the torch is held high – for brothers long gone; for those yet to come; and for the young Queen we honour today."

The loudspeakers strung along East Carriage Drive conjured mental images of Westminster Abbey as the dazzling pallet of colours took shape: gowns of white satin embroidered with rhinestones, silver diamante and pearls, flowing crimson robes trimmed in ermine, diamond-encrusted tiaras, miniver-edged trains that lengthened with rank, the distinct blue, green, rose-pink, white, and silver-grey robes of the Order of Chivalry, the scarlet of the military, the two blues of the Navy and Air Force, the judges splendid in red and ermine, the officers of the law, with full-bottomed wigs, in black-and-gold robes. There were the exotic costumes of India, Africa, the South Seas, and countries circling the globe – a copious sprinkling of princes and princesses, an amir here, a procession of sultans there, and, among them all, the statuesque Queen Salote of Tonga, her face beaming with warmth and good humour.

Down through the ages, since its founding in 1066, Westminster Abbey has been a source of great music and on this day it did not disappoint. For me, the overwhelming musical apogee occurred with the placing of the imperial state crown on the head of the new queen as she sat on the coronation chair with its Stone of Scone. There followed a succession of arpeggios that grew louder and louder as choir, organ, and orchestra launched into George Frideric Handel's two-hundred-year-old coronation anthem "Zadok the Priest."[13] The soaring phrases were sent heavenward to dance, swirl, and reverberate among the towering stone arches, swelling and swelling, again and again, in glorious triumphant joy, a sublime statement of the inexpressible! It was the first time I had heard this musical masterpiece. I was moved beyond words, a reaction that still clouds my eyes this half-century-plus later when, at the click of an Internet button, one is able to return to that historic crossroad.

I believe it may have been then that the dignified octogenarian, sitting three rows in front of us, rose from her seat in the teeming rain, raised her arms, and, looking heavenward, exclaimed in a clear, loud voice that was rich with emphasis and deep feeling, "Good Old England!" The throng around us cheered their approval of her sentiment and the rain offered a benediction as Dad, Mother, Alice, and I traded silent glances of loving appreciation for the privilege of sharing that moment. Three indelible images from that day rich in pageantry have accompanied me through the subsequent decades: the thirty-six scarlet-coated Royal Canadian Mounted Police riding six abreast on their matched black thoroughbred stallions, Queen Salote of Tonga, and, finally, the awe-inspiring gold state coach bearing the newly crowned Queen Elizabeth and Prince Philip.

The warmly beaming, 6'3" Queen Salote rode in an open coach. Although her red and gold gown was soaked through and water streamed down her face, she appeared completely oblivious as she waved to the cheering thousands with expansive, all-embracing warmth and evident joy. The more torrential the deluge, the more hearty her laugh and enthusiastic her wave. Her grace seemed symbolic of the human potential for transcendence. She left in her wake a flood of affection and lessons about both the irrelevance of pretense and the glorious joy experienced in celebrating the moment.

The fairytale baroque splendour of the gold state coach was arresting as it passed us, drawn by eight Windsor greys with four postillion riders flanked by members of the Queen's Yeoman of the Guard. Its gilded magnificence and profusion of allegorical carvings and painted exterior panels dazzled. And, on this overcast day, its brilliant transparency revealed the young queen remarkably energized and radiant in spite of the bone-rattling ride the coach provided owing to its ancient leather suspension.[14]

The palpable charisma of Coronation Tuesday lingered on through Wednesday when we returned to Buckingham Palace to view the nocturnal splendour of the Mall, spanned as it was, from the Palace to Admiralty Arch, by a magnificent series of towering illuminated arches, each carrying two lions rampant above and an enormous filigreed crown below. In addition, the full length of this historic carriageway was flanked on both sides by a stately procession of crown-topped standards, each doubly draped with floodlit banners.

Nearing midnight, after we had wended our way through the joyous mass of thousands upon thousands of late-evening revelers, a bobby at the Admiralty Arch informed us that we must return down the Mall past the Palace to reach Victoria Station for the train home to Croydon. The prospect of threading our way back through that endless sea of humanity was overwhelming.

It was then that the distant cheering at the gates of the Palace intensified to an ear-splitting roar as the balcony curtains fluttered. In an instant, my proudly indifferent, royalty-disdaining father sprinted past us, his face shining. First World War prejudices forgotten, he reached the Palace, his family trailing, as the queen and her prince made their appearance. It was in reflecting on Dad's radiant enthusiasm that I finally understood the full power of the magic we had shared.[15] We had witnessed "Good Olde England" fully embraced.

Crossing the Channel in mid-June, our compact British car bearing a Royal Automobile Club crest made its way through rural France and Flanders where the reminders of war frequently came in human form as the locals, especially the children, greeted us with a thumbs-up salute or a Churchillian V-for-Victory signal. Sometimes they were smiling – especially the young ones – but many remained formally sober-faced as they saluted, thus acknowledging a deeper allied bond. They were the citizens of Arras, Mont-Saint-Eloi, Lens, Vimy, Cambrai, Ypres, and Passchendaele and they remembered.

At first glance the land appeared blissfully intact, save for the scattered deep pockmarks, straggling barbed-wire remnants, commemorative monuments, and cemeteries, but as we drove on, Dad appeared to be looking for something. He pulled the car onto the shoulder of a deserted road. His expression was questioning yet intense. We were near La Targette Corners. The field across from us had gone to seed; the long-neglected fences were overgrown.

I followed him out of the car; Mother and Alice stayed behind. "Let's take a look over there," he muttered, pointing vaguely. "If I'm not mistaken, I think there is something there I'd like to show you." He was standing rigidly erect now; his gait had become purposeful. Arriving at a clump of underbrush at the edge of a field, he pulled back a tangle of branches to expose a black hole in the ground that was four or five feet across. The floor of this hidden tunnel quickly descended as it penetrated the darkness; fragments of decaying wooden beams protruded from the ceiling.

His gaze intensified, his face flushing with the rush of memory. Thirty-six years had passed since he last stood at this spot. I peered into the blackness as he described the night – or was it nights? – spent sleeping in the damp cave below us. His jaw was set as he added that it was here that thousands of Frenchmen died when gassed by the Germans.

We moved on: Cambrai, Neuville Sainte-Vaast, Vimy, Petit Vimy. He pointed out the field where he and his mates had played sports; the place where he considered cutting down the Canadian soldier who had been tied to a tree for failure to salute an officer; the church where his company had attended a worship service; and, finally, the towering Vimy Memorial with its memory-ladened inscription: "The Canadian Corps on 9th April 1917 with four divisions in line on a front of four miles attacked and captured this ridge. To the valour of their Countrymen of the Great War and in memory of their 60,000 dead this monument is raised by the People of Canada." At La Targette, a monument bore the name Neuville Saint-Vaast, the date of its liberation on 9 May 1915, and a plaque that read: "You, the living who pass by this torch, raised above the bloody battlefield, survey this ground replete with graves and think of our dead whose hearts were good." Within a radius of six miles of this site there were approximately 200,000 military graves, a testament to the utter madness of war. We walked in silence through the markers of the 44,533 graves of the Neuville Saint-Vaast German military cemetery and someone whispered, "How many Beethovens, Bachs or Mozarts lie buried here?"

On 10 July we stood huddled in the Zurich airport cloaked by awkward silence. Dad groped for words. "Time goes by so quickly. Only yesterday we were planning this trip." Each of us felt the emptiness. His flight home was called; he headed toward the gate and the patients waiting for him half a world away; Mother, Alice, and I returned to the car in silence and headed for Lausanne to take French courses. While our pursuit of enhanced linguistic skills was well intended, our classes were loosely attended; a golden opportunity was largely wasted, in part because I was suffering a lingering illness marked by fatigue, weakness, malaise, and nausea. The doctor called it hepatitis.

The weeks that followed involved further challenges as we headed home: a nocturnal fall into a roadside culvert (x-rays for fracture negative); a massive general strike in France that shut down trains, telephones, and stores, leading to a last-minute plan to sell the car in Paris; the sublimely haughty Paris gendarme informing Mother as she circled the Opera for the third time, "Madame, we drive on the right-hand side of the road in France," and Mother's exasperated reply, "I *am* driving on the right-hand side of the road!"; mounting strike-related risks, with three killed in Rouen riots; once again strike-induced change-in-destination plans from Calais to Le Havre; further transportation changes to enable us to reach Le Havre. That Mother missed Dad's collaborative input in meeting these adventures is certain, but, typical of her buoyant attitude, this was never evident or mentioned.

Early in the trip, I had done quick sketches of Mom and Al as we drove through France; later, a pen-and-ink sketch of Michelangelo's Moses, Mt Rosa, the Matterhorn, and some simple illustrations for my daily diary. Somewhere in this process, the joy of drawing from life and recording my impressions of new places took root. Memories were clearer, it seemed, when I observed the subject with sufficient presence to do a sketch. In this regard, our brief stop in Paris was dazzling. Most memorable was the Louvre with its apparently endless corridors of the masterworks – Leonardo da Vinci, Rubens, van Dyck, David, Van Gogh, Toulouse Lautrec, Frans Hals, Reynolds ... paintings I had seen copies of were now confronting me face to face.

LIFE AT FIFTEEN AND THEN SOME

Surrounded by my close-knit group of peers, I slid through my second year at Glebe with preoccupations largely social. Academic achievement remaining a nebulous concept; my only memory of those months involves the cruelty of classmates who repeatedly provoked startled responses from our teacher, a shell-shocked Canadian army veteran, by throwing carefully aimed spitballs or creating a sudden sharp noise by dropping a weighty book on the hardwood floor.

The following summer I was a YMCA camp counsellor. Two memories remain. The first concerns a mid-afternoon thunderstorm that featured an ear-splitting lightning strike that shattered the great elm directly above our tent and illuminated our canvas cube and its five or six occupants, the brightness rivalling a 1,000-watt light bulb. Campers and counsellor survived, the tree didn't.

Equally enlightening, in its way, was the waterfront campfire planned for a dark, moonless night. The highlight was to be a ghost story that would end the evening. It would be told by the camp director and was to feature, as a final touch, the appearance, far out on the bay, of a canoe bearing a legendary, long-deceased Iroquois chief brandishing a torch. I was to portray that aquatic spectre. The plan was to ignite a torch in response to a secret signal from the storyteller. To ensure the effect would be memorable, I made a last-moment decision to take with me in the canoe a pail of gasoline as backup for the already well-soaked would-be torch. It was going to be great! I watched for the signal in the blackness sixty yards or so offshore.

With a strike of the match, the torch burst into flame most impressively. At that same moment, however, the inferno jumped on a sheet of fumes to the pail at my feet, setting off a remarkable fireball as I dove for the water and the canoe flipped. I am told that the effect was spectacular. It was all that I had aimed for and more – well, sort of. As the flaming gasoline rocketed across the bay in all directions, I watched from below the surface. The flames soon burned themselves out, but I had some explaining to do.

Letters from home revealed things at 37 unfolding in predictable fashion. Mother wrote: "Dad is operating tonight. He has been very busy nearly every night ... Jim is working on his motorcycle, to sell. The clutch is broken. Betty is practicing the piano. ... Al writes that she has girls age 6 to 10 for summer school. She seems to be enjoying her work ... We had the Woodsides in for dinner and started to show transparencies but the bulb burned out, then movies, but the projector wouldn't work. They were all a fizzle!!" Dad's letter of 8 August read in part:

> I know you will contribute your best to the camp whether or not prizes, etc. come your way. We do things to be done to the best of our ability, not because of praise & appreciation from associates, but

because there is no other *right* way or satisfying way to do things. In the end and finally, son, we live with ourselves and we must account to ourselves for the way in which we do our job. We ourselves know when we have done a good job & that in itself is the just reward.

Son my spirit & love are with you now, daily and will be with you so long as you walk this earth whether I am here to see you in the flesh or whether I have gone the way of all flesh.

Looking forward to seeing you.

Dad

Dad brought to daily affairs an unshakable calm; Mother, on the other hand, consistently injected a special mix of warmth, goodwill, and a quirky capacity for inventive responses, particularly when her perceived rights, or those of loved ones, were ignored. An episode involving a belligerent neighbour illustrated this aspect of her character.

It wasn't that she bore our new neighbour malice. Indeed, she was determined to reach out in welcome when it became clear that the vacant lot beside us was to become the site of a new home. The chain of events that ensued, however, gradually eroded her charitable resolve. Excavation for our neighbour's house was complete and the foundation laid before I left for camp. My return in August thus provided a front-row seat as the ensuing drama unfolded.

First, there was the matter of the fence. City by-laws had been ignored when the massive chasm next door was extended to meet the property line. This resulted in our white-picket fence and adjacent trees toppling into the gaping hole. Mother's inquiries with municipal authorities met with a deaf ear. Our neighbour-to-be, Mr B, was indifferent. Mother's jaw became more firmly set, but she remained determined to be hospitable. The final test was yet to come.

Several months after our new neighbours moved in, fate smiled in a singularly ironic way. For whatever reason, the telephone company, in its wisdom, changed many phone numbers in our region. Suddenly, our telephone, which was already frenetically busy with the daily steady stream of calls from Dad's patients, became even busier. This was a serious issue. It could bring us to our knees!

With our newly assigned phone number, *additional* calls also poured in. They were for a local dry-cleaning establishment whose old phone number we now possessed. We were informed by one frustrated customer that our number appeared on the cleaners' stationery and statements of account. Ironically, the owner of the business in question was our new neighbour!

The phone company refused to change the number. The women at the cleaners were sympathetic but could do nothing without Mr B's permission. Mother phoned him, and, after identifying herself as his new neighbour, carefully explained her plight. She was pleasant, almost apologetic, but his response was swift and blunt. He had just purchased a large supply of stationary and we would have to put up with the inconvenience until it had all been used.

"But surely you could simply have your staff change the phone number as they make out the statement of account," Mother suggested in a friendly tone.

"It would waste too much of their time!"

"Surely it must be harmful for business to have your customers so inconvenienced."

"That's my business."

Mother was polite and controlled as she hung up the phone. She looked determined. I had seen that look before. As I recall, she did not discuss the matter further.

It was the next afternoon, I believe, when the phone rang and Mother called out cheerily, "I'll get it." Her "Hello," was buoyant, so I was dumfounded when the following pause was broken with a rather brassy, "What's that lady? Just a second! I can't hear a thing around here with all these boilers going!" Then, holding the phone away from her, "Hey Ralph, some old biddy here's calling about her husband's shirts!" Then into the receiver, "Sorry lady, you'll have to call back. Maybe tomorrow."

On the next call, an irate customer was demanding a dress shirt that was needed without delay. "Listen Mister," intoned Mother airily, "you'll be lucky if we find that shirt by this time next week."

After a moment, the caller responded, "This isn't the cleaner! Say, who *is* this?!!" Mother apologized and explained the situation in full. "Well I don't blame you a bit. I'd do exactly the same if I were you," he snorted.

The third call was to dispute a bill. "Don't worry about a thing, lady," Mother responded. "I'm sure we overcharged you. Just don't pay the bill." All calls stopped within forty-eight hours! The twinkle in Mother's eye lasted considerably longer.

The fall of '54 saw an increase in my awareness of the academic demands at hand, but progress was slow. Of more immediate concern, I must admit, was my purchase of Jim's motorcycle and the fact that grade eleven brought the opportunity to audition for Glebe's renowned choir, the Lyre's Club. Jim had been an enthusiastic Lyre under the founding director, Bob McGregor, and personal highlights of my first two years at Glebe had included savouring the rich four-part harmonies of this superb ensemble, not to mention the stories of their escapades during international competitions, concert trips, radio broadcasts, and their annual fundraising dance, the Harmony Hop.[16] The Lyre's Club theme song, "The Long Day Closes" by Arthur Sullivan, with its liquid phrasing and sense of transience, never ceased to draw both choristers and audience into the intimacy of the shared present.

Joining the Lyre's Club issued in a new dawn,[17] one that was soon followed by a second in the form of Judy Crain. Judy was bright, blond, delightfully authentic, and without pretense. Her face radiated a consistent cheerfulness that often gave way to an infectious chuckle. She was conscientious, hardworking, generous, open, respected, and liked by all. She and I thereafter juggled a joint social calendar during our final three years at Glebe. It was to involve a whirlwind of successive New Year's Eve Lyre's Club parties at 37, an endless succession of dances at one school or another, a weekend trip to Queen's with family in tow, Judy's chorus-line stint at Ottawa's 1956 May Court Ball, endless walks and discussions, hosting Germany's famed Obernkirchen Children's Choir, participating in a Newton, Massachusetts, student exchange, swimming and family time at the Crain cottage on Big Rideau Lake, and a low 1956 fly-past as Gord Larsen and I buzzed the Crain cottage in a Fleet Canuck which Gord had rented from the Ottawa Flying Club.[18] Judy was a breath of fresh air. During our final year at Glebe, the student body voted her head girl and our friend Dan Krupka head boy. The principal acknowledged their new roles by presenting them with gifts during a packed, full-school assembly. Dan was given a small, carefully wrapped box (a tie? a clock?) followed by the principal's formal handshake and a round of enthusiastic applause.

The presentation to Judy was next. In contrast to Dan's compact gift, hers was huge. Both presents had been sitting beside the podium as the assembly started. On being the centre of such attention and so conspicuously celebrated, Judy was feeling somewhat self-conscious as she was greeted by the appreciative students and congratulated by the principal, who then invited her to open her gift. It was difficult to imagine the contents. There was, as a result, a thunderous silence as she gingerly undertook the task at hand – massive ribbons, carefully taped gift paper, cardboard flaps closing the upper end. As the top opened there was a collective gasp and a muffled shriek from the new head girl as I sprang out of the depths. (It wasn't my idea.) The place was in an uproar, Judy jumping back with arms flying and flushed but managing her customary smile and laugh as the shock subsided.

Forty years later, I was approached by a stranger, a woman who identified herself as having been in grade nine during that assembly. She
wanted to tell me that Judy's surprise gift was the most romantic memory of her early years. It had left her in tears. Those final years with Judy
at Glebe were a privileged time for me, time filled with memories of her
and of our group of close friends.

SUNDAYS, BELIEFS, AND FAMILY ROUTINES

The weekly Chalmers Church service was Sunday at 11:00 A.M. The
minister until 1949 at this two thousand-member downtown centre of
worship was John W. Woodside. In my young eyes, the persona of this
distant figure was both vague and celestial, a state undoubtedly ensured
by the appellation "The Very Reverend" and the fact that he had served
as moderator of the United Church of Canada and as president of the
Canadian Council of Churches, leading me to assume that his status was
undoubtedly equivalent to that of the pope.

During the 1950s, Dr Woodside was followed at Chalmers by thir-
ty-year-old A. Leonard Griffith. To my pre-adolescent eyes, "This was
a man!" He brought rock-solid presence, a clear and thoughtful mind,
a challenging faith, and epic skills as an orator. Decades later, one of
his colleagues commented, "Leonard was probably the greatest preacher
Canada ever produced." Griffith combined forthright integrity, wisdom,
and a refreshing sense of humour. Soon after he and his wife, Merilie,
arrived at Chalmers, he informed the venerable congregation with a twinkle, "When Merilie turns forty, I plan to turn her in for two twenties."

Sunday dinner followed church. It was an important family time, a
reliable anchor in the weekly schedule. Betty would join us when Jim
was home from Queen's on "laundry weekends," thus making it a gathering of six around the spacious table. The dining room was an airy, open
space, with large floor-to-ceiling windows on two sides and easy access
from the front hall, kitchen, and adjacent flagstone patio and lawn.

Dad would sharpen the already dangerous stainless-steel carving knife
with several perfunctory passes over the accompanying file, and then
turn with a mix of surgical formality and evident pleasure to the ample
joint of beef that lay on the platter before him. He always stood during
this ritual, relaxed but intent. Generally, the medium-well-done roast
was ringed by browned potatoes, done to a turn. With the beef served,
each plate was passed to Mother's end of the table, where the vegetables
were waiting in their respective covered casserole dishes for her cheerful
enquiry about the appetite of each person.

The "good glass bowl" (it had been Grandma Henry's and came from "The Springfield Store" and thus had attained the status of a near-sacred relic) brimmed with Mother's trademark tomato relish. Various mustards, each with its own time-honoured pot, the special flowered butter dish, and the piping-hot sculpted gravy boat graced the linen tablecloth along with a scattering of small crystal salt-and-pepper shakers with silver tops. For starters, a small glass of tomato juice generally stood at each place beside the water glass.

With everyone served and the traditional "Oh, please, *do* start while it's hot!" dispensed with, the meal got underway with hands clasped around the table as grace was said or often sung – "Be present at our table Lord ..." This inevitably ended in a far from serious, baroque flourish of four-part harmony, egged on by Jim's cascading baritone run of eighth notes. If any semblance of sanctity was preserved, it was in the communal delight of a family tradition shared one more time. This weekly meal wasn't about form or formality. Rather, it was simply about being together, as a family, and being grateful for it.

Generally, early in the meal, Dad would initiate a discussion about the pressing issues of the day. I often resented these affairs. "Why can't we talk about what each of us has done today the way the Bensons do, rather than all this philosophy stuff?" To which Jim would offer a lofty retort that implied that someday I would grow up and learn to appreciate things I now could not understand. I would feel guilty.

There was no end to productive subject matter for these Sunday dinner gatherings: American civil rights (Is there racism in Canada?); the newly minted Canada-U.S. Distant Early Warning (DEW) Line to alert us to a Russian attack over the Arctic (Is there *really* a Soviet risk?); American Senator Joseph McCarthy's paranoid hunt for Communists (Dad's positive impressions of his Soviet Embassy patients); the U.S. test of a hydrogen bomb in the Pacific (Where is all this leading us?!); Jonas Salk's discovery of a polio vaccine (Descriptions of polio patients Dad and Mother had cared for on the Labrador coast); the brutal 6 December 1956 "Blood in the Water" Russia vs. Hungary water-polo game at the Melbourne Olympics, prior to the Russian suppression of the Hungarian Revolution (What is our responsibility to help the penniless folks now pouring into Canada from Hungary?);[19] the hero status accorded Martin Luther King and Fidel Castro ('Would *we* have the courage to speak up for the disenfranchised?); recent waves in the world of music as Maria Callas had her debut at the Met in Bellini's *Norma*, Arturo Toscanini died, and Elvis strode into our lives (reverence accorded the first two, curiosity the third, although Mother admitted finding him "interesting"

as she responded demurely when asked her opinion); murmurs of wonderment as the transatlantic cable-telephone service was inaugurated
("Think of it! Speaking live, directly to loved ones overseas!").

As I think back, I can't recall the exact topic that set me off one particular Sunday. Something from a Leonard Griffith sermon? The mono-
tonal congregational repetition of a creed? A theological point made by
Dad or Jim? Whatever it was, I clearly recall the volley I levelled across
the collective family bow, if not the precise wording.

> Who can go along with, let alone *believe* in, all that fantastic water-
> into-wine, three-in-one, head-in-the-sand, fairy-tale, mind-reading,
> heavenly choirs of angels, walking on water, original sin, miracle
> cures, immaculate conception, sleight-of-hand demons-into-pigs
> literalistic stuff?! And what about the archaic, magical-thinking
> creed that proclaims a human-like Father-God-creator, or Jesus
> his only son – *Only? Son?* Offspring of a *Holy Ghost*, through a
> *virgin* birth? Who descended into hell? Because of me? Then popped
> up again? And what about a communion of saints? (How do you
> define "saint"?) Resurrection? Life everlasting? (How do you define
> *life*, and how about *everlasting*?) And what about a creed that we
> must swear is the *only* lifeline to a bliss-ever-after existence? You
> can't be serious! The "don't-think," just "sign-on-the-dotted-line"
> or you'll-wish-you-had-ness of it all! The patent idiocy of pledging
> belief in the unbelievable, as the only way to win over an all-caring,
> all-loving, all-powerful, male God! Not to mention the premise that
> an all-caring, all-loving, all-powerful God is behind the unmerited
> suffering seen at every turn. And beyond that, how do we know the
> Gospels are accurate historically? And since they don't agree, which
> one shall we take as being historically reliable? And where did Jesus
> ever imply that he wanted to start a church anyway?!

My volley was met with supportive listening and openness, without
judgment but *with* debate.

An April 1955 dream gave rise to a very different memory.[20] It remains,
even now, the clearest dream I have experienced. It was around the time
of my sixteenth birthday. I would thus soon be able to obtain a driver's
licence. Indeed, I had been given several recent clandestine driving lessons by Mother on the back lanes of the nearby Experimental Farm. As
is so often the case, the dream had two parts. In the first, I was alone
in Mother's compact black Austin sedan, parked in front of 37, cau-
tiously experimenting with the clutch while changing gears back and

forth, from forward to reverse. Suddenly, I found myself stuck, off-road, part-way up the steeply inclined dirt path leading to the vacant lot adjacent to 37. The car had stalled. I climbed out to seek help. The scene changed, instantly; it was the second part of the dream. The stalled car was now nowhere to be seen and I was standing on the vacant lot facing the path descending to the street. I was now perhaps two or three feet above the spot where the car had been a moment earlier. It was a lovely bright day. There was a light breeze. As I looked down on the sidewalk in front of 37, two young men who appeared to be in their early thirties were approaching, chatting amiably. They were not more than twenty or thirty feet from me. They were tanned and had trim haircuts and open, friendly faces. They were dressed in light khaki slacks and shoes, and matching shirts with fabric epaulets at the shoulders. It was an outfit I had not previously seen.

As they approached, the fellow nearest the curb, the one with light sand-coloured hair, looked up at me with a knowing, somewhat amused smile of recognition. To my astonishment, I knew him immediately. He was Jesus. I knew him, not because he bore any resemblance to the long-haired biblical stereotype, but based on a deep inner certainty. It was him. I was astounded. Furthermore, I knew our recognition was mutual.

At that moment, I saw that he and his companion were turning to leave. I felt an overwhelming sense of loss, a soul-wrenching ache. No words were exchanged. They were unnecessary. In response to my inner anguish, his smile broadened slightly and through a direct eye-to-eye glance he reassured me wordlessly. "Don't worry. We shall meet again."

I awoke and sat up. I was left with a sense of indelible clarity and graphic reality that was totally unlike the lingering wisps of other dreams. I felt refreshed, excited, but filled with longing and a powerful sense of having had a profound personal encounter.

I realized it was not the sort of thing one could adequately put into words or share with others. Forty-five years would pass before I visited Israel and saw for the first time young army conscripts dressed exactly as in my dream. Its content and non-verbal dialogue has remained with me these six decades after our encounter.

DENNY F. AND THE WATER DEPARTMENT

During the summers of '55 and '56, I found myself working in the "real world" for the first time, as a minor contributor to the surveying team laying water mains for the Ottawa Water Department, particularly in Alta Vista and other new subdivisions. It was my first exposure to workaday life: from boredom to the joys and challenges of teamwork and the dilemmas created by contractors hungrily mapping regional urban development. Endless hours were consumed trudging on steaming summer asphalt under the blazing sun and days shivering through rain-soaked cold snaps. Based on the limited perspective gained through my lowly post, I *knew*, beyond any shadow of a doubt, that I did *not* want a career in engineering, *any form* of engineering.

My colleagues during those two summers were as varied as life can provide, but three overarching priorities reigned supreme across the ranks of my workmates, rendering all other topics of conversation irrelevant: cars, sports, and women. In that order. Cars ranked first, by a long shot. There was, however, some dispute about the ranking of the other two priorities and most agreed that to differentiate between sports and women was to split hairs. There were, however, rare exceptions among my confrères. For example, Clayton Ryan. Clayton was older than the others on the team. A quiet, hardworking, family man of grace and discernment, he was respected by all. A team leader, he exemplified life thoughtfully lived; he had no need to run with the pack. He made it clear that a man has the freedom to set his own course.

And then there was Denny F. He also marched to the beat of his own drum. Denny was a force of nature! In his early twenties perhaps, he was a free spirit, an impossibly charismatic, radiant light that naturally attracted all manner of moths. Denny was untamed. He had a limitless capacity to celebrate life, love, and himself. He would announce, wide-eyed, with an impish grin, "I wouldn't say that I'm the best looking guy in town, but what's my word against five thousand women?" He drove a long, sleek, pale-blue convertible – top always down. Denny was quick, insightful, and capable beyond most. He had untapped potential galore. His super-cool persona and appealing hand gestures (a come-hither wrist-flick beckoning motion of one or both hands, with first and second fingers extended) added a pseudo-Italian dynamic flare.

Denny called everyone, even his mother, "Jack," and prefaced all observations with "one thing about it." His rugged, tanned, open-faced good looks, sparkling eyes, tousled hair, and casual clothes radiated an appealing warmth that boosted the self-esteem and confidence of others.

We became friends and I felt certain that, if I could just get Denny to return to high school, there would be nothing he couldn't accomplish. Having talked him into my fantasy, I offered to run interference with the Glebe administration. They informed me that he would need a certificate attesting to grades completed. No problem. Denny came up with a document that appeared surprisingly crisp and newly minted. I expressed concern about its origins, but he just smiled at the secretary, and that was that.

Denny cut a wide swath through Glebe. The guys admired him; the girls were smitten. The school term was still young when, in a fit of enthusiasm, he decided to try out for the senior football team. Strong, fit, and full of enthusiasm, if completely inexperienced on the football field, he made the team. Things were going perfectly. That is, until the day we played at Lansdowne Park when, completely inebriated, he fell off the team bench on the sidelines. So ended his academic career. I suppose it was too good to last. Perhaps some spirits must remain unbroken. But ever since, when someone tries to define too narrowly all that is wondrous in the human spirit, I think of Denny and give thanks.

QUO VADIS?

What would follow high school? Where does my vocation lie? Ottawa artist and family friend Eleanor Williamson encouraged me to pursue my interest in art. Nothing else kindled a flame, but I recognized the limits of my talents and backed off without a fight in the face of parental shrugs suggesting that art would always be a good hobby but didn't carry much promise as a way to make a living. Medicine? The family business? Jim seemed to be enjoying his medical studies at Queen's: he would be graduating as I arrived in Kingston. The final-year medical students that Dad taught each year seemed to enjoy what they were doing. They came to 37 for dinner during their rotation and in the course of the evening Dad would give an illustrated lecture on the brain using the small blackboard in the basement playroom.

To some extent, medicine became my choice by a process of elimination, but on the positive side of the ledger three aspects of the profession seemed particularly attractive: the opportunity for service through direct personal contact; the obvious pleasure Dad derived from the profession; and the possibility of working with one's hands. Surely surgery, like art, could be a path toward creativity and fulfillment.

Grade thirteen, our final year at Glebe, fell into a daily routine: the walk to school with Bob or lifelong neighbour Eleanor, classes, homework, the Lyres Club, hanging out with Bob, Pritch, Dave, Gord, and the others, Judy, drawing, and exams. The annual prom that year, 1957, featured my inadequate assessment as a driver of icy streets, which led, in succession, to two head-on collisions – first with a snow-covered traffic island, then with Judy's father when I finally got her home. We had escaped injury despite the absence of seat belts.

With the last Lyre's Club concert on 1 March behind us, our year-end provincial examinations loomed large – algebra, geometry, trigonometry and statistics, French composition, French authors, English literature, English composition, physics, and chemistry. But space in the study schedule was demanded for one more blowout. On Wednesday, 3 April, I joined three male cronies and nine thousand others in a pilgrimage to the Ottawa Auditorium[21] for an evening that was heralded by the press as "the pop-culture event of the decade," the Ottawa concerts by twenty-two-year-old Elvis Presley.[22]

We arrived at the "Aud" to find a restless crowd milling, ant-like, about the building. The police were out in force. As showtime approached, a seemingly endless line of motorcycles – Harleys mainly – spread up Argyle Street, each leaning at its own proudly rakish angle, tightly slotted beside its neighbour, side by side. Each machine stood as an impressive backdrop for its carefully tattooed rider with his leathers, studs, and chains. Studiously coiffed hair, sideburns, and a silent, frowning sneer celebrated the unique *presence* of each man, while his leather-jacketed, bespangled, long-haired lady completed the tableau as she draped herself self-consciously over man and machine. The air was heavy with anticipation and the deep growling rumble of each new bike as it made its dramatic, sweeping entrance into the line.

Inside the arena the strutting, carefully choreographed tension bubbled, swelling with the growing throng as the minutes passed. Finally, the lights lowered, to a roar of approval. It was a raw-meat moment!

A band came out, to a sprinkling of applause. Then a singer. Poor soul. He was an Irish tenor. His first song encountered quiet restlessness; his second and third, frank hostility. Next, there was a dancer, perhaps a tap-dancer, and the music picked up in pace momentarily, holding the smouldering ambient angst in abeyance. Then, at precisely the right moment, the dancer gave a sort of Presley-esque gyration and the crowd went wild.

We were being played with.

Following a splendid introduction, the next act, Presley's back-up vocal quartet, appeared to a burst of thunderous applause. "Now this is more like it!" They sprinkled a few more Presley premonitions toward the sea of gaping mouths packing the stands, each tidbit provoking another eruption from the crowd. Excitement was building.

Finally, the announcer who was to introduce the announcer who would introduce Elvis was introduced. The continuing roar rose to new heights. Up the pecking order we went. Finally, it happened!

LADIES AND GENTLEMEN! ... [Roar] ... IT IS MY PLEASURE AND
GREAT HONOUR ... [Roar] ... TO INTRODUCE TO YOU! ... [Roar] ...
THE ONE ... [Roar] ... THE ONLY ... [Roar] ... ELVIS!! ... [Roarrrrrr]
... PRESLEY!!!!!

I noticed for the first time that there was an impressive cantilevered walkway running forward from the distant rear curtain. It sloped upward as
it approached the front of the stage. Blinding searchlights were playing
back and forth across the audience and stage in an apparently hopeless search for Elvis ... *Delay* ... *Delay* ... heart-stopping, breath-holding
expectations escalating. Sporadic weeping in the audience. "This is
unbelievable!"

Then, *he* appeared – gold-shimmering jacket, dark slacks, a gigantic guitar slung across his chest. He was a big man – taller than I had
expected – and hopelessly attractive with a childish grin. He walked
slowly up the ramp toward us and then descended the couple of steps to
the stage – *emotional chaos pulsating* – accompanied by an explosion of
flashing lights. Total pandemonium!

He reached the apron of the stage. He had a commanding stage presence! With everyone on their feet, cheering frantically, he reached the
mic; he cupped his hands over his eyes against the glare of the spotlights
and leaned toward us. Then, grinning, he exhaled a deep, drawn-out,
sultry, *Wwwelll!* ..., and the place went nuts. He played with the hyster-
ical masses a while longer – a strummed chord, another gravelly word
of greeting.

As I watched, a strange out-of-synch moment seemed to occur. I saw
it all from a fresh perspective. The carefully programmed manipulations
and interaction with the audience seemed to fade and beneath the sheer
lunatic madness of the charade and theatrics of the crowd I glimpsed
in Elvis a moment of authenticity. His mask dissolved. To reveal what?
The presence of a twenty-two-year-old peer? A hint of genuine puzzlement? A trace of youthful vulnerability? Though lasting only a moment,
it seemed real and touching. Then the moment was gone and it was on
with the show.

Last high-school moments: motorcycle sold, final exams written, the
marks marginal at best, application submitted to Queen's. Judy was
on her way to nursing at the Kingston General Hospital (KGH), as was
Eleanor Kidd, while Dan Krupka, the perennial gold medalist of our
year and head boy, was off to McGill. Bob was headed to the University
of Toronto, and so it went. Our gang of twenty, who had so memorably
shaped my Glebe years, was dispersing without fanfare. Hard to believe.

Then, on 25 May, the family celebrated Jim's graduation. Dr Wilder Penfield spoke at the convocation and Jim headed to Montreal for his internship at the Montreal General Hospital.

As August 1957 wore on, the time-honoured annual Mount family search for a summer cottage or farm spluttered into life, once again without success. Then, one balmy August weekend, Mother and I accompanied an affable young real estate agent in a small outboard runabout boat to an island on Grand Lake, forty minutes east of Ottawa in the Gatineau Hills. It was heavily wooded with old-growth cedar and towering white pines. Our agent headed the boat for the rambling forest-green cottage on the northern end of the hour-glass-shaped island "Here we are! Taft Island! It's quite special!"

We had not yet reached the makeshift dock when Mother and I silently looked at each other. It was one of those experiences of synchronicity that suggest the abiding mystery of *presence* in the lived moment. "This is the place!" she quipped, quoting Brigham Young. I nodded.

The sense of "coming home" to a place we had never been before was mutual, and the *Place* joined 37 in offering fertile roots for family comings and goings from that day on. The cottage and outbuildings dated from 1919 when Boston businessman W.A. Taft had purchased the island for $800.

The news finally arrived. I had been accepted into Queen's Meds '63. I assumed that it must have been my paternal and fraternal ties, since my average was 66 per cent – almost certainly the lowest in the class. High school classmates Earl Covert, Anne Porter, and Rich Kidd were all headed to Queen's Meds with me. Judy's mother wrote a warm note of congratulations. Judy suggested that to fully live our university experience we should date others as well. High school was definitely over.

Queen's, 1957–63

Oil thigh na Banrighinn a'Banrighinn gu brath!
Cha-gheill! Cha-gheill! Cha-gheill!

I daydream for a moment
and seem to see
a flash of Stewart plaid
and faintly hear the sound of bagpipes.

The strong smell of fresh beer,
limestone walls,
folksongs loudly sung,
the frenzied swirl of a tea dance,
blue leather jackets.

Recall those endless discussions and debates.
Professors of all sizes, with varying ability
propounding their beliefs.

Classmates,
their first blush of enthusiasm
later suffering to different degrees from the bite of the bug
called cynicism –
but each making a unique contribution to our year.

Six years flash past and we disperse.
Let's all return to drink together once again – at our
reunions.[1]

PRE-MED I, 1957–58

A cold drizzle – something between heavy mist and sleet – was blowing in off Lake Ontario as we drove into Kingston on that dismal, end of August 1957, morning. Slate grey waves were tirelessly attacking the bleached limestone shoreline just below the fifteen-foot-thick lakeside wall of Murney Tower, a solitary Martello fortress that had stood guard on that spot for a century, and I desperately needed a cup of coffee to wash the chill out of my bones.

"Welcome to Kingston," someone in my heater-less Morris sedan muttered bleakly.[2] "They say this is a *normal* fall morning here! Lord save us!" The final report I had submitted days earlier as summer inspector for the Ottawa Water Department seemed a distant figment of the imagination.[3]

My initial Kingston lodgings were spotty, at best. I left them after only three days at the insistence of Mother, who had arrived from Ottawa to check out her suspicion that the place I had selected might not be conducive to academic excellence; my second lodging was abandoned because of noise; the third was brief owing to my eviction for throwing classmate Al Mark through the bedsprings during a friendly wrestling match. Finally, true tranquility arrived with option four, an apartment I shared on 21 Sydenham St with a Meds '63 classmate and erstwhile Opeongo Road neighbour Richard Kidd.

Eating was a different story. Following a brief catch-as-catch-can period, I struck gold on being accepted for meals at a much-sought-after centre of excellence, a women's residence for ten and boarding house for many more, located a stone's throw from the campus. A local legend, "Ruth's" (or simply "164 Barrie"), was the prodigy of one Ruth Moore. A good-natured lady with an air of perennial youth, Ruth ran a tight ship. This scrupulously clean, highly organized institution was more than a business. It was her calling and life mission. Meals were taken together, two dozen or so at a sitting. Grace, a thrice-daily celestial pause in the hurly-burly of the day, was offered at each meal with gentle earnestness by Ruth herself following a reverential preliminary *All... riiiight ...* as we stood in expectant silence at our respective places.

Ruth's delicious home cooking, coupled with the opportunity to participate in a close-knit, family-like student community of thirty to forty peers from all faculties, provided a priceless foundation for university life. Her warmth and ready smile were catalytic in enabling the close friendship she enjoyed with each member of her extended student family. In my case, this bond was threatened only once. It was that unfortunate day I exuberantly and mindlessly responded to a request to pass the butter by delivering a frisbee toss of the butter dish to the other end of the table. Expulsion for that misdemeanour was mercifully brief.[4]

With registration on Monday, 9 September, 1957, we became members of the Aesculapian Society of Queen's University, a fraternity for faculty, students, and Queen's medical graduates founded in 1873. We had just embarked on a six-year program, two pre-medical years and four medical, that would lead to our becoming doctors of medicine, as preposterous as that seemed. Indeed, the likelihood of surviving the first week appeared to be slim. There were forms to complete, elective courses to choose, campus maps to study, faculty-information sheets to peruse, textbooks and instruments to buy, and, as dictated by our lofty second-year superiors in Meds '62, rigorous initiation demands to adhere to.

The Queen's University class of potential 1963 medical graduates, or Meds '63, met for the first time that Monday. There were sixty-five in the class, including seven women; each of us looked pale and awkwardly tentative as we took our seats. The dean, Dr G.H. "Curly" Ettinger, offered a warm welcome and introduced key faculty and administrative personnel. We were then invited to introduce ourselves to the persons sitting immediately to our left and right and informed that, at a minimum, one of each triad would *not* graduate. Perhaps, the dean continued, we would be interested in the predictive variables. Women were less likely to graduate than men; sons of doctors generally fared badly; parental income was relevant, with sons of blue-collar workers doing best; age was also said to be predictive – the older the better, with those who were over twenty on the day of that meeting being more likely to graduate. He ended with a flourish. "Blood, sweat and tears are no substitute for intelligence, but I'll take them every time!" The message could not be clearer. Having a terrible academic record, being eighteen and the son of a doctor whose income exceeded the blue-collar range, I blanched.

Our Meds '62 "big brothers" were then assigned. Mine was Peter McLean, who hailed from Ottawa. These higher-life forms were to act as personal advisers as well as a source of used textbooks. Furthermore, we were informed, the all-powerful Meds '62 Vigilante Committee would be our masters during Frosh Initiation Week.

Among the documents we received at registration was the "Time Table for First Premedical Year 1957–58." It brought an authoritative air and "this-is-it" reality with its daily 9:00 A.M. to 5:50 P.M. listings: calculus and statistics with Dr John Wilkinson (first term only), physics (second term only), general and qualitative chemistry with Dr Malcolm

Perry (lectures and labs), biology with Dr John Vallentyne (lectures and labs), physical education, and first aid (evening sessions, timing to be announced). I chose English II and Philosophy I (with lectures and a weekly tutorial) as my electives. It all felt surreal. A sense of overload and isolation prevailed; an outing with classmates at a Princess Street eatery didn't help. Getting in touch with Judy wasn't an option. *And I thought that university was supposed to be enjoyable!*

Adaptation to the new academic challenges took time. My reflections as the first term neared an end were summarized in jottings written under the heading "Midnight Wed. Nov. 27/57." I titled them "Desperation":

Oh, my brain is thick and hazy,
As I sit here almost crazy
Writing notes and reading poems on "The Flea"
as I sit trying to expound 'em
while my blood and brain are poundin'
and of everything around me I see three.

As I doodle and I scribble
from Chem. labs to Donne's drivel
I realize that I am sinking fast:
from the standard deviations,
to some "intuitive" equations,
Oh what the hell, I guess I'll never pass.

And just the thought of these titrations
and those tortuous gyrations
of the mind, while trying to cook another lab,
and longing for the times
when we could speak our minds
sans syllogistic form to drive us mad.

Then there's the Hexactinellida
and the Archiannelida
and thousands more with long fantastic names;
– when it takes words three feet long
to describe a mere micron,
I can't help think we humans are insane!

Now I'd like to thank you all
who have made this term a ball

with its dances and its songs and many a smile
for I'll truly miss old Queen's
after that party at the Dean's –
back to the books, but before I go, one thought, "Cha Gheil!"

In spite of it all, to my surprise, I had an unexpected inner sense of belonging. My first visit to Queen's several years earlier had been to watch cousin Don Connor (Meds '53) play for the Gaels' basketball team. Perhaps my unconscious experience of bonding with things Celtic dated from that weekend. But I think not. I believe it had taken root long before, through long-cherished mental images of Highland magnificence animated by the skirl of bagpipes, tales of swashbuckling bravery and independence, the tartan proudly worn. For as long as I can remember, there was something archetypal in all of that, something authentic, something deeply cherished. The fist-in-the-air allegiance suggested by the adage "Scottish by birth, British by law, Highlander by the grace of God" had always found resonance with me. I suspect that in all of that I found an admired windswept alter ego.

My enchantment probably dated from first hearing the pipes as a toddler and then was nurtured over the ensuing years as Dad read Robert Louis Stevenson's *Kidnapped: The 1751 Adventures of David Balfour*[5] to me and recounted First World War tales of Allied pipers striding "up and over the top" to lead their comrades into enemy fire, armed with only their bagpipes.[6] To my ears and heart, the Gaelic war cry *Cha Gheill!* – meaning "no surrender" – and the fighting song "Oil Thigh" were woven directly into the Stewart plaid, the limestone buildings, and the very soul of Queen's.[7] For me, these time-honoured, near-mystical essences were experienced most poignantly while walking through the campus on a silent, clear, moonlit night or, equally, during the unexpected descent of a lashing storm. They were undoubtedly also kindled by the sense of community, history, and grandeur of spirit that made Queen's a special place.

As a Tuesday afternoon biology lab was coming to a close early that fall (we had been unsuccessfully trying to see something – *anything* – through our new microscopes), I glanced at my neighbour, whose ocular lens was about to fall to the concrete floor. I caught it in midair and handed it over, making a note of her name in the lower-right corner of my new timetable – *Faye Wakeling*. She was, I learned, rooming with my former Glebe classmate Anne Porter. It was admittedly an odd approach but, I enquired, did Anne think Faye would be interested in going out for coffee that evening? The message came back that she already had a date with her sophomore "big brother" but would be interested any other evening. It was arranged for Wednesday, 16 October.

Four years later, on 12 August 1961, my toast to Faye, my new bride, on our wedding day ended with a recollection of that first date. We had gone to a movie, Frank Sinatra in *The Joker Is Wild*. My wedding toast on that joyous 1961 afternoon ended with: "Four years ago two kids went out on their first date – to a movie. The movie they soon forgot, but the song from it became theirs from that night on, and today dear, four years later, 'Who knows where the road my lead us / Only a fool would say / But if you let me love you / It's for sure I'm going to love you all the way, /All the way.'"

Faye was from Dundas, Ontario. We compared notes about family, home, and high school. (Like Judy, she had been head girl.) Why had we chosen medicine? Why Queen's? She had an older brother. Her parents loved curling and the Tiger Cats. She enjoyed swimming and diving. She was bright, articulate, forthcoming, honest. She was granite-certain of her carefully constructed opinions and would be happy to defend them at the drop of a challenge. And did I mention lovely? She radiated self-confidence. There was a lot of laughing and sparring about political views, as we walked, ran, and danced our way to the lower campus after the film. So *many* topics to explore! Who would have thought life could *be* so amusing, delightful, full, rich? It was a crisp, invigorating Queen's September evening. And somewhere nearby a lone piper was practising. Perfect. There was a sense of opening; a world filled with possibilities. Our dizzying hand-in-hand tour of the lower campus was filled with rapid-fire exchanges of opinions and rollicking debate. Intoxicating. High octane. Faye was completely stunning in every possible way.

Half a century later, when an honorary doctorate of divinity was bestowed on her by the Faculty of Religious Studies at McGill University's United Theological College, her presenter would comment, "If one wants to leave one's feet up on the sofa, rather than have them planted onto the real soil of the earth, one would do well to avoid Dr Faye Wakeling. She is a passionate, articulate, collaborative enabler, a stirrer of passion within, and a provocateur to all who meet her." All of that was evident during that first luminous evening. I walked her back to Muir House, the stately old home that served as one of the on-campus women's residences. That good night had become a good beginning. For the next twenty-eight consecutive evenings, we saw each other for at least a quick coffee, usually more: a night spent sitting on the rocks by Murney Tower with Lake Ontario stretching away and away in the moonlight at our feet; the time I pulled off the highway at a quiet spot for a moment of togetherness only to find I had chosen the garbage dump and the Morris was now up to its axles in mud; the day at the gym when Faye introduced me to her basketball skills.

Faye's introduction to family and 37 Opeongo came later that fall. It was accompanied by my delighted refrain, "I've got Faye in Ottawa," sung ad infinitum to the captive carload audience as we drove into town. On meeting her, brother Jim commented appreciatively, "Well, she's certainly pretty," and he later added, "And she's very quick too!" as he emerged from a gruelling weekend of debating Faye on a horizon-stretching variety of topics. As one who prided himself on the Socratic method, Jim was humbled. The family was impressed. So was I.

Two paths toward experiencing community seemed well trodden in this campus town: partying with unlimited booze, and alternatively, bonding with those of like mind through common interests. I found the second route more tempting. It took very little stirring of the pot to get together a group of ten to twelve classmate choristers to sing the old favourites – "Kum ba ya," "The Saints," and all the Weavers' standards – and soon we were serenading the women's residences on campus and at the hospitals.

It was a few months later that Faye and I found ourselves huddled in my car, immersed in a searching discussion with our Meds '63 classmate Harley[8] about the role of religion in our lives or, more specifically, the role of Christ. We dissected the differences between mere cultural conditioning and something more. We puzzled over the role and nature of faith and the evidence for and against the various creedal notions. We reflected on the probability of an existence after death. Here was an opportunity to share in-depth questioning. We raked through the glowing spiritual coals, probing here, adding a log there. The hours flashed past, as did the fall. In due course, Harley and Dutch Reformed Church stalwart Hans Verbeek[9] launched a Meds '63 Bible study group that included seekers of all faith traditions and none at all, and a year or so later they formed a Queen's chapter of the American-based Christian Medical Society (CMS).

I had previously experienced the Christian narrative as a comfortable social, moral, and cultural context through which to consider life. Through the CMS, I met men for whom it was something more, much more: their reason for living, their guide in each decision, their ever-present absolute. These were men of calibre in the academic world, critical thinkers. The New England regional CMS meetings we attended attracted colleagues from Boston University, Tufts, and Harvard. They were not religious fanatics conditioned by rigid scriptural dogmatism, but clear-thinking leaders, teachers, scientists, and clinicians grounded in their own experience, men who claimed "a personal relationship with Christ" and lived lives of service to others. Thought-provoking.

Meanwhile, back in the world of endless lectures and studying, one Pre-Med I memory shines brightly amid the continuing all-pervasive grey angst generated by attempting to stay afloat. It happened in the early fall. The leaves in the Medical Quadrangle were splendidly gold, red, and a fading yellow; the breeze, when it blew, had the first hints of the brisk chill that lay ahead. With the deepening heaps of scribbled notes taking on epic proportions, someone suggested we form a discussion group to tease out the relevant issues in recent biology lectures. There were perhaps six classmates in the group when I asked if I might tag along. Soon, we were eight or ten. Each of us took the responsibility for one cloudy issue and we agreed to reconvene in the Meds Quadrangle on the following Saturday afternoon to present our findings to each other.

At the appointed hour, we sat on the grass shaded by the spreading autumn splendour above. One after another, we presented our new-found insights. I don't remember my contribution to this scholarly onslaught on our collective ignorance. But I *do* recall the thrill of experiencing my first sweet taste of self-directed learning. Learning for learning's sake. It was an eye-opening experience. We never met again for that purpose, but the seed had been sown.

What with new lodgings, Ruth Moore's, Faye, adjusting to Queen's and to Meds '63 contexts, spiritual debates, occasional drawing, Ottawa weekends, and the concerns of daily life, the term passed with little room for studies. Exam results were predictably dismal. I was discouraged, anxious, and quick to rationalize when the letter from Dad arrived.

January 1958

Darling Son:
There have been a few times in my life when I have longed for the ease of speech and freedom of use of the English language which was enjoyed by such as Wordsworth or Longfellow, Byron or Shakespeare. One such time has been the hours since you, our son, left us on Sunday. Do you ever feel that there is so much to be said and yet you experience difficulty in giving expression to that which fills you & is bursting to be said? Or again, hesitate to say things fearing that it might be misunderstood? I have not slept properly Bal my son, thinking of you and I'm going to try to put on paper what I would much prefer to discuss.

The written word is so final whereas one can discuss things & banter ideas back & forward as in a game of tennis. But there is never time for us to sit down and talk. I feel so guilty about going out to fly as soon as you arrived. I should really have cancelled the time there so that those golden minutes may not have been lost. You see, we usually fail to appreciate the thing we have that is ours, regardless of its value, whereas we can see so much of value in that which is possessed by the next one. Always the grass is greener, the music is better, the laughter more hilarious and youthful just over the way. And so we, I, lost that golden hour with you. It can never be regained for it is gone forever.

I think you should come home Bal (and please come alone, much as I enjoy your friends ... We – you and I, need that). You and I should become acquainted – go fishing, go to a meeting, or better, play chess or checkers so that we can share that which each has & which will be lost to each – and oh! how soon!

Bal, son, I can see in you & your reactions so many of the ideas (spoken or unspoken, realized or unrealized, conscious or subconscious) which were mine at your age. As we grow up, in our climbing, we grow through different stages. In late teens we feel the vigour and urge of life surging through us, the urge to sever contact with home, or feel the environment there is not just up to the mark – (It is OK but !!!!). We haven't time for it, except to meet our physical needs. And where there is over-concern for our welfare & urging to do this or that, we, in our teens, fail so often to realize that it stems from love such as we shall never again have showered upon us and also from experience in this art or job of living & it is well worth listening to. [Instead,] we must follow the urge & surge of youth which is in us pushing us on we know not exactly where, but certainly pushing us on.

Bal Dear, frankly, I think you need to put on the brakes, hold back, sit & listen, travel a little slower & control the bubbling, surging force of youth. I want you to be full of life, happy, carefree to an extent but have a definite control over that urge to life. Control your temper. Make a decision now not to lose that temper. I have done so – that is lost my temper, so often. Around the Civic hospital I have lost respect & prestige because of losing my temper. We need to learn the control which comes from playing sports (where one may learn to take life's spills on the chin without reacting). Those of us who are not athletic have to learn that lesson elsewhere, in the school of life, but often we learn it too late. So we try to pass this lesson on to our sons, but the fact is, experience is the only real teacher & so I know these word from me will have little effect – or will they?

Bal, I'm frankly disappointed in your term standing at Queen's. No, don't get hot. I know what you planned, you told me and you did just what you planned. But it is not & was not enough. You should have made a better showing. No, not for me who am instructing Queen's medical students, not for Jim, for yourself. You should learn at once to place the proper emphasis on work & on play, on the females of our race & on your confreres – the males of our species.

Please do not think I am scolding, far from it – but I do want to put across some points. I want you to come home & talk these things over. You see you have no desire to come home unless you go immediately out to do something else. And I am not criticizing that aspiration. If any criticism were due it would be my failure to develop over the years the bond of shared interests which would make it otherwise. Now, you have reached manhood, but in that attainment I am anxious to see you make a bit of modification & perhaps rearrange to some extent your values.

(Jim is coming home this weekend so think of coming next, and come alone.) I want to see you with no one else here. Son, I'll stop now. All my love goes with this to you. God bless you my boy & bring you ever closer and under His guidance.

Love, Dad

P.S. Mrs. Crain called to offer Maude a ride to the meeting of the Board of the Protestant Children's Village tonight. They went together. I have not yet bought another plane!!!

Additional letters were exchanged. The planned visit home occurred. Although it was much briefer than desired, helpful dialogue took place. Clearly, I was not working hard enough. Furthermore, I read slowly and had poor time-management and organizational skills. I had never developed studying habits or the capacity for prolonged concentration, *unless* I was drawing, and then I could focus on the task at hand for seemingly endless hours.

Dad, on the other hand, was working too hard (long hours daily and too frequently nights spent in the OR). He was exhausted much of the time and was experiencing asthma attacks. Mother's letter of 13 February 1958 illustrated the point. "Dad went to Toronto and was supposed to arrive home at 1:15 a.m. but the plane was diverted to Montreal because of weather. He arrived home by bus at 5 a.m. and was at the Civic at 8 a.m., then at the office for 9 a.m., and St Louis-Marie de Monfort at 12:30 to do a gastric resection." In a letter written the same day, Dad noted, "Have been working terrifically hard & the coming week looks worse than ever – I love it though!"

This led us to discuss how Jim was finding residency. Dad noted that he also was working too hard (episodic high blood pressure, not enough exercise or sleep, poor diet, and, according to Betty (7 February 1958): "Jim seldom gets home before 8:00 p.m. on his nights *off*, sometimes not 'til 10:00 p.m." Betty added a P.S.: "Sure you don't want to change your mind regarding your choice of career, Bal?!"[10] As our discussions concluded, our personal challenges seemed clearer, but whether either of us could chart a more prudent course would remain to be seen.

The January 1958 term got underway with heightened academic resolve and high expectations surrounding a forthcoming concert by Glenn Gould in Grant Hall on 12 February.

The twenty-five-year-old Toronto-born prodigy was already recognized as one of the foremost classical pianists of the era, a renowned interpreter of J.S. Bach, and a man of wide-ranging interests as well as eccentric ways. The hall was sold out. Faye and I had balcony seats next to the stage, which, given the Lilliputian dimensions of Grant Hall, were just above Gould's right shoulder, less than twenty feet from the keyboard.

He opened with sonatas by Mozart and Beethoven. The Mozart had just been underway for a few minutes – skipping, dancing, sunlight in sound, wondrous – when I heard it. I was horrified. Someone close by was humming. And there was nothing subtle about it. Having read about Gould's unpredictable ways, I feared that if he heard this mindless interference he might storm off the stage in a rage. I shot a withering, soul-destroying glance at each of the most likely culprits seated nearby. The humming continued. If anything, it seemed louder. I cannot now recall whether he had moved on to the rollicking Beethoven, but suddenly I realized that it was Gould himself who was responsible for that infernal droning continuo. He, however, appeared to be completely unaware as he carried on, deeply focused on the task at hand. The applause was generous.

As he returned following the intermission, a reverential air of stillness hung over the house. Gazing down at his feet and apparently completely unaware of the audience, the tousle-haired figure made his way to his remarkably low, well-worn, rickety chair. In the audience, backs had straightened and all breathing seemed to have stopped. There was a palpable sense of expectancy. Heads tipped back, or to the side, many with eyes closed. We were about to hear J.S. Bach's *Goldberg Variations*. Glenn Gould's Columbia recording of this masterwork three years earlier had elevated him from unknown to global phenomenon.

He sat hunched, head low, massive hands, and those powerful, long, spider fingers suspended. The grace-filled opening notes were offered up with a sense of calm that was wrapped in deliberate inevitability. His body was swaying, his mouth moving as if talking to the keys. Three minutes later the tempo quickened and we were swept along. In his own world now, swaying, dancing, singing to the keys, rocking side to side in the flow of the world he and Bach were creating. More swaying. Trance-like. Every fibre of his being focused in supple dynamic hyper-attention, his craggy head sometimes almost touching the keys as, cobra-like, he wove a hypnotic spell. Totally focused, he was inhabiting that other world with complete grace, unity, and certainty. His fingers were flying now, hands a-blur, each finger a jack hammer striking the keys, flying, swaying, talking, hands crossing, his free arm now slowly sweeping the air over his head in a graceful, perhaps dismissive, wave. On and on, and on, and on. We were in sure hands. Twenty, thirty, forty minutes. A final majestic statement of the theme progressing with triumphant certainty – and it was finished. How long had he been playing? Irrelevant. Time had nothing to do with it. This was outside the recognized time-space continuum. Silence followed. Silence. The audience knew what it had heard. Then, the silence gave way to thunderous applause. But he was in his separate universe. He rose from the piano with a lurch and strode off the stage, without so much as a glance at the audience. The applause continued; he did not return.

Pre-Med I rushed on in a torrent of didactic lectures. The end of the term was approaching with freight-train inevitability. To miss even one session was to fall behind by page after page of near-illegible scribblings. In such a case, one joined the line of classmates asking to borrow Bob Vaughan's brilliantly complete, artfully organized notes, each line recorded in a flowing, strikingly clear, hand.

The final exam schedule was posted, copied, and pinned over my desk. Mercifully spaced, these life-determining tilts were grouped over the Easter period, a grim symbolism that was not lost on me. Notes were compiled and summarized and a study schedule pencilled into the dwindling available hours.

On 23 February, I joined other student invitees for Sunday afternoon tea at the home of the Queen's chaplain, the Reverend A.M. Laverty. Attendance seemed prudent under the circumstances! My personal invitation had been addressed to "Dear Bal" and was signed "Padre," a warm gesture that was in keeping with his remarkable instant recognition of essentially *all* Queen's students. In even the most fleeting passing on the street, Padre would extend a cheery greeting, acknowledging the student by name while, time permitting, asking a personal question.

"Hi Bal, what's the news from Jim and Betty? They're in Montreal now, aren't they? ... and your parents? Do give them my best wishes."[11]

On 4 April, Good Friday, Mother wrote: "Alice home for the weekend from Western. Last night she and I went to a Tremblay Concert – Glenn Gould. In spite of his gymnastics he is a wonderful player." She closed a hastily scribbled note: "Give up worrying and make up your mind to do what you can & that to the best of your ability and you'll do fine. For goodness sakes tidy up too Bal. Don't go unshaven. Heaps & heaps of love Darling, Mum." In a brief note a day or two later she wrote: "Dad says take 1/2 of one of these Dexedrine tablets. I wouldn't take it too late or it will keep you awake all night. Must rush this to the P.O."

Pre-Med I was over. Faye and I had both passed; a half-dozen or so of our confrères did not and a few from Meds '62 dropped back to join our ranks. The fact is, however, that I managed to get through only after writing a supplementary examination in chemistry and my overall average was perilously low. Faye and I spent the summer working at the Ottawa Civic Hospital.

OCH SCRUB NURSE, AND THE *PLACE*

The summer of '58 enabled an unexpected renaissance when I was hired as a scrub nurse in the OCH operating rooms. It was a duck-to-water experience. OR Director Mary Armstrong assigned Holly Hollingsworth to be my personal instructor; the surgeons were patient and encouraging. Indeed, most felt I was getting the feel of it rather quickly. My nemesis, however, was Joe Samos.

Dr Samos gave all OR nurses a hard time. He was a prickly character during even the most straightforward cases, and so his scrub nurses soon developed strategies to allay his edginess. "Just bring up his daughter Ruth, or the Conservative Party and you'll be all set," I was told. In my case, nothing worked. The critical comments he levelled at me on my first day soon became cutting, then personal, then belligerent. With things going swimmingly with all other surgeons, I was mystified. Others were assigned to his cases whenever possible, but each time the need to scrub with him arose, the torrent of abuse recurred.

I did not mention the problem to Dad until the summer was drawing to a close. He listened with care, teasing out the details of each situation and asking for a verbatim account of our exchanges. He knew Samos as a colleague and was familiar with his foibles. He was silent for a minute or two as he considered the options, then opined, "Well son, I'll tell you what you should do. The next time this happens go with him to the surgeons' dressing room after the case and hit him as hard as you can with a single punch to the solar plexus." Those blazing eyes confirmed his seriousness. It was the only advice he ever gave me that I intentionally ignored.

During that summer, the family christened the "Place," also to be known as "the Island" or simply "Grand Lake." This three-acre, boat-access-only,

hourglass-shaped hideaway quickly acquired an atmosphere of secluded
safety. There, we found ourselves set apart from workaday cares by the
water and winds surrounding us. We were treated to an unpredictable mix
of blazing sun, ever-changing cloudscapes, and intermittent showers to
accompany the woodland scent of the great white pines at the north end
of our new-found Shangri-La, and the warm fragrance of the old cedar
forest at the south. There was no electricity. Coal-oil and propane lamps
lit our island world.

On the heavily forested northern shoreline, the weathered forest-green
cottage melted into the surrounding foliage, becoming almost invisible
to those passing in motorboat or canoe. "The Point," a rocky outcrop-
ping a few yards from the front door, commanded a sweeping panorama
of the sparsely populated northern end of the lake, while a homemade
dock gave shelter to our modest flotilla: an aging rowboat, a modest
four-seat outboard for waterskiing, my Laser sailboat, and the old Taft
canoe that lay upturned on the lakeside retaining wall. A sandy beach
and rocky shelf at "the Narrows" halfway along the island path would,
in due course, give rise to lasting memories of hours spent with wading
infants. And there were, of course, visits to the outhouse, or "do-some
house" as one grandchild christened it. It was a two-seater, and its tattered screen door strategically faced an opaque tangle of underbrush
while a collection of tacked-on pictures cut from magazines brightened
the bare-plank walls within.

Lasting images would come into being as the years passed: family
reunions, especially the annual gatherings for Mother's 14 August birthday; heavy downpours that seemed diabolically timed to soak groceries
and other perishables during transportation from the mainland car park;
the mind-boggling unpredictability of outboard motors and their fuel
supply; perilous night crossings without a flashlight in spite of all precautions; the semi-liturgical daily carting of water from lake to kitchen
where the elderly bucket and matching ladle reliably stood in for more
refined urban water sources. And then there was the rich ambience of
the post-swim barbecue; Nettie baking fresh bread on the wood stove;
fishing from the Peterborough rowboat; lying out to windward with
shoulders touching the water when running with the wind in the Laser;
Dad's harmonica and Faye's guitar accompanying evening singsongs by
the fire; northern lights sweeping from horizon to horizon in silent pastel shock waves; epic surround-sound thunderstorms experienced with
awe from the nestled woody dryness of the screened in porch. Heaven
on earth.

PRE-MED II, 1958–59

Genetics with Dr Elof Axel Carlson and his fruit flies, organic chemistry with Dr Malcolm Perry, physical chemistry with Dr Bob Wheeler, physics with Dr Roberts, and psychology, including child and abnormal, with a series of lecturers. It was to be a challenging year.

In his letter of 21 September, Dad wrote:

Well here we go again: I start my weekly letters to my son who is away from home. It is the life cycle repeating itself & so it continues to do without regard for feelings. As I think back, I have never been able to bring myself to the place where I could believe that my going away – even in the army, meant to my people what it means to me to have you even go off to Kingston to university. But of course, how could I know? How are you to know ...?

Sincerely, Dad

My centre of gravity remained blissfully non-academic: joining the Queen's cheerleading team, serving on the class executive committee (eventually as social convener, vice-president, and president), and seeing Faye regularly. It was a social focus that soon led to my being invited for Socratic chats with Dean Ettinger and Dr Perry. Both expressed concern regarding my slow-to-bloom prowess in chemistry and recommended due diligence while offering support. Their personal interest impressed me, but sadly I do not recall any radical trimming of my sails as a result. It would not be the last time that I experienced the remarkable commitment to student nurturing that was so typical of the Queen's medical faculty.

At the same time, Mother and Dad applauded my interest in trying out for the cheerleading squad, on the grounds that "there is nothing so good for a young person as good hard sports, enough to make one a little tired, so as to produce a keen mental attitude. It helps you control your thinking and will help you study," a hypothesis into which I read a plea for a diminishment in "the life-surge of youth" that Dad had cautioned about earlier. Along that line, he added, "Regardless of social activities do accept my constructive criticism this year & keep up with your work. Don't let Faye or anyone or anything prevent you from keeping each day's problems faced squarely and properly dealt with." He closed that letter with good wishes for Faye, Richard, and Judy, noting once more, "I do so want to be of any & every assistance possible."

The 24–26 October football weekend in Toronto, featuring the Queen's Golden Gaels versus the Varsity Blues, was a whirlwind! The

Queen's engineering students had organized a "Queen's Marathon" (or "Quarathon") as a prelude to this annual tilt. It would entail a marathon run by Queen's students down the main highway from Kingston to Toronto.

"And, in addition to running the 165 miles, we'll push a bed the whole way!"

"Perfect! And we'll have a Queen's co-ed in the bed – a series of them actually, since this will be a relay!"

"Fabulous!"

"We'll need a police escort, I guess."

"I'm sure they'll go along with it, if we make it a fundraiser."

"O.K. and before the game, when we arrive at U of T, we'll read them a formal proclamation reminding them of Queen's perennial superiority! *Then*, at game time, Queen's celebrated track star Al Hyland, wearing his distinctive golden Queen's track suit and trademark winning smile, will carry the game ball into Varsity Stadium! He'll be the icing on the cake."

"And he will be accompanied by the pipes and drums of the marching band."

"And the strains of all of us in a gigantic kick line hundreds strong, singing 'Oil Thigh' as we enter the stadium."

"Great!"

"But the Queen's Superiority Proclamation *must* be read somewhere special, say, Hart House!"

"Excellent!"

It all happened pretty much as planned. Fortunately, the Queen's engineering students had anticipated multiple breakdowns en route to Toronto and trucked along spare runners, beds, and co-eds.

Standing on the Hart House steps, I read the Queen's Proclamation on behalf of our beloved alma mater. It was graciously heard by University of Toronto President Claude T. Bissell[12] on behalf of the assembled dignitaries and onlookers, all to the accompaniment of the Queen's pipe band, and at the stadium Al completed the Quarathon run on schedule.

We had planned it perfectly. Well, not quite. I well recall my stunned amazement as we entered Varsity Stadium, singing lustily, only to be confronted for the first time with its immense size and the vast throngs of Varsity fans. They extended up and up, apparently forever. Cheerleader volume sufficient to shatter glass in Kingston simply dropped to the turf in front of us. How small we seemed. The final score was Queen's 0, U of T, 44.

One afternoon that fall, as I walked through the pediatric ward during a pre-clinical visit to Kingston's Hotel Dieu Hospital, I noticed a short, chunky boy sitting defiantly on his bed, his right arm – or perhaps *both* arms – in casts. He returned my benevolent glance with a stare that was indifferent, if not sullen. Intrigued, I waved my way into his room with a cheery greeting. No response. I commented on his colourful pajamas. No response. I asked about his arms. Again, no response. Instead, I received an evaluative look that conveyed something between disinterest and disgust. Joe, it turned out, was from Wolfe Island, directly offshore from Kingston. Had I done some digging I would have known that he was a deaf-mute lad who attended the School for the Deaf in Belleville. A bright boy, about ten years old but small for his age, Joe had injured himself while playing with his mates. He would soon be going home and then would return to the residential school. In that first meeting, Joe taught me an important lesson about the need to understand the context of the person I wished to reach out to. We became friends. I visited with his parents and brought him to Ottawa for a few days the next summer so that he could see the sights of the capital and collect players' autographs at an Ottawa Rough Riders practice.

With the 1959 New Year, Dad invited Jim and me to join him in attending the Joint Canadian and British Medical Associations meeting to be held in Glasgow that summer. The studying seemed to be going better, although I *had* started drawing again in my spare time.

Letters received in late February and mid-March suggested that my current sense of equilibrium was not universally appreciated.

Dr. H.T.R Mount
276 Elgin St.
Ottawa, Ont.
25th February, 1959

Dear Mr. Mount:
On the envelope of a letter received recently from you, a note was seen to the effect that you needed money urgently.

I am certain that just a few months ago the matter of finances was discussed and after your careful estimate you were provided with funds which were adequate to carry you through the year. I am, therefore, concerned at this situation which has apparently arisen and shall be interested to have an explanation.

Yours very truly,
HTR Mount,
MB, MS, FACS

A letter from Mother during the same period opened with comments relating to church communion cards, the recent bad weather, and the stresses resulting from Dad's secretary being off sick. It then continued:

We were glad to receive your letter and to hear that you are beginning to concentrate better. I am looking forward to getting started again at art and hope I can do plenty this spring and summer. I do think you are improving tremendously in technique, but I have been thinking over your suggestion that you show the last drawing of the girl to Dr. Carlson. I don't believe it would do you any good but rather *harm* – even if he *might* be the kind to appreciate suggestive or vulgar things. I really feel it is *very unbecoming* and harmful to your reputation as a young man to draw and exhibit such vulgar drawings Bal. If my classes and drawings created this idea in you I am more sorry than I can say. Believe me the people in that life class never exhibited their drawings & I can see I shouldn't let them be seen at home. The bone structure is necessary for proportions in portrait work, and that is the purpose of those classes. Besides they consisted of much older & married people or pupils. You surely aren't so familiar with the female anatomy to take pleasure in drawing it and putting it up in your room. Please don't Bal. It is not good for *your reputation* nor any who see it. Believe me it is not smart – nor would Dr. Ettinger think so. There *should* be almost a sacredness, not to mention a modesty, for girls' anatomy, and it *grieves* me beyond words to see this familiarity in you Bal ... please take those nudes down and *dismiss it from your mind.*

Financial matters were discussed with Dad; the choice of magazines as a source of models for my figure studies, with Mother. Our apparent lack of agreement as to whether my improving drawing skills outweighed considerations of propriety was discussed, as was my surprise at her strong reaction, given my view of her as my mentor in issues artistic.

The Pre-Med II final exams were upon us before I knew it.

April 30, 1959
Department of Chemistry
Gordan Hall

Dear Mr. Mount,
I have just finished reading your paper and I would take this course of events if I were you. I would go to England *BUT* I would also take

my Physical Chemistry notes with me and spend a few leisure hours reviewing them. I am sorry to be the harbinger of bad news, however I do wish you a pleasant trip.

> Yours truly,
> R.C. Wheeler

Travel plans shattered, I said goodbye to Jim and Dad and began studying for my supplementary exam in physical chemistry.

At summer's end, the family dispersed. I returned to Kingston for my Med I year, with expectations running high. Jim was off to the Massachusetts Eye and Ear Infirmary in Boston for a subspecialty residency in neuro-ophthalmology under the attentive eye of Betty and their two delightful young ones, Heather, a talkative, seemingly all-wise, two-year-old who consistently charmed all and sundry, and Howie, three months old. Alice and her church-choir singing companion, Peter Knewstubb from Cambridge, England, remained in Ottawa, working in an office and research lab respectively. (Peter had been awarded a research fellowship in physical chemistry by the National Research Council of Canada.) Mother was busy fundraising for the Ottawa Children's Village. Dad was enthusiastically "active in the profession" and loving it. As we parted, each of us found our personal anticipations tinged with a sense of loss in leaving the *Place*, as we tasted the suddenly chill winds and Grand Lake whitecaps that announced another early September exit from our island home. My supplementary-examination passing grade showed improvement but I remained in the bottom half of the class.

MED I, 1959–60

"First Year Medicine. Finally!" It had a nice ring to it and I plunged in with enthusiasm. Anatomy and neuroanatomy with Drs John Basmajian and colleagues, biochemistry with Dr Jim Beveridge, histology and embryology with Dr John Orr, physiology with Dean Curly Ettinger et al.

As the days became weeks, became months, a new sense of order seemed to evoke a rhythm, direction, and purpose. On 16 October, at the Meds formal, I surprised Faye with an engagement ring. It was two years to the day since our first date. On Sunday evening, 18 October, Dad wrote: "I'm so sorry I was not here when Faye phoned. Maude told me she seemed very pleased and happy and her happiness must have made you happy. Bal, keep a keen & real understanding between you & do not allow anything to come between you which might mar your future. Make your lives together that ideal life which I know is possible & neither of you be guilty of any act which might tend to make your lives together a business relationship & void of that close union which is possible. I am most anxious for your complete happiness." And at Queen's the following day, Padre Laverty wrote:

19 October 1959

Dear Bal,
Let my first word reiterate the pleasure I had in your and Faye's engagement and let me wish you well most sincerely.

I know how interested you are in your year and what a good job you have done as President [of the class executive committee] but I write to issue just a cautionary word in the hope that you will not overdo things in that area so that your work suffers. There is a general recognition among your senior friends around here – among whom I am pleased to number myself – that you have distinct ability, but there is some concern lest you dissipate your efforts too widely and be too prodigal with your time which really your studies should claim.

With the assurance of my regard and with renewed good wishes for you both,

Sincerely, Padre

At about that same time, Professor John Basmajian of the Queen's Anatomy Department held introductory meetings with each member of the class. We had been impressed that he already knew each of our names and appeared to be aware of our individual academic records. My meeting with him was brief and to the point.

"Well, Mount, I think that if you apply yourself you *may* get through. You'll never do much, but perhaps there will be a place for you as a GP in some small town."[13] I felt his tone regarding family medicine was uncalled for but then recognized with a shudder that the object of his derision was me, not those in family practice.

Comments from Dad were similar in tone and wonderfully direct. "You have a very heavy year and it will take all your energy and time to make the standing that you *must make*. To be forewarned is to be forearmed!"

Countless hours spent in the anatomy dissecting room offered an immersion experience that for me was soaked through and through with symbolism. We were leaving the societal norm and entering a sanctuary that provoked conscious and unconscious reactions in many of us.

Anatomy wasn't just another course, like English, statistics, or chemistry. We didn't *take* it. It took us. We were *becoming*, and the initiation rite lasted a full year. Each cadaver – our table hosted a lean middle-aged male – was attended by a quartet of students whose collective persona emerged as the months passed. Our individual styles varied from plum-the-depths-pondering to skim-the-surface and get-on-with-it, from reductionist "just-the-facts-Ma'am" to searchingly philosophical. We were guided in our dissecting endeavours by reference texts that varied from the voluminous *Grey's Anatomy* (used with liturgical solemnity by Harley) to the standard coil-bound Queen's bookstore dissecting manual used by the rest of us. My partners on this journey were David "Sneaker" Sutton, Mickey Sole, and Andy Simone, colleagues whose paths would eventually lead them to hematology, family practice, and dermatology (coupled, in Andy's case, with mission work alongside Mother Teresa), respectively. Gifted by the deceased stranger among us, we painstakingly scrutinized the minutiae of our own physical nature and that of all whom we would care for in the years to come.

My Med I concern was biochemistry. Though it was more palatable by far than its predecessors, thanks to its obvious link to life, it was nevertheless still *chemistry*! Histology, embryology, and physiology were a different matter. *Their* relevance to life was staring us in the face! But even with them there was a problem. Systems-based block teaching (where the anatomy, embryology, histology, biochemistry, and physiology of a given organ or system were considered conjointly) was a yet-to-be-discovered notion of future medical teaching, and thus we were confronted with a hodgepodge of dissociated factoids.

Compulsive editing and reviewing of daily lecture notes had become an essential prerequisite for survival, as were the weekly letters from home, both input streams attempting to inculcate life values perceived to be critical for success. In letters written on the same mid-November weekend, Mother admonished, "Don't miss an opportunity to go to church and witness for Christ by your example Bal dear" (for mother, this was a *highly* atypical appeal), while Dad advised, "As soon as you reach twenty-one years I think you should open a bank account in Ottawa at a bank and branch of your choice and establish a relationship there. It is of great value to you throughout life to be known well by some banking establishment and the sooner you commence this the better." He closed with "Good wishes to you. I think of you and pray for you daily. Give my love to Faye, 'My new daughter.'" Mother also ended her letter, "Love to Faye." That same week, the object of their affection participated in an intercollegiate diving competition during which she struck her head on the diving board yet learned, following her groggy exit from the pool, that she had still managed to finish fourth.

Given Mother and Dad's respective parenting roles during my childhood, it was hard for me to visualize how our family would function if Faye and I *both* had medical careers that were as demanding as Dad's. Would she consider changing her career path? Was that suggestion a logical extension of my parents' example? A product of male chauvinism? Anxiety born out of immaturity and insecurity? Or did it arise out of attention to the uncertainty that Faye expressed regarding her future in medicine, in the wake of the sweat and tedium of the two pre-medical years? Perhaps all of the above?

Whatever the dynamics, Faye decided that on completion of the Med I year she would switch career tracks from medicine to physiotherapy. Enquiries clarified that McGill would credit her three years at Queen's as sufficient to require that she complete only one further year of training to obtain her degree. She could live with cousins Bill and Joanne Bewley while in Montreal. Such a plan would enable us to get married in a year and a half!

Had Faye been pressured? Yes. Would she have come to the same decision on her own? Possibly.[14] But maybe not. In any event, the decision was made and jobs secured for the summer of 1960.

MARIAN ANDERSON

A Queen's Concert Series notice caught my eye. Renowned sixty-three-year-old contralto Marian Anderson was to give a concert at Grant Hall – a perfect birthday present for Alice. I scooped up four tickets before they sold out. Faye suggested that Alice bunk with her. Monday, 22 February, 1960. Remarkably, Faye and I had seats that were front row-centre, with Alice and Peter two or three rows back, in our section.

The capacity crowd welcomed the gracious soloist and her accompanist with evident respect. Her five-part program opened with songs by Handel and Haydn. A section of Schubert lieder followed, ending with "Der Erlkonig," which earned my pencilled program note, "terrifying," in spite of my lack of German. Her impact did not simply depend on the talent of a polished professional. What she embodied seemed deeper than that. Tall and stately, she had a quiet presence that carried with it both ethereal transcendence and breathtaking immanence. Her voice was arresting – from the exquisite upper range to the rich, mellow, soulfulness of her lower register. She radiated openness. She led us to an inner place defined by total presence. Next came the arresting Samson and Delilah aria "Mon Coeur a Ta Voix," which was programmed to take us to the intermission. Enthusiastic applause, however, brought her back for a mid-concert encore, "Comin' through the Rye," which she rendered in a delightfully lilting Scottish brogue.

The fourth section featured four contemporary songs. They led to her final offerings, the Negro spirituals "Go down Moses," "O What a Beautiful City," "He's Got the Whole World in His Hands," and "Roll Jerd'n, Roll." My note was brief: "Superb!"

"He's Got the Whole World in His Hands" evoked profound stillness. She was standing directly in front of Faye and me, perhaps ten feet away – not more. She had moved to the stage apron, her eyes closed as she journeyed inward – in a fashion similar to Glenn Gould playing Bach a year earlier. As she continued, I began to realize, *This is what she believes.* Then, *No, not that. It isn't about "belief" at all. It's about experience. She is singing out of her lived experience.*

It was an awakening. It was clear that *her* world was in safe hands! And that was so, she informed us, for everyone and everything, for "the wind and rain, the sun and moon, the gamblin man, the lyin' man" and "the crap shootin' man." Then, with voice little more than a whisper and filled with compassionate mellowness, she extended her hands, palms up, her eyes still closed, her face radiant, and continued, "the little bitsa baby, you and me bruddah, you and me sistah," and finally, slowing, eyes still closed, "He's got everybody ... *here* ... right ... in ... His hands ... He's got ... the ... whole ... world ... in ... His ... hands." There was a collective holding of the breath as the spiritual ended. As with the Bach a year earlier, it was followed by total silence. Once again, we knew what we had heard; what we had witnessed. We had been on sacred ground. It was just that simple. There were two encores: "There's No Hiding Place down There" and the Bach-Gounod "Ave Maria." My note, scrawled along the side of the program, read: "The encores spoke for themselves. There followed a standing ovation [a hollow term for the spontaneous uncorking of pent-up emotion and appreciation that her artistry and outpouring of self had produced] and those who didn't have tears in their eyes had large lumps in their throats. And she was humble."

As the audience filed out into the crisp night air, Faye and I were invited by our classmate Anne Porter to attend the small reception for Miss Anderson. She greeted us near the door. I awkwardly mumbled my appreciation, feeling the inadequacy of words. Her gentleness and warmth were calming. A brief cup of tea, and we made our way home.

Alone in my room at 21 Sydenham, I relived the gift we had been given that evening and felt compelled to attempt one more expression of thanks. What *was* that moment of awakening, that sense of wonder and profound presence? I believed we had experienced the transparency of an open soul.

Reading the rough draft of my letter to her these many years later, I find its inadequacy painful, glaring. It spoke of creeping cynicism, spiralling doubt spawned over the previous three years of medical school and the mounting uncertainty regarding issues of the spirit, and then noted, "I felt tonight an awakening and new access to an answer to those questions." It was not difficult to guess the hotel where Marian Anderson was staying; I slipped my letter under the door of her room.

Back to the books, with the next exams commencing on 18 March. Thankfully, the studying paid off with good marks in biochemistry, anatomy, and the others, save for a rough time with physiology, regarding which, in her letter of 12 April, Mother reassured, "Harry agrees with you that it's a bugbear of a subject."

The final exams were looming: 9 May, anatomy-lab final; 16 May, anatomy; 17 May, biochemistry; 19 May, histology and embryology; 19 May, histology and embryology lab; 20 May, physiology. Happily, I made it over the hurdles and once again my ranking in the class climbed a little. Alice and Peter were married in a splendid family celebration on 18 June, with Faye a bridesmaid.

Having no supps to write, the product, it seemed, of enhanced clarity of focus, both academic and social, I moved on to my summer position as an orderly at the Civic, while Faye was off to a poolside summer of new relationships at Merrywood Camp, located between Perth and Smiths Falls in eastern Ontario. It was a summer characterized by unexpected estrangement on both our parts, reactions that should have been explored at greater depth.

I purchased a copy of Yousuf Karsh's book *Portraits of Greatness* and ordered a print of his magnificent 1945 study of Marian Anderson from his Ottawa studio. My only previous contact with the great photographer was decades earlier when he had taken Dad's photo and mine as a long-haired infant. I was thus surprised when we crossed paths as I settled my account with his secretary. He remarked with warmth and a sly smile, as he passed, "Well Mr Mount, it *has* been a while. We *both* had more hair when I last saw you!"

Since Dad and I planned a trip to New York during the week of 24–31 August, I sent a note to Marian Anderson to enquire whether she would be kind enough to sign the Karsh photograph as we passed through Connecticut, stressing that I did not wish to bother her in any way. Her response, postmarked Danbury, Connecticut, 25 August 1960, was on personalized stationery.

Aug 25, 1960

Dear Mr. Mount,
It was pleasant to hear from you again. We did reply to your previous letter only to have it returned to us because the Syclenham St. [sic] address was not correct.

It happens that we have been able to spend only an occasional day or so at the Farm this summer and cannot be certain that we shall be here during the week of August 24–31. Most of our time is now spent in Philadelphia because of our Mother's illness.

However, if you cared to mail the portrait (as others have done), we would be happy to autograph it. May we suggest, however, that you give us an address that would be certain to reach you.

Every good wish for a pleasant holiday.

Sincerely,
Marian Anderson

Her earlier letter was enclosed:

July 16,1960

Dear Mr. Mount:
May we sincerely thank you for your kind words of February 22, 1960. We do hope you will understand that it was not until our return from a prolonged concert tour that your kind words were brought to our attention.

One is always happy to hear from one's friends and your particularly warm and comforting letter was most rewarding. One can well understand that through strain, worry and stress one might become a bit discouraged and feel he has been "overlooked." That is human! But we must remember that it is easy to have Faith when the world is bright; it is when darkness creeps in that we need it more than ever. Through constant prayer, one finds that strong Faith casts away the shadows and lets in the light.

With the fervent prayer that you may have a long and happy career in your chosen field,

Most sincerely,
Marian Anderson

A further note was attached to the signed Karsh portrait when it arrived.

September 15, 1960

Dear Mr. Mount:
It is with pleasure that we advise you that we have returned to you under separate cover the Karsh portrait with our autograph.

   May we take this opportunity to thank you for your kind words. Also, we are happy to say there has been a marked improvement in our Mother's condition.

With kind regards,
Sincerely,
Marian Anderson

A half-century later, Marian Anderson's portrait faces my desk. To glance up from my work is to find her lost in reverie and I recall Karsh's comment, "With her, I was convinced the harmony of music came from the harmony of her being."[15]

As with a Rembrandt portrait, his photograph offers a window on an open soul. When Karsh clicked the shutter, she had just started to hum to herself, in response to her accompanist's soft playing, at Karsh's whispered request, the accompaniment to the American spiritual "The Crucifixion." In capturing that moment, Karsh preserved what I had seen and heard that evening these decades past, a person transported to the timeless connectedness of the radical present and with that, her Lord.

MED II, 1960–61

Bacteriology with Dr N. Hinton, pathology and clinical microscopy with Dr R. More, pharmacology with Dr H.D. McEwen, physical diagnosis and physiology with multiple lecturers, psychiatry with Dr B. Sloane.

   Hallelujah! There appeared to be a significant curriculum thrust toward clinical issues: bacteriology and pathology promised to be interesting, physical diagnosis and psychiatry stimulating and enjoyable, physiology, in all likelihood an extension of the demanding Med I course, and pharmacology an unknown. How quickly the mass of material to be covered was growing! I scrawled a late-September list of urgent reminders across the envelope of a letter from home: "1) Get Pathology lectures, 2) Catch up on notes, 3) Finish Physiology lab, 4) Answer Pathology question, 5) Write up Path lab, 6) Read Davidson."

Meanwhile, the advancing fall brought unsettling news from home: Mother bedridden with a Ménière's attack[16]; Uncle Morris Rogers dying with a presumed heart attack, leaving Aunt Veda and family; Dad's hurried trip to Toronto for his funeral; Aunt Millie's previously stable Parkinson's disease now progressing; Alice and Peter preparing for their move to England. Writing to Faye in Montreal became a daily anchoring point.

Taking a history and carrying out a physical examination were, they informed us, skills that we would continue to hone throughout our professional lives. Our powers of observation and deduction must be equal to those of Sherlock Holmes, or so it seemed. I was supposed to examine that frail-looking elderly woman, though I had no idea what I was doing. I was all thumbs, shaking more than she was. Uncertain if my hands were too cold, too wet, too rough, or simply too uncertain. My whispered request, "Now, would you please take a deep breath," was almost completely inaudible. I definitely looked more drained than she did.

Mastery of the physical examination seemed an elusive goal: the art of picking up the most subtle variations in the human condition: changes in scleral tint ("best seen in a natural light"), skin hydration and texture, a variation in muscle tone or the brittleness of the finger nails, changes in gait or tendon reflexes, minor aberrations in cognition or speech. The list of easily missed findings that would be evident to the astute clinician was endless.

"Appreciate the nuanced evidence available with auscultation," admonished one clinical tutor. "Listen. Focus. Did you hear that split-second heart sound? That faint systolic murmur? The intermittent slight rub over the left base, posteriorly? What about the succession splash in her abdomen? I thought not! Now, young man, tell me about the information available in carrying out a rectal examination."

It rapidly became clear that physical diagnosis had more to it than the uninitiated might suppose. But no matter, one mustn't lose heart. I, for one, was eagerly anticipating my upcoming introduction to psychiatry. Indeed, it seemed possible that my future might well lie in that direction, some distance from the endless hair-splitting of indiscernible physical findings.

On my highly anticipated first afternoon on the psychiatry service, I was assigned to Dr J. Robert Smithers, a British registrar who was at Queen's for a one-year stint as a senior fellow.[17] Between puffs on his massive briar, he informed me – somewhat condescendingly and with a distinct note of imperious self-satisfaction – that we would be going out on a house call. We were, he proclaimed, helping to pioneer a new program. "It's a trial community-based initiative in, as we say at the

Tavistock, 'Community Liaison Psychiatry.' The latest thing, you know. Very progressive!" I followed him in descent into his faded blue, 1955 MG convertible with its worn leather seats, large shining spoked wheels, and polished chrome accessories. Community psychiatry; I was thrilled.

We were, J.S. informed me, on a fact-finding mission. The consultation request concerned a lad who lived in Odessa, an inauspicious cluster of humble dwellings ten miles or so northwest of town. It seemed that eleven-year-old Johnny had been running away from home recently.

"Truancy, fights, minor pilfering, that sort of thing," J.S. puffed importantly. His tobacco had that rich, intoxicating, caramel, and old-saddle-leather scent that invariably tempts me, even now, to acquire a pipe. Someone was burning leaves nearby, and what with the pipe and the leaves and the breeze as we tore by, it all seemed too good to be true. We were taking health care *to* the people! Ambassadors of wellness, as it were.

"They send him up to bed at night, and sometime later, he goes out through the window and shinnies down the drain pipe. He may be out all night. Three or four times, some weeks. Been going on for over a month."

"Where does he go?"

"Well, it seems there is a new resident in town. Recently moved in from Toronto. The local women say she's ... well, a prostitute. She's young though ... Hymenoptera, old chap: Hymenoptera – bees to pollen ... bees to pollen! That sort of thing. Quite." He puffed on in silence while consulting a pocketed scrap of paper bearing the scribbled address.

We pulled into a dirt yard on our left, slurring to a stop with a cloud of dust and a final throaty growl from the engine as the dust and noise settled into the protesting squawk, scurry, and flutter of two or three mangy hens.

We headed for the once screened-in porch that ran across the front of the cottage. The two front steps were in poor repair. The porch itself was filled with depressing mounds of refuse – the tattered remains of a canopy swing, boxes, rags, a door-less fridge hived up with rust and dirt, a roll of rotting carpet, a stack of old newspapers, the remains of a wooden chair, and two old tires. To our left there were bottles of what may have been crankcase oil, another jumble of rags, and an assortment of tools.

J.S. knocked with brisk intentionality on the plank door. When there was no reply, I experienced a momentary sense of relief, but the door then burst open to reveal a massive beefy presence. She was perhaps 5'7" but appeared taller. Her bare arms were muscular; there was a tattoo just below her right shoulder. Her bulging T-shirt and jeans were concealed by the dirtiest apron I had ever seen. She wore a perpetual snarl as she scanned us questioningly.

Introductions by J.S. identified us as visiting from the Kingston General Hospital. She stepped back without a word of welcome and we stumbled into the twilight greyness within.

In the single room that was the totality of this modest dwelling, there was only one piece of furniture, a table. It was fashioned from two saw-horses across which lay three, maybe four, two-by-eight-inch planks. An unfinished bench lined each side. We sat.

As our eyes became accustomed to the dim lighting, I noted a single piece of reading material, a somewhat encrusted, well-thumbed comic book which had clearly served as both library and fly swatter. She peered at us vacantly.

"Mrs. ...?" J.S. offered hesitantly, his voice trickling off into a whisper. Her eyes narrowed threateningly. He attempted a dialogue, his tone somewhere between formal interview and apology, his style becoming increasingly ill at ease with each halting query. The story was more or less as J.S. had said.

I watched as communication fragmented before my eyes. The musty room began to feel uncommonly warm; my clothes felt tight. Were those beads of perspiration forming on J.S.'s forehead? I recall only two of his lines of enquiry.

"When Johnny requires correction, which one of you usually disciplines him, you or your husband?"

"Whichever ones of us gets to him first!"

"Hmm ... yes... I see ... And what method of correction do you and your husband employ?"

"We kicks the shit out of him!"

Our exit was awkward. More of an escape, really. As I recall, no treatment plan was outlined, no follow-up visits offered.

J.S. remained silent on our trip back to the hospital. A career in psychiatry now somehow seemed to me to be much less likely.

THE QUEEN'S TELEGRAM AND OTHER MISSIVES

In the Canadian Football League (CFL) that fall, Queen's Golden Gaels alumni Ron Stewart, Lou Bruce, and Gary Schreider were members of the Ottawa Rough Riders team that qualified for the annual championship Grey Cup game, to be held 26 November in Vancouver. They would be battling the Edmonton Eskimos. The approaching Canadian Classic provided moments of trivial diversion from our toing and froing to class and burning the midnight oil while brewing just one more "cuppa" to keep weary eyes open.

Then, it occurred to me as I dashed off to classes one early November day that we had in front of us a superb opportunity to rally the old Queen's spirit from its pre-exam doldrums without distracting from the grinding bookish task at hand.

Why not conjure up a game-day telegram to our ex-Gael trio of CFL all-stars? I drew up the text and asked the Queen's radio station to get the word out and fellow students to arrange for sign-up locations at the campus store, library, the Student Union, the various residences and administrative buildings, and so on. Each spot was equipped with an official log-in sheet and a can in which to drop the minimal fee required to have your name added. The telegram read: "Stew, Lou and Gary, Congratulations all-stars. We are proud of you. Beat Edmonton. Oil Thigh."[18] The signatures followed, including those of Principal W.A. Macintosh, the deans of each faculty, the university registrar, Jean Royce, the Golden Gaels coach, Frank Tindall, and each of the players, members of the Arts '61 and '62 executive committees, the Queen's *Journal* editor and staff, various campus clubs and residences, Meds '63 classmates, the Queen's band, countless professors, and then the students, hundreds upon hundreds of students, single file, so to speak, a goodly sample of one Canadian university generation.

Two of us huddled in a bare room. I read out a name while the Canadian National Telegraph stenographer typed it, off it went into the night, then on to the next name. It became the longest telegram ever sent from Kingston. Our task commenced at 9 p.m. Friday; by 11 p.m. both Kingston radio stations had the story and a newspaper reporter called for an interview. Television cameras and a photographer arrived to shoot the completion and measuring of the final product – 2,071 words, 30 feet, 6 inches in length.

By 1:30 A.M. Canadian Press had the story. When the whole thing was in the bag at the other end, the word came from Vancouver. "It looks fine. You better get some sleep or you'll miss the game. We've had photographers here filming this stuff as it comes in." Our greeting was delivered to the Rough Rider dressing room two hours before game time, Saturday.[19]

The Riders defeated the Eskimos 16 to 6 that day. Gary Schreider scored a field goal in the first quarter; Lou Bruce delivered a punishing hit on the Ottawa two-yard line, causing an Eskimo fumble and an Ottawa recovery for a touchdown. Ron Stewart was named the Most Valuable Player of the game.[20] A good day all around.

Dad's letter written Sunday evening, 4 December, was full of nostalgia at the impending departure of Al and Peter.

Dear Bal:
Son! How are you? Why have you not been home today?
Why will you not be here next weekend? What excuse have you?
Guess you'll have to change to Ottawa U. to complete your medical degree! ...Today was White Gift Sunday & I saw you as a child walk across the front of the church to deposit your gift. I'm operating tomorrow. Two big cases – one at St. Louis & one at the Civic ...
    Good wishes son. I love you. Have a happy & full life in service of others.

Dad

In mid-December, Alice and Peter left for England. Feelings of loss were mitigated by the escalating pressure of pre-Christmas exams and by the knowledge that Al would return in the summer for our wedding.
    The January back-to-the-grindstone transition merged into February snow and plunging temperatures, with the family pursuing our respective daily tasks in Kingston, Montreal, Ottawa, Boston, and Cambridge. Faye was now only a few months away from being a full-fledged physiotherapist. I signed a 1 May lease on our first home, a third-floor, one-bedroom walk-up (with fireplace) in a stately old King Street limestone landmark by the lake.[21]
    Letters from home continued to convey shadows of transience:

Sunday February 26. Maude and I are sitting in the library at a card table. She is similarly employed. Nettie has gone out, Beau [the family collie] is out & the house seems very quiet indeed. As I came downstairs this morning, I found myself wondering what it was like when we had three children here in the house with us! The wheels of time roll on!

Thursday, March 16. Alice's birthday on Saturday; Jim's tomorrow. Time is going too fast. Harry is very busy operating at Civic and St. Louis, plus the office full as well as his desk. I wish he'd cut the days shorter.

Easter exams had yielded good marks, but trouble lay ahead. The finals came and went and June brought the denouement of the Kingston life

I had lived over the past four years and, with that, an unexpected sense of loss. The finals had been challenging but our wedding plans offered hope for the future. I packed the contents of my 21 Sydenham digs into a few boxes, said goodbye to Ruth Moore and 164 Barrie, and ruminated about each of the recent final exams.

The exam results were disturbing. While my overall class standing showed further improvement, pharmacology was an exception. Once again, I had to write a supplemental exam, a disaster during what should have been a summer filled with joyful anticipation. It was back to the books as I returned to 37.

And there was more. On 22 July Mother and Dad, accompanied by Al who had returned for the wedding, were transporting cottage supplies to the Island when, with a misstep between boat and dock, Mother's left leg was crushed. The head of the tibia was fractured and displaced into the knee joint and the lateral condyle was sheared off. Characteristically, she remained stoic, even positive. Open reduction and pinning of the shattered remains occurred next morning at the Civic and a hip-to-foot cast followed. Her presence at the wedding was now clearly in doubt.

Letters written to Faye during those pressure-cooker days revealed my respect for the challenges posed by pharmacology.

Friday July 21.
The work is all around me, with mountains ahead and only the
foothills behind. I have been over the lectures since Christmas and
a third of the earlier notes, but that is only the first time through,
and, of course, I have long-forgotten dosages, routes of administration, physical and chemical properties, absorption rates, metabolism,
toxicology, cross-intolerance with other meds, etc. from those early
months – and only two weeks to go.

July 30[?].
I have just finished going over the course for the second time and it
seems absolutely hopeless.

August 1.
I so want our marriage to be a success. We are both such selfish
people that it will take all our love and all your patience with me to
overcome some of the rougher moments that lie ahead. Let's always
keep a sense of humour ... I want our marriage to be one of those
rare unions that all admire and few attain. It worries me to think
that *everyone* gets married with these hopes and yet something

happens to take the shine off life, the relationship becomes chilled with use rather than richer. I hope I can always remember to think of your point of view, rather than trying to make you see mine ... We are starting with *so* much. Let's always keep the tremendous love we have now.

The letter from Queen's was dated 8 August 1961: "Dear Balfour, This is to notify you that you were successful on the supplemental examination in Pharmacology. So congratulations and best wishes for the events of next weekend. Very truly yours, H.D. McEwen PhD, Secretary, Faculty of Medicine."

The wedding on 12 August at St Paul's United Church, Dundas, was all we had hoped it would be, with Mother gamely attending on crutches, leg in a cast, the Reverend Malcolm Johnston officiating, and Harley at the organ as family and friends celebrated with us. Telegram greetings arrived from Ruth Moore and Dr Donald Balfour at the Mayo Clinic. We felt richly blessed, if somewhat dazed, as we left for our Gaspé honeymoon.

131 King Street East, our apartment at the upper reaches of three flights of once-elegant winding stairs, was a stone's throw from the lake and overlooked Sir John A. MacDonald Park with its imposing statue of our first prime minister. Our tiny loft was a locus of stability for studying, a place of welcome and hot chocolate for friends after a winter skate on the lake, in short, a safe lair in which to adjust to married life. It was also a place of spontaneity as we invited in a lecture-tour-weary childhood hero, American/Argentinian adventurer and "tigrcro" (hunter of jaguars) Sasha Siemel for an evening chat.[22] Brimming with adjustments and challenges galore, it was, above all, our home.

MED III AND IV, 1961–63: THE CLINICAL YEARS

Faye was the architect of a calming ambience that carried us through Meds '63's two clinical years. Logician and strategist extraordinaire, she was a shrewd analyst who instinctively calculated the shortest distance between any two points. While medical school has been described as being divisible into two parts – the *pre-cynical* and the *cynical* years – that was not to be my experience. The load was staggering and the path uphill, but the way forward was made straight by Faye.

The two clinical years confronted us with a robust ensemble of teachers who provided a flood of information coupled with a surfeit of urgent reading. Abstract concepts gradually came alive at the bedside and in the lecture hall as *diseases* were transformed into *experienced illness* on acquiring a human face. Med III and IV were an introduction to the triumph and tragedy of life on the edge, for patient, family, and caregiver alike, as revealed by professors who exemplified the full range of luminosity: from the encyclopedic knowledge of the young specialist fresh from fellowship exams to the burnished presence of the Ancient Mariners – the awe-inspiring masters of the Art of Medicine, demonstrated when knowledge is tempered by wisdom, skill by gentleness, facts by insight, stature by humility, and hard news by compassion. In due course, each of us experienced that thrill of recognition when, for the first time, the truth in the research paper or textbook paragraph becomes evident in the person before you, and you can name it, give it a context and meaning, and diminish the fearful power of uncertainty through a caring presence and appropriate therapy.

The accumulation of medical wisdom is, however, never linear. It more closely resembles the drawing together of an elegant, infinitely complex, woven fabric. Working with countless information strands of all colours, textures, strengths, and degrees of relevance, one moves toward an imagined seamless whole that, if you set your sights high enough – that is to say, on the suffering of the whole person rather than simply the disease – is never quite realized. Thus, one's reward becomes the process of constantly moving forward, rather than achieving a hypothetical complete understanding.

FORD CONNELL

It was early in the fall of '61 when the realization hit me: internal medicine *is infinitely bigger than I am!* Over coffee with a huddle of classmates, I expressed my angst, and Penny, a fellow Meds '63 traveller who seemed particularly tuned in, responded with an air of assuredness.

"Well, Bal, you know what you might do is link up with Ford Connell. He makes Sunday morning rounds with his residents and he doesn't mind it if you tag along. I've found it really helpful."

"General Bullmoose?" I asked in disbelief.

She chuckled. "Don't let that gruff facade fool you! His bark is much worse than his bite. He's a sweetie. Just ask if you might follow him around Sunday mornings. You'll see."

Later that week, as Medical Grand Rounds offered up its final golden nugget of wisdom and the front-row seats were, in turn, offering up their august occupants, I approached Professor W. Ford Connell, cardiologist and chief of medicine.

His starched, unbuttoned lab coat swung threateningly as he spun to peer down at me, arms akimbo, great bushy eyebrows knotted, his riveting gaze radiating total attention. He had, that very same second, managed to pick at his nose, utter a violent blasting sneeze that shook the whole room, and swivel his assessing stare to register each nearby soul. Nothing escaped him. Now *I* was the subject pinned on his visual dissecting table. "Dr Connell, I wondered if I might join your team as you make rounds Sunday mornings." There was a pause as he considered the request.

"Well, Mount, don't expect any teaching!" he roared.

"Oh no sir, no teaching," I nodded, knowing full well that it would be impossible for Ford Connell to let any opportunity to teach pass unheeded.

From then on, I made rounds with Ford each week for two years. Wes Boston, a Meds '57 classmate of Jim's and at the time senior resident on Ford's service, told me decades later that their team wanted to kill me. "We had Sunday rounds down to forty-five minutes before you arrived," he recalled. "But when you came along, it soared to an hour and a half, often two hours."[23]

Ford Connell. How can one adequately convey that larger-than-life phenomenon? Much of it had to do with his sharp, discerning mind, his capacity to be fully present, and his vast store of medical knowledge. But there was more. He carried himself as if on a mission – erect, purposeful, apparently always in a hurry. But you instinctively knew that the hurry wasn't to escape *from* but to enter more fully *into*.

My General Bullmoose metaphor related to this charged aura, his appearance of being on the cusp of either an insight or an explosion. It was an impression that was infinitely heightened by his thrusting head, flying tufts of thinning hair, and piercing eyes, as he peered at you from behind those periscope glasses, and, of course, his readiness to question each wary student. He questioned. But then, before you could get your brain in gear, he would be off down the hall with a giant stride, and you were left childishly stuttering – in both step and speech – at his heels, trying to keep up.

Keeping up with Ford, however, was, by design, impossible. For example, when John Ruedy was his resident, he discovered to his dismay that if he arrived at 8:00 A.M. to get on top of overnight developments before Ford arrived, the chief was already there. Thus, John started to arrive at 7:30 A.M. Within days, Ford had adjusted his routine. "I've already seen him," Ford would mumble in a gruff, offhand manner when John reported an overnight crisis in patient care. And so it went. Before long, John was arriving at 6:30 A.M. It was then that he received the phone call. "John, it's Mrs Connell. I'm calling to ask if you would please let him win, just once."[24]

During our last two years at Queen's, we were confronted with an overwhelming, yet invigorating, smorgasbord of medical, surgical, obstetrical and gynecological (OB/GYN), psychiatric, ophthalmologic, pediatric, and radiologic topics. Comprehensive lectures, attended by the whole class, were complemented by small-group teaching regarding the specifics pertaining to particular patients and their families as we rotated from one specialty to another.

The rudiments of obtaining a history and physical examination were gradually being refined. Late in our second pre-clinical year, with some degree of pride, I had presented the documentation recording my first history and physical to Dad during a weekend visit to Ottawa. It was twenty pages long. He supportively named it the most complete he had ever seen, and managed to do so without smiling or referring to its novella length. Now, on the wards, when we worked up a new patient, we were learning to winnow wheat from chaff as we ploddingly made our way through the history of present illness, functional enquiry, past medical history, family history, occupational history, psychosocial history, and, where relevant, sexual history. Then it was on to the step-by-step, detailed physical examination and urinalysis. Finally, there was the task of writing it all up and pondering the selection of relevant orders: the chest X-ray, screening blood tests, and other investigations needed in this particular instance.

The comprehensive one-and-a-half to two-page (maximum) note by the intern filled us with admiration, the less-than-one page note by the resident, with awe, the precise half-page masterwork of the fellow or member of the attending staff, with something close to reverence. Should you be the one who was expected to present the new case to the team of six to eight students, interns, residents, attending staff, nurses, consultants, and visiting professors during ward rounds next morning, the cascade of relevant data had better be organized, complete – *and* concise!

The Queen's standard of teaching was high, the clinicians committed, and the patients and their relatives remarkably trusting. The latter were always the first to mistakenly address us as "Doctor" as we scurried about the wards.

Memorable images from those foundational months remain clear all these years later: the faces and needs of our patients, among them the muscular young psychotic lad seated before us in the small lecture room, who scanned our class with wild, wide eyes and a smile while noting with excitement as he shifted in his chair, "Things are beginning to speed up now! They're beginning to buzz!" (as each of us hastily checked the location of the nearest exit); the post-fellowship-examinations hyper-acuity of the recently minted young specialists (Les Valberg, Jack Parker, John Fay,

Peter Morrin) – each *so* observant, discerning, articulate, and ever-ready
with a nuanced remark in discussing the current literature; the relaxed,
easy-going senior internists, Gub Kelly and John Milliken; the aloof, aristocratic Malcolm Brown and the prices paid by his ulcer-prone, hyper-
tensive residents; Larry Wilson's organized competence as clinician and
administrator; the niggling saltiness of neurologist Denis Naldret White
(or, as he was wont to say, "not Dennis; it's DEEnis, as in penis"); the
Scottish brogue and contagious passion of Edwin Robbie Robertson as
he led us through OB/GYN mysteries ("She had a *terrrrible! burrning!
seeearing* exudate, poor lassie!"); the lithe, youthful, brush-cut professor
of psychiatry Bruce Sloane pensively starting his lecture with the observation, "That's strange. I have *just now* had *two* colleagues go out of their
way to greet me with a smile. Always be suspicious when that happens";
the usefully organized Highland gruff of Andy Bruce's lectures in urology
and his well-aimed piece of chalk that could silence an inattentive student
at eighteen paces when it ricocheted off his head; the nurturing kindness
of pediatricians Alex Bryans and Don Delahaye ... and so many others.

DLCB, THE CHIEF

Standing somewhat aside from all of this was the fiefdom of General
Surgery. While it was indeed an integrated part of the carefully laid out
curriculum, this voluminous course, in contrast to Internal Medicine
where lectures on each subject were presented by a specialist in that
area, was given by *one* man, the chief of surgery, Dr Dermid Lockhart
Cameron Bingham.[25] DLCB, as he was commonly known, had claimed
this right to exclusive presence at the undergraduate surgery lectern for
ages, perhaps decades, as if by feudal precedent.[26] Meds '63 was the last
class to experience this remarkably unified, old-school, somewhat pon-
tifical masterclass.

Dr Bingham was every inch the feudal lord – in the operating room,
on the ward, in the lecture hall, driving home in "The Bentley," at the
elegant stone Bingham manor-house in its tranquil Highway 15 setting
just beyond the edge of town, in his book-lined library with its oak
pulpit reading stand, when seated at table with formal dining room
aglow, or when passing through the estate's country kitchen with its
old-world charm.

Feudal lord. The term here does not imply arrogance, aggression, or
overweening self-satisfaction, nor a need for power or the fawning attention of others. Instead, it simply reflects the lived-out natural order of
things as he saw it, the appropriate assignment to oneself of each task

and standing as the one who was, in his considered opinion, most capable of meeting the need.

The chief's perception of his place in the world was evident in his bearing. Below that receding hairline and broad (intelligence-implied) forehead, his penetrating gaze reached you through slightly hooded eyes that peered over the top of his reading glasses, his head tilted slightly forward, his eyebrows mildly raised in evaluation, as he assessed the quality of your last assertion. His hair had a perpetual trimmed-earlier-today appearance; his discrete tie was carefully selected (reflecting its old-school UK academic origins), muted, conservative, and confident; his white shirt spotless, and the gold, shield-emblazoned cuff links, just so.

The rumours made the rounds through our class. "That proud cuff-link crest undoubtedly belongs to the International College of Surgeons. He's an Honorary Fellow you know! Has been for years. I've been told he is close to that other surgical Scot, Ian Aird – chair at Hammersmith and author of *A Companion in Surgical Studies*. DLCB and Aird were with Monty and the Eighth Army in North Africa, you know. We must get him to tell us his 'Desert Fox' stories."

A freshly pressed three-piece suit alternated with his immaculate, starched lab coat, depending on the setting. Razor sharp, parade-square trouser creases and polished shoes completed the picture, yet all of it somehow managed to remain understated, bearing as it did an unmistakable suggestion of British reserve, a conceit underscored by his soft, precise diction with its faint hint of supercilious indifference. He carried the day behind a shield of quiet authority.

Like Ford Connell, DLCB was about six feet in height, give or take an inch or two, but if you were a disciple, you could be forgiven for believing that either man was a head taller.

The "Bingham Lectures" in surgery had the advantage of continuity and flow. As the weeks became months we came to understand his perspective intuitively. We could weigh his assessment of significance, risk, and treatment options against the wording, tone, and descriptors used in earlier lectures. His undisputed skill as a surgeon and depth of experience in war and peace were things we could count on.

In my case, I had accepted all of that long before arriving at Queen's. The summer I was eleven years old, I was at home when Dad hung up the phone following a brief, matter-of-fact telephone conversation informing us that Alice, who was at Camp Oconto north of Kingston, had been thrown from a horse, suffering an ugly laceration extending some ten inches down the medial aspect of her right thigh. She had been transported to the Kingston General Hospital where Bingham would tend to her needs. Consent for surgery was requested and given. "She'll be fine; he's a good man," was Dad's only comment prior to bundling us into the car for our trip to Kingston.

The Meds '63 appreciation of Bingham's preachments was sharpened by his steady flow of aphorisms and prodding wit. He seemed amused by, and not a little disdainful of, our juvenile habit of writing down every word he uttered. Thus, when he came out with, "The common bile duct is approximately the size of a goose's quill," this line was delivered while peering over his glasses to see who would transcribe it. Most of us did. (*In God's name, how big is a goose's quill?*) DLCB's pithy maxims were always quick to come to mind in moments of need:

> "If you don't put your finger in it, you'll undoubtedly put your foot in it."
>
> "Seeing is believing, but feeling is the naked truth."
>
> "The published mortality rate for that procedure is generally around 2.6 per cent; however, in One's personal series it is 1.1 per cent.[27]
>
> "That sort of thing is a sin against the Holy Ghost." [This pronouncement was offered by DLCB in reference to a medical error of omission, the chief being a man who claimed to be "a third-generation atheist."]
>
> "Odd sort, internists; curiously limited. Now, on the other hand, surgeons are internists who also operate."
>
> "A rectum that cannot blow its own trumpet is unworthy of the name."
>
> "What colour is the healthy gall bladder? It is Cambridge blue, gentlemen."
>
> "Attention to detail, that's the essence of it! While One was a Clinical Tutor at the Royal Infirmary, Edinburgh, One knew men of the calibre of Sir John Fraser who would sit at the bedside observing the obstructed abdomen for twenty minutes or longer, at a time."
>
> "Surface anatomy, that's the thing. It is said that Lord Moynihan might palpate the local tissues for up to fifteen minutes prior to making his incision."
>
> "One has operated on the king of Syria at his palace. Now the latrines there – even in the palace – consist of a simple hole in the floor. This requires a position that appears to reduce the probability of hemorrhoids."

On one fine fall occasion, as the class enjoyed a memorable evening of food and drink at the Bingham estate, a group of us found ourselves cloistered in the sumptuous leather-bound library as we scanned, in awe, the elegant furnishings and extensive collection of textbooks and journals. A copy of *Gray's Anatomy* lay open on the reading stand. Dr Bingham joined us. "Consulting Grays's, sir?" queried Roger, one of our more forward classmates. "Hmm," nodded the chief, his eyebrows arching imperiously, "Why, yes. I read through Gray's once a year. Do you?" That ever so gracious evening, hosted specifically for Meds '63, ended with a fine fireworks display in the Bingham gardens.

Another sample of Bingham largesse involved Harley during his student surgical rotation. Late one afternoon, a young woman with a hot appendix was admitted and soon found herself on the way to the OR. "Come along Smyth. We shall do this together." And they did. With infinite patience, the chief became the assistant as he guided his later-to-be neurosurgeon clerk through his first appendectomy. On completion, with the patient safely in the recovery room, it was, "Come now Smyth, you must be hungry. Let us have some supper." They made their way out Highway 15 in "The Bentley" and later, after a delicious meal courtesy of Catriona,[28] Harley was delivered back to his Barrie Street rooms in the same fashion.

Like Dad, Bingham had been trained in the vanishing era of the surgical generalist. While he had stopped doing chest and orthopaedic surgery prior to our arrival on the scene, in addition to abdominal and pelvic surgery, he was still engaged in surgery of the thyroid and parathyroid glands as well as radical head and neck procedures.

Meds '63 classmate and legendary Golden Gaels captain and corner linebacker Dave "Skener" Skene was on-service when a woman in her forties with a locally advanced cancer of the floor of the mouth was admitted. Cervical lymph nodes were involved. Eating, drinking, and speaking were seriously compromised, the area was infected, and the prospects grim. What to do? The options included, at one end of the treatment continuum, simply offering her nursing care while struggling with the control of pain and other symptoms, or, at the other extreme, the radical head and neck surgery commonly referred to as a Commando Procedure. The latter would involve an "en bloc" resection of her jaw, floor of the mouth, and part of the tongue, as well as wide removal of the lymph nodes and tissues on that side of her neck. Not a happy choice. A half-century later, Skener still recalls the sensitive weighing of the various pros and cons, Dr Bingham's support of the patient, and the challenging surgery that ensued once mutual agreement had been attained. Such situations may confront patient and surgeon with a lose-lose roll of the dice. To Skener's discerning eyes, DLCB came through with high marks as both surgical technician and supportive communicator.

In March 1961, unknown to Meds '63 at the time, Dr Larry Wilson, chair of the KGH Interns Committee, established a subcommittee to review the academic health of the Queen's hospitals.[29] The committee found that KGH and the Hotel Dieu were functioning as community hospitals rather than academic centres of excellence. Beds were controlled by family physicians and any specialty involvement was largely at their behest. There were no designated "teaching beds" and the Outpatient Department was essentially non-existent, as was specialty training in family medicine. There were no trained emergency physicians. Indeed, students rated the bedside teaching at the Ottawa Civic as better than that at KGH. Of the twenty intern positions available at Queen's hospitals in 1961–62, only seventeen were filled and, of those, only five by Queen's students; the remainder were foreign graduates. Following extensive consultation, sweeping changes in the staffing and functioning of the Queen's teaching hospitals were agreed to on 22 November 1962.

In the spring of 1962 Dr Bingham retired as chief of surgery. Over the following months, all of the review committee's recommendations were implemented and a new dean appointed. In addition, new division heads for Medicine, Surgery, and OB/GYN were named.[30]

In the midst of these radical reforms, Meds '63 named Dr Bingham our honorary president for the Med III (1961–62) year and later, as our days at Queen's were drawing to a close, followed up by naming him permanent honorary president. The medical-school forces for change were outraged. Dr Bingham was quietly pleased.[31]

Though retired, DLCB doggedly soldiered on during his remaining months at KGH in the face of intermittent intergenerational academic chess matches. Following the arrival at Queen's of orthopaedic surgeon Dr Michael Simurda, a Surgical Grand Rounds was devoted to "March Fractures." Also known as a stress, or fatigue, fracture of a metatarsal bone, these injuries are the result of recurrent stress in persons exposed to excessive, or suddenly increased, standing or walking. The Grand Rounds in question featured one or two recent cases of this humble, yet potentially troubling, injury as an introduction to a discussion of the problem led by our new chief of orthopedic surgery. The tone of the presentation was appropriately low key (a "here's something you need to keep in mind" sort of thing), and in his comments our new service chief did himself proud. All present seemed pleased with this debut. Dr Bingham, however, who was in his customary front-row seat, had said nothing. At the conclusion of the Rounds, someone high in the academic pecking order stood and, by way of courtesy, asked DLCB if he had anything he might wish to add. In response, Dr Bingham paused momentarily, then quietly rose to his feet and turned to the audience of this well-attended coming-out party. "Yes well, you see, in North Africa, during the Eighth Army offensive – Tobruk, El Alamain, that sort of thing – One tended to see rather a lot of these fractures. For instance, One's personal experience consists of 248 cases." And with that, he sat down. The scales had been adjusted; perspective achieved. There was a deafening silence, a clearing of throats, and a shuffling of suddenly restless feet as, in sustained silence, we filed out of the amphitheatre.

SKENER AND TORT DO US PROUD

The Wednesday, 22 November, 1961 Queen's *Journal* headline proudly proclaimed in gigantic bold lettering, YATES OURS. On 18 November the Golden Gaels had won the coveted Yates Cup, symbol of Canadian intercollegiate football supremacy, with a convincing 11–0 victory at Richardson Stadium over the defending champion McGill Redmen, to whom the Gaels had fallen a week earlier in Montreal – their only defeat that season. It was the first Yates Cup for the Tricolour since 1956. All Meds '63 eyes were on our two all-star classmates, Skener (the Gaels' captain that year) and Terry "Tort" Porter. It would be the last game they played as Gaels, having decided to hang up their cleats in deference to the academic demands facing them. Corner linebacker Skener was at his opponent-crushing best; Terry was, as usual, tough, solid, and richly deserving of the Queen's *Journal*'s accolade noting that he "has played every position but pitcher [and] has always been a fierce and able competitor." Ex-Gael and future CFL Most Outstanding Canadian Ronnie Stewart, who was on hand, commented, "If you want to win badly enough, you win." The *Journal* observed, "Queen's wanted to win badly enough."

MILESTONES

Happily adjusting to married life, immersed in our clinical years as medical students, winning the Yates Cup: the milestones celebrated were effervescent. The letter from Dad was addressed to 131 King Street East, Kingston. To each his own milestone.

Sunday April 8, 1962

My Dear Ones,
This is a beautiful afternoon. It is 4:45 p.m., I'm sitting in my room thusly employed, have taken Nettie to [her friend] Dot's & driven

out to the airport. Carl Tapscott Singers are on the air & I love their work. I'm experiencing a strange feeling. Is it "nostalgia"? I don't fully understand that word & when I hear it I see a horse, well fed, but which has just tasted something extremely distasteful to it & its head [is] thrown [back] with its upper lip drawn well up in an expression of disgust and incredulity. No, that isn't quite what I mean. It is a feeling of slightly pleasant aloneness & a further question as to what life really is. You see, no one knows where life started or why.

Nostalgia – it brings to mind April 8th 1917 when I attended my most impressive church service. It was in an old building in Écoivres beside Mont-Saint-Éloi. You may recall it Bal. I pointed out the building as we drove thru the village in 1953. There were an indefinite number of troops, all young men 17–24 yrs – few older, & we all knew that before 14–16 hrs had passed an indefinite number of those present would be dead or wounded. Who would be alive? I suppose was in most of the minds as we listened & took part in the service. Perhaps the recollection of that incident serves to give me that indescribable feeling today. The singers have just sung "Keep Right on to the End of the Road." Harry Lauder sang that song to us & continued to sing it after his son had been killed. How could he do it? ...

Darling ones, good wishes to you both. I'm with you every minute.

Love,
Dad

DONALD CHURCH BALFOUR

May 1962. The Med III year ended with no supplemental exams and Faye, Mother, Dad, and I headed to Rochester, Minnesota, so that I could meet my namesake. While elderly and somewhat frail, Dr Balfour was a gracious host. In the course of an afternoon filled with reminiscences, he took us on a tour of the Mayo Clinic and told us about the Balfour family home and his pipe organ, recalling that, because of its great size, on their giving up that residence, the organ was reconfigured into two instruments. He then took us to hear the larger of the two in Christ Methodist Church, its new home.

Later that evening, following a superb dinner for five in the dining room of his current stately lodgings, we had coffee in the drawing room. With only the increasing shadows of that soft, early-summer evening to light the room, Dr Balfour sat at the grand piano and played one rollicking piece after another, most of them Scott Joplin rags. As the evening came to a close, his voice drifted to me across the near-total darkness. "Now, Balfour, I want you to see if you can name these last two pieces." The first was "The Maple Leaf Rag," but the second I couldn't identify. It was an upbeat rendition of something I had never heard before. He played it once more with less improvisation. Still no success. Finally, with great patience, and I'm sure a twinkle in his eye – although we were long past the hour when the lighting permitted such a diagnosis – he played it again. It was our national anthem, "O Canada." Our common Canadian roots, his history of support for Dad and Mother, and my link to him thus joyously celebrated, he bid us goodnight.

Dr Balfour died a year later at the age of eighty, on 25 July 1963. What a privilege it was to have met and been hosted by that gracious and gifted leader in the development of academic surgery whom I was honoured to call my namesake and now friend.[32]

On 10 December 1962 Queen's held a special convocation to present Marian Anderson with an honorary doctorate, thus marking the anniversary of the 10 December 1948 United Nations adoption of the Universal Declaration of Human Rights. In her convocation address, Anderson spoke of her friend Eleanor Roosevelt, who had died a month earlier. Describing her as a dedicated worker for the great cause of human understanding, she noted, "Her heart was always open to the best of all music, the still sad music of humanity." I heard her comments as a reminder to be alert to the daily suffering around us. She spoke of her voice as "the gift of a kind Providence which has allowed me to interpret to a kindly world some of the joys and sorrows and immortal longings of my own people." Personal ability seen as a gift, gift as an opportunity for service, service as a natural response to suffering.

FORD, THE QUINTESSENTIAL HEALER

I had long since seen through Dr Connell's apparent brusqueness, in spite of the prevailing colourful if not apocryphal tales. A colleague related: "Just the other day Dr Connell was waiting for the Watkins elevator. When the doors finally opened, a medical student inside announced to those waiting that the elevator was full. Without warning, Dr Connell reached out, collared him and spun him out on his ear with the comment, 'It isn't now,' as he himself stepped in."

I also was aware of his legendary diagnostic skills. Another colleague commented: "One day on his service I'd been up all night with a new admission, uncertain of the cause of her acute abdomen. We had done everything and couldn't be sure. When Ford arrived, I took him to see her first thing.

As we went through the door he took one look at her and said, 'acute gall bladder.' I hadn't even told him her story." He was, of course, correct.

One overcast Sunday during my final months as a medical student, Dr Connell gave his residents a dismissive wave of his hand prior to the completion of their regular Sunday morning patient rounds. They had been hurrying all morning in the hope of attending a mid-morning chat over coffee with a visiting professor. I trailed after Ford to see the last two patients.

He swooped into the first room, lab coat flying. "Morning, Charles!" he proclaimed, with a crisp bellow and a perfunctory nod of his head as he took his place in the bedside armchair. "How was the night?" Without waiting for a reply, he added, "By the way, have you seen the listings today? There's a significant decline in several sectors."

Charles nodded as he put down his newspaper. He was a businessman, an executive in an international shoe company that was known for its habit of chewing up its senior executives and spitting out the bits. "I saw that, Ford, but over and beyond that, did you notice the movement in the oil sector?" They were off and running.

During those Sunday morning sessions I carried with me a pad where I kept a running tally of the things I needed to read up on as a result of those "no teaching, Mount" rounds. The list was long. I now jotted down, "stock market trends." I knew *nothing* about the stock market! Surely this was yet another thing I'd have to bone up on.

Ford was sitting erect. There was an air of mutual respect as their staccato exchange continued. One business leader to another. It was hard to know what to write on my pad, so I just added an exclamation mark after the word "trends" and underlined the whole thing in desperation – "Stock market trends!"

As I was still processing all this, Ford suddenly stood up (I backed against the wall) and, in one almost imperceptible motion, he took Charles's pulse, checked his sclera for pallor, looked at his tongue, listened to his heart and lungs, palpated his upper abdomen with a quizzical raise of the eyebrows that silently asked Charles if his former epigastric pain was continuing to improve (Charles nodded), and checked for residuals under the breakfast-tray cover. The stock-market torrent continued for a moment, then, with a perfunctory parting handshake between two knowledgeable investors, we were out the door as Ford bellowed, "Keep it up, Charles. Progress. Things are improving nicely!"

The last patient on that rounds was in the next room. Both were private rooms that overlooked Lake Ontario. Ford sailed through the door and I slid into the background against the wall. To my utter amazement, Ford slouched into the over-stuffed easy-chair that he had dragged over to the bed on entering, and then, leaning back, he swung his long legs onto the bed, crossing them just above the footboard. He casually clasped his hands behind his head and rocked back even further.

"How's she goin', Gordon?"

"Not so bad, Dr Connell."

Ford gave a great honking blow into his tablecloth-sized handkerchief as he peered across the bed at the threatening sky outside.

"Have you spoken to Molly this morning, Gordon? Might be a good idea to give her a call. Might be good to check that the boats are secure. We could be in for a blow."

"Good idea, I'll do that."

"Why don't you do it now? I'm in no hurry." And he did.

Gordon had been admitted with a cardiac problem, but I don't recall the details. What I clearly remember is that I was watching two fisherman, for Gordon was a fisherman who lived on Wolfe Island. There they were, discussing the weather, recent squalls, the problems with one of Gordon's boats, his son's health, and the help available to him in doing the heavier work when Gordon returned home. One fisherman to another.

We finally made our way back into the hall, but not before Dr Connell had listened to Gordon's heart, reassured him, and chatted about plans for discharge. Ford had spoken quietly in this dialogue. He seemed particularly relaxed. So did Gordon.

Back in the hall he waved me off as he marched on to see his father, "Dr W.T.," now a chronic-care patient in another wing.

"Get along now, Mount."

As I watched him disappear down the corridor I wondered if he was *at all* aware of what he had just done. Or was his rural-Ontario facade simply unconscious reflex interacting as he moved through his busy day?

Suddenly, it was late April and my last Sunday rounds with Ford were rapidly approaching. Medical school was quickly morphing from present to past tense.

What an outstanding exemplar of the art of medicine Dr Connell had been! Over my long career, I would rarely enter a patient's hospital room without recalling Ford's visit to the bedsides of Charles and Gordon. But had the quality of his presence to them been purposeful? Was he conscious of what he was doing?

I think he bought coffee for the team as rounds ended on that last Sunday, but it ended up feeling like an awkward formality, a delay in getting on with the day for the residents, for me, a painful delay in the inevitable parting with my mentor.

Ford walked with me to the front door of KGH. Neither of us spoke. The walk through the silent halls seemed both endless and too short. I tried to comment on the patients, the weather, but anything that came to mind seemed meaningless.

We reached the foyer with its vaulted ceiling and stopped. What could I say? Neither of us could look the other in the eyes. He stared fixedly up at the chandelier above us as we pumped each other's hand. My voice croaked out in spurts, "Dr Connell, I, don't know *how* I can ever thank you, how I can ever express ..."

"Well, Mount, you may not have learned much medicine, but I hope you learned something about how to talk to patients." My mind raced. He *did* know! He knew *exactly* what he was doing.

We still could only look obliquely past one another. My eyes were brimming. He was still gazing awkwardly up at the ceiling fixture. I loved that man.

The letter from Montreal contained good news. I had been accepted for internship by McGill's Royal Victoria Hospital (RVH). I was delighted. There had been another factor at play in selecting my first choice for internship. In passing through the Vic's imposing front doors, during my visit to Montreal for interviews, I had walked alone, somewhat intimidated, down the long marble hallway from the front door toward the imposing white marble statue of Queen Victoria. As I approached her, the hospital operator paged "Dr Moseley, Dr Moseley" ... then, "Dr Mason Cooper, Dr Arthur Elvidge, Dr Joseph Luke, Dr Arthur Vineburg." My mind was made up. Through my student days I had used Moseley's *Textbook of Surgery*. These were the names I had lived with, the men I had learned from. If they would have me, I was theirs.

PETER MORRIN AND MALCOLM BROWN
AT THE ELEVENTH HOUR

The finals had arrived. The *final finals*, after six years. I was filled with an odd admixture of feelings – relief on the one hand, but fatigue and a variety of fears on the other. I recalled psychiatry professor Bruce Sloane, or perhaps it was George Laverty, mentioning "free-floating anxiety" and my current unrest seemed to confirm that this was something I must read up on.

The problem was, my internal-medicine oral exam was to consist of completing a history and physical on an unknown assigned patient, *a patient who could have anything in the world*, followed by a grilling on his or her medical condition by none other than Malcolm Brown,

THE Malcolm Brown. I had certainly drawn the short straw! People have been known to *die* from far less lethal circumstances!

I walked into the screened-off KGH sunporch and was introduced to my patient, a local farmer named Smith. He looked more fit than I did. I wondered if he had any idea what was at stake here. So I told him.

"Mr Smith, I am glad to meet you and appreciate your taking part in this interview today. I think you should know that whether or not I become a doctor rests on my figuring out what ails you, so anything you feel might be relevant ... well, don't hesitate to let me know." And off we started.

Things were going quite well when, a half-hour later, the door opened and in walked Peter Morrin, the "Oral Examinations Co-ordinator" for internal medicine. It was his job to recruit the patients, ensure an optimal environment, sort out any problems that might crop up, and generally make sure that the student (and patient) had a high probability of surviving the ordeal.

"Well now, Mr Smith," crooned Peter with his usual pleasant but matter-of-fact intensity and telltale undertone that suggested Dublinesque origins, "Is this young fellow treating you alright?"

"Oh, yes, Doctor!" enthused Smith with all the ardour of a blushing bride. "Absolutely! Best Doctor I've ever had!!"

Now, to appreciate fully what happened next, I must tell you a little about Peter Morrin. Peter, an Irish internist with an unmistakable lilt to his speech and twinkle in his piercing eyes, had arrived in Kingston with his delightful American southern belle bride two years earlier at the age of thirty. He had just completed three post-fellowship years at a nephrology unit in St Louis, Missouri, and was razor sharp. Indeed, he was at a rarified peak of academic preparedness that few attain, even when fresh from writing the Royal College Fellowship exams. For example, in chatting with Peter on one occasion, a member of our student group cited a scientific article to support a clinical observation. Peter immediately jumped in. "No! No! *Never* cite the literature like that! You *never* say, 'I read somewhere that someone found such and such!' Never! What you say is, 'A recent study has shown ...', or, better still, 'As Schultz and Jones recently reported in the New England Journal ...,' and even better, 'the boys in Boston – Shultz and Jones, at the Brigham – reported in last month's New England Journal that, in their lab' ..." Peter was a breath of fresh air. A dazzlingly, bright, ebullient spirit, a great storyteller, and the possessor of an overflowing, sly, ever-sparkling Irish wit.

And so, as Mr Smith began waxing eloquent about my celestial powers, Peter began to smile, his eyes dancing, and with a delighted guffaw he interjected, "I'll bet!! You know, you two remind me of my classmate in Dublin! He was a good fly fisherman, but not much of a student – rarely attended lectures. Anyway, when *we* sat *our* final examinations in medicine, our examiners were professors from London. Imported for the occasion, they were. A haughty bunch! It was an ordeal feared by us all."

Peter, was in full storytelling mode now. "Anyway, when my classmate met *his* patient it turned out the man lived near his very favourite fishing spot. The two men were enthralled. 'I can't believe it! You know that stream that runs into the cove, by those great rocks?' one exploded. 'I do indeed, m' lad. One of the best spots – m' favourite in fact,' responded the other. 'I can't believe it, *mine* too!' And so it went. Then, suddenly, the door opened and in walked the visiting professor from London. 'Well now, doctor, introduce me to your patient and tell me what is wrong with him.'" Peter continued:

My friend was aghast. They had been so into the fishing that he had never even asked his new friend what was wrong with him! But of course, he knew he could never admit that, so he blurted out, "Well sir, I'd like to present Mr Murphy. He's here with angina pectoris; presented with a heaviness in his central chest and a pain that ran down his left arm." The professor checked his notes. The card clearly said, "Murphy, peptic ulcer." He turned to the patient. *Very strange! Very strange!* "Murphy my good man, would you be good enough to tell me why you are here?" "Well yer Honour," Murphy replied without hesitation, "I had this heavy feeling here in the middle of me chest, and this great bleeding pain right down me lef' arm." "Hmm, I see," grumbled the disgruntled professor crossing out the diagnosis on the card and writing down *angina pectoris*. Then, turning to my classmate, he growled, "Tell me what you know about angina pectoris."

"Well," Peter added, delighted. "You see, it was the only thing my friend knew anything about – other than fishing of course, so he squeaked through. But the end of the story," he said, with a satisfied grin, "is this. After the examiner left the room my friend turned to Murphy and said, 'My good fellow, how can I *ever* thank you? You have saved my life!' 'Well now,' Murphy responded with a shrug, 'I wasn't going to let you down, especially in front of a bloody Englishman!'"

Smith, Peter, and I laughed. And we were still enjoying the moment a second later when the door to the sunporch swung open imperiously and in floated Malcolm Brown. The strange thing was, I was completely relaxed. Peter's warmth still filled the room. I turned to face Professor

Brown, who was, in fact, much more gentle then I had expected, and the oral went well. Peter Morrin and Mr Smith, not to mention Malcolm Brown, had just managed to get me successfully through medical school.

My final marks were less than brilliant – an average of 73.9 per cent, but my rank in the class had crept up to eleventh. It seemed a satisfying continuation of a trend that I hoped augured well for the future. Of interest were my A in psychiatry and C in urology.

From our first days at Queen's in September 1957, Meds '63 had proven to be a remarkably united body. This seemed somewhat surprising, given the disparate character of its members. Generally speaking, the feelings were not so much bonds of affection but, instead, the bonds forged out of mutual respect, tolerance, and sense of earned brotherhood. We were a classic example of the whole being greater than the sum of its parts. The students in the years preceding and following us were at times intimidated by our brazen sense of unity in sports and campus activities. There was cohesion in our ranks. We could count on each other. An interesting example of that occurred in early March 1963 when final exams were upon us. Our landlord, a graceless lawyer known in town for anatomical reasons as "the one-armed bandit," evicted Faye and me from 131 King Street for having called the fire department concerning worrisome electrical problems. He was furious, saying that we should have called him instead. With our call, the fire department had what they had long desired, the grounds to have the building inspected and rewired. Our eviction date was 1 May, only days before final exams. The potential for catastrophe was averted when a handful of classmates moved us to temporary new quarters in a period of three hours.

Fifty-four members of Meds '63 graduated in our Grant Hall convocation on Saturday, 25 May, 1963.[33] It was a memorable opportunity to applaud one another, congratulate our prize winners, and bid farewell to the class for one last time. The class elected DLCB permanent honorary president and the Binghams convened a reception at their home later that afternoon. In his farewell message to us Dr Bingham wrote:

In the years that have passed, the goal was graduation, but in the years that are to come the prize is less sharply and clearly defined. Perhaps for some it is material wealth and the acclamation of the world; for others, a quieter life in a narrower circle; and for others still, a life seeking and looking on the frontiers of knowledge. But whatever way and mode of life you choose, have cause to be proud of what you are and do; be gentle with the sick, the poor, the very humble people; be patient with those who are afraid; learn of the greatness and courage of so many human beings; keep your word and do to others what you would want done to you; serve your Country and her people both in peace and war. Also, as important as anything else in your lives, do not become so engrossed in your work that you neglect your own home and families. Don't imagine that because you give them bread and lovely things that they can do without your presence and your love.

When you leave, you take with you the best wishes, the affection, and the hopes of your instructors, but also when you go you leave as a legacy to us memories of six years which will blend with and become part of the tradition and spirit of Queen's University.

Good luck!
DLC Bingham

Internship and Residency, 1963–68

Never, no never, did Nature say one thing and Wisdom say another.
                                                            Edmund Burke

To be uncertain is uncomfortable; to be certain is absurd.
                                                                Lao Tau

Truths do not conflict.

                                                                   HTRM

THE ROYAL VICTORIA HOSPITAL, MCGILL

The move to Montreal was yet another life-shaping crossroad. What is it about islands? And why is that question important to me? Oddly, I have always thought of Montreal as an island. Reasonable enough, it *is* on an island. But that is my *sense* of it as well. Is it because, as an anglophone, I am part of an island within an island, a minority within a minority and thus somewhat freed from the sense of pre-eminence so common in Caucasian North America, with a certain humility prompted by knowing how it feels to be on the other side? That is perhaps part of it. After all, on the "mainland" there is nothing to stop us. We can charge on and on with an illusion of entitlement – running before the wind, as it were. But if home is on an island, we must learn to tack early and often, to *make short boards*, as our sailing ancestors would say, if we are to escape being blown onto our lee shore.

Another aspect of home as *island* may be symbolic, the degree of unconscious comfort to be found in returning to *water*, our individual and collective original security. Whatever the reason, I have felt at home at 37 Opeongo overlooking Dow's Lake, at the *Place* on Grand Lake, at Queen's on the shore of Lake Ontario, in Montreal with the St Lawrence and Ottawa rivers at hand, and, in due course, in New York City on the Hudson, then at L'Abri on Lac Mercier at Mont Tremblant. Perhaps peace is found in opening to the presence of our inner sea.

Our new home port was to be 4965 Côte-Saint-Luc Road, a sturdy, beige-brick, four-storey structure, situated mid-hill on the north side of that busy, steeply sloped thoroughfare. Our apartment was just to the left on the ground floor as you entered the nondescript front door, its small balcony thus commanding a southwest view – perfect for watching the desperate sliding vehicles (once, a city bus executing a perfect 360-degree spin) as they descended the icy winter pavement in front of us. The apartment consisted of one bedroom, a dining/living room, a kitchenette, and a bathroom, and it was ideally located for our purposes: our new church home, Dominion Douglas United, was only three or four blocks away (uphill), and it was fifteen minutes or so by car across the upper slope of Mount Royal to the Royal Victoria Hospital, also known as "The Royal Vic," the RVH, or simply "The Vic."[1]

My internship was to start on 1 July 1963. The last days of June were spent unpacking, setting up bricks-and-boards bookshelves, and hanging pictures on empty walls while listening to radio reports of President Kennedy's visit to West Berlin. It was almost two years since Soviet-sponsored East Germany had erected the Berlin Wall to prevent its citizens from fleeing the deteriorating conditions in their beleaguered land. Now, we found ourselves watching JFK's speech on the steps of Rathaus Schöneberg in Berlin before a cheering crowd of a half-million. He radiated hope, youthful vigour, and confidence, his hair, like the German flag behind him, blowing in the wind. In those memorable moments, my boundless admiration for JFK was easily transferred to the Vic and the journey that lay ahead. His capacity to find opportunity and community in adversity and the unknown profoundly impressed me. Drawn by his open manner and elegant rhetoric, we witnessed extraordinary leadership and courage, the courage to speak with resonant clarity in the front yard of the adversary.

INTERNSHIP

We newly recruited and name-tagged Royal Vic interns, dressed in standard white shirts, slacks, and shoes, with pens and notepads at the ready and stethoscopes on standby, assembled in the J.S.L. Brown Amphitheatre to get our marching orders. My rotation for the year was to start with general surgery, including a stint in the ER, then OB/GYN, then, after Christmas, internal medicine for the final months of the year.

Copies of the RVH Interns' Manual, containing essential telephone numbers, lists of normal lab values, and other useful in-house information,
were distributed. We were on our way.

The McGill graduates seemed more sure of themselves. For one thing,
they appeared to have no difficulty finding their way from pavilion to
pavilion through the bewildering maze of corridors, whereas I feared I
would never find my way back to a given pavilion, let alone a particular
location within it.

We were to be on call (which meant sleeping in the hospital) every
other night and weekend, causing me to remember Betty's letter asking
me how sure I was that I didn't want to opt out of a medical career.
Thankfully, we would have a couple of weeks off in August when Faye
and I could go to the *Place*.

My inaugural Emergency Department weeks proved to be an experience best described as getting one's feet wet at the deep end. I enjoyed it.
There was a sense of teamwork and mutual support. Rachelle "Press"
Presseault was one of the nurses.[2] She was competent, dynamic, and,
as Mother would say, "full of beans." She could be relied on for useful
advice that would see a rookie intern through any unexpected tight spot.
Perhaps it was through Press that I first learned, "When in trouble, ask
a nurse."

With the arrival of August, I rotated from the ER to surgery. Each
morning, hurried rounds with the other residents started at 7:00 A.M.
Our tour from patient to patient amounted to troubleshooting concerning overnight developments and the delegation of duties to the junior
ranks before the senior members of the team headed to the OR for an
8:00 A.M. start.

We underlings were left with the "scut work," the grease that kept the
wheels rolling. Typical instructions were as follows:

> Once the bloods are drawn, you'll need to do the dressings. In Room
> 387, check the amount of discharge from her drain; culture it, if
> you're concerned. With Mr Johnson in 381, you'll need to review
> the intake and output sheets with Nancy for the past week. Find out
> where we stand with his fluid and electrolyte balance. Also, have a
> look at his recent films and lab values before rounds with L.D.
> [Dr Lloyd MacLean] this afternoon. And, oh yes, ask Nancy where
> things stand with Social Service regarding placement for Mme Pinot.
> We need that bed. And one last thing, the Jelansky family, or at least
> the wife, has been anxious to speak to L.D. Tell her he'll be around
> this afternoon.

It was during those early August days that I made my mind up. I would become a urologist. Why? Although my respect for Ford had led me to consider internal medicine briefly, there was never any real doubt about becoming a surgeon given my enjoyment of drawing and creating with my hands. Furthermore, Dad and Jim were both surgeons. It seemed a no-brainer. But then what? *General* surgery? If not, which subspecialty? I wanted a specialty that would offer both a clearly defined area of expertise and a broad variety of surgical techniques. Urology included radical abdominal, plastic, bowel, vascular, pelvic, transplantation, perineal, and transurethral surgery. It was perfect.

I made an appointment to meet with the urologist-in-chief at McGill, Dr Kenneth J. MacKinnon (or "K.J."). He informed me that to pursue that path I would need to follow internship with two years of general-surgery residency, then urology training. We left our early fall 1963 first meeting with a mutual understanding that I would take that route. From then on, he became my mentor and confidant.[3]

Our island paradise on Grand Lake was awaiting. It was at its best that August. Skiing, swimming, camp fires, Mother's birthday on 14 August, drawing, short canoeing jaunts for picnics. We talked of the future. While my career path was now clear, an unexpected concern repeatedly came to mind. Surgery as a child had left me with one testicle. What if further delay in starting a family was to find us beyond a point of no return and unable to have children? It seemed a needless fantasy – a mindless worry, really. There was no reason for concern, but there it was. We decided that the time had come to delay no longer, and when we headed back to Montreal, Faye was pregnant.

The 1954 British film *Doctor in the House* explored the growing pains of medical student Simon Sparrow (Dirk Bogarde) and his classmates as they endured the rigours of medical training at fictional St Swithin's Hospital, London. One line from that hilarious romp (or perhaps one of its six sequels) has lived with me since first hearing it at age fifteen. Sparrow and his quaking peers were being cross-examined by the bombastic chief of surgery, Sir Lancelot Spratt. On presenting them with a disastrous medical scenario, he bellowed at them, "What would you do?!" One of the students responded, "Call a doctor."

"You *are* the doctor!!" roared Sir Lancelot. The audience laughed. *I* didn't, even at fifteen!

Fast forward a decade, *I* am the young would-be doctor in that scene, and the weight of responsibility for the well-being of another still seemed an onerous thing. I might, therefore, have predicted the dream conjured up by my well-primed unconscious during that internship surgical rotation. On the night in question, four of us interns were sleeping in the cramped on-call room deep in the bowels of the Royal Vic Interns' Residence. I was in a bottom bunk which I hoped would facilitate a rapid response should an urgent phone call come in. This, then, was the setting for my *Doctor in the House* encounter.

In my dream, I found myself caring for an unconscious, critically ill, middle-aged woman who required constant observation. My job was to monitor her pulse continuously, but I was totally exhausted. This led my dreaming self to conclude that I simply *had* to lie down, even for a moment. Perhaps, I thought, if I lay along the very edge of my patient's bed it would be alright and I would be able to continue to follow her status without contravening propriety to any great extent. So I moved carefully onto her bed – lying on my side, still monitoring her pulse – just along the edge, mind you – while resting my head on the mattress, all the while reassuring myself, *It will only be for a few minutes – just until my head clears – surely that will be* OK. It was at that precise moment in my dream that the telephone in our on-call room rang. Leaping to my feet, I reached it at the second ring. My three roommates were still unconscious, snoring. Stunned, and still more or less asleep, I croaked, "Hello!" into the receiver.

"DR MARTIN RAFF, TWO, THREE – FIVE CARDIAC! DR MARTIN RAFF, TWO, THREE – FIVE, CARDIAC!" the locating operator bellowed in my ear.

This is impossible! I thought. *How can I follow this woman's pulse and answer the phone at the same time?!*

"You have made a mistake!" I shot back, adding, "You've got the patient's room!" I slammed down the receiver. But in that instant, just before the line went dead, I heard the operator's distant, bewildered voice, "I can't understand it! I can't understand it!"

My head hit the pillow just as the phone rang for the second time. Instantly, the dream had dissolved. I was awake, knew where I was, and what I had just done. *Horrors!*

"Hello," I growled gruffly, an octave below my normal range in an attempt to disguise my voice.

"DR MARTIN RAFF, TWO, THREE – FIVE CARDIAC!" She roared.

"Hey Marty, it's for you!"[4]

To my relief, with the passing weeks, the surgical routine began to fall into a rhythm. Working up the new patients was beginning to take less time, the norms of patient assessment and care were becoming second nature, and my rare opportunities to act as second assistant in major abdominal cases were richly rewarding. There was always something new to learn by observing basic procedures from the perspective of a surgical assistant rather than that of summer scrub nurse. On the other hand, my family time was non-existent. Faye was working as a physiotherapist at the Vic and would have enjoyed it had it not been for our work schedules and her ghastly first-trimester nausea.

We were buoyed by the unexpected news that Alice and Betty were also pregnant. Remarkably, Mother and Dad were about to have *three* new grandchildren, roughly the same age. Peter and Al were now settled in Cambridge and Peter's research lab at Clare College was up and running. Jim and Betty were enjoying Boston, with Jim working at the Massachusetts Eye and Ear under Neuro-Ophthalmologist David G. Cogan. And there was no grass growing under Mother and Dad's feet that fall. They were visiting cousins Don and Norma Connor in Kampala, Uganda, and living at an Anglican mission station at Entebbe while Dad did surgery at Mengo Hospital. Their eagerly anticipated letters offered detailed descriptions of their many adventures.

Dad's surgery in Uganda included abdominal cases, correction of orthopedic deformities, and a variety of minor procedures. His letter of 20 October noted, "I have been to only three wards [today] & have actually outlined Rx for only a couple, one of these is a meningocele which I hope to fix tomorrow p.m."[5] Mother wrote (24 October), "Harry is carrying on as usual and has quite a lot of surgery," then added, concerning her own activities, "I have just marked another batch of entrance to nursing papers which were very very poor. I am really quite nauseous with these papers & am now glad to start on those on shock, administering injections, etc., etc." Their letters to "Dearest Faye & Bal & '1/4'" expressed their joyful anticipation of our baby.

WHERE WERE YOU ON THAT DAY?

Shortly after starting my OB/GYN rotation, I retrieved an ancient Royal Vic rocking chair, a discarded relic of earlier practice norms, from a basement storage area in the Women's Pavilion. With a plan to refinish it for Faye, I started stripping off the countless layers of paint, using as my workshop a vacant nook adjacent to the on-call room. It would be a perfect Christmas present for an expectant mother. Things were becoming less hectic clinically and the clinical pressures promised to slow even further as Christmas approached. With a little luck and a lot of elbow grease, my gift would be ready on time.

It was a Friday afternoon and I went to see a new admission on the gynecology ward prior to planned rocking-chair restoration time.

Having completed my patient's history and physical, I needed to draw some blood for her baseline tests and strode out of her room to collect the necessary tubes and syringes. As I passed the nursing station, a voice shouted – or maybe I only *heard* it as a shout. Maybe the universe didn't really stop. Maybe the whole shuddering planet hadn't frozen. But I *did*! Someone beside me was yelling and all time stopped in midstride.

"Kennedy has been shot! President Kennedy has been shot."

"How serious is it?" "Is he badly injured?" "Will he be OK?" The fog of uncertainty clouded in! Impossible!! Kennedy shot? Not possible!! Indescribable. Then, the news came. "President Kennedy died at 1 p.m. CST, that is, 2 p.m. EST." The Montreal *Star* printed a postscript edition at 4:17 p.m. that same afternoon, with the headline: "Friday, November 22, 1963, Assassinated in Dallas, President Kennedy Killed. Governor of Texas Also Shot."

Like everyone else, I recall *exactly* where I was the moment I heard. *Exactly!* For their part, Mother and Dad, still in Uganda, commented later that in Entebbe there had been a particularly charged sense of shock and grief as the news swept their way. Somehow, there had been a feeling of being personally involved. Cousins Don and Norma – Don was teaching pathology at the medical school – were hosting a dinner party for friends at their home in Kampala when the news reached their dining-room table, provoking a profound sense of immediacy and identification with the events in Dallas. A member of the U.S. Secret Service was one of their guests. He and his wife excused themselves and left the gathering. Hours later, the Kampala *Argus* headline carried the simple dyad, "Kennedy Assassinated."

Alice and Peter were in Cambridge. It was early evening. Peter had been helping with meal preparations. Alice was tending to eight-month-old Wilfred. Suddenly, the news from Dallas! Stunned! They reported "an immense sense of loss reverberated across England."

In Boston – in *Boston* for heaven's sake! Why, JFK was a native son! – Jim and Betty were speechless: Jim at the hospital, Betty at home with Heather Lynn and Howie. For both of them, their already highly developed sense of personal responsibility gave way to something like confusion, then a need for distancing and for refocusing on their individual tasks at hand.

It was a world fast-frozen in a universal ground-zero experience. But *I* knew! I knew for sure! The *real* epicentre on that dreadful day had, in fact, been in Montreal! It had been on the gynecology ward at the Royal Victoria Hospital, and my overwhelming thought was, why couldn't it have been me rather than him? It wasn't simply emotional whiplash born of the shock of the moment. It was a sustained response erupting from the recognition of the catastrophic eclipse of urgently needed leadership during desperate Cold War times. And, in its place, a sense of cruel emptiness, a vacuum, had replaced all that might have been, a dark, pervasive, oppressive, crushing weight. Why couldn't it have been me?

Next day the tributes reached eloquent heights as world leaders, governments, and private citizens attempted to express their agony. In the Montreal *Star*, a full-page black-bordered photograph of the president at his desk was accompanied by a simple unreferenced quote, "There Hath Cast Away a Glory from the Earth."[6] The prime minister of Canada, Lester Pearson, noted: "The world can ill-afford his loss ... [It] is one of the great tragedies of history, but for us now, it is something more, it is a great, heartbreaking, personal tragedy. There are millions of people tonight throughout the world who will feel they have lost a friend ... He was a man of generous mind, of generous instinct. He had a quality of mind and a quality of spirit far surpassing the usual quality even of men who become leaders of great nations ... I feel I have lost a friend."[7]

PERSONAL ENCORES

Vapid attempts to move on filled the days that followed. A letter I wrote to Mother and Dad two weeks later ended with a query. "If a person 'A' is affected by things such as art, music, literature, or anything beautiful, and has stronger feelings emotionally (i.e. a mature emotion) than a person 'B,' does 'A' have a fuller overall enjoyment of life on looking back at its end?" Dad replied in, for him, an unusually large and flowing hand, "Yes. Why do you ask?" I responded with a brief note suggesting that we continue this exploration at Christmas. That plan was to be cut short.

During the week that followed, I detected a testicular swelling and went to see Dr MacKinnon. Given our earlier discussions about my joining his urology-training program, there was no hesitation on my part. I felt that I was consulting a friend. He concurred with my suspicions and on Thursday, 19 December, he operated while Faye, Mother, and Dad waited in the OR family waiting room, updated by progress reports through the kindness of my thoughtful fellow intern, Peter Hacker.[8]

As promised, K.J. came to see me in the recovery room. I was swimming upward toward consciousness when I heard his voice. "Yes, Bal, it's malignant. It's an embryonal cell carcinoma. We'll talk a little later."

In the days that followed, he added, "Bal, I want you to do something for me. Should you have any questions, any at all, I want you to ask me rather than going to the literature yourself. You can call me anytime. I will be happy to interpret the literature for you. I'll give you the facts as they are, but it will be easier for me to extract a balanced perspective." It was a deal.

I was in a private room in the Ross Pavilion. My fragmented thoughts came in bunches – questions mainly: the implications of the pathology report; treatment options; prognosis; issues around the gaping uncertainty about my future. Would I live to see our baby? That became my immediate goal.

While Faye, Mother, and Dad were close by and I had the support of my extended family and friends,[9] I had an intense sense of being alone. What seemed particularly strange was the degree to which Faye, Mother, and Dad appeared to be relatively unconcerned, calm and at peace with the whole thing. And yet I knew the fact was that many in my situation didn't make it. Didn't they care? How careful they were to conceal their anguish. It belonged, they thought, in the halls, not in my presence. Anguished debates and tears, yes, but never in my presence.

The full weight of the aphorism "There are no atheists in foxholes" sank in. But what about God? What about miracles? What is the place of prayer? To what end? I have never believed in a divine diddler, a God that would interfere at whim with natural law. Such thinking just doesn't lie within my comfort zone. On the other hand, I realized with a grim smile, neither does the alternative! "There's Mother again," I thought. "She always does manage to see the irony and humour in a bleak situation."

Faye's cousin, Montreal Alouette place-kicking all-star Bill Bewley, came to visit. It was such a shot in the arm to see his bright, vibrant smile come through that door and the easy grace in his firm handshake. He was one of those people who make you feel better just being in their presence. His comrade-in-arms grip offered reassurance. "Bal, we have a saying in the Alouette's dressing room. In the midst of a tough game, when our backs are against the wall, we have a motto. I want you to have it. *When the going gets tough, the tough get going!*" Trite perhaps, but a source of unimagined support during the weeks that lay ahead.

Two issues impressed me from the outset. First, I was struck by my unexpected presentment months earlier at the *Place* that Faye and I should no longer delay having a family. It had been remarkably prophetic. Second, I could never ask "why me," never feel sorry for myself. A few weeks earlier, on 22 November, I had said, and meant it with all my heart, "Why him? Why *not* me?" Now, lying in this bed, how could I possibly ask "Why me?" I had to smile again as I imagined Mother saying, "I told you to be careful what you wish for!" It seemed I must simply recognize and accept the way things are. That had to be my starting point. There would be tears, fears, and uncertainty, and the potential for loving attachments lost, but *no* self-pity or questioning. To the contrary, what *did* go through my mind was the 1953 plane crash. Getting out of *that* had seemed a miracle. And what about family, friends, and home? Frankly, I had been fortunate, blessed beyond measure, in fact, and I knew it. Dad's oft-repeated motto, *Of him to whom much is given, much will be required*, struck home. It always *had* impressed me but never more forcibly than now. Instead of "why me," the more pertinent question seemed to be "Why shouldn't it be me?" And part of me realized that I had once again been blessed, for I was aware of how formidable the "why me" hurdle is for many. It wasn't for me.

On a particularly empty late afternoon, after the last visitor had left for the day, a sense of quiet but determined desperation gelled. No panic. I was dead calm, present, aware of the survival data, and by then had agreed to abdominal surgery at Memorial Sloan Kettering Cancer Center (MSKCC) in New York. I lay looking up at the ceiling of my hospital room. Everything was still, totally still. The clicking of a clock seemed deafening.

I suspect the challenge that I expressed to the empty room may have been spoken aloud. "God, I don't know if you exist. But if you do, now's the time to step up. Now's the time to make yourself evident." There was absolutely no sentimentality in this, no theatre, nor any clear underlying expectations. My words *were*, however, in dead earnest. I was as serious as I have ever been.

Reaching over to the bedside table, I picked up the inevitable hospital Bible. Never having been a biblical scholar, I thought it appropriate to let it open where it might. If there was a comment relevant to my situation, let it speak for itself. There was an edge of challenge there – certainly a sense of bleakness. It opened at Psalm 116, a prayer of thanksgiving for deliverance from death, which I had never read before. I read it. I was astonished and somewhat embarrassed at the magical-thinking notion that this Ouija Board response might have personal relevance to me. Could it be the promise of a cure? The implication that I might be "chosen," as the psalm suggested, when Tom Dooley and countless others were not was completely unpalatable.[10] Absurd. Dooley was a star. His brief life of service had blazed a glorious path across the mediocrity and self-interest that most of us leave behind. To me, Dooley appeared to be one "whose sandals I am not worthy to untie." His 1958 brainchild, MEDICO, was a visionary experiment in whole-person care. He had undergone surgery at Memorial Sloan Kettering, where I was now headed, then died of his disease, but he lived through his illness. His tough-minded yet gracious response suggested a deeper meaning in the psalmist's suggestion that bonds had been loosed. One could imagine Dooley finding sustenance and grace in its words to the very end of his journey.

Like Kennedy, Dooley was a man of action, a man on the move. He wore around his neck the St Christopher's medal of a traveller, and on its back he had engraved Robert Frost's words, *The woods are lovely, dark and deep, But I have promises to keep, And miles to go before I sleep.* Taken together, the memory of JFK's death and Tom Dooley's grace-filled life enabled me to see that the real miracle at the edge of being is the unexpected experience of being accompanied and supported.

A day or two prior to my discharge from the Vic, the door to my hospital room swung open and in strode OB/GYN Chief Resident Ted Roman. He held something in his outstretched hand. Given the great size and strength of this Canadian Football League retiree, it seemed a small object, perhaps a toy. It took me a moment or two to identify it and understand what it represented. "Here," he tossed off, in a typically dismissive growl, "Thought you might have some use for this in the next few days." With that, he delivered Faye's Christmas present, the now pristine rocking chair. He had finished the stripping and refinishing himself. How remarkable for a frenetically busy chief resident to invest the time and effort to undertake such a demanding project, especially in those over-crowded pre-Christmas days! How remarkable for anyone, at any time!

A change in Christmas plans was called for. We would gather in Boston with Jim, Betty, and family en route to New York and my 3 January admission to MSKCC. It was wonderful to share in the grace and community conjured up through Betty's sunny presence and careful stewardship, a gift for us to share the magic and wonder of Christmas with Howie, Heather Lynn, Betty, Jim, Mother, and Dad. The meaning of family was deeply felt.

At "Memorial," *all* the patients have cancer. While it sounded depressing, I once again encountered a paradox. On walking through the door, one recognized, "I am not alone." There were hundreds there who shared my plight and not all of them would die. In addition, however their personal journeys might end, the potential for victory of the human spirit was evident on all sides. It was uplifting, inspiring, hope-filled. My roommate was a man in his sixties. He might have been Italian. He looked as if he had been involved in manual labour all his life. While we never spoke, for he was occupied by the demands of his own difficult journey, he was aware of my joining him and offered a wordless welcome as I came on board. I was impressed by his attitude. He met his crisis with what William Osler would term *aequanimitas*, implying a centred calm. Although he died during our few days together, I remember him still. He taught me as much as has any man about grace in facing adversity, Osler's prerequisite for being a complete physician.

On completing my MSKCC baseline admission tests on Saturday, I had no obligations prior to my surgery Tuesday morning. Faye and I set off to see our first opera. The Metropolitan Opera House stood proudly at 1411 Broadway.[11] A few last-minute seats were available, and so we joined Charles Gounod, Marguerite, Méphistophélès, Dr Faust, and friends for an afternoon date with destiny. Wonderful. Captivating. We were hooked.

"Did you notice, there is an evening opera as well?" The evening performance was sold out, but, we were informed, if we were willing to take our chances, we could join the line for evening standing-room tickets the moment the curtain fell on Faust. We did, and in return, the evening was spent with Giuseppe Verdi, Rigoletto, Gilda, the Duke, and the gloriously fiendish Sparafucile. With the sublime quartet of Act Three, we were transported well beyond the concerns of the day. An immeasurable gift!

Tuesday morning at 7:00 A.M. a dynamic, tanned, life force wearing a dazzling white custom-tailored scrub suit beamed his way into the room, a couple of assistants at his heals.

"Hey, Dr Mount! Willet Whitmore! Glad to see that you made it alright." He simultaneously patted my shoulder and shook my hand. "Great! Great! Look," he nodded his head supportively while giving me a warm, evaluative, and hope-inducing physical once-over. "We're going to take care of this for you this morning and you'll be on your way. Don't worry about a thing." The buoyancy of his step and the warmth and confidence in his demeanour were contagious. I felt sure that he had just come from winning a couple of sets of tennis. He probably had.

I realized I was grinning. I couldn't help it. *Absolutely!* I thought, *Exactly! Right! Let's get this taken care of!!*

On the wall of the MSKCC chapel are the words, "Come to me all you who are weary and burdened, and I will give you rest." They spoke to Faye during her hours of solitary vigil.

YET MORE

By early February, my activity level was returning toward normal. There had been no cancer in the lymph nodes.

On 7 February, Faye and I were visiting Mother and Dad at 37. When the phone rang, we thought of Betty and Jim in Boston. Would this be news of the baby? I picked up the ground-floor phone just as Dad did the same upstairs. It was the Harvard obstetrician. Betty, ablaze with life, talented, vivacious, brilliant twenty-nine-year-old Betty, had just died in childbirth. Jim's Betty?! Our Betty?! No!! No!! No!! The message was impossible to comprehend.

"Would you repeat that?"

"What happened?"

Something about aspiration, something about an intracranial bleed. Betty gone. "Where is Jim? He asked *you* to call? Is he OK?"[12] The baby, David Bruce Mount, was a fine little fellow in good health. We were being engulfed in, repeatedly swept under by, a maelstrom that threatened from all sides: JFK's assassination; my malignancy; Betty's death. And the swirl of events continued.

Within a week there was another phone call. It was Peter in Cambridge. Al had just been hospitalized with an antepartum hemorrhage. Mother flew to England, and Margery Alice Knewstubb was born on 22 February. A week or two after that, Mother underwent excision of a recent facial blemish. It was a squamous-cell carcinoma. She barely rated an honourable mention on the current family-crisis scale.

Meeting treatment protocols of the day, I entered a chemotherapy program and the cascading side effects quickly undermined the post-operative gains I had made. Radiation therapy followed.

On 26 May our son was born. Christopher Balfour James Mount was a lovely, healthy, sturdy boy, weighing eight pounds, fifteen ounces. Finally, a note of joy!

But within days, Faye's temperature soared with an infection. It reached epic heights. She became listless. Her obstetrician drove to our apartment and, finding her drowsy, carried her out to his car as I looked on. He drove her to the Vic where she was admitted. In the weeks that followed, Chris began to lose weight and was admitted to the Montreal Children's Hospital (MCH) for a battery of gruelling tests that led to the diagnosis of Coeliac's disease.

It had been a dizzying, numbing, deadening six months. It provided me with a glimpse behind the glazed eyes and expressionless faces of those I would encounter in years to come as they journeyed through their personal valleys of the shadow. But, with those mists lifting, life as a family emerged as a precious gift; we had Chris. Faye designed an announcement card, with a stylized illustration and the announcement, "Now we are three."

With the utmost patience and support of Dr Philip Hill and the Department of Medicine, I started to rejoin the clinical ranks as a Royal

Vic caregiver sometime in February and in my 13 April letter to Dad I noted:

> I am on the most amazing service at present!! The Metabolism Dept. runs what they call the Metabolic Day Centre for persons with endocrine problems. They are admitted for the day for work up & discharged that p.m. The white haired boy of the Royal Vic is Dr Martin Hoffman – very clever & nice to work with/for. He is responsible for this centre. I am running it this month. I work 8:30 a.m. ... to 4:30 p.m. five days a week, so it fits the type of reduced schedule I feel up to at present.
>
> I've been doing a good deal of sketching lately. We have driven into the country and around Montreal, drawing. I'm using conté. It gives the soft rust & brown tones often seen in figure studies. I have done several nudes and like the medium tremendously ... One of my recent works that I would like you to see is a large portrait of Christ ... just the head; done while he is on the cross. I did it Easter weekend and we have it in the hallway – rather bold style. I can't tell you how much pleasure I derive from drawing.

CROSSROAD

As my internal-medicine rotation was ending, I received a call one morning from Dr MacKinnon's secretary. He wished to see me and wondered if I could drop around that afternoon. "What about 2:30 P.M.? Would that be convenient?" Was this to be bad news? Had there been evidence of further disease on my follow-up x-rays? The intervening hours dragged by.

"Hello, Bal. Come in. Have a seat." K.J. closed the door and returned to his desk, pulled out a pipe and lit up. "How are things going? ... How is Faye? ... The baby?" I broke into a cold sweat. This didn't look good. What was on his mind? Clearly, he was having trouble getting it out. I started to fidget.

"How is Howlett's service working out?"

He finally got around to it. "Bal, I'm planning for the future of the Department. We need to build our subspecialty strengths. As you know, Doug and Yosh are bringing new expertise in their areas of interest and I'm examining our further needs. We need someone to specialize in urologic oncology and I would like to suggest you think about being that person. What I am suggesting is that you complete your internship, the two surgical-residency years, then our urology training program, and after that, the two-year Memorial Sloan Kettering Fellowship program with Dr Whitmore. You would then return to a position here at McGill. How does that sound?"

I was speechless. We talked. The next seven years of my life had just been mapped out. I immediately agreed.

Dr MacKinnon followed me to his office door, "Oh, and Bal, I think you'll agree that it would probably be wise not to mention all this to anyone other than Faye. You have a long road ahead. There's nothing to be gained by making it more complicated than it needs to be." The message was clear. His trust required a response of redoubled effort and focus. Just when I thought I was giving my best, I found I could ratchet it up another notch or so. However grim the months past, there were now suggestions that the years ahead held promise.

The extended family gathered at the *Place* that summer and found in community the mutual support, busyness, spontaneity, laughter, and tears that were the by-product of Chris, Margery, and David, our three new additions, the still-fresh grief over Betty's death, the numbing residue of our various medical crises, and the pragmatic demands of the toing and froing of island life. How much had changed since Faye and I last sat on the rocky point contemplating our future. Could that really be just one year ago?

It was a time of learning to let go through entering the immediacy of wind, water, sun, rain, and the scent of the pines and cedars. And in all of that we found the challenges and healing connections that enable new life. A time to swim, sail, and sit on the dock, with feet dangling in the water, mesmerized by the sunlight on the waves, a time to draw and read, a time to retell old tales and spin new ones, a time to relish Nettie and Peter's fresh wood-stove-baked bread.

SURGICAL RESIDENCY, 1964–66

The two years of general surgery included rotations on urology, the Vic's surgical Intensive Care Unit (ICU), and the general-surgery services of the Queen Mary Veterans' and Montreal Children's hospitals. The every other night and weekend on-call schedule with sleeping at the hospital, coupled with the hefty twelve-hour-plus schedule during days *off*-call, continued, but on the brighter side, there was less scut work. Furthermore, I was now in the OR every day. The routine was rich in challenges, rewards, and new additions to my compulsory reading list, a list that would be tended to *When?! This evening? Not likely! I'm on call tonight and will likely spend half the night in the* OR *with emergencies, then I'll be making rounds at*

7:00 A.M. *and in the* OR *until afternoon rounds, then, tomorrow night, I won't get home to see Chris and Faye until after 8:00 P.M. ... Reading? Great! When?!' But, I must admit, it is* so *stimulating and satisfying. Totally exhausting, but satisfying – maybe addicting.*

The total number of hospital-based hours spent on-call in a week could be brutal. There was the week Senior Resident John Duff and I covered the Department of Surgery while the other residents were out of town attending an international surgical meeting. As the week wore on, I started to keep track of our accumulated hours of sleep. From Sunday until the following Friday evening, John logged an average of 2.5 hours daily, while I got several hours more. I felt guilty about John being first call for emergencies, but in typical John fashion he argued that, if a decision for or against admission or surgery was necessary, his assessment would be required and he thus could see no merit in both of us being called.[13]

The junior resident was second assistant on the major cases but first assistant on uncomplicated appendectomies and hernia repairs, as well as, before long, straightforward gallbladder surgery. Supervision was consistent, constructive, and encouraging. We practised tying knots in off-hours and were active participants in going in, sucking, sponging, and closing. Motivation was high and progress rapid. We quickly became skilled in anticipating the surgeon's next need and in assuring a dry, clearly visualized operative field. As weeks became months, we developed confidence and sure hands. We began to feel comfortable with it all. But, as in everything else, pride goeth before a fall. Life seems to be designed to keep us humble.

A year earlier, I had been one of the interns in the Emergency Department the night a stabbing victim came in, a young fellow in his early twenties. He had an upper abdominal wound that was bleeding profusely. He smelled heavily of beer and was agitated and terrified, but, in spite of the apparent major, perhaps life-threatening, injury, his blood pressure and pulse were normal. He was stable. We cut away the blood-soaked clothes and notified the operating room that he was on his way up.

"Looks like you'll need to explore the upper abdomen to rule out organ injury and internal bleeding." But, as we cleaned him up and re-examined the wound, it became evident that the bleeding, though brisk, was coming from a tiny perforating branch of the left internal mammary artery.

"Give me that hemostat." The field was instantly dry! The wound was completely superficial. Amazing. Our major trauma case had suddenly become, well, trivial at best (or worst). The knife had struck the xiphoid process – the bony lower end of the breast bone – and had ricocheted off. A little irrigation, a couple of sutures, and that was that.

A year later, I was at the Queen Mary Veterans' Hospital and was about to do my first gallbladder under the watchful eye of the chief resident, the attending surgeon in the wings. My spirits were high.

The call to go to the executive director's office came as I was on my way to the surgeon's dressing room. *Should I send a message that I'll be there after the cholecystectomy?* I wondered. *Perhaps not. There was a come now!* tone to that message. I sprinted upstairs.

"Dr Mount, do you recall someone by the name of Jean-Pierre Legault?"

"No."

"Well, the police claim your name is on his hospital record and they're on their way here to pick you up sometime between 10:30 and 11:00 this morning to testify at the trial."

It was the stabbing case from the year before. "I'm afraid I can't possibly go. I have a gallbladder to do," I announced, in a tone that implied that such a schedule was a regular occurrence.

"Well, I suggest you go with them. If you don't, they'll just issue a subpoena and you'll have to go anyway. You won't have achieved anything, but you *will* have irritated the judge." I could see the gallbladder slipping away.

During the ride to the courthouse in the squad car – my first squad-car ride – I began to get into it. I had a blue corduroy jacket on over my white junior resident shirt and slacks. My stethoscope was crammed into the pocket.

The courthouse was hot, humid, and depressing. An endless succession of slouching floor-level figures with blank, grey faces lined the dimly lit corridors, lending a definite Dickensian atmosphere to the whole scene. A stale, dank odour hung in the air – my first courthouse. The policeman issued me into a packed courtroom – my first courtroom – and gestured to the bench where I should park myself.

The proceedings were in French and I struggled to follow the gist of the animated testimony. The courtroom was stifling, the long dead air heavy and motionless. I slid out of my jacket and sat it beside me. A few minutes passed. The judge was becoming irate. He was now almost screaming.

Good Lord! Is he screaming at me?!

Now everyone had turned to stare in my direction. I was confused. I shook my head in puzzlement.

"Put on your jacket, you!" roared the sergeant-at-arms, or at least the hulking fellow who looked like he might answer to that title, "or you will be in contempt of court."

I put on my jacket and started to perspire. Soon great rivers were running down my neck and back.

Finally, the case before the court ended and the dramatis personae silently shuffled out a side door while a sullen lad was issued into the prisoner's box as the next case was called to order. My patient was in the ragtag group that followed him into the courtroom.

After an embarrassing display of my linguistic limitations, the judge switched into English.

"Doctor, please tell the court about the injuries sustained by M. Legault?" There was a hush. Ah, this was more like it. Providing *official* medical testimony! I described the location of the wound, the bleeding, our concern about internal injuries.

"Doctor, would you say that this was a life-threatening injury?"

"Well, no, actually it was very fortunate. You see, on entry, the knife struck the xiphisternum and was deflected off, and ..."

There was a commotion. The woman furiously typing the transcription was speaking to the judge.

"Doctor, how do you spell that word?"

"What word?"

"Xiphi – something."

Now, under other circumstances it is possible that I could have spelled it. What had been "perspiration" became "sweat" in any man's vocabulary. "Z, I, P, H, no ... X, I, F, I , no ... Z, I, P, H, no ..."

"Thank you, Doctor."

Any credibility accorded me in the wake of the jacket incident had now permanently evaporated. I can't recall anything further about the trial. The squad car dropped me at the front door of the Veterans' Hospital and I trudged up to the recovery room to see my now post-op gallbladder.

MY FIRST HOCKEY GAME

The last quarter of that first year of surgical residency was spent on the urology service, an introduction to endoscopic procedures and my first opportunity to evaluate the relevance of my new-found surgical skills to my chosen specialty.

One of our patients that spring was from New Brunswick. Tom was a big, soft-spoken, unassuming fellow who, having soldiered through the trials of chronic renal failure, had undergone a kidney transplant during an earlier Royal Vic admission. Sadly, the initial success of the procedure was followed by rejection of his new kidney and Tom had now been admitted for its removal and management of his unstable condition. While a second transplant remained a distant possibility, each step of his journey was marked by further complications and his outlook was bleak. What could be done to bolster his sagging spirits?

Tom was a lifelong supporter of the Montreal Canadiens. He had followed the fortunes of his beloved Habs since early childhood but had never attended a National Hockey League (NHL) game. Dr MacKinnon phoned a friend, Canadiens' general manager Frank Selke, Jr, to explain the situation.[14] "By any chance, might it be possible to obtain two tickets so that Tom could realize his dream of seeing a Canadiens game?"

It was April and the playoffs for the Stanley Cup that year were between Montreal and the Chicago Black Hawks. "I'll tell you what, Ken, if there's a seventh game, it'll be in Montreal and I'll get you two tickets."

"The final game?! Of the *Stanley Cup*?! Why, that would be wonderful – simply wonderful!"

The Canadiens were coached by the legendary Toe Blake[15] and featured the likes of Jean Béliveau (captain), Henri Richard, Ralph Backstrom, Bobby Rousseau, John Ferguson, Dick Duff, Yvan Cournoyer, Claude Provost, Jacques Laperrière, J.-C. Tremblay, and Jean-Guy Talbot. The Black Hawks included such notables as Bobby Hull, Stan Mikita, Phil Esposito, Pierre Pilote, Chico Maki, Eric Nesterenko, and Kenny Wharram. The Habs had won the first two games in Montreal. The series then moved to Chicago where the home-ice advantage was again evident. Back in Montreal for game five, the Habs were victorious, but with game six in Chicago, the series was again tied at three games apiece. The stage was set for a seventh game, to be held at the near-sacred soul of the city, the Montreal Forum. Fingers had been crossed that this would happen. Tom was to have his dream come true.

He would need to be accompanied. Sue, the urology head nurse and arrangements coordinator for Tom's grand evening, asked if I would consider accompanying him. Thus it was, that on that balmy Saturday, 1 May, 1965 evening, Tom and I were off to the Stanley Cup final, the first NHL hockey game either of us had attended – *ever!*

We were, in fact, sitting in the Selke family seats – third row of "the reds," near the north end of the rink, the best seats in the house. As we emerged from the dimly lit passage under the stands into the shimmering brightness of the shrine itself, I experienced a hyper-brilliance of enhanced focus, colour, speed, and sound. Everything was enlarged! The atmosphere was electric, super-charged, and pulsating with anticipation that extended down from rafters to ice. The players were loosening up at each end of the rink. They were much closer, larger, and faster than I had expected. We were helped to our seats. Tom looked pale; he seemed weak and unsteady.

The puck was dropped. The game was underway, to the roar of the standing-room crowd. We were only a few feet from Tom's heroes as they shot past us, as if filmed in fast-forward, their level of concentration, focus, and determination magnified beyond my wildest imagining. Tom was seated at my left, the Selke family and their guests farther along. A large, boisterous woman in a fur coat was ensconced to my right. She was screaming, her train-announcer voice bellowing a torrent of encouragements or invectives at each player as he shot past. "Come on, Henri!"... "Go Yvan!" (It was Cournoyer's first season with Montreal) ... "Give it to em, Jean. Hit the bugger!" ... "*Hull*, you big blond bastard!! ... "*Esposito*, you son-of-a-bitch!!!" ... "*Mikita*, you bum!!"

They were so close and she was so loud that my immediate fear was that the players would leap over the boards and come at us. More than that. As Bobby Hull roared in on the Habs net, the puck a blur on his stick, my neighbour's elbow jabbed me in the ribs as she checked me hard into Tom. *I'll soon be black and blue if this keeps up.*

My further angst related to the suspicion that I probably had a *first game he's ever seen!* sign pasted on my back and forehead. I was reminded of watching a chess match once when I was surrounded by experts. Everyone around me picked up nuances of the game that I couldn't see – they groaned, they gasped, they nodded approvingly, in unison, and I had no idea what they were in spasms about.

As the first period ended, Tom whispered, "I need to go back to the hospital."

"What? *What* did you say?!" I couldn't believe it.

"I need to go back to the hospital?"

I felt a rush of concern – *two* concerns actually: concern for Tom, concern that I might kill him myself.

"Leave?! ... Now?!"

I looked at his pasty complexion and took his pulse. He really was not likely to tolerate another period. Now I *was* concerned, and it was for my patient!

Just as I was determining how we could make it to the nearest exit, Sue appeared. Unknown to me, she was seated several rows behind us.

"I've been watching him. I'll take him back to the ward," she offered. I protested.

"Don't be silly," she tut-tutted. "I've seen hundreds of games. Besides, I can be back here by the time the second period starts." With that, she led Tom away. Then, I noticed that my neighbour in the fur coat had also disappeared in the milling intermission throng.

Tom would be cared for. I sat basking in a too-good-to-be-true technicolour dream. Dazed. The last two periods of the seventh game of the Stanley Cup finals lay ahead!

At that point, the man in the seat behind me tapped me on the shoulder. "You don't know who you're sitting beside, do you?"

"No, I don't."

"That's Mrs Blake. You're sitting with Toe Blake's wife!"

The last two periods were adrenaline-soaked as the ecstatic crowd celebrated great hockey. The roar was unending! The Habs triumphed, 4–0.

As the final minute ticked down, everyone was standing. The roar was now deafening. With the final buzzer, there was a riotous explosion of joy as the Habs flooded over the boards to storm goalie Gump Worsley. Pandemonium!

Mrs Blake whirled around to engulf me in a massive bear hug. As we embraced, cheered, and slapped each other on the back, J-.C. Tremblay, down on the ice, swept Toe's fedora off his head and tossed it into the air.[16]

What had the evening meant to Tom? Had the joy of anticipation added quality to his pre-game days? Tom did not live to return to New Brunswick but we hoped that evening with the Habs had added a few transcendent moments, and that it had somehow eased his journey.

JUNIOR-RESIDENT CONSCIOUSNESS RAISERS

That spring our various individual efforts seemed trivial when measured against the dogged determination of the 1965 Selma-to-Montgomery, Alabama, civil-rights campaigners who, on 7 (Bloody Sunday), 9, and 16 March, under the non-violent leadership of the Reverend Martin Luther King, encountered brutish Governor George Wallace and his Alabama state-trooper thugs as the world watched state-endorsed terrorism against non-whites. These consciousness-raising confrontations resulted in the passage of the Voting Rights Act, which became law on 6 August. As fate would have it, that same day, in London, the Beatles released "Help" and in due course Faye presented me with the album as a study aid for my upcoming Royal College of Physicians and Surgeons fellowship exams. I was more than aware of the challenges facing both the civil-rights protesters and those taking "the Royal College Written Exams" and "the Orals." The Beatles' lyrics struck home.

"Help" became my theme song during the endless hours of studying that lay ahead. Cousin Bill's slogan *When the going gets tough, the tough get going* and the image of the against-all-odds civil-rights victory provided encouragement, as did my new tradition when needing a study break – recruiting Chris from crib or playtime to "do our tricks." Lying on my back on the floor, I would then throw him in the air and catch him on my extended feet. He would whirl around high above me, his eyes sparkling, with an eruption of giggles and balancing skill, until we collapsed in a tumble of laughter, tickles, and squeals of "Puff me, Daddy" before I got back to the books.

SURGICAL RESIDENT AND MOMENTS WITH THE CHIEF

My second year in surgery brought increasing responsibility and exposure to our attending surgeons, each with his own distinctive quality: the sound judgment, leadership, enthusiasm, and dry humour of the chief of surgery, Lloyd MacLean; the deft head-and-neck surgical skills of Eddie Tabah; the mutual old-crony dance of Mason (the "Silver Fox") Cooper and his Second World War colleague Harry Morton; the unflappable calm of chest surgeons Tony Dobell and Dag Munro; the bluster of Shorty Long.

Shaving early one morning, I glimpsed the slight suggestion of an unexpected shadow in the mirror. I palpated the area. There was a two-centimetre mass in my left neck just above the proximal end of the clavicle. I was astounded. I was certain that it hadn't been there the day before. Picking up the phone, I called the Vic and paged Eddie Tabah. We met in the ER. I was admitted for surgical exploration. The mass was within the thyroid gland, part of which had to be sacrificed to get good margins. The pathology showed it to be an inclusion cyst with no evidence of malignancy. Another roller-coaster ride.

On Christmas Eve that year, I was on call in the Emergency Department at the Children's Hospital. We had been busy earlier in the day but, as night fell, things were quiet. Well, not quite quiet. As the hours wore on, I needed to diagnose and sort out an acute abdomen. Not in one of our small patients, but my own. Intermittent pain had become constant as frustration deepened to concern. I did my own white-blood-cell count. It was modestly elevated. My temperature was normal, pulse a little fast, but that was to be expected. It was now nearing midnight. Nick, my more junior colleague, examined me, noting diffuse tenderness and some rebound tenderness on the left side. An acute abdomen for sure.

I lay down in one of the examining rooms to wait it out. By 2:30 A.M. it was definitely worse. What to do? The casual snowfall of the early evening had hardened into a driving snowstorm, mixed with sleet. The roads were slippery and I was uncertain of my ability to make it to the Vic in my trusty Volkswagen. It was now approaching 3:00 A.M., Nick couldn't drive me – *one of us* had to cover surgical call! At 3:30 A.M. I decided to phone the Royal Vic's chief of surgery, Lloyd MacLean.

Looking back, I can't imagine why I didn't simply phone the Royal Vic's telephone operator and have her connect me to his home. Perhaps it was my preoccupation with the pain, but it simply didn't enter my mind. Instead, I chose the Montreal telephone directory. I had not imagined the number of MacLean listings, but by focusing on those with the first initial "L." and assessing the probability of each address, I selected the most likely candidate and dialed. I was all too aware that it was now almost 4:00 A.M. on Christmas morning.

"Helloooh ..." crooned a soft, melodious male voice on the first ring. I was aghast! I had no idea who this was, but I was positive it *wasn't* the chief!

"I'm very sorry to bother you, but is this the MacLean residence?" I croaked, by this time doubled up with pain.

"Yes it iiisss ..." the voice crooned. This was *definitely* not the chief! No chance! I was desperate.

"Is this Dr MacLean?"

"Yes it iiisss ..." came the infinitely patient, soporific response. Whoever this was, it sure as hell *wasn't* L.D.!! Of that, I was certain! But, what else could I ask? "Look," I pleaded, "Is this L.D.?!" There was an explosion.

"YA!! Say, who IS this anyway?!" Now *that* was L.D.! I explained my plight.

L.D. walked through the Children's Hospital ER door at 4:30 A.M. Natty and freshly shaven in his tweed jacket, plaid vest and slacks, scarlet scarf, and fedora worn at a jaunty angle, he was nevertheless all business.

"BAL," he enthused, "What's going on?!" He always said my name like that – an up-beat, explosive, semi-shout, full of dynamic energy and cheer, with an emphasis on the "BA" and a twinkle in his eye! This time, it was toned down just a touch.

He examined me, then, "Bal old buddy, you have an acute abdomen, alright. But on a night like this I can't transfer you to the Vic, so I'll tell you what I'm going to do, I'm going to admit you right here."

"To the *Children's*?!!" I was dumfounded and somewhat puzzled. "I didn't know that you have admitting privileges here."

"I don't, but my wife does. I'll admit you under her name and by the time they figure it out we'll be out of here."

· I spent the night on the adolescent ward with intravenous fluids running. By morning, the storms – both on the streets and in the abdomen – had settled. I spent the next few days of watchful waiting at the Vic before being discharged for a delayed Christmas at home with Faye and Chris.

It was two or three months later when the problem recurred. This time I was admitted directly to the Vic under L.D. It was 8:30 next morning when I first saw him. He breezed into the room with John Duff, then a senior fellow, in tow. John was carrying a covered tray.

"BAL," L.D. erupted, "how was the night?" He was still entering the room and there was that distinctive glint in his eye as he continued without waiting for my reply, "Now old buddy, do you recall those Christmas concert skits when you impersonated me?! Well, for some reason they came to mind this morning as I was coming up here and I've asked John to bring along a colonoscopy tray."

Once again things settled without surgery; it was to be my last admission for that problem.

L.D. ran a tight ship. He had a clear vision of what an academic Department of Surgery should be. On being recruited as department head, he reviewed all existing research projects and closed those that did not meet his standards. The responsible colleagues were outraged. He ruled with a fair but firm hand.

I loved scrubbing with the chief. Each case could be relied on to entail one or two memorable moments. For example, there was the complicated day when I was paged on the wards and informed that I should immediately go to the OR to scrub in on an abdominal procedure that had been started by an attending surgeon who had been called away. L.D., I was informed, would join me as soon as he was free. It was about noon.

As it happened, he arrived first, so I was curious about the full story of that problem-fraught morning.

"Everything OK?" I blandly called from the adjacent scrub basins, holding the OR door open with my foot. He shot a glance at me over his mask, his eyes dancing. "It's been an *unbelievable* day!"

"Oh really?" I prompted, as I entered the room to gown-up.

"I got to the hospital about 7:00 A.M. and wanted to check things out in the lab before heading here for my eight o'clock case. Well, I got to the lab and opened the door and there was this couple making love – in *my lab! In MY LAB! MAKING LOVE!* – and at 7:00 A.M.! Can you believe it?!"

"Who was it?" I prodded mischievously as he continued. "And the day has gone downhill from there!" He did not mention the event that had led to his having demanded the departure of the initial surgeon on the procedure we had inherited, but in due course it became clear that

L.D. wasn't the only one having a bad day. The scrub nurse, a rather large, slow-moving person, had not worked with him before and so was not accustomed to his routines. The problems came to a head when he started the anastomosis that was to join the remaining stomach remnant to an adjacent loop of small bowel. L.D.'s usual practice was to lay in place perhaps twenty silk sutures along the proposed anastomosis line and then, when all were in place, to tie each of them, one after another in rapid succession. Next, his assistant would cut all twenty of them in equally rapid succession. With his regular scrub nurse at the helm, it was poetry in motion. Each suture was placed with a flick of his wrist and the instrument holding the next would be slapped into his extended hand while his eyes remained glued to the operative field. No need to divert his gaze. No need to request the next suture. It was teamwork at its grace-ful best. On this occasion, however, the nurse was flustered and poetry in motion had been reduced to one awkward stuttering mishap after another. The usual wrist flick / suture application / flick / application / flick had ground to a halt.

At first, L.D. did not comment but then he quietly remarked, "Give me a pack of 3–0 silk." Confused, our slow-moving scrub nurse retrieved a full package of silk sutures and the chief carefully set up his own modest, modified "high stand" adjacent to the operative field. He was back in business!

When ready for his next suture, he was happy to accept what the scrub nurse offered if it was ready. Otherwise, he would prepare and use his own. Remarkably, he was humming along at close to his usual speed.

Minutes later, however, our ill-fated nurse hopelessly tangled her total supply of sutures. They now lay in a spaghetti heap on the high stand, completely unusable! Seconds later, I caught my breath as I saw the nurse's hand surreptitiously approaching L.D.'s supply. His rejoinder was instant, "Hold on, baby, you can play in *your* sandbox, but you *can't* play in mine!" And *that* was the end of that!

That isn't to imply that L.D. was impervious to the needs of colleagues. There was the night I assisted him and chest surgeon Dag Munro as they carried out Canada's first lung transplant. History in the making! A privilege to be scrubbed in! Quite so, but, after countless sleepless hours, I fell asleep in mid-procedure while holding a retractor. It was 3:00 A.M.; L.D.'s quiet response was, "Bal, we're doing fine here. Why don't you grab a few winks in the dressing room. We'll call you if we need you."

He was sensitive to the concerns of his patients as well. During my stint working in the surgical ICU, I cared for Mr Panandopolous, a post-operative Greek gentleman with *very* little English whose recent chest and abdominal surgery had been extensive. It had been tough going, but, in spite of all he had been through, his original cramping abdominal pains had returned. To make things worse, he was surrounded by this strange, frightening, completely foreign, English-speaking, surgical ICU with its whirring machines, flashing lights, beeping alarms, and endless tubes issuing from every orifice, not to mention three other *very* sick roommates, all crammed into this compact, high-energy, pressure cooker. The poor man's eyes were wide with bewilderment and fear. As we made rounds together, L.D. questioned me about his status over the preceding twenty-four hours and then turned to the man with a sympathetic shrug.

"Look!" he reassured emphatically from the foot of the bed (L.D. was at heart an empathic man and his keen desire to be supportive was directly proportional to his decibel level). "Mr Panandopolous! Everything is going to be OK! You're going to be alright! You're doing fine, and anyway, if all this persists, we'll take you back to the operating room and I'll shorten your loop!" I'm not sure what Mr Panandopolous thought his loop was, or even if he knew he now had one, but his eyes widened even further, which I would not have thought possible.

L.D. never missed a shrewd clinical observation or the chance to celebrate the moment in his own inimitable style. On one occasion, in preparing for a particularly formal and high-profile inter-hospital Surgical Grand Rounds, he informed me that I was to present the history and physical findings, an account of the surgery undertaken, and the resultant recalcitrant hospital course relating to a patient I had cared for on the ward. She was a woman in her early forties with a complicated bowel obstruction and grim prognosis. For there to be *any* chance of even modest improvement in her condition, her management had required frequent manipulation of the nasogastric tube that ran from her nose to a network of bottles beside her bed. In response to the patient's eagerness to assist in any way she could, L.D. had offered a detailed description of how she could gradually withdraw the tube herself, inch by inch, on an hourly basis, over the following days. She had agreed and with uncomplaining determination she had participated according to his instructions. Progress had been gradual. Regrettably, it was at times two steps forward and one step back, and in the end the outcome was disappointing. Nevertheless, she took it all in stride. I was greatly impressed by her courage, grace, and stamina.

Thus, it seemed to me, that in addition to the admittedly interesting physiological, surgical-anatomical, and management-related conundrums we had encountered in her care, the transcendent human element needed airing at this prestigious academic gathering. I spared no details in presenting her case to the packed amphitheatre crowd of surgical staff and esteemed visitors. In my eyes, here was evidence of a laudable human spirit and unusual fortitude.

Looking back, these decades later, at the stillness that hung over the packed amphitheatre at the conclusion of my presentation, I should have guessed that it indicated dumbfounded shock rather more than appreciation of the existential subtleties I had found so moving. After all, case presentations at formal Surgical Grand Rounds were *always* crisp, dry, concise, to the point, and exclusively physiologically focused.

As my presentation finished, I sat down with a sense of satisfaction that I had more or less presented the critical elements of her triumphant story as I saw them. A moment of total silence followed. Then L.D. stood up and staggered to the microphone. "BAL! – thank you for that unforgettable saga." He grasped the sides of the podium as if fearing he might swoon. "Now, if we could perhaps take a few moments to collect ourselves, I'll ask our visiting professor to make a few comments."[17]

UROLOGY TRAINING, 1966–67

1 July 1966. With internship and two years of general surgery completed, Ken MacKinnon, heretofore my personal cancer surgeon and mentor in career planning, was now my daily clinical tutor. His unwavering assessing gaze, chiselled features, trim 5'11" stature, and distinctive erect posture conveyed his thoughtfulness and perennial interest in others. Focused yet relaxed, attentive and encouraging, he was a widely respected advocate for quality patient care and hospital-wide inter-professional bonding. His hair was black but greying at his prominent sideburns. A natty, yet muted, dresser, he was not averse to a highlighting dash of red or plaid. His trousers and lab coat (or kilt on special social occasions) were always compulsively pressed, his shoes shining.

Ken MacKinnon was a gentle, wise, caring man. "Dr MacKinnon" to the world, "Ken" to his wife, Ann, and his peers, he was "K.J." to us, his respectful trainees. His clan of nine children knew him as "Dad," and in due course he became "Pop" to his twenty-plus grandchildren. A by-product of fathering this goodly flock was his capacity to meet every situation, from trivial happenstance to world-shaking crisis, with measured tranquility. He bestowed a palpable calm on any room he entered and was memorably present at each encounter. He had time for everyone, whether the hospital chief executive officer or the newest member of the cleaning staff. He was a perpetual calming presence.

A man of staunch Catholic faith and Nova Scotian Celtic roots, K.J. brought a rich enquiring mind to his many interests. And there *were* many! Family, countless patients and their worried loved ones, fishing, the pursuit of academic excellence, urology as an evolving art and science, medical education, the well-being of his numerous students, more fishing, the challenges of hospital administration, cultivating roses, the plight of people engulfed in poverty or other forms of unrelenting need, the production of noble wines (the MacKinnon product was described as "well-rounded and sophisticated, offering an honest warmth when properly experienced"), the rare essences found in subtly blended pipe tobacco, single-malt Scotch: the deliberately shaped contours of a well-ordered life. His oldest grandson observed tellingly, "Pop and I would just sit in the reeds and cattails, our fishing lines lazily hanging in the water and he would tell me stories ... Inevitably, these talks came back to the familiar themes of service, medicine and God."

The Royal Vic's urology service involved twenty semi-private and sixteen private inpatient beds, a cystoscopy suite with general anesthesia for endoscopic surgery, the main Royal Vic operating rooms, an outpatient clinic, and a consultation service to the nine-hundred-plus patients located in the sprawling maze of Royal Vic pavilions. It was a bountiful learning environment. Each year, McGill took on three new urology trainees. The two colleagues entering the program with me were the ebullient, Iranian-born enthusiast Homa Khonsari and the more pensive Mohawk First Nations Canadian Sid Snow.

The first year of urologic training fostered progressive refinement in a host of nascent skills: more nuanced history taking and physical examinations; specialized abdominal, pelvic, and endoscopic surgery, as well as renal and ureteral plastic and vascular surgery; and assessment of the complex interwoven mix of issues arising in the sufferer's body, mind, and spirit that *always* defines one's experience of illness.

Time-tested axioms that became evident over that year included: apparently simple challenges merit the same careful assessment as life-threatening nightmares; potential disasters can morph into triumph, if foreseen; excessive busyness may result in irritability, avoidance, and defensiveness; chronic fatigue carries a deadening weight; arduous rewriting (with four colleagues) is involved in preparing one's first published paper ("Arteriovenous Fistulae for Haemodialysis: Advantages with Cadaver Renal Transplantation"[18]); and, for me, the rich reward that is gained when one confides to a frightened young patient, "I too have found myself on this path that you are on. I made it through just fine, and I am confident you will."

As 1967 dawned, we applied to adopt our daughter, Lauren Faye, and joined Canadians across the land in marking the centennial anniversary of Canadian Confederation. Since my 1967–68 second year of urology training was scheduled to be at Queen's working under my former professor Andy Bruce, Lauren, Chris, Faye, and I would be leaving Montreal in June.

Seasons of Our Discontent: Kingston, 1967–68

The moving finger writes; and, having writ, moves on: nor all thy piety nor wit
shall lure it back to cancel half a line, nor all thy tears wash out a word of it.
Omar Khayyam

KGH UROLOGY

Our return to Kingston in late June had a "coming home" feel to it, but now, with children in tow, a one-year time limit on our stay, and Royal College fellowship exams pending in the fall of 1968, there was an added sense of urgency. I was ever-aware of the clock ticking.

Our compact Collingwood Street bungalow with its small play area out back provided just the right space for the four of us. The tranquil neighbourhood offered playmates for Chris, private time for Faye and Lauren (usually referred to by her Daddy as Wrennie or Wren), and, for me, an opportunity for quiet study sessions that stretched well into most nights. Happily, the Kingston General Hospital urology practice was a fraction of that seen at the Vic, thus allowing fortuitous blocks of red-eyed cramming on a daily (and nightly) basis.

Andy Bruce had not changed. He was a capable clinician and a good teacher, and his perennial air of intensity fostered an impression of physical stature beyond his actual height. Lean, lanky, and brusque, with evaluating eyes that peered at the world from beneath bushy black brows, he had neat, close-cropped hair and a receding hairline that, coupled with a full-brush moustache, underscored a somewhat confrontational demeanour. Though he smiled easily, one sensed an edginess just beneath the surface. A man always on the move, he made his expectations abundantly clear and was not given to small talk or pleasantries. It was not difficult to imagine a royal lineage back to Robert the Bruce lurking within. Our relationship was cordial but never close.

The summer and fall of 1967 fell into a dependable rhythm shaped by my clinical work and studying – with an occasional smidgeon of family time on the side. We did not anticipate the tumultuous events that the New Year would bring. Perhaps we might have seen it coming, what with festering Quebec nationalism, the Vietnam War, the blossoming Hippy "Summer of Love" restlessness, the Arab-Israeli Six Day War, and the increasing violence of the American civil-rights struggle that had led to the introduction into the lexicon of the phrases "black power" and "burn, baby burn." But in the after-glow of Expo, our centennial celebrations, and the arrival of our daughter Lauren, the future generally looked sunny.

TRUDEAU

On 14 December 1967 Prime Minister Lester B. Pearson announced his retirement from politics. It was to be effective on the appointment of a new leader of his Liberal Party. As 1968 dawned, a number of strong candidates were considering the job.

Pierre Elliott Trudeau, Pearson's minister of justice and attorney general since 4 April 1967, had, over the intervening months, given priority to constitutional review and reforming the Canadian Criminal Code. Rather than favouring "special status" for Quebec, or a "confederation of ten states" formula, Trudeau supported a bill of rights within the constitution.

In the New Year, Pearson named Trudeau to the principal seat at the upcoming critical Federal-Provincial Constitutional Conference – an assignment that included a politically valuable pre-conference visit by Trudeau to each of the provincial capitals. The Federal-Provincial Conference provided a national forum through which many English Canadians encountered Pierre Trudeau for the first time.

Daniel ("Equality or Independence") Johnson of Quebec's Union Nationale party had anticipated having Prime Minister Pearson as his debating opponent as he argued on behalf of Quebec sovereignty at the conference. Instead, he found himself facing Trudeau, whose agile mind, biting rejoinders, and flawless logic mesmerized the national television audience, as did his apparently boundless confidence, poise, and sharp-eyed persona.

As I watched those spellbinding televised federal-provincial sessions, I found myself developing the condition journalists soon labelled "Trudeaumania." On 20 April 1968 Trudeau became leader of the Liberal Party and thus prime minister of Canada. He called an election for 25 June. In the campaign that followed, Pierre Elliott Trudeau, who was unmarried, kissed the ladies not the babies.

Who was this man? A Montreal-born gold-medalist law graduate from the Université de Montréal and holder of graduate degrees from Harvard and the London School of Economics, Trudeau had many sides, which included world traveller, journalist, political philosopher, pro-secularization devout Catholic, modernist, and social democrat. He was known for the rose in his lapel, his Mercedes sports car, and his celebrity dating (actors Barbra Streisand, Margot Kidder ...). He was a long-time friend of Fidel Castro and invited John Lennon and Yoko Ono to visit him on Parliament Hill as part of their world peace crusade.

Trudeau didn't take himself too seriously but wasn't above responding to opponents with a pointed "fuddle duddle!" Volatile and enigmatic, he was capable of both elegant formality and sliding down the bannisters at both Buckingham Palace and Marlborough House, as well as executing an impish pirouette behind the back of Queen Elizabeth II. He was a superb skier, excellent swimmer and diver (his highly conditioned body clothed in a minimalist bathing suit), judo aficionado, expert canoeist, and experienced outdoorsman.

But Trudeau stood for more than charisma. He would help to shape Canada through his vision of a unified, bilingual, multicultural, just society. Here was a forty-seven-year-old constitutional maven who said, "There's no place for the state in the bedrooms of the nation." He planned to decriminalize homosexual acts between consenting adults, allow for easier divorces, and permit abortion if the woman's heath was in danger.

Suddenly it appeared that, thanks to this internationally celebrated liberal-thinking intellectual, Canada was no longer a stodgy, vaguely retrogressive, backwater. We were on the cutting edge of progressive and democratic thought.[1] One Sunday afternoon that spring, Trudeau made a brief campaign stop at the Kingston airport. I was among the hundred or so who turned out to greet him.

LA FÊTE NATIONALE DU QUÉBEC

As the Liberal incumbent for Mount Royal, Quebec, Pierre Trudeau was in Montreal on 24 June 1968. It was Saint-Jean-Baptiste Day, the annual "Fête Nationale du Québec" celebrating the patron saint of French Canada. The Canadian federal election was booked for the following day, 25 June.

During the Quiet Revolution of the 1960s,[2] Saint-Jean-Baptiste Day had become a rallying point for an increasingly strident expression of

Quebec nationalism and, in due course, a nationalistic crossroad for the emerging separatist movement. The venerated statues of the saint that were prominent in the parades of an earlier era had largely given way to a sca of blue and white Quebec flags, raised on high in an acknowledgment of the "maîtres chez nous" (masters in our own house) philosophy of the day.[3]

Prior to the 1968 Saint-Jean-Baptiste parade, Pierre Bourgault, leader of the Rassemblement pour l'Indépendance Nationale (RIN), explained that since Trudeau refused to recognize Quebec as a French nation, he had no right to attend the celebration, noting, "His celebration is on July 1st; ours is on June 24th … He is not welcome and we will protest."

That Saint-Jean-Baptiste evening, thousands of demonstrators shouting anti-Trudeau slogans and waving placards reading "Trudeau the Traitor!" assembled in Parc La Fontaine across Sherbrooke Street from the municipal library where the official parade review stand had been erected. Protestors were confronted by police on horseback and motorcycles pushing into the crowd in an attempt to control an event that was rapidly becoming a riot. As a would-be Quebecer and a hard-core Trudeau supporter observing these events from Kingston, I was both stunned and mesmerized by the unfolding television images. So was the nation.

Prime Minister Trudeau took his place with Mayor Jean Drapeau and the other invited guests on the elevated blue-and-white-draped stand. When the crowd saw Trudeau, they were enraged. Surging out of the shadows of the park, they broke through the police cordon and charged the review stand, screaming and throwing a shower of stones, bottles, and eggs at the assembled dignitaries.

The passing celebratory parade halted in confusion. Brawls between demonstrators and police erupted and became violent, both in the park and on Sherbrooke Street. The Canadian Broadcasting Corporation (CBC) cameras began to swing back and forth from viewing stand to park, revealing fires set by the rioters, aggressive clubbing of protestors by the police, people trampled by the horses, and cars being set on fire. Chaos reigned.

Security officers, both in the review stand and on the street in front, were now urging the dignitaries to withdraw to the safety of the municipal library behind them. Those sitting around Trudeau were struck with a shower of projectiles as the level of hostility escalated. The swarming protestors were getting closer and some were breaking through to reach the reviewing platform. Mayhem was escalating as Canadians from coast to coast to coast watched with horror.

In Kingston, I couldn't believe what we were seeing. Could this really be happening? In Canada?! In Montreal?!

The dignitaries in the bunting-draped stands were now standing, uncertain what to do. They hurriedly collected their belongings and began to stream into the safety of the building behind them. Their confused, uncertain, tentative movements provided a striking contrast to the darkly threatening advancing mob battling to get at them.

Trudeau was being urged to leave the reviewing stand by the alarmed security guards. With evident anger and disdain, he forcefully shook off their hands, shoved them back, and returned to his front-row seat. He was defiant! Resolute! He leaned forward over the guardrail, arms folded, staring defiantly at the screaming throng just feet below, rejecting all attempts to move him. Across the country, any lingering doubt about the calibre of the man evaporated. The next day his party won 154 seats, including 56 of the 74 seats in Quebec.[4]

TINDERBOXES WE HAVE KNOWN

During these months many other cauldrons of discontent and violence were simmering across the global landscape. It was early January 1968 and we had just cleared away the holiday decorations when the first murmurings of further escalation in the conflict in Vietnam came our way. Opposition to the Vietnam War in the United States had grown over the preceding year. Indeed, by 1967, most Americans felt U.S. involvement had been a mistake.

On 31 March 1968 President Lyndon Johnson announced the cessation of bombing of Vietnam, called for peace negotiations, and stated that he would not seek re-election. Two weeks earlier, on 16 March, Robert Kennedy declared his decision to run for president, stating that the United States was, in his opinion, "on a perilous course."

I found RFK's candidacy galvanizing – the old Kennedy magic had injected an instant source of optimism into American politics – but that optimism was now mixed with a gnawing, five-year-old undercurrent of Dallas-generated apprehension. "Bobby," for that is how I thought of him, ran with characteristic upbeat Kennedy determination on a platform of non-aggression in foreign policy coupled with racial and economic justice. My pulse quickened with both the thought of another Kennedy in the White House and the rapidly diminishing number of days prior to my upcoming Royal College fellowship exams.

My gruelling sprint through the complexity of the medical material to be covered in preparation for the exams was capped each night by burning the midnight oil into the early pre-dawn hours. The pressure was unending; the mountains to be scaled were forbidding. Against that perspective, Bobby's brash determination to run *his* uphill course against an incumbent president struck a chord. I penned a sign for the wall over my desk and there it stayed through the arduous months that lay ahead. It read: "I Am Now in the Race and I Am Running to Win. Robert Kennedy, March 1968."

On Thursday, 4 April, we had an early supper, and then I descended to the isolation of my basement desk and the mountain of data to be digested before bed. When it was time for the late-night CBC news, I felt ready for a break. I had just reached the living-room door as the announcement came that Martin Luther King had been assassinated in Memphis, Tennessee. The announcer looked drained, stunned. Looking up from the prepared text in front of him, he noted that, in Dr King's last speech, delivered just the day before, he had spoken about his own death. His words had been: "Like anybody I would like to live a long life, longevity has its place. But I'm not concerned about that now. I just want to do God's will. And he's allowed me to go up to the mountain. And I've looked over. And I've seen the Promised Land. I may not get there with you. But I want you to know tonight, that we, as a people, will get to the Promised Land. So I'm happy tonight. I'm not worried about anything. I'm not fearing any man. Mine eyes have seen the glory of the coming of the Lord." Later, in speaking about those prophetic words, Coretta King, Dr King's widow, remarked, "The mantle of prophesy descended on Martin's shoulders."

The death of the thirty-nine-year-old Nobel Peace Prize laureate, clergyman, and leader of the American civil-rights movement was devastating. The waves of disbelief, anger, grief, and numbness seemed all-encompassing. Two aspects of the sickening news struck me as I attempted to understand the enormity of the loss for all who value sanity, human rights, and the remarkable gift of Dr King's courageous and enlightened leadership – the remarkable accuracy of his prophetic vision of death, and the obligation facing those of us who continue to be challenged by the opportunities he had been denied. Once again, the familiar childhood prod came to mind – "of him to whom much is given, much will be required." For me, it wasn't about an ethereal trumpet call, nor was it a recurrence of my "why couldn't it have been me rather than him" reaction generated by the death of JFK. Instead, it was a rekindling of my awareness of being the consistent recipient of unearned privilege. If Bobby had added a note of determination, hope, and encouragement as I slogged away at the books, Dr King's loss reawakened an old sense of indebtedness and obligation.

Rather than an altruistic awakening, it was a cold-bath reminder of the ease of my path when compared to that of others.

On Wednesday, 5 June, at the Ambassador Hotel in Los Angeles, Bobby was assassinated. Once again, I felt engulfed by a sense of bewilderment, anger, frustration, disgust, and meaninglessness. I felt a reactionary sweep of fury at our American brothers and their bizarre love affair with guns – JFK, Martin Luther King, and now Bobby! A country that held the Second Amendment to its constitution, a creed written for another time and circumstance, to be more precious than the continuing army of lives it appeared ready to snuff out needlessly; a country that smugly proclaims that it is "the greatest country in the world." That Saturday the world gathered at St Patrick's Cathedral in New York City as Ted Kennedy delivered the eulogy for his brother.

When the Democratic National Convention convened in Chicago during the last week of August, all the elements for conflict were in place. Day after day during the four days of the convention, the world watched with a sense of collective disillusionment and sadness the unequivocal evidence of a broken democratic system.[5]

It was sometime in those grim weeks that I found myself in the Kingston General Hospital surgeons' lounge between cases, dressed in OR greens. My heavy plastic cystoscopy apron reached from chest to knees. One other surgeon was in the room. I did not know him well and we had not spoken. Then, as Andy Bruce walked through the door, our colleague asked me how the studying for the fellowship exams was going. In response, I mumbled something vaguely non-committal, but it was Professor Bruce who took the opportunity to wax eloquent on the subject. "Oh they're not anything to speak of, you know. Very straightforward really, these Canadian exams. They're nothing like the Royal College of Edinburgh exams that *we* had to write. Now *they* were a different matter! THEY were exams worthy of the name!"

Without speaking, I took off the apron, wound it into a ball, and threw it at him with all my strength. He was not more than ten feet from me. It caught him in the chest. By the time they realized what had happened, I had left the room and phoned Ken MacKinnon in Montreal to say I was not prepared to work another day with Andy Bruce. Ken asked me to wait until they had discussed the matter.

Later, Professor Bruce and I exchanged half-hearted apologies and I stayed for the remaining weeks prior to leaving for New York at the end of June.

The experience with Willet Whitmore at Memorial Sloan Kettering awaited. So did the Royal College fellowship exams.

Memorial Sloan Kettering and the Jackson Labs, 1968–70

It helps a man immensely to be a bit of a hero-worshipper,
and the stories of the lives of the masters of medicine do much
to stimulate our ambition and rouse our sympathies.
Sir William Osler, Aequanimitas

New York, like a scene from all those movies
But you're real enough to me, but there's a heart
A heart that lives in New York.
Simon and Garfunkel
"A Heart in New York"

Winston House, 430 East 67th Street, was our destination. We found it with surprisingly little trouble. "It's at 67th and York; can't miss it!" turned out to be just about right. "Just across the street from the hospital" was also true, "the hospital" being Memorial Sloan Kettering Cancer Center.

Winston House was a twelve-storey subsidized apartment building for MSKCC residents, fellows, and others.[1] "Mount, yes, we have you in 2K – end of the hall, second floor, turn right as you leave the elevator."

By early evening, we had disposed of the rented van, unpacked most of our belongings, settled Chris and Wren in the bedroom nearest the living room, and set up our bedroom (which was to double as my office) across from the bathroom at the end of the short hall. It had been a warm day and the air-conditioning unit in our bedroom was humming away. With the door closed, it offered a sort of white noise that screened out all other sound. I found it encouraging. In fact, it was perfect. Cocooned in that relative isolation, I could hit the books with no trouble at all.

Bricks-and boards bookcases were our specialty. We had brought along the boards from Kingston. "Now, if I can rustle up some bricks we could get the bookcase together and put away the books, records, and odds-and-ends tonight; we'd be completely settled! I'll pop over to the hospital and look around in the basement. I've never seen a hospital that didn't have some old bricks lying around somewhere." I was on a roll. It had all fallen into place more quickly than we had anticipated. We were established in our new home and ready for battle with a day or two to spare prior to fronting up for Dr Whitmore on Monday morning.

I entered Memorial by the East 67th side door, facing Winston house. All was quiet, deserted in fact. Sure enough, down the darkened basement corridor to my left I found some bricks stacked against the wall. I even managed to find an old wheelchair to use in transporting them. I was beginning to feel like a genius.

Getting to the door with my loaded wheelchair, I was heading out into the warm 1 July New York night air when something hard pressed into the centre of my back.

"Keep your hands on the chair, and stay just where you are. Don't move. Fine. Now, tell me what you think you're doing."

"New urology fellow" ... "Canada" ... "Dr Whitmore" ... "bricks-and-boards book case" ... "wife and children in Winston House" ... "No, *really!*"

We decided I should leave the bricks and wheelchair where I had found them and put further plans for imports to Winston House on hold until morning. And, yes, nearly as I can recall, he really *was* armed! Polite, but armed, and very sure of himself. It really was a revolver pressed into my back.

I retreated to 2K. "Toto, I've a feeling we're not in Kansas anymore!"

"Shhhh, I think the kids have just drifted off ... What was that about Kansas? ... Did you find any bricks?"

"Well, sort of."

Welcome to New York! As cousin Lou (that's Central Park West pioneer of group-psychotherapy Dr Louis Ormont) liked to say about New York City, "There's a lot of energy here!" Indeed, two years later we had reached the point where, if we didn't leave soon, we would never leave. New York had become home. Who knew that might happen?!

A night or two after the bricks-and-boards caper, I went to the corner store to pick up some milk. It was after midnight, perhaps 1:00 A.M. On reaching the corner (67th at First Avenue), I was amazed to see several hundred people silently making their way along First – a crowd. A *big* crowd! I was sure there must be an emergency – a crisis of some sort. A fire? An accident? All these people! Then it dawned on me. There is no crisis. There just happens to be several hundred people walking down the street at 1:00 A.M. Welcome to New York!

On entering the small store, I felt an unexpected sense of delight – I belonged! A New Yorker. Presenting my carton of milk at the counter, I smiled broadly at the grizzled apparition at the cash register. "Hi!" I offered. He stiffened, eyes narrowing, and he said nothing. I gave him a five; he slapped down the change – no words, no answering smile. As I left, I entered the passing crowd. *No, not Kansas anymore, but there sure is energy here!* Shortly thereafter, the twelve-year-old son of a Winston House colleague was robbed at knifepoint – the take was twenty-five cents. When the police were informed by his alarmed parents, the officer asked, "Well, where was the kid, exactly?"

"67th, between First and Second."

"Oh! ..." exhaled the cop with a shrug of understanding, "You *never* walk on that block!"

Back at the books, I taped the aging study schedule over my desk and beside it the small sign that had kept the motor running in recent months: "I Am Now in the Race and I Am Running to Win. Robert Kennedy, March 1968."

· Andy Bruce's dismissive words notwithstanding, the Canadian fellowship exams had a high failure rate, and I knew it. Notification from the Royal College of the fall- examination schedule provided a sharp focus to each ensuing hour.

The written examinations were slated for 16 September (surgery), 17 September (clinically applied pathology and bacteriology), and 18 September (clinically applied basic sciences, including anatomy, physiology, biochemistry, "and other appropriate basic sciences"). They were to be written at the Royal College of Physicians and Surgeons of Canada headquarters at 74 Stanley Street, Ottawa.

Candidates who were successful in the written examinations were to register for the oral and clinical examinations, which would take place at the Toronto Western Hospital on 21 November at 8:00 A.M. (clinical examination) and 2:00 P.M. (basic science). There was a final ominous note: "You are to report at 6:45 P.M. in the Auditorium, main floor, Toronto Western Hospital, to receive the results of your examination from the Chairman of the Examining Board."

Several factors offered a glimmer of hope for the crunch weeks that lay ahead. First, following a weekend visit to the *Place* on Grand Lake, Faye and the kids stayed on for an extended vacation while I returned to the quiet of Winston House. Second, Dr Whitmore was in my corner.

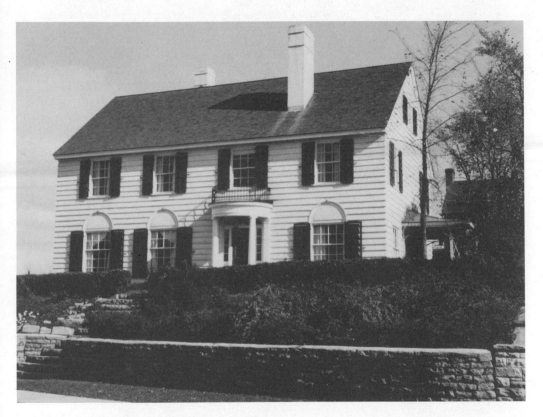

37 Opeongo Road: where it all began.

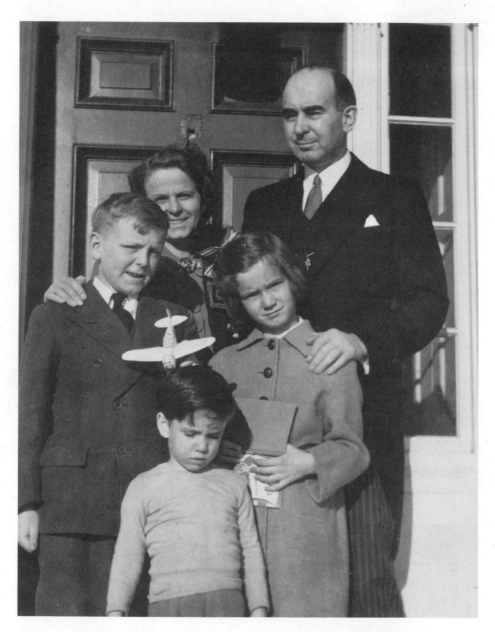

Wartime years: Dr and Mrs H.T.R. Mount with Jimmy, Bal, and Alice.

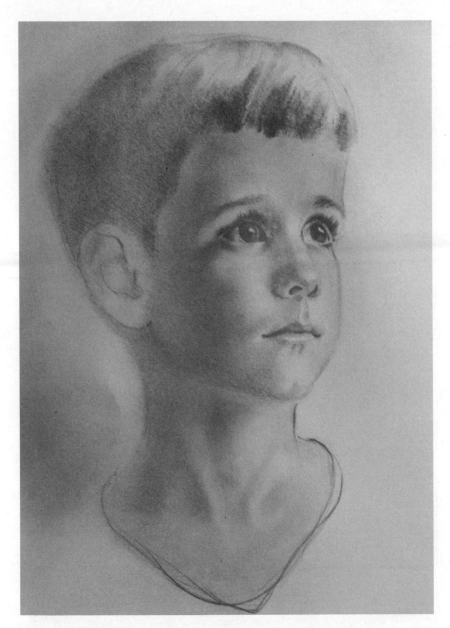

My 1945 introduction to the artist's craft through Winston Elliott.

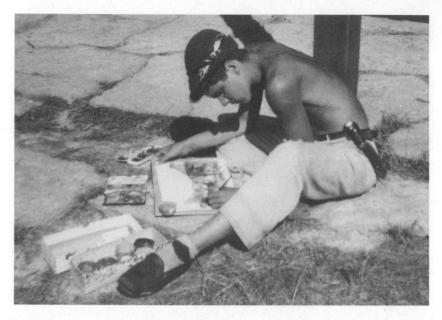

Watercolours: limitless discoveries at the end of a brush.

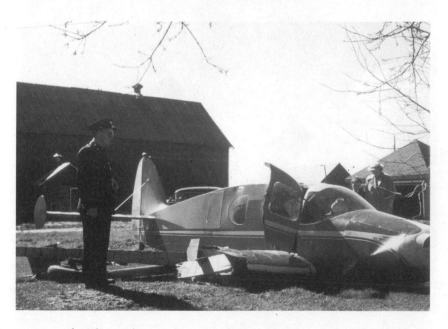

CF-EQL after the crash.

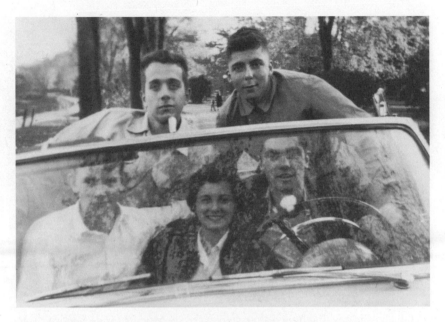

Denny at the wheel, with Phyd and (L to R) Pritch, Dave, and Bob.

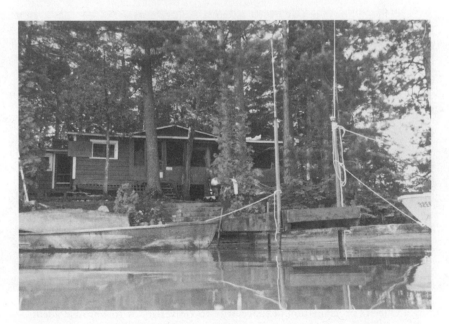

The *Place*, our Grand Lake Island paradise.

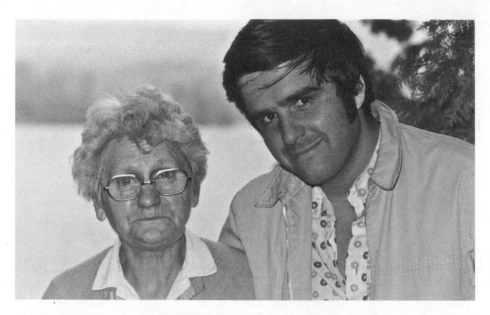

Nettie joined us post-war and thereafter there were six Mounts for decades to come.

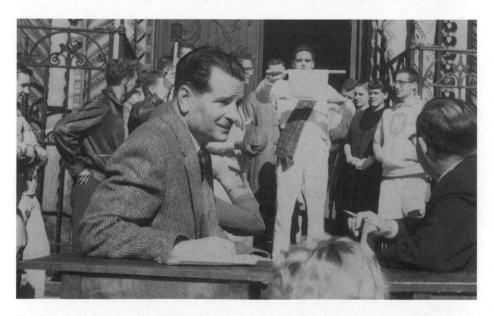

Reading a Queen's proclamation of superiority to University of Toronto President Claude T. Bissell.

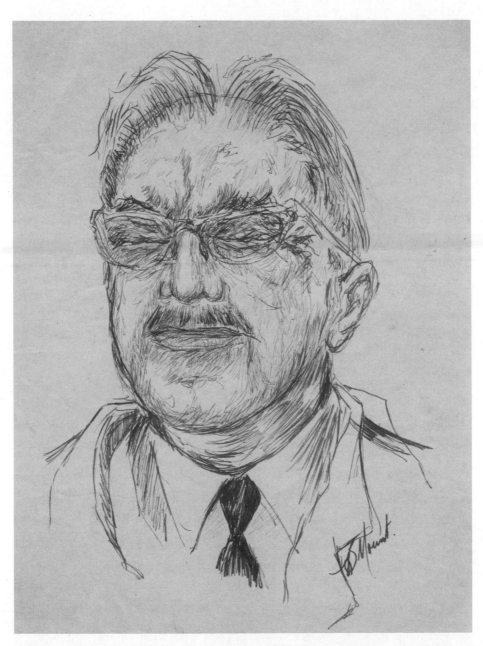

Ford Connell: from my Medical Grand Rounds lecture notes that week.

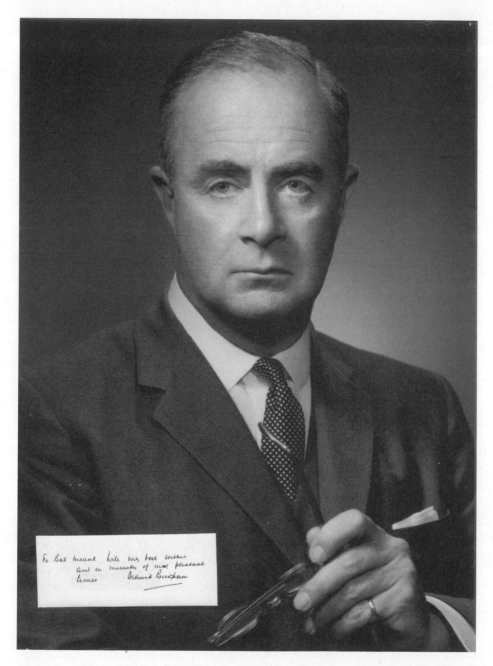

D.L.C. Bingham: professor of surgery, Queen's University. (Photographer unknown.)

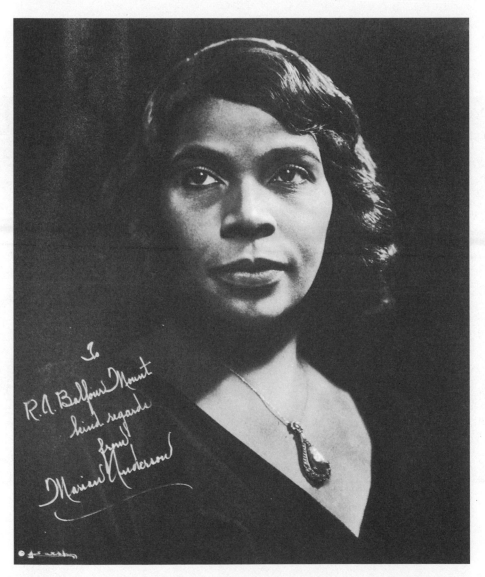

Marian Anderson: the transcendent realized. This is my personal copy of the photograph of Marian Anderson by Ottawa's Yousuf Karsh. I purchased the photograph from Karsh, who, at the same time, signed my copy of his landmark book *Portraits of Greatness*, "To Balfour Mount, with the hope that through his chosen profession he may serve humanity and thus find joy and satisfaction, Yousuf Karsh 1960." This treasured volume lies at hand these sixty years later.

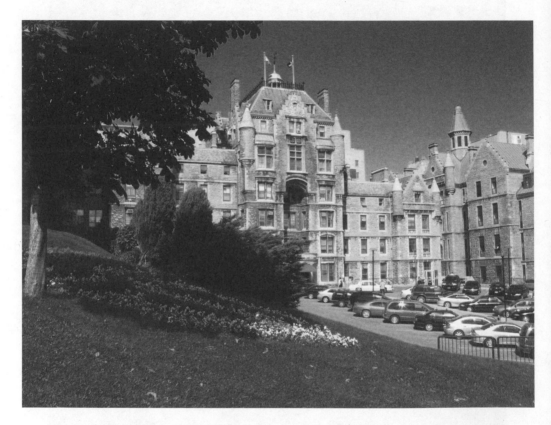

Montreal's Royal Victoria Hospital: my permanent professional home.

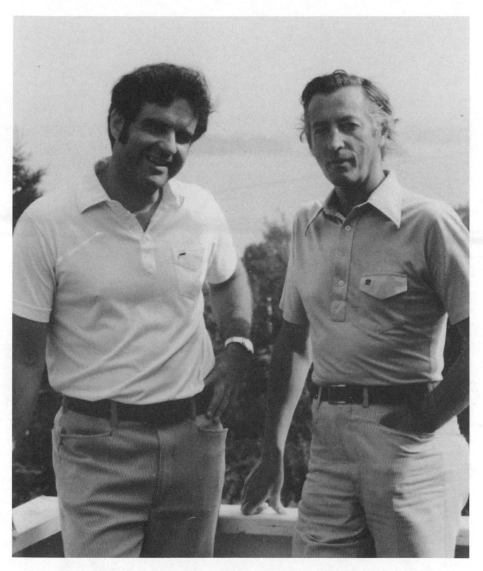

With K.J. (Ken) MacKinnon: surgeon, mentor, designer of my life path, and friend.

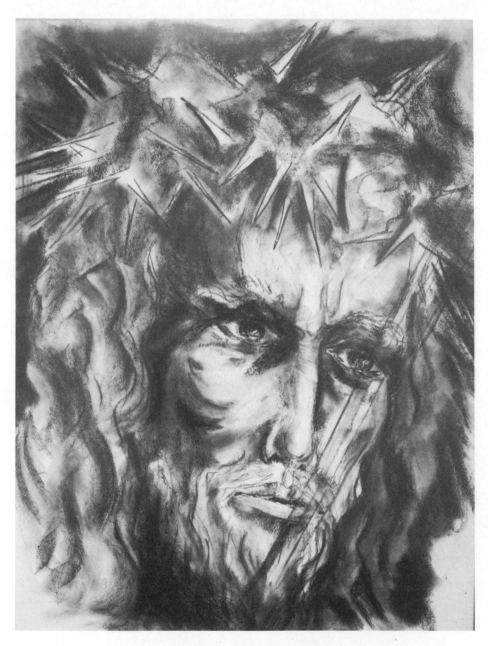

Easter 1964: a personal confrontation with life's assumptions.

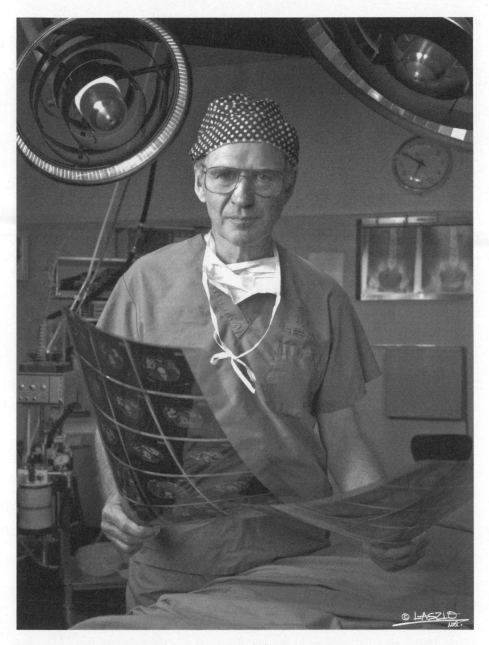

Lloyd MacLean ("L.D."): the Royal Vic's chief of surgery and dynamic presence.
(Courtesy of Lascio, Mtl.)

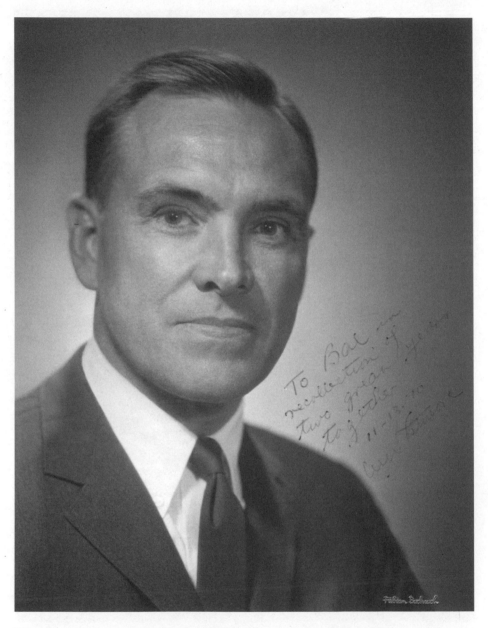

Whit: Renaissance man in all he undertook. (Courtesy of Fabian Bachrach, New York City.)

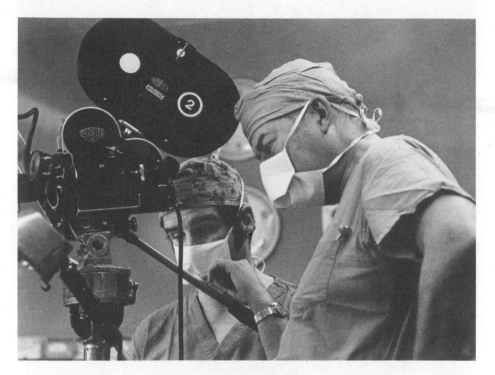

Creating teaching films at Memorial Sloan Kettering.

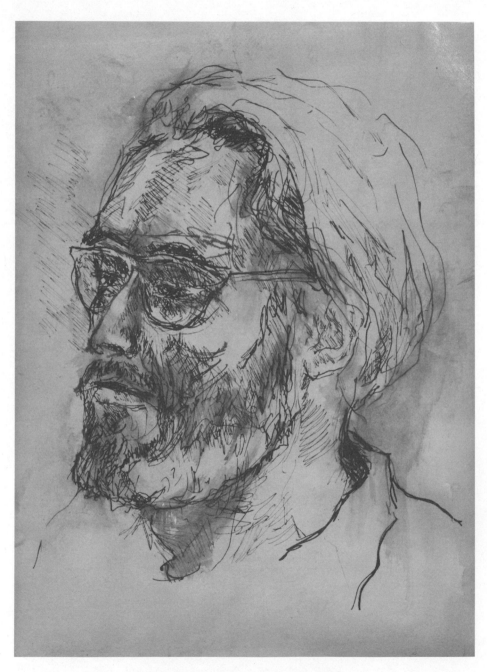

John Francis Williams: gifted pilgrim on the road less travelled.

In response to my letter a year earlier, he had written: "I can understand your anxiety about writing your Canadian Fellowship exams next September and wish to assure you that your schedule could be so arranged that you could start your program on July 1, 1968 as planned and count on a light schedule to permit you ample time for study." Third, I soaked up the regular weekly rounds with Drs Whitmore and Harry Grabstald at Memorial as well as those chaired by the illustrious Victor Marshall, chief of urology at the New York Hospital–Cornell Medical Center across the street. And fourth, Urologist Mike Laplante, who had completed the McGill urology training program and fellowship exams a year earlier, was in New York on scholarship and needed a place to stay during the coming weeks. Excellent! With Faye and the kids at the island, he would move into 2K with me and do the cooking. Each day thereafter, as I studied, I prepared a "Mike Sheet" that listed urology topics that required our in-depth discussion over dinner that evening. A man of unflappable equanimity and encyclopedic knowledge, Mike was a godsend! I taped a new sign to the wall over my desk: "W. Whitmore Jr. / K.J. MacKinnon / V. Marshall / L.D. Maclean / A. Bruce: 5 of 6 good reasons why."

A letter posted 23 August arrived from Dad. He was seventy-two.

Tuesday, 5:45 p.m

Dear Son,
It is difficult to book patients so that one is kept busy and yet not overloaded. Now, at this hour, I am free from patients but with more to come & so I shall get busy with a reply to your letter ... I am working away, frankly about as hard as ever. Tomorrow I plan to do two or three epidurals for lumbago ... [News of Faye, Chris, Lauren, and the extended family at the Island followed, and warm wishes for my studying filled the following six pages that preceded his closing words.] I look forward to the opportunity of talking with you about life; the now & the hereafter; mankind's life on this earth which in fact has been but a moment in the existence of this earth. Truly, how can we grasp the meaning of it all – the place of the All Powerful Father of Life, – What is man that Thou art mindful of him & the sons of men that Thou visited them? What about the old hymn? "We shall know as we are known never more to walk alone?" Shall we know each other, or is this life – the soul of man, the living thing that is in all life & living things – just in this life? Let us put off further discussion until later. In the meantime good wishes to you son ... Dad

The "Writtens" came and went, leaving an inevitable cloud of uncertainty. Two Western Union telegrams were delivered to Winston House at noon on 28 October. I read the first words of the one left at my door – "I regret ..." – and then noticed that the telegram was addressed to a colleague who had written the exams with me. He had failed. Running up the stairs to his door, I intercepted my telegram. I had made it through. The "Orals." I checked into the Toronto hotel; the night was fitful. At 7:30 A.M. next morning, Thursday, 21 November, I joined the silent cluster of fellow victims at the Toronto Western Hospital. They were pale (some bordered on pasty green), mute, wan, clearly unwell, perhaps critically ill! The appearance of these, my fellow lambs to the slaughter, had a curious effect on me. Their distress ameliorated mine, leaving me with the thought that, however grim I might feel, I was in better shape than they appeared to be. I concluded that I could do it! The unexpected wave of confidence was still lingering when my name was called and I left that cell of discontent to confront the panel of examiners.

At 6:45 P.M. in the hospital auditorium, the envelopes were handed out. Rather than euphoria, success felt more like relief-tinged disbelief. In the weeks to come, the disbelief evolved into an increasing sense of letdown and meaninglessness, in spite of now being immersed in a busy, rich-to-overflowing clinical life with Drs Whitmore and Grabstald. The surgical volume exceeded anything I had ever seen or imagined, but an undercurrent of emptiness remained. Was my overwhelming fatigue physical? Psychological? Social? Spiritual? A need for renewed connection to Self,[2] family, and other core sources of meaning? As the weeks passed, family and the clinical feast surrounding me slowly seeped into the newly liberated spaces.

WHIT

Willet F. Whitmore, Jr moved through life fully engaged and with evident grace. The Bard would have said he was "quick mettle." His warmth, enthusiasm, and insight called those around him into dialogue and unimagined personal capabilities. His ever-buoyant positive attitude, as I said earlier, was infectious. To be with him was to come away with broadened horizons and new certainty that undreamed-of potential was at hand. The historian Cornelius Ryan, a patient of Whit's, described him as the "Cary Grant of medicine" – not, I suspect, based on his comely appearance and perennial smile, but because he *was* the highly evolved man that the actor so admirably portrayed in countless films.

He was Leonardo, a polymath of rare stature, a superbly skilled surgeon to be sure, but he was so much more than that. Hours spent in the
OR with him were a special privilege. He was a surgical artist. Tissue
plains appeared to open spontaneously; his every move seemed effortless
as the most complex distortions of anatomy surrendered to his attentive
eye. His operative reports were instructive. Unlike the usual word sal-
ads that clog patient charts, the records Whit left us are memorable as
lessons in surgical anatomy, process, and the fine art of writing tightly
phrased eloquent prose.

A man of unusual intellectual ability, Whit was a discerning analytical
thinker. Fred W. Stewart, the noted pathologist who had initiated Whit's
recruitment to Memorial as chief of urology at the age of thirty-three,
put it simply, "I thought he had a lot more intelligence than did most of
the Hospital's staff."[3]

Willet Whitmore embodied the ideal of surgeon as scientist, philosopher,
and humanist in the constant search for "why" and "how," a search that
fuelled both his careful critique of published research data and his deep
concern for his patients. For example, he defined the crux of the prostatic
cancer-management problem in a single elegant sentence: "Is a cure possible in those for whom it is necessary, and is it necessary for those in whom
it is possible?" In this, he led the charge in recognizing that radical surgery for prostate cancer is often recommended when not indicated, given
the idiosyncrasies of the epidemiology of the disease. While his criticism
could be blunt, his reasoning was always flawless and his rhetoric never
stooped to personal attack. This, coupled with his disarming charisma,
enabled him to speak with rare candour in criticizing the field he was so
instrumental in creating. Indeed, he was widely considered to be one of
the outstanding urologic surgeons of his time and the undisputed father of
urologic oncology. His "Whitmoreisms" became the beacons that illuminated and shaped critical thought in the field.

"When the results are good, we tend to say, 'That's a good treatment.' When treatment fails, we shake our head and say, 'That's a
bad cancer.'"
"Let's try to replace heated opinion with cold facts."
"The current state of prostate cancer may not be good medicine
but it sure is good business. There are more people making a living
from prostate cancer than are dying from it."

Whit treated colleagues at all levels of the team as equals. In like manner, he was ahead of his time in his attention to patient quality of life

when weighing treatment options and in placing a high priority on frank yet supportive reality-based dialogue with patients and their families.

He was also an attentive naturalist and his interests, from entomology and herpetology to astronomy, led him to assemble monuments as varied as the observatory on the roof of his country house and the museum of carefully labelled specimens that lined the shelves in the basement and garage of his home in town.

An admiring scribe noted, "An intensity of spirit, health, charm [and] vitality radiated from the man ... There was a quiet authority about him as though he needed no trappings to set off his distinction." In a similar vein, distinguished former students Jim Montie and Joseph Smith observed: "Certain individuals are held in sufficient esteem by their trainees that even a subtle indication of disfavour is sufficient to make a strong point. When faced with what he considered a substandard effort, Dr Whitmore's sole comment might have been, 'mediocre.' From someone who perceived anything less than full effort a failure, this was a horrible commentary. There was no need for him to raise his voice or engage in a personal attack or public display. This one word represented a searing indictment."

On fronting up for 7:00 A.M. rounds one morning, I learned that during my night off there had been a crisis in the Intensive Care Unit involving one of Whit's patients. A new experimental antibiotic had been prescribed and the precautionary restrictions placed on its use demanded that the fellow on call administer the injection. Unfortunately, when my colleague, Dr S., was summoned at 2:00 A.M. to carry out this humble task, he refused. One thing led to another and the chief of surgery, Edward J. "Ted" Beattie, the person ultimately responsible for the ICU and an old-school *surging* surgeon known for his volatile temperament, was contacted by the head nurse for advice. Dr Beattie arrived on the scene from his home at approximately 3:00 A.M. In a rage, he phoned Whit.

"Whitmore, your fellow has refused to get out of bed to care for one of your patients. I had to come in! I can't see any reason why *I* am here while *you* are at home sleeping, so get in here!" Whit came in without a word.

Whit and I were booked to do a cystectomy at 8:00 A.M. that morning. I arrived in the surgeons' lounge just as he was phoning the locating operator to have Dr S. come to the Ewing Pavilion OR. While I had found the reported details of the ICU drama of the night before more than sobering, I was also intrigued to see how our unflappable leader would handle the unacceptable insolence from both Beattie and the fellow, so I busied myself with the coffee machine in the corner, with the curiosity of one unable to avert his eyes from an impending disaster.

Whit turned to face Dr S. as he arrived. "S," he said in his usual quiet, unhurried tone, "you dropped the ball. That's twice. Once more and you're out of the game." With that he excused himself and left for the OR. That was the only comment he ever made about the events of that night. His *aequanimitas* was legendary.[4]

Shortly after that, I witnessed the legendary Whitmore cool once again. Whit and I had flown to Kingston for a one-day Queen's University seminar at which he was to be the featured visiting professor. The medical amphitheatre was packed. Unfortunately, with what organizers had intended to be respectful deference, Whit had been asked to chair the question-and-answer session that addressed an aspect of urologic oncology concerning which he was the recognized world authority. As a result, the invited panelists were considerably less well informed than their moderator.

Whit was at his diplomatic best as he fielded the questions from the audience and skillfully drew in one panelist after another while eliciting a comprehensive response. He succeeded in transforming the potentially awkward situation into a triumph in collegial medical education. All was well. Indeed, an afterglow of satisfaction pervaded the hall thanks to the rich content of the session. That is, it pervaded until one last questioner stood.

"I know Memorial Sloan-Kettering Cancer Center! You believe in barbaric, aggressive treatment until the very end, no matter what! Your protocols are the only thing you care about! Well I don't think it's right! Now what do you have to say about that, Whitmore?"

All were aghast! The room was engulfed in embarrassed silence. I felt deeply offended that someone would speak to Whit like that! In *Canada*! where he was our guest! ... *my* guest ... or *anywhere else*, for that matter!

It had been a long day. Whit was still at the podium. His voice was measured but easygoing, his expression relaxed but intent. "Well now, it would be difficult, in the time available, to discuss the guidelines underpinning each of our treatment protocols, but let me say that we attempt to offer our patients treatment options based on the most recent research, the stage and grade of their particular problem, and a careful assessment of their individual medical status, so as to balance treatment risk and potential benefit. Let me add," there was the trace of a smile as he continued, "if you are ever in the neighbourhood, come on down and I'll show you how it's done."

In a similar vein, there was the exchange Whit had with a patient some months later. The man had refused Whit's recommendation of potentially life-saving surgery for his locally advanced cancer, preferring instead homeopathy and an exercise regimen. Whit responded patiently and discussed the probable outcome of such a course of action at length, but the man insisted. When their protracted dialogue ended, Whit gave him an appointment for three months later.

"Why," I asked after the patient had left the room, "did you give him a follow-up appointment rather than simply sending him back to the referring doctor?" I was thinking of colleagues who preferred not to follow patients who had not heeded the advice given. Whit nodded thoughtfully, then noted quietly: "Bal, there are a couple of reasons behind my offer to follow the patient in this situation. First, it gives me an important opportunity to learn more about the natural history of untreated disease, and secondly, it means that I will be there to lend a hand when the need arises."

Perhaps my most indelible memory of Whit's grace under pressure relates to one busy day during my final months at Memorial. That morning we had two retroperitoneal lymph-node dissections booked, in addition to his weekly clinic. Each node dissection was demanding and time-consuming, taking three or more hours to complete. Between cases, Whit left for the clinic while I closed, my aim being to join him briefly prior to starting the second operation. It was a pressured schedule, but I appreciated the rare privilege of being a silent observer as he interacted with his clinic patients – the chance to witness a master clinician at work. His inevitable welcoming smile as he greeted each person consistently spread a glow of optimism before him.

"Hey, Mr T., great, great! How's it going? Let me have a look at you ... By the way, did you ever get away on that hunting trip you were planning?" As such informal chats with his patient continued, Whit would slide his hand under the loose gown and gently checked the neck, shoulder regions, axillae, chest, and abdomen. It was so deft, gentle, and fleeting that the patient hardly noticed. But it was, I knew, a virtuoso examination of the potential trouble spots. Depending on the needs of the case, this baseline exam was supplemented, as required, with an appropriate extension of the same unobtrusive attention to detail.

Thus it was that I silently entered the examining room behind Whit just as he went to see his next patient – a tanned, retired lawyer from Florida in his mid-seventies. Whit had just reviewed the man's lab tests and was turning to greet him when he was cut short by an indignant shout. "Whitmore, where have you been?! My appointment with you was booked for a half-hour ago and I've been waiting all this time! I want an explanation!" He was in a rage.

I couldn't believe it. My desire to protect Whit from such offensive nonsense was overwhelming. I undoubtedly flushed as I thought to myself, *Who does this jerk think he is?!*

Whit smiled with his customary welcoming warmth. He appeared not to have heard him. "Terrific, great; well, here we are. Now, Mr G., tell me how things are going. Let me see ... yes, it's been three months since ..."

"Whitmore," roared the man, "I asked you a question and I expect an answer! Where have you been?!" (At this point I was ready to attack!)

In response, Whit simply shrugged and, with a winning smile, patted the man on the shoulder. "Just trying to make a living, Mr G."

As the kids would say, Whit had endless "cool"! A colleague at Memorial, Robert Donohue, a 1964 graduate of New York University and, like Whit, a western rivers rafting enthusiast, tells the story of the day they, with a group of sixteen friends, were preparing to camp for the night mid-way down the spectacular Colorado River through the Grand Canyon in northern Arizona. Suddenly, the tranquility of their breathtaking surroundings was broken by the shout of the alarmed senior boatman urging them to hurry to the raft.

"Go now!" he exploded. "There's a rattlesnake in the campground!"

"How many of them are there?" responded Whit, unfazed.

"One," shouted the boatman.

"Give me a moment," murmured Whit heading up to the campsite from the beach.

Alarmed, Bob informed the senior boatman, "You need to know, that if anything happens to that man, you're dead! Do you have *any* idea who that is?! He is the father of urologic oncology!"

Minutes later, Whit returned to the group. Bob recalled the moment with typical candour. "The stunned silence was now shattered by the heart-stopping high-pitched sound of the menacing rattle of the pissed-off creature curled around Whit's neck, it's eyes bulging and rattles trumpeting, or whatever it is that rattles do!!"

The snake's head protruded from Whit's left hand, his thumb and index finger firmly clamped behind its gaping jaw.

"Bob, have you got a credit card?" Whit asked casually.

"What the hell are you asking me for?" stammered Bob, a man rarely lost for words. "He can charge whatever he likes on my card, just keep that damn thing away from me!"

"Bring it here," continued Whit. "I want you to shove the card into the corner of his open jaws on both sides." Bob did and the venom poured all over his hand.

"My right hand helped steady my left hand, which contained the card. Staying conscious with my hands shaking that much and getting into the corners of the snake's mouth were the real challenges," Bob confessed.

Don't worry about the venom," Whit murmured calmly. "Just wash it off. It won't hurt you as long as it isn't internal."

Whit stood there for a moment or two contemplating his de-venomed adversary with the unhurried focused attention that was so characteristic of the man, and then added, almost absentmindedly, "It will take two days for the venom to reaccumulate. In the meantime, he isn't dangerous. I'll be back in a few minutes. I'm just going back up the trail a ways to release him."[5]

"NOO YAWK" MAGIC

On one clear, crisp New York evening in Advent, Faye and I accompanied Chris on the cross-town bus. Dressed to-the-nines, with Chris's eyes shining, we blended in with the elegantly turned-out finery of the New York intelligentsia who climbed aboard at each stop. The city's sparkling lights, seasonal decor, and, for many on that bus, the anticipation of an evening filled with toy soldiers and sugar-plum fairies had conjured up a festive sense of community that transformed the usual workaday New York City bus ambience into something approaching that of a horse-drawn carriage. Welcoming warmth prevailed. We smiled discreetly as our fellow travellers joined us in their jewellery and gowns, dark suits – some tuxedos – and upturned collars. The bus was filling rapidly. We were, it became evident, all bound for the same magical treat, the much-heralded annual Lincoln Center performance of Tchaikovsky's *Nutcracker Suite*.

A young gentleman smiled and stood up as we headed down the aisle, offering his place so that Chris could stand on the seat and look out the window at the shimmering city twinkling in all its splendid holiday red and greenery: taxis and streaming cars; celebrants hurrying to and fro into the closing shops; warmly lit eateries; brownstones; festive apartment doorways with their bundling doormen standing proud in the fresh dusting of snow. The chill blast of night air at each stop seemed to add a tingle of excitement rather than cold. Second Avenue. Third Avenue. We were just crossing the next broad thoroughfare when our vista suddenly opened dramatically. There, directly in front of us as we gazed out the side window, was the Park Avenue median spreading south in all its grandeur, as far as the eye could see. The closely placed Christmas trees, each dazzling with countless white lights, stretched on and on, the elegant buildings framing the scene quietly and underscoring the stately grandeur of it all.

Chris was astonished! Enraptured! "Twee! ... Twee! ... Twee!!" he gasped at the top of his lungs, in disbelief and wonder. Just four and a half years old, he was completely overcome. We all were. Viewed afresh, thanks to Chris, the scene we had almost taken for granted captured the attention of the busload of instant converts. who stared with new awareness and silent appreciation at the magic of it all.

The unassuming, neatly dressed gentleman with greying hair and moustache sitting next to Chris bent toward him as we neared Madison Avenue. He was sixtyish and spoke with a soft voice, "And you, young man, where are you off to tonight? It is getting a little late, isn't it?" Chris attempted something about, "a special time with Mommy and Daddy." His new friend said how much he hoped Chris would enjoy it.

At Fifth, the bus turned and we made our way into the mysteries of Central Park and on to Central Park West, then to Lincoln Center.

The theatre was resplendent in its plush upholstery, gilt decor, and air of excitement. Our seats were front-row centre. The members of the orchestra were making their way to their places in the pit as we arrived. The violinist next to the concert master seemed familiar as he quietly slid into his seat. And, as he did, he noticed Chris and offered him a wink and knowing smile as the house lights dimmed. Then, Chris's moustachioed bus-mate friend escorted us into a land of wonders – a massive Christmas tree that grew before our eyes, toys, and children – mystery and magic, music and dance. Oh, such music!

With the New Year, we had an undeniable sense of delight in being New Yorkers, if only for a brief time: Central Park strolls with the kids; evenings at the opera; visits with cousins Joan and Lou; the radio perennially tuned to WQXR – "the Radio Station of the New York Times"; fabulously predictable New York drivers (if there's the mere suggestion of a space there, they'll swerve effortlessly into it – every time! Depend on it!); the streaming yellow cabs; the dynamic 24/7 flow of humanity; the cacophony of horns and sirens; the museums, galleries, and street-corner food vendors. A person could walk down Broadway, as Faye and I did one evening, and, on passing his restaurant, between 49th and 50th streets, bump into world heavyweight boxing champion Jack Dempsey and exchange a handshake and brief chat.

With a chuckle we watched the New York City closed-circuit TV coverage of the fundraiser staged by the entertainment industry in support of John Lindsay's quest for re-election as mayor. It was the eve of the election and suddenly it looked as if Lindsay might lose to his right-wing opponent, who promised cuts to the arts. Coretta King spoke in Lindsay's support, as the candidate sat in the front row, beaming widely. Then, Woody Allen strolled to the microphone. "Hi, I just want to say that I support John Lindsay. Now you may not care what I think, but I represent a segment of the vote ... the pervert vote. And it matters who gets in! After all, the mayor of New York has the second most difficult job in the country. The most difficult is the one Mrs Agnew has to do when she goes to bed every night." Lindsay won.

Our New York City included Central Presbyterian Church at Park Avenue and 64th Street, with our new-found friends Ginny and Doug Medin, who arrived at "Central" battling against a background steeped in the conservative theological right of the American Mid-West, even as we arrived questioning our background in the theological left of the United Church of Canada. Thus, as couples, we had acquired totally opposing senses of the imagined ideal that lay at the summit of the road less travelled. At "Central" there was also the young organist Richard Westenburg, on his way to prominence with all-star renderings of Bach's *St Matthew Passion* and seventeenth-century masterpieces by Claudio Monteverdi, Giacomo Carissimi, and Heinrich Schütz.

New York! The Big Apple! I eventually had to face up to the fact. I had come to love New York, plain and simple!

The stream of celebrities passing on the street and encountered at Memorial seemed endless. For example, there was the day Whit called his answering service to pick up the weekend messages. "No calls, Dr Whitmore – well, there were one or two on Saturday, but they said it wasn't urgent and I suggested they call Poppy [Whit's secretary[6]] on Monday. Oh yes, there was one more – Mrs Onassis called. She said she would like to speak to you, but I told her you weren't available."

"I see. Well, make a note of it. In the future, if Jackie calls, I am *always* available!"

In my own case, I once bumped into a guy on the corner as I made my way to a concert at "Central" one evening; he looked very familiar – like an old friend – so I said, "Hi" – and he said, "Hi," and smiled, then we chatted about the weather, and I thought, *Just the way he always did when ... When was that? ... Where do I know him from?* Then I realized it was Jack Lemmon. He was in New York filming *The Out-of-Towners*.

At first, I had to do some soul searching. Was there a fawning component to my reaction on these occasions? I think not – well, maybe an iota with the *Piano Man*, Billy Joel. With Jack Lemmon, it wasn't so much fawning as the fact that in person he seemed to be the same ordinary good guy I had come to know on the screen.

All of which brings me to the day I became concerned about one of my post-op patients. I went to see her on rounds that afternoon and didn't like the way she looked. She was a big woman; early fifties; her pressure was very low, pulse rapid and thready. She felt hot; she was drowsy. Asking the nurse to check her vital signs, I reviewed her chart. *She needs a central line, blood culture, cross-match, antibiotics, and lots of fluids stat!* Requesting the specific kind of central line I preferred, I re-examined my patient.

After what felt like an eternity – by this point, my patient had spiralled even lower – the nurse returned to say that she would have to order the line I had specified from central supply. It would take at least half an hour. I suggested she get one from the recovery room several floors above us, but then told her to forget it, saying, "You stay with the patient. I'll go for it myself," as I sprinted down the hall.

Arriving at the elevator, I thanked my lucky stars. Unbelievable! It was already waiting there, door open, the white-gloved operator looking like he had been summoned for me. *Amazing!! Perfect!* I was in full flight.

"Take me up to Recovery and wait for me. I have to pick up something; I'll come right back down. Lord, I'm glad you're here!"

He didn't move. It was then that he said, with a slight break in his voice, "Sorry, this elevator is taken."

Taken!?! How in God's green earth does an elevator get to be "taken"? I asked myself.

Several things then happened simultaneously. I realized the elevator operator was actually ignoring me and staring straight ahead at the wall of the elevator, his posture rigid. Furthermore, I noticed that he and I were not alone. Indeed, standing side by side at the back of the elevator were two of the largest men I had ever seen. They were from India – perhaps they were wearing turbans. They, too, appeared to be ignoring me. Indeed, they were staring past me – straight through me, as it were!

At that precise moment, they took one step toward me. All was silent. Nothing made sense. I turned.

There, less than three feet from me, was Indira Gandhi. We were face to face. Smiling graciously, she offered a slight bow of her head as I commented with a respectful grin, bowing from the waist, "I guess it *is* taken." I stepped to one side and she entered. My mind was rushing. The news reports hadn't mentioned she was in town. Later, I learned that one of her colleagues was dying on the ward. When Prime Minister Gandhi had been informed, she had flown from India to say goodbye. The media had not been informed. Happily, the central line was soon placed and my patient recovered.

One celebrity contact lingers with me as having been special yet marked by a less than distinguished reaction on my part. Rudolph Bing, general manager of the Metropolitan Opera since 1950, had telephoned Whit.[7] L.M. (pseudonym), one of the Met's leading soloists, had been diagnosed with kidney cancer.

Poppy paged me to say that L.M. was being admitted and would bring with him his x-rays and the results of recent investigations. Whit had already booked the radical nephrectomy for the following day.

Faye and I had relished performances at both the Met and the New York City Opera – with their galaxy of stars that included Franco Corelli, Joan Sutherland, Monserrat Caballé, Marilyn Horne, and so many others. Mountaintop experiences in abundance! I looked forward to meeting this patient.

L.M. was sitting up in bed when I entered his room. On our initial greeting, the room shook as his volcanic bass-baritone "HELLLOO!))))" reverberated to fill each corner.

Could that be real!? An affectation? I had never heard a voice like it. I was flabbergasted as he rumbled, "GLADD TO MEET YOUU!))))."

Dumbfounded, I found myself inexplicably balling up a hand towel and then, unceremoniously, tossing it in his face from my position at the foot of his bed. This was not an Andy Bruce hardball fired out of frustration and anger; instead, it was perhaps, a spontaneous, disbelieving, "that-voice-of-yours-is-hard-to-fathom" gesture of astonishment, awe, and wonderment. *Let's face it, it's hard to rationalize stupidity!*

It is uncertain who was more surprised by the towel in the face. We parted laughing and shaking hands.

The surgery went well. But could anyone *really* have a voice like that? Could that thunderous resonance *possibly* be real? I headed up to the recovery room to see how our patient was doing. L.M. was still asleep. He was stable. But the whole room, and everyone in it, shook with his moaning: "UUHHHHHHH))) ... AHHHHHHH))) ... UUUHHH)))) ..." He was completely asleep, and yet the volume, the resonance, the rich thundering cascades, the table-rattling impact, they were all there in spades. No pretense! It really *was* his gift! Amazing![8]

Whit was both a surgical innovator and a perfectionist. He would refine an operative technique and then carry it out with compulsive, near liturgical, attention to detail. The same way – always the same way! Exactly, precisely, reliably the same sutures, the same hand movements, the same precautions, the same minute safeguards. Always – "until a better one comes along." While open to further technique modification in the interest of efficacy and diminished patient risk, there was never change by chance, or change for the sake of change, and each fellow soon learned to reproduce Whit's carefully developed "surgical Whitmoreisms" – "until a better one comes along."

His meticulous two-layer technique in joining ureter to bowel when fashioning the patient's new ileal conduit after removing a cancerous bladder is a good example. "It's a fool-proof anastomosis," he would quip, leaving no doubt about the good-natured double entendre that implied that his assistant fellow was the fool he had in mind.

One such surgical Whitmoreism intrigued me. He had devised an ingenious method for removing the male urethra, from one end of the penis to the other, without leaving an obvious scar – the short incision on the perineum soon becoming invisible. He deftly turned the penis inside out – *really!* – in a slick gesture, then returned it (minus the potentially pre-cancerous lining) to its normal position and appearance. All in just a few minutes! I was fascinated. His ingenious trick, for it was really that, a sort of surgical sleight of hand, wasn't described in any of the textbooks.

With a little prodding, I convinced him that his innovation should be written up. The resulting article was published in the journal *SG&O*. It was my third publication and a source of some delight since, during my childhood years, row upon row of the esteemed *SG&O* volumes had lined Dad's office shelves in our home.

That success led to another idea. Why not a teaching film? Whit's inverted-penis procedure had to be seen to be believed. We discussed the idea briefly. He liked it and, in his customary nurturing style, urged me to run with it. He would supply the required funding and recruit award-winning medical-documentary filmmaker Warren Sturgis of Sturgis-Grant Productions to do the job.

The final edited 16-mm. film version, *A Technique for Urethrectomy in the Male*, with soundtrack text refined by Whit and read by me, was eighteen minutes long. It became a valued teaching tool which we could take on the road – and did. Marvellous!

With completion of the urethrectomy film, a series of further projects seemed obvious. Working with Warren Sturgis and his film crew had been a delight, a taste of New York cinematic excellence. Warren had become a friend and the urethrectomy film had provided a vehicle for easily disseminating Whit's surgical concepts beyond the small circle of privileged fellows. A banquet of possibilities lay before us. Whit wasn't hard to convince. He did the surgery; we worked together on the soundtracks which I read for the final film versions: *Technique for Radical Cystectomy in the Male* (twenty-three minutes), *Technique for Ileal Conduit Urinary Diversion* (fifteen minutes), *Technique for Retroperitoneal Lymph Node*

Dissection (twenty minutes). The American Cancer Society-sponsored *Cancer of the Urinary System* (twenty minutes) followed, as did a splendid gourmet evening for Faye and me at Warren and his partner's wood-beamed and panelled New York townhouse.

The films proved to be a perfect length for use in weekly rounds, teaching seminars, and one-hour lecture slots. The interactive discussion they generated was always lively and there was also the advantage of having a portable, ready-made session up one's sleeve, with no need for slides or preliminary preparation, during a "visiting professor" session.[9] I was greatly impressed by the power of the visual image as an effective teaching tool. My career had been changed in the production of these surgical films with Whit.

By the summer of 1969, we had acquired a "urology yellow" Dodge Dart (a personally appealing, but soon discontinued, shade) for an eagerly anticipated two-week return to the *Place* and the full therapeutic magic of family time and island life without electricity, running water, neighbours, or indoor plumbing but rich in the sound of wind in the pines and waves on the rocky point.

Of course, we knew about Apollo 11. I think we had heard somewhere that the 16 July liftoff had gone without a hitch. Neil Armstrong, Michael Collins, and Buzz Aldrin were on their way. But, somehow, the lapping of Grand Lake had largely lulled all that out of consciousness and it came and went, much like the other days in our blissful island-induced cycle. What we *did* keep in mind was that we would be driving to Ottawa that Sunday to attend a concert by Joan Sutherland at the National Arts Centre.

On that very special Sunday afternoon, the renowned coloratura soprano was at the peak of her extraordinary powers and all present felt profoundly privileged as we experienced her magnificent cascading voice and gracious presence. At concert end, the applause was deafening.

Returning to the stage from the wings, she walked to the apron, slightly raising her hand. With that unexpected signal that she was about to speak, a sudden silence fell on the house. "Thank you so much. You are very kind. But I want to tell you that the Americans have just done something far more wonderful than anything I could do. They have just landed men on the moon." Once again there was a roar of applause, this time for Armstrong, Collins, Aldrin, the National Aeronautics and Space Administration (NASA), our American cousins, *and* Joan Sutherland. It was 20 July 1969.[10]

It was, however, Wednesday, 13 August, 1969 that would live on in my memory. A series of separate images and sounds remain: our vantage point in the crowd on First Avenue near the United Nations Headquarters; the large hand-printed sign "Welcome Home Apollo 11 Astronauts" in the store window across the street; Chris sitting on my shoulders and Wren plucked out of her stroller to be held high by Faye; the cheering thousands of beaming faces on all sides; the growl of the escorting police motorcycles; the proudly waving and erupting energy of the ecstatic crowd; the snowstorm of paper joyously raining down on us from surrounding near-celestial windows across the street; the echo in my mind of JFK's words eight years earlier, when he had pledged that before the decade ended the United States would land a man on the Moon and return him safely to Earth; Armstrong, Aldrin, and Collins, arms raised in something between a wave and a salute, perched triumphantly on their flag-draped convertible.[11]

"BAH HAWBA" AND THE JACKSON LABS

While the three-month period allotted to research during Whit's MSKCC two-year fellowship program was too brief for a groundbreaking original study, it might be sufficient, he reasoned, to plant a seed, stimulate an inquiring mind, or inculcate the notion that critical thinking is an essential ingredient of clinical practice.

Anticipating my upcoming research period, Whit suggested I review the work of Leroy C. Stevens at his lab in Bar Harbor, Maine, with an eye to establishing his model for inducing testis tumours in mice at Memorial. Stevens had shown that grafting the genital ridge (primordial testis) from a twelve-and-a half-day-old mouse embryo into the adult testis of the same inbred strain[12] resulted in the development of testis tumours in 80 per cent of the male grafts. Thus, for the first time, there now existed a reliable model for producing and studying an unlimited number of germinal testicular cancers with the aid of specimens that pathologically resemble that human cancer.

My late-fall, flying visit to Bar Harbor found the sleepy coastal community hunkering down for winter in the wake of the annual exodus of summer tourists. I headed for the Jackson Laboratory, an impressive complex of buildings sheltered from the vicissitudes of the sea by a sloped headland bordering the property. Founded in 1929, this sprawling campus had attracted a remarkable faculty dedicated to biomedical research and education. The Jackson Labs were renowned for the inbred strains of "JAX® Mice," a product they developed for export to research centres around the world.

Dr Leroy C. Stevens greeted me with a somewhat tentative, averted gaze and retiring manner. "Call me Steve." This informal, rather rumpled, colleague spoke quietly; his straggly head of hair and dark, generous eyebrows topped a perennially enquiring, vaguely quizzical, expression. Modest in height and demeanour, and an introvert by nature, Steve possessed an overflowing generosity of spirit, a winsome humility, and low-key openness. The light in his eyes was a giveaway indicator of his delight during research discussions.

Testis tumours in mice? My fascination grew as we both relaxed. I was an all-thumbs neophyte in a strange land. No problem. He would be happy to make himself available as needed. Like Whit, Steve drew you in with his apparently unquenchable interest in the mysteries uncovered by his work.

We toured his lab then the vast, spotlessly clean, environmentally controlled, mouse breeding and housing facility. Row upon row of catalogued, shelving units were stacked six or eight shelves high, the rows separated by commodious aisles. It was a veritable supermarket of carefully developed inbred strains of mice – thousands of strains – each having been developed to investigate the genetic basis of cancer or a host of other diseases. Each was categorized by phenotype, genotype, and gene expression.

Steve introduced his assistant, Don Varnum, and the three of us ambled through the building as Steve described their technique for determining the exact age of mouse embryos, the surgical preparation of the twelve-and-a half-day embryos, the technique for surgical exposure of the paired genital ridges, their extraction by pipette, and the method of grafting them into the exposed testes of an adult of the same inbred strain. We then inspected mice that had been grafted by Don over the preceding week or two and he demonstrated the harvesting and preparation for study of the resultant tumours.

What was the feasibility, I asked, of my setting up a similar colony of strain 129 mice at Memorial? Steve's eyes sparkled. "I don't see why not. We can advise you along the way. It will be great to have your observations as things progress." While the project was appealing, if daunting in scope, the available time was hopelessly limited.

"Steve, since I will be doing all this over the next six weeks or so, is there any way I could do it here, in your lab? I'm sure that after my time with you and Don I would be in a better position to set things up at Memorial. Would there be some place here in town where Faye, the children, and I could stay?"

"Well, we have students here every summer, but I've never had anyone over the winter. However, I can't see why you couldn't stay in one of the summer cabins. A couple of them have space heaters and they are right here on the property."

Within the week, Faye, Chris, Lauren, and I were packed. We planned a 6:30 A.M. departure next morning.

We reached Bar Harbor late that night, invigorated by the stars, the crisp November night air, the sense of the sea close at hand, and the rustic simplicity of our small cabin.

The weeks became a happy tumble of work, family time – including skating on the pond (not enough snow for building snowmen) – reading, and sustenance shopping in the small store. And with *no* need to be on call!

We explored the local community and church in the anticipation of joining in the holiday spirit of this picture-postcard New England town, but there was a sense of exclusion by the taciturn, polite but distant, locals. When we four "outsiders" attended the Christmas church service, no one in the small congregation acknowledged our presence! "You aren't a true *Mainiac*," a lab colleague explained, "unless you've been here at least six generations." There was no ill will, that was clear. We recognized that these sturdy souls had learned frugality in relating as a consequence of the personal rites of passage found in many isolated communities, particularly those subjected to torrents of seasonal tourists.

The week the immense storm hit the coast, Faye and I knew there was something unusual occurring. *Both* of us had a local townsman *initiate* a conversation – and that was a first!

"Been out along the shore road? Allows how you might find that worth a look."

The winds had been impressive, but our little cabin, tucked behind the headland, had been shielded from the ferocities of storm and sea.

Picking our way along the deserted, debris strewn road, we drove to the crest of the hill and watched in awe as the waves broke *over* the hundred-foot-high cliffs of the neighbouring headland up the coast, sending massive sheets of spray a full mile inland with each wave, while the immense sixty- to eighty-foot grey-brown churning waves threw boulders the size of bowling balls across our road. Meanwhile, at the small sandy cove near town, the fury of the storm exposed a legendary shipwreck long buried under the beach, though its remains, we were told, had not been seen in the lifetime of anyone now living in Bar Harbor. We were awestruck by the power of nature.

Toward the end of our Bar Harbor adventure, I returned to our cabin one day for our customary lunchtime soup and sandwich. Faye motioned to me, "Lauren is talking! It started this morning."

Squatting on the floor beside Chris, Wren (they were now almost six and three, respectively), and toys, I jumped in.

"Wrennie, Mummy says you can talk now. That must feel good. Was it frustrating before, not being able to say what you wanted?" Wren was bright, active, happy, responsive – she clearly understood everything said to her but until then couldn't be bothered speaking. As the pediatrician put it, "She'll speak when she needs to." I wasn't, however, prepared for her first words.

"Yes, now I can speak. Before I couldn't say what I wanted to, but now I can. It feels good." It was a foreshadowing of the independence that would always be our precious Wren.

It was time to head home to New York City. This wonderful oasis on our two-year MSKCC journey had provided exposure to an academic centre of excellence,[13] introduced us to Steve and his research model, enabled the setting up of the Stevens testis tumour model at Memorial (Steve's line of investigation would lead others to the holy grail of stem-cell research[14]), and fostered memorable family times.

Whit invited Steve to present research rounds at MSKCC. It was an opportunity to repay my friend and mentor in small measure for his exceptional generosity. Dinner and an evening of theatre – something low-key but memorable, a real New York experience seemed called for. I phoned the Vivian Beaumont Theater at Lincoln Centre.

"Do you have anything on next Friday evening?"

"Yes, we do. How many tickets would you need?

"Three."

"You're in luck. We have just had three tickets turned in and they're front-row centre."

"What's the event?"

"Simon and Garfunkel."

"*Who* or *what* is Simon and Garfunkel?!" I asked with considerable misgivings.

"Singer-songwriters. Local guys, from Queens, actually. They're pretty good."

"Thanks I'll think about it."

Could an evening spent with something called "Simon and Garfunkel" have anything to recommend it?! I opted instead for something that sounded safer. It was an off-Broadway play of long-forgotten name. Steve, Faye, and I settled in our seats, noting with concern, as the lights dimmed, the large number of empty seats. A large black fellow barged through the curtains to confront us. "Hello, you motherfuckers!" he roared.

Simon and Garfunkel?! These many decades later I still have recurring nightmares about that missed opportunity and have long since become a dedicated S&G fan.[15]

Our New York days were drawing to a close. The McGill job offer was on the table, but Dr MacKinnon had encountered bureaucratic delays in finalizing the details. Furthermore, I was increasingly concerned about moving the family back to Quebec. It was during these days of indecision that Whit left me with one more "Whitmoreism!"

"Bal, you're good. You're no Willet Whitmore, but you're good. If it wasn't for Ken, I'd offer you a job." Translation is required. First, I had managed a passing grade, nothing more. Second, in Whit's always discerning assessment, his personal track record still set the ideal height of the bar. (His evaluation of himself did not represent an inflated ego but, instead, his habit of calling it as it was.) Third, should it not work out at McGill, I had a job at MSKCC.

Why not Quebec? La Belle Province had continued to be a cauldron of increasing, restless change. The Front de Libération du Québec (FLQ) had been responsible for many bombings between 1963 and 1970.[16] Their targets included anglophone homes and mailboxes in Westmount, a federal-government bookstore, McGill University, and the Montreal Stock Exchange, where twenty-seven people were injured, one person killed, and another permanently maimed.[17] In addition, two armed FLQ members with plans to kidnap the Israeli ambassador had been arrested in late February. Then, in June, with our final decision overdue, a raid on an FLQ home unearthed firearms, ammunition, three hundred pounds of dynamite, detonators, and a draft ransom note to be used in kidnapping the American ambassador. Anglophones were feeling increasingly uncomfortable in Quebec. By 1970, "the great Anglo exodus" had started. (By the early 1980s, 20 per cent of anglophone Quebecers had left the province.)

News that Royal Vic surgical peers would be attending an annual conference in New York at this critical juncture seemed providential, a chance to get the latest word from the front lines. I headed to the downtown hotel to meet with Jean-Guy Beaudoin and other recent surgical residents.

"What are the risks?" Opinions on all sides were aired. Nothing conclusive; it was even somewhat encouraging. "No reason to change horses in mid-stream."

"McGill isn't going anywhere." And so it went long into the night.

A day or two later, Chris was looking out our apartment window toward East 66th when he quietly commented in a wistful tone, "Ohhh ... there's a beautiful sunset over 'P.S.183' [his public school]." In fact, the heavy grey sky with the low-lying sullen clouds showed only a faint grey-mauve smudge across the black underbelly of one particularly threatening cloud just above the huddled buildings. A "beautiful sunset"? It was definitely time to head north out of the city.

When McGill came through, we made our move, becoming the proud owners of a brick, three-storey, semi-detached house at 600 Victoria Avenue. Only minutes from the Royal Vic as the car flies, a two-minute stroll from the highly praised Roslyn Public School, and blocks from our church, Dominion Douglas United, it seemed custom-made. A promising new life lay ahead. Ken MacKinnon extended a warm welcome. We were home.

Joining the Royal Vic Team

How noble it would be ...
to erect an entirely new set of buildings ...
upon some suitable site where it would stand as
a monument of benevolence and munificence
to the inhabitants of this prosperous city.

Dr Palmer Howard,
dean, Faculty of Medicine,
McGill, 1870

... a hospital for the reception and treatment of sick and injured persons of all
races and creeds, without distinction; for the advancement of medical science,
and for the establishment of a training school for nurses.

R.B. Angus, president,
RVH Board of Governors,
RVH Opening Day, 2 December 1893

Chris was six, eager and exploding with life, with a new friend, his trusty bike, and the summer sun tantalizingly at hand. Lauren, three, was inventive, inquisitive, and reflective. She soon would transform her spacious new room into her own personal, very secret world. The summer weeks flew past with days of unpacking and rearranging at home interspersed with precious time swimming, boating, and gathering around campfires at the *Place*.

Most urology colleagues at the Vic were committed to developing a strong integrated academic team under Ken MacKinnon's leadership. Doug Morehouse focused on urethral reconstruction, voiding dysfunction, and stone disease; Yosh Taguchi, on micro and vascular surgery. My arrival added a focus in oncology. Ken's vision was to build a salaried partnership that would foster academic growth rather than the earlier norm that emphasized private-practice income. Yosh and Doug were a gift – capable surgeons, effective teachers, and warmly welcoming colleagues. On the other hand, another member of the department, who was a decade older than I, resolutely opposed my recruitment as well as Ken's plan for subspecialization and financial partnership. His destructive and aggressive oppositional stance would persist while Ken and I remained in the department. "It is in pardoning, that we are pardoned," Dad would remind me. How did we do in measuring up to that standard? Ken, pretty damn well; me, not so much. Nevertheless, my plate in those first months was filled to overflowing with establishing office and surgical routines, creating a urology chemotherapy clinic, sharing in night and weekend clinical coverage, participating in student and residency teaching, preparing research-grant applications, and presenting Grand Rounds at the various McGill-affiliated hospitals and beyond.

A three-year Medical Research Council of Canada grant in the summer of 1971 enabled my recruitment of Miriam Husk, a talented research assistant from Sherbrooke. She was a rare find. A natural team player, Miriam was bright, insightful, and a "self-starter." She visited the Jackson Laboratory, set up the Royal Vic Strain 129 mouse colony, and carried forward our testicular-tumour research with the Stevens genital-ridge graft model while initiating a variety of other projects. As the pace picked up, so did speaking commitments at rounds, society meetings, and seminars in Canada and the United States.

THE OCTOBER CRISIS

In October 1970 a sea of provincial and national angst suddenly swamped our personal anguish as we found ourselves living in moment-to-moment uncertainty laced with disbelief as headlines out of Montreal circled the world.

Monday, 5 October: British diplomat James Richard Cross was abducted from his Montreal home by the FLQ, the terrorists who had killed six, wounded twenty-seven, and committed two hundred bombings and robberies in Quebec over the preceding seven years. My mind was *churning – Unbelievable! I pass Cross's home each day as I drive home from the Vic. What in the world has happened to the liberal-democratic values we have cherished in Quebec? How safe is my family living in this province?*

Prime Minister Trudeau and Quebec Premier Robert Bourassa declared that they were unwilling to negotiate with criminals. *Good for Trudeau and Bourassa. They had no choice. Negotiating with terrorists who threaten the rule of law through violence and blackmail would only further undermine civil order and place democracy at greater risk.*

Saturday, 10 October: Quebec Labour Minister Pierre Laporte was abducted by "bandits" (as Trudeau referred to them) claiming to be the "Chénier Cell of the FLQ." Laporte had been playing ball with his nephew on the front lawn of his home in Saint-Lambert at the time. *How many of them are there, for heaven sake? What and who are the Chénier Cell? The FLQ seems to be able to strike at will. When a franco-phone elected representative of the people can be kidnapped at his home, how safe is anyone in this province?*

Tuesday, 13 October: Journalists intercepted the prime minister on the steps of the Parliament Buildings, expressing concern about the risk of Canada becoming a police state, given the deployment of troops on Parliament Hill and in Montreal under the National Defence Act the day before.

"Sir, what is it with all these men with guns around here?" Trudeau was asked.

He answered that soldiers were being used "as peace agents in order that the police could be more free to do their job as policemen." He continued, "I think it is more important to get rid of those who are committing violence against the total society and those who are trying to run the government through a parallel power by establishing their authority by kidnapping and blackmail."

The journalist pushed further, asking again whether Trudeau risked producing a police state. In the context of a seven-minute discussion, Trudeau replied, "Yes, well there are a lot of bleeding hearts around who just don't like to see people with helmets and guns. All I can say is, go on and bleed, but it is more important to keep law and order in the society than to be worried about weak-kneed people who don't like the looks of ..."

"At any cost?" the journalist asked. "How far would you go with that? How far would you extend that?"

Trudeau's response made headlines. "Well, just watch me."

Absolutely! It's not about becoming a police state; it's about protecting a democratic society.

The global media was instantly awash in accounts linking the phrases "bleeding heart" and "just watch me" and Trudeau was branded a "gunslinger" by many. *Gunslinger?! Let me watch that film clip again! Was he cool-headed or short-fused in his response? Is this sensationalistic journalism? I saw coolness under pressure and determined responsible leadership on behalf of the elected Quebec government and, indeed, on behalf of the country beyond.*

While my reaction to the FLQ violence and support for Trudeau and Quebec Premier Bourassa was shared by most, as the days passed the response across Quebec and beyond became divided, confused. Should there be confrontation or negotiation with the anarchists?

Wednesday, 14 October: A petition signed by sixteen "eminent personalities" including René Lévesque and Jacques Parizeau of the Parti Québécois (PQ), *Le Devoir* editor Claude Ryan, and union leaders called for negotiation with the terrorists and the release of Cross and Laporte, who were referred to as "political prisoners." *Madness! "Political prisoners"?! Such a petition gives implied support to the terrorists rather than siding with Bourassa's newly elected democratic government. Mind you, if negotiations were seen to take place, it might forestall anything happening to Cross and Laporte. It's an unstable, treacherous situation; I am with Bourassa and Trudeau.*

Thursday, 15 October: The Quebec government, with the unanimous support of the leaders of the three opposition parties in the National Assembly including Camille Laurin of the Parti Québécois, called for reinforcements from the "Van Doos," the fabled Quebec-based Royal Twenty-Second Regiment of the Canadian Army, to assist Quebec authorities in countering the kidnappings and call to violence. The Canadian soldiers would at all times take orders from, and report to, the chief of the Sûreté du Québec. Later in the day, Laurin reneged his support for the request for troops.

Why did Laurin back down?[1]

Friday, 16 October: the War Measures Act, legislation originally passed in 1914, was brought into force by Trudeau at the request of Montreal Mayor Jean Drapeau and the Quebec provincial government, thus enabling increased powers of arrest and detention in the face of what Trudeau termed an "apprehended insurrection." Four hundred and sixty-seven people were arrested and held without charge.

The War Measures Act was called for! There must be a clear line in the sand. This call to anarchy must be met with clarity and the full weight of democratically elected governments.

That afternoon, coming around a curve on the Boulevard in Westmount as I drove home from the hospital, I was confronted by armed Canadian soldiers approaching in full-alert stance. It was a sickening, overwhelming experience.

Can Quebec nationalism run wild have driven us to this?

Saturday, 17 October: Pierre Laporte's strangled body was found in the trunk of a car near the Saint-Hubert airport.

Madness!

Thursday, 3 December: James Cross was released in return for safe passage of the perpetrators to Cuba.

Where are the sentences for these murderers?!

Those unjustly incarcerated under the War Measures Act were afforded the right to an independent review before the Quebec ombudsman and received compensation of up to $30,000 from the Quebec government. Only 18 of the 467 arrested were convicted of being accessories to the FLQ.[2]

As these events unfolded, the overwhelming majority of Quebecers supported the actions taken by Bourassa and Trudeau. But, as time passed, opposition to the War Measures Act grew and historical revisionism gained wide acceptance. The murderers were cast as "victims"; the murder itself as "an accident."

A CAREER IN QUEBEC: TO BE OR NOT TO BE?

Confidence in the stability of Quebec and its future in Canada had been eroded. Ken MacKinnon and I discussed the possibility of moving together to a new academic centre. In the closing months of 1970, we visited the University of Wisconsin, at Madison, and the University of Western Ontario in response to invitations to join their programs. A similar offer came from McMaster University.

Quebec's October Crisis was not our only concern. In December 1966 the Canadian Parliament had passed comprehensive Medicare legislation that became effective in July 1968. While Ken and I were in favour of the legislated changes, there was strong opposition from many colleagues and the future of health-care reform was far from clear. Anglophone colleagues were leaving the province in significant numbers as the 1970s arrived. The political and economic future of Quebec, the possibility of further social unrest, the status of Medicare, and a continuing low referral rate of oncology patients all remained considerations to ponder.

On the other hand, there was reason for encouragement. In addition to the usual range of open and endoscopic urologic procedures, during my first months back at McGill in 1970, we had completed a retroperitoneal lymph-node dissection and two radical cystectomies, with a third pending. In addition, our new chemotherapy clinic was providing positive results. During that first year, one young testis-tumour patient who had presented with lung metastases had a complete response. When this had been sustained for six months, we proceeded with the surgery to remove residual retroperitoneal disease and he subsequently remained disease-free.

THE SIGNIFICANCE OF PRESENCE

Two patients referred to me during 1970 were to remain etched in my mind with unusual persistence. Both young men had testicular cancer. On referral, one had extensive cancer spread, the second, a tall, gentle fellow who seemed particularly vulnerable, had no evidence of remaining cancer when first seen by me. In both cases I intervened with a retroperitoneal lymph-node dissection and chemotherapy. Both men remained cancer-free on long-term follow-up following these treatment interventions.

While this result was gratifying, it was similar to that of other patients under our care. Why, then, were these two, in particular, etched with such clarity in my thoughts? Both lads had found it reassuring to hear that I had experienced a cancer journey similar to theirs, yet I sensed that our persistent bond was not dependent on our shared experience of illness. There seemed to be something more, and that "something more" seemed relational at its core. The underlying reason, however, remained unclear.

On further reflection, it appeared that the *quality of presence* one brings to, or finds in, an interaction comes in at least three forms: "casual," "functional," and, finally, what I came to think of as "radical." *Casual presence*, I concluded, was an apt description for interactions characterized by what was little more than transient physical presence, as in the chance proximity of two people on a bus, an elevator, or in passing on a busy street. In contrast, *functional presence* described the collaborative relating that is generally required for diagnosis, therapeutics, or any other shared enterprise, however trivial. It may involve presence that is interactive, analytical, sequential, and linear, a presence that appears to be largely left-brain-generated; one that involves intentionality. It became clear, however, that there was a third *level*, or perhaps *quality*, of presence and I came to think of it as *radical presence*. It seemed to occur less frequently and not necessarily as a product of conscious intent. Could it be the factor responsible for my sense of bonding with those two patients? That deeper level of connection appeared to entail body, mind, and something more – something more deeply focused, something less concrete, something that might be unconscious, something involving that less easily defined variable thought of as "spirit," however that term is understood. My contact with these two young men appeared to exemplify this third category of relating. Perhaps identification was a key unconscious determinant. It seemed that, when this deeper connection occurs, it takes one to a different place, a place with an enhanced potential for a sense of wholeness, support, and acceptance, *whatever* the treatment outcome. It appeared to offer a sort of "brothers-in-arms" experience of *union* with the other.

As already noted, I had, on occasion, experienced such radical presence and its sense of silent, focused depth while drawing or listening to music. Indeed, such unexpected moments had, on occasion, gifted my life from early on: as a teenager, on seeing – really *seeing* – the Rocky Mountains in all their breathtaking majesty for the first time; on *seeing*, as a teenager, a lone stranger sweeping the floor at the Ottawa train station; on *seeing* the totally arresting expression on contralto Marian Anderson's face during her Queen's concert, and subsequently, on viewing the arresting photograph of her taken by Yousuf Karsh. Years later I would witness radical presence in experiencing Jean Vanier's demeanour as he *listened* to a critical questioner; and again in the ethereal grace of a solitary long-distance runner on the shore of Norway's Nordfjord.

For me, Canadian songwriter, poet, and novelist Leonard Cohen expressed radical presence with his customary deft turn of phrase in his song "Love Itself." He had found himself immersed in a state of profound realization on encountering the morning sun coming through his bedroom window. He saw the arresting mystery of the moment. He was describing the awakened awareness I had felt that morning as a teenager when I wakened to find the sun streaming through *my* bedroom window. Cohen wrote:

The light came through the window,
Straight from the sun above,
And so inside my little room
There plunged the rays of Love.

In streams of light I clearly saw
The dust you seldom see,
Out of which the Nameless makes
A name for one like me.[3]

Perhaps it is particularly when the experience is unexpected that we find such a personal confrontation with the transcendent potential at hand, a focused awareness that can move us into unconscious identification, timeless silence, and sense of union. Perhaps the underlying mechanism has to do with leaving ego behind and thus an unanticipated shift from *self* toward *Self*.[4] Enhanced right-brain processing appears to account for this cognitive shift, but it has been suggested that such perception can be purposefully developed.[5] The recognition of such levels of perception and an accompanying sense of "truth" has been documented from as early as the writing of the Upanishads in 800–500 BCE.[6] A final observation is that radical presence tends to dissolve with an attempt to analyze it.

JEAN VANIER

A brief newspaper item caught my eye: "Jean Vanier to Speak at Loyola Chapel." Shortly before that, I had come across a magazine article that opened breezily with the assertion, "If you don't worship Jean Vanier, you have never met him." *That's a little much!* I thought, with more than a touch of skepticism bordering on disdain.

The son of the nineteenth governor general of Canada,[7] Jean Vanier had, as a young man, served in both the Royal and Canadian navies, obtained a PHD in philosophy at the Institut Catholique de Paris, and taught philosophy at the University of Toronto. In 1964, at the age of thirty-six, he started the first L'Arche community for persons with intellectual disability, in Trosly-Breuil, France, and in 1971 he co-founded Faith and Light, an international movement for people with disabilities and their families and friends. Over the ensuing years, this universally revered Catholic theologian, philosopher, writer, and humanitarian had been a catalyst for transformation and awakened living in countless lives. I cannot recall how much of this I knew as Faye and I made our way into the already crowded Loyola Chapel.

Perhaps six hundred people had already gathered in the roomy, high-ceilinged sanctuary as we took our seats halfway up the centre aisle, on the left. There was an air of anticipation, a faint but happy buzz. Twenty or so animated jean-clad youths in their early twenties were clustered on the floor between the front row of seats and the simple wooden chair and table awaiting the speaker. You could feel a quiet energy in the room.

Our speaker entered accompanied by two or three others who, a few steps later, had melted into the crowd. A hush swept across the room as he slipped onto the chair behind the table. It was then that the young people on the floor in front of him started to sing – softly but joyfully. He had glanced out at us in the audience, a faint smile forming, but with those first notes his head turned to gaze down at the source. They had taken him by surprise with their L'Arche song. His expression conveyed delight and warm recognition, indeed, a profound presence and the tenderest love. In that interaction, they and he had clearly become the only ones inhabiting their world. It was a moment filled with unexpected grace. His radical presence was evident.

Jean Vanier appeared to be about 6'3" or so. He was stooped, an acquired posture one suspected, earned through a life-time of listening attentively to the words of those of more modest stature. His large, wonderfully craggy features were crowned by unruly white hair. His clothes were worn, his shirt open at the neck to reveal a shapeless T-shirt, his cardigan baggy and threadbare, his smile infectious, his clear eyes totally engaging.

He spoke without notes, telling us about L'Arche and the friends with whom he lived in community. He spoke about the plight of the handicapped who have been marginalized and who desperately need to feel loved and appreciated. He described their work together, and their play, the lessons they had taught him, the challenges they have faced together. He laughed about his own feet of clay, the bubbling up of anger which on occasion has confronted him with his limitations and reminded him of his own frailty. He reflected about the occasion he was mistaken for a panhandler in the Paris Underground.

There was no evangelical grandstanding, no bombast from on high. On the other hand, there was no watered-down liberal vagueness of belief. Everything about him made it unmistakably clear that his daily guide was the Christ, the risen Jesus of Nazareth. It was as though he was talking about his partner on a travelling-light backpacking journey through life. He was joyful but deadly serious, humble yet self-assured, openly a seeker yet certain of his path, simple of speech yet brilliantly articulate.

I unexpectedly found myself realizing that I would follow this man anywhere. I trusted his judgment and the depth of his insight. I felt the nakedness of being exposed by the real thing yet fully accepted for who I was. Having attended the session with no particular expectations, I was totally amazed.

His comments complete, we were invited to take part in an open dialogue. When Jean had been speaking, I was struck by the all-pervasive ambience of caring and intimacy that is enabled when pretense leaves the room. Now, in the question period, it was the same during several brief exchanges.

At one point, the man across the aisle from Faye and me stood up. He disdainfully waved away the proffered microphone and with blazing eyes and pulsating temporal arteries shouted, "Vanier, I know you!" (He may *not* have been shouting but it felt like he was.) His tone was vicious and completely unexpected. He continued, "I know you Christians! You think the rest of us are damned! Now what do you say to that?!"

There was total stunned silence in the room. I suddenly felt cold.

Now, I must admit that, being such a highly evolved person and all, my reaction was *kill!* I mean, the *idea!* – the very *idea!* – that someone, *anyone*, would *dare* speak to *my friend* like that! Yes, it is true, I suspect that even then I had already presumed myself a colleague if not part of his inner circle! In my mind, he had already moved from total stranger to a friend I would risk everything for. My withering gaze spun away from the questioner and returned to Jean. I was enraged, yet fascinated. How would he respond?

He was looking at his questioner. Deeply. *Looking!* He was, it seemed, radically present. He wasn't looking at his buttoned-down suit, or his face, or his apparent culture of origin. None of that. He was looking, it seemed, at his soul. The rest of us in that crowded room had disappeared. I realize now how misguided, romantic, or perhaps plain daft that sounds. But I had never seen one person look at another like that. Totally calm, but with the respectful intensity of one who takes seriously and respectfully an accusation levelled at him. He remained silent. It was similar to how he had looked at the young folk sitting around his chair when they began singing softly to him as he arrived. It was, it seemed, the second out-of-time moment of the evening. Then he spoke.

"Well" ... he paused, bringing us all into his present moment of non-judgmental calm (that was the sense I had of it), "let me comment on that by saying that in India we have a number of l'Arche communities. They are run by a friend of mine whose name is Dr Reddy. He is a Hindu. When we are together one of the things we like most to do is to pray together ... Does that answer your question?" My neighbour had returned to his seat.

The next question was from a lovely young woman across the aisle and near the front. I remember her near-black hair. She looked serious, earnest, somewhat distressed, intent. It was clear that she felt she was having a private conversation with a trusted mentor. And she was.

"Please tell me about prayer. I pray but I feel no one is there. Nothing happens. I feel I am making something out of nothing. I'm simply making it all up."

Again, Jean looked at her. He *looked*, at depth, in silence. I don't know how long it was – a second? an eternity? He answered using the metaphor of making coffee in a percolator. He reminded us that at first the water is clear and then, slowly, the colour deepens "until it is that full rich texture that we treasure and had hoped for." The gathering ended and we returned home surrounded be a sense of newness; refreshed by the experience of the unique blend of faith, intellect, assuredness, and humility that we had witnessed. I wondered when our paths might once again cross.

Years later, having become a close friend of Jean's over the intervening decades, I would be humbled by a deeper understanding of the woundedness that invariably affects us on our journey as we make our way from ego-dominated self to the full potential of our imagined Self which, we pray, will reflect a fuller union with the transcendent, in spite of our innate brokenness. In 2019, at the end of Jean's remarkable life, disclosure of details regarding his personal neediness raised universal concern and widespread disillusionment. In coming to grips with this devastating drenching in unanticipated reality, I found that it brought to mind the Nazarene who, observed, "Let him who is without sin cast the first stone." And again I saw the expression on His face as Jesus made His way through the thronging crowd west of Capernaum and suddenly paused to ask, "Who touched me?" and then looked back over His shoulder at the woman with menorrhagia who had just "touched the hem of his garment." I imagined that His eyes were deeply focused on her, even as, centuries on, they would be focused on Jean, on me, indeed, on each of us, as we attempt to deal with the infirmities that haunt our uncertain path in the face of all-too-limited personal coping resources.

A LITHUANIAN TRANSURETHRAL PROSTATIC RESECTION

It was in the fall of 1971 that a phone call was relayed into my office by the secretary. "Dr Mount," said a heavily accented voice, "I am Dr Petras Tulevicius, a urologist from Vilnius, Lithuania. I am here in Montreal visiting my uncle Jurgis Janavicius. You will remove his prostate tomorrow. I would like to ask you if I could attend you to watch. I would be very grateful." Indeed, Mr Janavicius was booked for a transurethral prostatic resection late the next morning. I invited Dr Tulevicius to my office for a cup of coffee.

An outgoing, sturdy man, my height, but half a decade older, with open Slavic features, alert watchful eyes, and an unkempt field of rust-brown hair, pumped my hand. "I am Petras. You call me Peter."

Born in Lithuania, where he now practised, he had trained in Moscow. A relaxed chat about his work revealed that, although his training was highly regarded in both Russia and Lithuania, he had never seen a transurethral prostatic resection. Their surgical equipment, he explained, was simple, their resources limited. He would, he stressed, greatly appreciate observing his uncle's surgery. To his utter fascination, that took place the next day and we became friends.

Before he returned to Vilnius, Peter and I watched all the MSKCC films and shared in an animated discussion in response to the stream of questions they generated. A visit and meal in our home led to a day trip to Ottawa together and my procuring for him a copy of the current standard urology textbook. Our friendship had deepened.

As we discussed his years in Russia, I mentioned that Faye and I would be visiting Moscow in the coming year. We would be travelling with an adventuresome ad hoc group calling itself the Geography Club of Montreal. It included Meds '63 classmates Don Pringle and Terry Porter, their wives, Bev and Andrea, and the Wiegands, Fred, a Royal Vic surgical colleague, and his wife, Helen.

It was 1971. The mere idea of visiting Russia was exotic. The Cold War was at its height. None of us knew *anyone* who had actually visited the Union of Soviet Socialist Republics (USSR). The trip promised to be exciting, if not a little daunting. We had jumped at the chance.

"But, Ball," Peter exclaimed, "that is wonderful. You must speak at the Moscow Cancer Institute where I trained.[8] I will meet you in Moscow and take you there. And, Ball, I will arrange for you to show your films and I will translate the soundtracks into Russian. You will show them. They will be amazed. Ball, they have seen nothing like them."

WHIT CALLS

It was Wednesday afternoon, 1 March, 1972. I was working my way through a light office schedule when the secretary asked if I could take a call from Dr Whitmore. We spoke briefly and then hung up with a promise to continue our discussion by mail. He had just offered me a position at Memorial.

From a purely professional standpoint, the privilege of working with Whit would be unrivalled. Harry Grabstald described joining the MSKCC attending staff and working with Whit as being "the best fifteen-year residency anyone has ever had."[9] Furthermore, the low rate of oncology referrals generated to date, the uncertainties around Quebec nationalism, and the questions generated by the newly implemented Medicare system all added weight to Whit's offer. Collaboration with Whit on several research and writing projects continued over the ensuing months. I promised him a final decision by February 1973.

MY SECOND HOCKEY GAME?

The official announcement was in late April 1972. Canadian negotiators returning from the International Ice Hockey Federation (IIHF) meetings in Prague announced that the Soviets had agreed to play an eight-game hockey series that would, for the first time, feature the best Canadian (NHL) players against their best players, the initial four games to be played in Canada, then, during September 1972, the final games in the USSR. In the past, IIHF rules had prevented Canada's best from international competition on the grounds that they were "professional" (the best in the USSR were indeed equally "professional" by all criteria but considered "amateur" by the IIHF). Thus, it had been twenty years since Canada had won an Olympic gold medal and eleven since winning a world hockey championship. During that same interval Soviet teams had won three gold medals and ten world championships. The near-mystical Canadian belief that we develop the finest players in the world would be tested for the first time.[10]

THE PERENNIAL UNEXPECTED NEWNESS OF THE *PLACE*

How invigorating to be creeping once again along the rutted road winding through the trees toward our mainland boathouse. It had been a year. The car, packed to the roof, was caressed by the branches at each spruce-scented curve. My companions smiled expectantly, in silent anticipation: Wren sitting beside Faye; Chris beaming excitedly as he peered in all directions simultaneously; Czar Nicholas, our Samoyed, with nose out the window, drinking deeply of this new world. The pungent summer air brought a personalized mix of memories to each of us.

We pulled into the overgrown parking area. The trusty Glaspar bobbed lazily at the dock. Out of the corner of my eye, I caught Nicki studying a grass snake slithering noiselessly under the weathered boardwalk at the boathouse and a small frog retreating onto a lily pad. The boat key and barn swallows were in their habitual resting places. The Island was waiting.

How blessed we felt. Gulping air and spray, we sped toward the island, then, leaning to the left in a great sweep, we arched playfully past the guesthouse before making a graceful turn to the right around the point. The motor roared and cavitated in exuberance as we kicked up a glorious wake with that last tight turn and then wallowed in our own backwash, coming to a sudden stop at the dock.

The *Place*. Joy. Jim, as promised, had put out the full "three section" dock that summer. A rush of familiarity overwhelmed as each minute aspect of this beloved reality told us that we were home. I glanced at my life-jacketed children, everyone smiling, lost in thought. Chris manfully secured our mooring.

This is what Canada is all about: this mysterious, living lake with its shimmering array of ever-changing blues and sparkling diamonds;

this symphony of shadow and light streaming from the brilliance of the sky; this lovely tapestry of a thousand greens. To be surrounded by this peace-filled tranquility again: it seemed all-new! We would be there for two weeks.

Cutting down the towering great white pine out back with my chainsaw seemed the thing to do. It would cure the dampness in Mother and Dad's icehouse bedroom, I argued. (Boys with new toys *must* be boys!) Two options confronted me: to stand "here" or "there" for the execution. I chose "there." Watching it all with her usual assessing eye, Faye stopped me, and the roaring saw, with a single index-finger stroke across her neck.

"What?"

She suggested I move from "there" to "here." Prior to finishing the last cut, I did.

Two seconds later, the massive severed trunk lay quivering in the locked-in confines of "there," exactly where my head had been. Faye had just saved my life. She always was a careful observer.

"Where Were You in '72?"
A Cold War Experience

Nyet ... Nyet!!!

Russian hosts (repeatedly)

Da, Da, Ca Na Da!! Nyet, Nyet Soviet!!

Canadian fans

English is *such* an ugly language!

Professor Marinbach,
Moscow Cancer Institute

Ball, one must learn to be a strong Soviet man.

Petras Tulevicius

The precedent-setting Canada–Russia hockey series of 1972 lay ahead: four games in Canada to be followed by four games in the USSR.

As any Canadian hockey fan that summer would tell you, "It isn't *just* a game, you know! It isn't only about who invented it, or who does it best. It's a battle of two ways of life *and* two ways of playing the game. It's about our system against theirs, and, for once, it will be our *best*, against their *best*! It isn't about diplomacy. The cards are on the table: we don't trust them; they resent us. They dislike everything we stand for – *greedy, spoiled, lazy capitalists*. We're going to show them! And it will be history! Years from now our grandchildren will probably ask, 'Where were you in '72?' They call this a Cold War! Well, I suspect it'll get a lot hotter come September!"

How seriously did both sides take it? Prime Minister Pierre Trudeau dropped the puck for game 1 in Montreal and met the plane when Team

Canada returned from the USSR as the series ended. Communist Party Secretary Leonid Brezhnev, Soviet Premier Alexei Kosygin, and Soviet President Nikolai Podgorny as well as a large Red Army contingent in dress uniforms attended game 5, the first game on Russian ice. Years later, Canadian team leader Phil Esposito commented, on looking back, "I'm not too proud of it, but there's no doubt in my mind that I would have killed those sons of bitches to win. And it scares me."[1]

Miraculously, the dates for this historic showdown dovetailed with our existing Geography Club of Montreal plans to visit the USSR. We would attend game 5 of the series, the first game in the Russian leg of this international showdown!

Sportswriters were in awe when the names of Canadian team members were announced. The lineup was breathtaking. Superstars all! "Perhaps the best hockey team ever assembled," most agreed.

As the neatly coifed, blue-blazer-clad Russian players deplaned to file quietly into Montreal's Dorval airport on 30 August, they looked somehow vulnerable, like schoolboys. The official Soviet statement was, "We have come here to learn." The long-haired, super-cool Canadian team was relaxed and confident, with perhaps a hint of arrogance.

An estimated twelve million Canadians watched game 1 on 2 September in Montreal. With the final buzzer, it was Russia 7, Canada 3. The country had been rudely awakened. Humbled! Shocked! We had learned some new words in Russian: Tretiak, Yakushev, Mikhailov, and Kharlamov, among others.

Team Canada won a rough-and-tumble game 2, but sportscasters accused Canada of poor sportsmanship if not "attempted manslaughter." Game 3 ended in a tie. In game 4, at Vancouver on 8 September, emotions were running high. The final score was Russia 5, Canada 3. The four games played in Canada had ended with Russia leading by one game, and as the Vancouver game ended more than fifteen thousand Canadian fans heckled and booed our team, shouting obscenities.

Friday, 22 September. Our cramped Montreal–to–Moscow Aeroflot flight with its indifferent and scowling stewardesses lasted a tedious, submission-inducing, eight-and-a half sleepless hours. It was ghastly. We arrived stiff-legged with swollen feet and ankles at 2:30 P.M. and were herded to an austere room featuring a platoon of grim-faced customs officers. All interactions with customs agents were intentionally threatening: their expressions fixed; their demeanour rigid. My urology teaching films for use during my lectures at the Moscow Cancer Institute were confiscated. "Nyet!!" I could not take them with me. The formal letters of invitation were of no use. It was, after all, the Cold

War. Distrust if not frank dislike met us at every turn. This gruelling rite of passage lasted two hours, managing in the process to strangle slowly all vestiges of endemic Canadian humility, largesse, and "after you, Alphonse" goodwill. Indeed, our host's unmistakable hostility was numbing and the most benevolent among us gradually acquired a frosty, subdued mien.

Any lightening of mood was dampened further in motoring from airport to city as we gazed at the grim bleakness passing us in the gathering shadows. Row on row of unlit tenement buildings dotted the fields at random. Even the apparently "new" buildings, with their stark, dirty-yellow unpainted concrete walls, appeared to have aged five to ten years in construction. The near empty road carried an occasional ancient grey green, snub-nosed truck but very few cars. An occasional wood-frame cottage with wooden fence and water pump in the yard passed below our darkened windows. Bent women of a certain age worked alongside men as labourers. Uniformed soldiers in high black boots stood in random groups, ignoring the drab, faceless, but warmly dressed citizens who stared blankly at us as our bus rolled endlessly on, a sense of decay and overwhelming decrepitude permeating everything.

Moscow. The imposing Hotel Russia faced St Basil Cathedral on Red Square. We were dispersed to our rooms and then regimented into a cavernous dining room for a rapid-service supper that included cabbage salad, cold meats, light beer, and kafé or ché, at tables set for four to six. In the wake of our hellish flight, we were convinced it was the best meal we had ever tasted! Now, on to the Luzhniki arena.

Game 5: 22 September, Moscow. "Can you believe it? We're in Moscow for game 5! Can this be real?!"

Night had fallen as our bus stopped at a deserted park. We disembarked to see an apparently deserted building shrouded in darkness. Could it be the fourteen-thousand-seat Luzhniki Palace of Sports? No crowds, no lights, no one selling scalpers' tickets or team jerseys. It all seemed somewhat disorienting in that brisk, rather cool night air as we headed into the shadows.

We reached the arena to find hundreds of Canadians milling at the locked doors chanting GO CANADA GO! Outraged army officers appeared from nowhere, shaking clenched fists on high and roaring, "Nyet!! Nyet!!!" No one listened. The chanting continued.

Once inside the nondescript building, the solemn attendants examined our tickets and nodded at our Intourist chaperone as the world of empty shadows became a well-lit hockey arena, full to capacity, expectant, but unlike anything we could have imagined.

We had entered near one end of the rink. There, beginning to our immediate left and sweeping around the end of the ice and along the far side to round the distant end, each numbered plywood seat was filled with an immobile, silent mass from rink to roof – a sea of motionless heads. *Are they alive?* They were all clothed the same, with ties and olive green (or was that grey?) overcoats. Few women. If alive, they seemed to be waiting obediently for permission to breathe, or perhaps a signal of some kind. They were expressionless. *Strange! Not a sound, not a movement. Very strange!* We later learned that they were Communist Party officials who had displaced the *real* Russian hockey fans.

In contrast to that amorphous mass, which accounted for roughly three-quarters of this Alice-in-Wonderland gathering, the image in our Canadian quarter (or less) of the stands was startlingly different.

The silent, stolid mass across from us was replaced by a gyrating, throbbing, flag-waving, screaming, trumpet-blowing (*Bra da ... da da da ... da da, da da, ... da da!!*), sign-thrusting ("Ville de Laval"; "Together"; "From Timmins to Moscow"; "Go Frank and Pete"; "Sarnia Is Here, Whitey"; "Mission Impossible" ...) crowd, with an explosion of red and white and red again, scarlet maple leaves on white *Go Canada* shirts, rainbow streamers on hats, and a chorus of shouts and anthems that kept erupting at near-pain-threshold volume in spurts of inebriated enthusiasm: *O Canada, our home and native* ... The trumpet began again (*Bra da ... da da da!!*). I felt a passing spasm of guilt, a feeling that we should meet our hosts with a solemnity that matched their own. *Goodness! This is embarrassing! Heavens, we are our country's ambassadors. We are Canadian!*

It was when the trumpet next sounded that I realized we were headed for trouble. Individual army officers took a careful fix on the solitary trumpeter and made their way into the stands to silence him. The scowling officers arrived in haste, but the trumpet had already disappeared, to re-emerge farther along and several rows back. *Bra da ... da da da ...*

They now were furious, roaring, "Nyet! Nyet!" as their numbers increased and they closed in, to a chorus of boos and yells from our Canadian section. An inebriated defence force of Canadian fans started to close in around our musician. Cooler heads reminded each other that we were supposed to be goodwill ambassadors, but few if any heeded the call to reason.

The Red Army caught "trumpet-man" and disappeared under the stands. (Later inquiry revealed that in a back room he was significantly roughed up and his ample head of hair shaved off.) The Canadian response was now loud and clear, TO HELL WITH YOU! LEAVE HIM

ALONE, YOU BASTARDS. YOU MAY LIVE IN A PRISON, BUT WE DON'T! The atmosphere was raw with tension and the game hadn't started.

Rumours of discontent and low team morale had accompanied Team Canada to Moscow. Three disgruntled players had quit, others seemed to be taking the whole thing too lightly, causing teammates to react. There was a suggestion that some Team Canada players seemed to miss the fan adulation experienced at home. All in all, things didn't look hopeful and we Canadians in the stands were well beyond taking all this objectively. It really *was* war and it didn't look promising from our vantage point.

Studying the faces in the stands across from us, it was not hard to see contempt and something else – an accompanying sense of veiled fear and hostility. Another trumpet! The army started up into the stands once more, causing three thousand Canadians to stand as one and give a spontaneous full-volume rendering of the national anthem. O CANADA, OUR HOME AND ... It was a moving moment.

While some of us were embarrassed at our collective behaviour, there was tacit agreement that they weren't going to take another Canadian from the stands without a serious discussion!

At this point, the official pre-game opening ceremonies got underway and things calmed down. Young girls with flowers for each player skated onto the ice as the players on both teams, standing in lines that stretched across the rink, were introduced. It was Phil Esposito's turn. Our leader! His name rang out and he began his out-and-back bow, caught his skate on something in the ice surface, and unceremoniously fell flat on his face. The audience gasped. The enemy laughed. It was embarrassing! Excruciating! *Dear God, Espo!* For a moment, we Canadians hoped the earth would open and swallow us. Our leader! He sprang to his feet and, in front of both teams and some fourteen thousand others, made an elaborate, exaggerated, sweeping bow before Brezhnev! The Canadians stood, cheering Phil, applauding, each of us pretending that it wasn't one of the worst moments of our life.

I like to think that was when the momentum came back. We were a long way from home. The eleven thousand Soviets were now shouting encouragement to their team, but they were drowned out by the three thousand Canadians, "GO CANADA GO," and it was game on!

An energized Team Canada was on the ice that night: working as a seasoned unit, forechecking, backchecking, forcing the Soviets into mistakes. At the end of the second period, it was Canada 3, Russia 0.

During the intermission I noticed the legendary, thoughtful, ever low-key sports commentator and philosopher Howie Meeker walking pensively back and forth alone and walked over to where he was pacing. He looked concerned.

"Hi, Mr Meeker, Bal Mount from Montreal. What do you think? You look concerned."

"Well," he responded, "Golly, I'm afraid we're easing off. The Russians are coming on. If this continues we could be in trouble."

"We'll keep our fingers crossed," I responded. "Great to meet you." He waved, still looking pensive.

With the end of the third period it was Russia 5, Canada 4. Howie Meeker had called it. The Soviets were now up by *two* games! The whole thing had slipped away from us! We would have to win *all three* subsequent games! *Yah, right!! To date we have only won one of five!*

Peter Tulevicius was flying in from Lithuania expressly for my Moscow Cancer Institute lecture. Thus, following a day filled with failed attempts to make contact, I was delighted to hear his sonorous "BALL" ringing from the balcony above us during the intermission in Saturday evening's performance of *Rigoletto* at the Kremlin. He had guessed that we might be there.

Our Geography Club group was booked to depart on Sunday, the next day. With the assistance of the Moscow Cancer Institute's chief of urology, a Professor Marinbach, plans for us to retrieve my films from the customs agents were finalized while Faye and I rebooked our departure to Leningrad for late Monday.

The Institute of Experimental and Clinical Oncology, USSR Academy of Medical Sciences, is impressive in its size and imposing formality. Peter and I were greeted by Marinbach and eight or ten colleagues who joined us for morning ward rounds. Another thirty or so planned to participate in the film discussions during my afternoon lecture and film session. They all knew some English; Marinbach was fluent; several colleagues interpreted, as required.

Ward rounds were to include visits to several four-bed rooms and two open wards with approximately twenty beds each. With initial hallway introductions to my Russian colleagues complete, we got off to a somewhat rocky start when Marinbach asked how we had enjoyed *Rigoletto*.

"A fine production," I enthused, then adding, "My wife and I were interested to hear it sung in Russian. In Canada, we generally stage operas in the language in which they were written, so I have previously only heard it in Italian." The comment was innocent enough. I was truly interested in performance traditions in Russia and thus wasn't prepared for Marinbach's response.

"I can understand you preferring other languages," he intoned with obvious condescension, "English is *such* an ugly language!" His colleagues' attention sharpened, betraying both their understanding of English and their interest in how I would respond.

"As for that," I laughed, "I believe our rationale lies more in a concern for the composer's original intent than other considerations. Nevertheless, your comment brings to mind my other reaction to last night's performance. 'English is ugly?' I must say, I found it rather unsettling to have Rigoletto charging about the stage exclaiming, 'Nyet!' 'Nyet!'... Ha Ha."

Was my response an example of emotional contagion spreading from the Luzhniki arena? I couldn't be sure but Marinbach's barbs continued all day, making for a particularly lively visit.

As we were about to enter the first ward, Miranbach stopped. "By the way, Dr Mount, when we are with the patients please do not mention the word *cancer*. Many of our patients understand English and it would upset them. For example, one of the men in this room is a shepherd from the mountains and his English is very good."

"Professor Marinbach, you surprise me. Are you suggesting that these men and women have been admitted to a facility called the Moscow Cancer Institute, yet don't know their diagnosis or recognize even the possibility of having cancer? Do you not feel that it would ease their anxiety if you could talk to them openly and supportively about their condition?

"They should not be told."

"Dr Marinbach, if *you* had cancer, wouldn't you want to know?" He blanched.

"No. I would want my doctors to know, but I would not want to know."

"You know, Dr Marinbach, I find that hard to understand. Uncertainty breeds anxiety and anxiety paralyzes coping mechanisms, whereas *lessening* uncertainty supports coping. I had testicular cancer when I was twenty-four and found it important, critical in fact, to be able to talk to my doctors about it."

The circle of colleagues around us was intent but silent. Marinbach paled even more. With an expression suggesting something between shock and frank fear, he responded, "Oh, Dr Mount, you must not say that. Don't ever say that."

At the bedside, I felt dismayed as I chatted briefly with the intelligent shepherd, sensing his isolation as he played a game imposed on him by his fear-filled doctors.

With Peter providing a Russian translation of their soundtracks, our four MSKCC films seemed well received. Having trained at the Moscow Institute, Peter was familiar with their lagging surgical approaches and limited resources. Each of these films, he had assured me, would present dazzling new ground and I looked forward to having the rich exchange of ideas that had followed similar sessions in Canada, the United States, and Germany. Regrettably, that was not to be. Within minutes of starting the first film, Marinbach commenced a running commentary in Russian. Only later did Peter inform me of the critical, clearly defensive tone of his remarks. Any meaningful dialogue with his underlings had thus been prevented. Peter was embarrassed.

Game 6: 24 September, Moscow. With our Geography Club friends now in Leningrad, Faye and I watched game 6 at the hotel with a group of Czech factory workers and a handful of Russian hotel guests who drifted in as the game proceeded under the scrutiny of the officious, unsmiling czarina for the floor whose task it was to survey all comings and goings. The Czechs were cheering for Canada prior to the Russians joining us, and, to the Russians' surprise and our delight, that continued through to the hard- fought 3–2 Canadian victory. We were congratulated on the win by our new Czech friends and gave them our Canadian flag, to their delight.

Time spent with Peter in Moscow and Leningrad afforded a glimpse of Russian life that extended beyond the controlled Intourist perspective that was otherwise our prescribed norm. On the positive side, the stunning Moscow subway system left us humbled. Cathedral-like stations were scrubbed clean and rich in red, white, and grey marble, their vaulted, frescoed ceilings resplendent with murals of heroic figures at work, war, and sports. Their halls displayed larger-than-life bronze statues: women and girls, men and boys, championing their country's socialist values. The escalators ("Stand to the right; pass on the left, нравиться") that transported us down to these monuments to national pride were near-vertical, fast, and very, very long. The trains were solid and, like Montreal's, quieter than those in New York, Paris, and London. Passengers sat quietly reading, without making eye contact or talking. "It is considered rude to interrupt the thoughts of others."

In Leningrad, we were taken to the austere October Hotel. At the registration desk, Peter spoke for the three of us and Faye and I were given a room without delay, though clusters of semi-petrified humanity who had been there long before our arrival remained immobile in the lobby. Asking Peter why the others were left waiting. He replied, "Ball, you are so naive. You must learn to be a strong Soviet man."

Passing his room en route to ours, he stopped, "Here is mine. I shall leave you here, Ball. I shall knock on your door in a few minutes and we shall go for a walk."

The door to Peter's room stood ajar. The ends of two single beds were visible through the twilight within. Two shoeless feet protruded over the end of the bed closest to us. He was a man of colour, a giant of a man, judging by those legs. He was snoring heavily. "But Peter, there must be some mistake, the room is already occupied."

"Ball," Peter smiled, pushing his bag past the man's feet, 'You are so naive!"

Our room was simply furnished but clean. Faye decided to stay behind, writing cards to family back home while Peter and I set out on the walk he had planned.

Stepping into the murky shadows of a cool September Leningrad night, Peter stated meaningfully, "Ball, you will see everything." His student years in Moscow were less than idyllic; he was proudly Lithuanian. But his comments on Russia and the Communist system were always circumspect. He believed, it seemed, that the walls had ears and he was particularly guarded when we were in a building, *any* building.

Peter was a practising Roman Catholic and his time-honoured Lithuanian practice of his faith involved a mix of smoke and incense, confession and indulgence buying, candles and veneration that I, as a Canadian Protestant, found foreign, if not bizarre. We relished these differences between us and they became an enjoyable jousting point in our growing mutual affection. "Peter, you Lithuanians pray too much! That rosary of yours isn't a rabbit's foot you know!"

"Ball, if we have time, I shall teach you to pray, but I expect it might take a long time."

We soon found ourselves on a broad, deserted street lined by old stone buildings in total darkness. Two very drunk students weaved past us, then stopped. My London Fog raincoat had given me away. They were anxious to talk.

"You speak English? We speak English. Talk to us in English. Where are you from? … Ah, Canada. Canada good. Have you ever seen New York City? What is it like? What do you think of our politics? What about Czechoslovakia and Hungary? USSR is like this," he drew a circle in the air. "We shall never be able to leave. USA and Canada are very good."

Peter was restless. He interrupted, suggesting that we must leave. "Come, Ball."

"But, Peter, I should talk to them. It is important." Now Peter was visibly agitated.

"Ball, come! You do not understand. You cannot help." He chuckled, "The funny thing is, they think I am KGB, sent to keep an eye on you."

We came to an open square in semi-darkness. It was lined by more large, stone, shadow-encased buildings. There were a few more people than before – alone, and in twos or threes. Many of them had been drinking. I found myself filled with a sense of oppressive heaviness. It was about 10:30 or 11:00 P.M. Peter took me by the arm, "Come Ball, I want to show you something."

He led us down the cobblestone alley that skirted the hulking building in front of us. As we rounded its distant corner, the scene opened unexpectedly. Directly in front of us was a train station with several sets of railway tracks disappearing into the distant blackness. Each was lined on both sides by a twenty-foot-wide asphalt walkway. These endless paths had been transformed into vast islands of humanity. Teeming thousands, it seemed. Silent and immobile. Most were sitting, a few were threading their way through the motionless crowd. Many were very old. All appeared stooped – with age, or cares, or poverty, or hunger, or alcohol. A few were muttering sporadically among themselves. One or two youths were softly singing – one had a guitar. Everywhere there were bundles of food in net sacs – cabbages, potatoes, I could not make out the other contents. A few carried scrawny, subdued chickens. And here and there, a bundle of clothes or a battered suitcase had been tucked away.

A ponderous antique steam engine bearing a red star was parked on the track just beside us, its elephantine procession of empty cars trailing off into the darkness. It was green, the wheels and cow catcher, red. *Straight out of Doctor Zhivago!* I expected to see Julie Christie and Omar Sharif descend the worn stairs of the nearby coach ... or at the very least Boris Pasternak. It looked as though it had been parked there for decades. The apparently carved-in-stone throng seated along its sides was motionless, frozen in time, oblivious, ignoring or unaware of its improbable presence.

To our left, the ground floor of the dimly lit building was open, revealing a vast waiting room containing row upon row of benches, each filled with elderly, grimly silent, waxy grey figures; they, too, stretched on and on. *This is a railway station, for heaven's sake*, I thought, as if repeating the obvious to myself would make this silent tableau more believable.

Crumpled and unshaven, with matted hair, mended fraying clothes, and vacant stares, they were waiting. We made our way through the cavernous room. Peter leaned to my ear: "Ball, do you see? Every month it is the same awful food they buy and line up for, hours on end. Endless lines for expensive goods. They have to come. There is no food for them in the country. Use your eyes, Ball. Use your ears and nose. Think. Ball, you are so naive! See that strong Soviet man." He was small, elderly and frail, gnarled like an old tree. "It is good for him to sit up waiting hour after hour. He must be strong ... And, Ball, look at her." Just beside us as we passed through the rows was a bulky, stooped, white-haired woman, heavy-set, bundled, expressionless. She looked to be in her eighties but may well have been much younger. She sat hunched, staring vacantly straight ahead. "Ball, it is good for her to sit up all night on that bench. It will make her strong. You must learn to suffer, Ball, learn to endure. Don't worry about the drunks. They are everywhere. The police take them away ... and the young people have nowhere to make love. Ball, you must be a strong Soviet man."

Silent and deep in thought, we emerged back onto the station platform. At that moment a massive steam engine slowly pulled in, with its red star and all its time-worn green and red significance exuding a sense of restrained power and overwhelming fatigue as it uttered its final chugs, then exhaled. One last shudder, blast of steam, and squeal of brakes gave way to silence.

All was quiet, the stillness deafening. Then, slowly, the silent mass of waiting humanity rose as one and oozed further out onto the platform, only to wait once more, and wait again, for this long-cursed and prayed-for monster to take them home.

It was Tuesday; game 7 was pending. But first, a flying "group visit" to St Petersburg's State Hermitage Museum on the banks of the Neva River. The former residence of the Russian tsars, the Hermitage was now home to one of the world's most important collections of priceless art. "Unfortunately, we have only time for a brief visit," our Intourist guide cheerily proclaimed, "but it will give you a taste." The collection, she explained, was initiated in 1764 by Empress Catherine the Great and comprised close to three million paintings, sculptures, and other artifacts. Housed in this vast maze of corridors and halls was art from across the world and down the centuries, from ancient Egypt to twentieth-century Western Europe. The paintings included a dizzying array of masterpieces. Among those of personal interest, I knew from my earlier reading, were works by Titian, Veronese, Raphael, Leonardo da Vinci, Tintoretto, Valázquez, Michelangelo, El Greco, van Dyck, Rubens, Rembrandt, Bruegel the Elder, Ter Borch, Gainsborough, Reynolds, and, in addition, stunning works by seemingly countless Russian artists that I, in my ignorance, had never heard of. And there were also Impressionist and post-Impressionist works by Renoir, Monet, Manet, Van Gogh, Gauguin, Pissarro, Cézanne, Sisley, Degas, Matisse, and Kandinsky. Sadly, however, we saw only a handful, and then only briefly, in passing. "We must move on!" we were told. The notion of racing past this stunning feast was dizzying. I was agitated and told Faye that I needed to leave. A "brief visit," the guide had said?! *Brief?!* This rushed sacrilege was total madness! "We must move on," we were told.

Game 7: 26 September, Moscow. Tense, we settled in front of the TV provided by the hotel. Silence. Apprehension. We were informed that the Team Canada dressing room was papered with telegrams from more than 50,000 fans back home (9,281 well-wishers from Moncton alone). Back and forth: the first period 2–2; the second period scoreless; goals by Gilbert and Yakushev in the third, then a brawl leading to major roughing penalties to Bergman and Mikhailov. It looked as if the game would end in a tie, but, with 2:06 left to play, Paul Henderson scored. Canada 4, Russia 3. It would all come down to the last game. Canadian assistant coach John Ferguson predicted, "The Soviets will use every trick in the book, on and off the ice. It will be a well-played chess game."

Leaving Leningrad, a 430-mile Wednesday afternoon bus trip southwest through gently rolling countryside dotted with trees and cottages took us to Ukraine and its capital, Kiev. Thursday morning was commandeered by a propaganda-rich tour of the city under the stern leadership of our stridently Communist, bourgeois-capitalist-hating guide who spewed an uninterrupted tirade describing the virtues of Communism. Who could argue with the logic that suggested that a labourer deserved a higher wage than a doctor? After all, the physician is reimbursed in part by the pleasures found in his work, and thus the worker earns 180 rubles per month and the physician 120, our guide explained. He went on to note that all citizens in the Soviet republics were loyal only to the Soviet Union. None, he said, had nationalistic ties to their republic. I responded that I was surprised by that claim since Ukrainian Canadians were strongly nationalistic.

"They are our worst enemies," he snarled.

On we went to the venerable St Sophia Cathedral, now a museum. Closed during our visit, it served as a reminder of the eclipse of Christianity in the USSR. A 900-year tradition of worship on that very spot had simply vanished. The few remaining centres of worship we glimpsed in the USSR were attended by a tiny, elderly, remnant of a once-flourishing faith.

A few days earlier, I had watched as a guide herded a large group of bright-eyed attentive children past a painting depicting a religious procession. With a smirk, he debunked religion as mythical nonsense. The children listened, respectfully absorbed, and moved on. I felt a sense of despair at the evident drive to devalue the inner life and wondered whether our Christian brainwashing was less dangerous than this secular form. But perhaps, I concluded, the more important question is whether the child has been left with a recognition of the presence and power of mystery that surrounds our deepest attachments. *And yet, and yet*, I told myself, with a sense of unexpected delight, *Lighten up a little. The human spirit will out!'*

This sense of reassurance was, in part, the legacy of a remarkable encounter a member of our group had in Moscow. On wandering alone into a hotel restaurant late one evening, he noticed that a man sitting alone at a table by the far wall was beckoning to him. The hotel staff seemed to be watching this interaction with considerable interest. Our colleague hesitated, but, concluding that there was nothing to lose, he walked over to the table.

"Sit with me," said the stranger in fluent English, "I want to talk to a vulgar Canadian." It was clear that the waiters were particularly amused.

"The waiters are laughing because you don't know who I am," the man continued. "I am Yevtushenko. Sit with me and have a drink."² As their conversation wore on, the renowned Russian poet, novelist, dramatist, actor, film editor, and director invited our friend to his apartment, stating, "I like to hear my poetry read in English."

The apartment was spacious and comfortable, the walls lined with paintings, including several by Picasso. The great man spoke of his poor reception by the press in New York during a visit to the United States "at the time of the Czechoslovakian problem."³ He then turned the discussion to the Canada-Soviet hockey series and spoke with interest and enthusiasm about the Canadians singing "O Canada" at the first game. He had been very impressed. Finally, he asked his guest to read him his poetry. The readings and the wine continued into the night.

"Where were you in '72?" Now, I must admit, fewer grandchildren ask me that today than I had predicted back then. And that isn't the only surprise to have come along. For instance, who, during game 8, would have thought that before long we would be adding other new words to our Russian vocabulary, words like *glasnost* and Gorbachev? Game 8 was, however, a landmark in its day. It may not have been Vimy, but it *was* a nation builder in Cold War times!

Game 8: 28 September, Moscow. Ferguson was right! Game 8 *was* a chess match that started before they dropped the puck! The Russians made the first move by announcing that there had been a change in referees for game 8. The two incompetent Germans from earlier games would now be officiating. The Canadian response was, "If the Soviets insist on those two referees, the eighth game will not take place." The Soviets did insist but then undertook prolonged negotiations that led up to game time. The conclusion was that Kompalla, one of the questionable German officials, would still work the game. Meanwhile, the Montreal Geography Club flew one thousand miles south to Sochi on the Black Sea. As we arrived the temperature was 78° F and the Soviets were leading 2–0.

Tension mounted as we were ushered to a room furnished with carefully arranged rows of just enough chairs to meet our need. They were grouped around a colour TV and, as we hurriedly took our places, we were updated on the action so far. Play had been intense. J.-P. Parisé had been given a minor penalty by Kompalla. He had questioned the call, thus earning a ten-minute misconduct penalty. In response, he threatened Kompalla with his stick and was given a game misconduct. Mayhem had broken out. The Canadian equipment manager threw a chair on the ice. Coach Harry Sinden joined the ruckus. Chaos ensued. Emotions were running high. The play finally resumed and as the period ended the score was 2–2. We sent up a roar of applause. *Da, Da, Ca Na Da!*

It was then that we noticed that, following our arrival, we had been joined by a silent row of burly, somber Russians, arms folded, unsmiling. They stood behind us in an unmovable line from wall to wall. We were surrounded. Each of us carried out a stealthy assessment of the nearest exit door and windows.

The Soviets scored three times in the second period, Canada once, and the period ended with the Soviets leading 5–3. They were playing great hockey, but Canada had a strong period as well.

With two Team Canada goals in the first half of the third, the game was tied at 5–5. But the light to signal the second of those goals had failed to go on, setting off a near riot as members of Team Canada clambered over the boards and onto the ice shaking their fists.

What was going on?! The Russian fans behind us could not explain. Nelly, our Intourist guide, translated the Russian broadcaster's comments, "This is *not* the sort of hockey we came to play!" The turmoil settled when Team Canada combatants were escorted off the ice by teammates, thus avoiding the intervention of a squad of military police.

The clock was winding down and a tie seemed inevitable, but then, with only thirty-four seconds remaining, Henderson scored and *the series of the century* ended, Canada 6, Russia 5. Pandemonium. The Russian fans behind us once again melted away in silence. We were delirious!

The Needs of the Dying

Two roads diverged in a yellow wood,
And sorry I could not travel both
And be one traveler, long I stood
And looked down one as far as I could
To where it bent in the undergrowth;

. . .

I shall be telling this with a sigh
Somewhere ages and ages hence:
Two roads diverged in a wood, and I –
I took the one less traveled by,
And that has made all the difference.

Robert Frost,
"The Road Not Taken"

One fall afternoon in 1972 I agreed, with some reluctance, to attend a specially scheduled lecture at McGill's McIntyre Medical Sciences Building. I remember feeling considerable indifference about the whole affair. Only vaguely, if at all, could I recall having heard of the speaker. Elisabeth Kübler-Ross was to discuss her work with the dying. It seemed, at best, an odd topic.

Dr Kübler-Ross had already been introduced to the overflow audience when I quietly slid in through the entrance at the rear of the Palmer Howard Amphitheatre, McGill's largest medical-lecture hall. I was amazed. Not only were the four hundred seats filled, but, standing behind the last rows of seats, faculty members were stacked three or four deep across the entire auditorium.

Closest to me in this packed throng of standees was Francis McNaughton, known to all and sundry simply as "St Francis." He was at the very back, balancing on tiptoe in an attempt to see. Professor

McNaughton had been neurologist-in-chief at the Montreal Neurological Institute from 1951 to 1969 and was highly revered as a teacher, clinician, and administrator of unusual grace and depth. I was profoundly impressed to come upon this great man at the back of the standees, striving to see and hear with such evident attentiveness. My attention was now galvanized. Who *was* this speaker? *Why* this remarkable crowd?!

As I scanned the packed room more carefully, my astonishment grew. Fire regulations notwithstanding, the three Palmer Howard stairways were packed with huddled figures sardined together – a mix of faculty and students on each step from my sixth-floor vantage point down to the fifth-floor podium. In addition, across the front of the hall several dozen students were sitting cross-legged on the floor surrounding the speaker. I estimated that there were at least six hundred of us crammed into the room, something I had not seen before, or ever would again.

What of Dr Kübler-Ross? Clad in slacks and a turtleneck, she had ignored the podium and chosen instead to perch on a lab table facing her audience, legs dangling, microphone in hand. All were mesmerized. The scene had the feel of an epic Cecil B. de Mille moment!

Unknown to me at the time, this Zurich-born Swiss-American psychiatrist had been catapulted to international prominence by the publication of her book *On Death and Dying* three years earlier, in the fall of 1969. A few weeks later, her public adulation had increased to rock-star proportions when *Life* magazine published a feature article detailing her discussions with dying patients, in particular a candid conversation with Eva, an attractive twenty-one-year-old woman with incurable leukemia.

The response to her book and the *Life* magazine cover article seemed self-generating. *On Death and Dying* would soon be translated into twenty-six languages. A bright light had been focused on the needs of the dying and on our societal and professional taboos associated with death. Professor Marinbach's deep-seated fear of discussing death with his Russian patients came to mind as our speaker weaved her galvanizing narrative.

She described the highly personal individual experiences of people who are dying, the unexpected insights of young children at the end of life, and the psychological adjustment process she had observed among those nearing death. Her work had led to teaching seminars on death at the University of Chicago's Billings Hospital and her breaking through the *nobody-dies-here* barrier that had been the long-standing norm prior to her arrival at that highly regarded six-hundred-bed centre of academic excellence.

I had never heard a more effective communicator! Wherein lay her impact? Her observations were fascinating and her relaxed self-assurance unmistakable. She delivered her message with an appealing "Switzerdeutsch" accent using brief, to-the-point sentences. But there was more to it than that. Elisabeth Kübler-Ross, or "EKR" as she was widely known, was a skilled storyteller. Each account was coloured by an openness and compassion that took the listener into the *lived experience* of those involved. She offered phenomenology at its essence-revealing best. She spoke of the transformative experience she had as a teenager after the war in visiting the Nazi concentration camp at Majdanek, Poland, where 960,000 children had been murdered, and her own experiences with illness as a child. All became grist for her mill.

She spoke with unshakable conviction as a champion of the vulnerable and in that sense an archetypal voice of her time. While her words were lilting rather than strident and often accompanied by a twinkle in her eye, they reflected deeply held convictions about the needless injustice faced by those whose spokesman she had become. She echoed the student protesters of 1968, the rising tide of Western feminists, the opponents of the Vietnam War, the advocates of gay rights, and so many others who were speaking out. While her Palmer Howard audience would usually have had little time for an argument that was not substantiated by sound quantitative data, EKR's powerful anecdotes struck home. In her stories we encountered ourselves and the patients we cared for.

Her ability to engage the listener was exceptional! Years later, a colleague returning from an annual meeting of the American College of Surgeons described his amazement when attendees sprinkled through a Kübler-Ross plenary-session audience of several thousand repeatedly offered spontaneous answers to her rhetorical questions.

"And vat do you tink he vas telling me, ven he said dat?" she asked.

"He was afraid," a man at the back of the room responded, leaning forward, clearly believing he was in a private conversation.

Within twenty-four hours of hearing her, I had the humbling experience of recognizing that there was considerable room for improvement in how I was meeting the needs of two men with prostate cancer who were under my care.

An invitation to act as chairman for a planned January 1973 adult-education evening "On Death and Dying" at our church had no evident weighty significance. It was simply one of those things that one is asked to do. You say yes, of course. It didn't occur to me that this might be a life-changing crossroad. Nor did I realize that I knew absolutely

nothing about the topic! I was a doctor, a surgical oncologist; surely I
must know all about such things.

The program that evening was to include the CBC film *To Die Today*
featuring EKR. The invited panelists for the discussion following the
film were Mrs Leah Park, assistant director of nursing at the Montreal
General Hospital, Dr Dag Munro, thoracic surgeon at the Vic and
the Royal Edward Laurentian Chest Hospital,[1] and the Reverend Mel
McDowell, chaplin at the Vic. The handout given to those attending the
session was the anonymously written piece, "Death in the First Person."
It set the tone for the evening and for countless teaching sessions and
workshops in the years to follow.

Death in the First Person
Anonymous

I am a student nurse. I am dying. I write this to you who are, and will
become, nurses in the hope that by sharing my feelings with you, you
may someday be better able to help those who share my experience.

I'm out of the hospital now – perhaps for a month, for six months,
perhaps for a year ... but no one likes to talk about such things. In
fact, no-one likes to talk about much at all. Nursing must be advancing, but I wish it would hurry. We're taught not to be overly cheery
now, to omit the "everything's fine" routine, and we have done pretty
well. But now one is left in a lonely silent void. With the protective
"fine, fine" gone, the staff is left with only their own vulnerability and fear. The dying patient is not yet seen as a person and thus
cannot be communicated with as such. He is a symbol of what every
human fears and what we each know, at least academically, that we
too must someday face. What did they say in Psychiatric Nursing
about meeting pathology with pathology to the detriment of both
patient and nurse? And there was a lot about knowing one's feelings
before you could help another with his. How true.

But for me, fear is today and dying is now. You slip in and out
of my room, give medications and check my blood pressure. Is it
because I am a student nurse, myself, or just a human being that I
sense your fright? And your fear enhances mine. Why are you afraid?
I am the one who is dying.

I know, you feel insecure, don't know what to say, don't know
what to do. But please believe me, if you care, you can't go wrong.
Just admit that you care. That is really what we are searching for.
We may ask for whys and wherefores, but we don't really expect

answers. Don't run away ... Wait ... all I want to know is that there will be someone to hold my hand when I need it. I am afraid. Death may get to be routine to you, but it is new to me. You may not see me as unique, but I've never died before. To me, once is pretty unique!

You whisper about my youth, but when one is dying is he really so young anymore? I have lots I wish we could talk about. It really would not take much more of your time because you are in here quite a bit anyway.

If only we could be honest, both admit our fears, touch one another. If you really care, would you lose so much of your valuable professionalism if you even cried with me? Just person to person? Then, it might not even be so hard to die ... in a hospital ... with friends close by.

Our committee had gathered to discuss plans for the session and over coffee we recalled examples of inept care at the end of life that each of us had witnessed. It was our pragmatic colleague Dag Munro who then challenged us with his customary incisiveness: "You know, rather than relying on galloping anecdotes, someone needs to do a study to determine how people die in our hospitals."

Why not? I thought. *The question is important; it sounds to me like a straightforward project; should lead to interesting and informative data. Of course, the study would need a high-priority rating across the hospital if one was aiming to garner adequate multidisciplinary response rates to an "attitudes toward death" questionnaire. It would need a sponsoring committee with gravitas.*

The RVH Task Force on Grief, later renamed the RVH Ad Hoc Committee on Thanatology, came into being.[2] The first meeting was on 28 February 1973.

We would need interviewers and data crunchers. A research grant of $2,000 was awarded by the McGill Subcommittee on Grants in the Social Sciences. Two second-year medical-student assistants were recruited for the summer.

Who were the patients whose needs we were attempting to assess in this study? We used the term *critically ill patients*, defining them as "those for whom treatment aimed at cure or prolonging survival is no longer relevant, but who may or may not be terminally ill." Three research goals were clarified: to determine the nature of the emotional and physical needs of the hospitalized critically ill; to identify existing deficiencies in meeting these needs; and to propose means of improving their care.

Strategies we adopted to achieve these goals included: enlarging our committee to include representatives of all hospital departments; developing the 1973 "RVH Questionnaire on Death and Dying"; interviewing selected critically ill patients and their families; carrying out a literature search pertaining to end-of-life care; surveying RVH staff regarding current deficiencies in care and their recommendations for its improvement; consulting Dr Kübler-Ross regarding our procedures and strategies; and, finally, visiting St Christopher's Hospice, London, England. The last tactic was added based on the impressive publication record of its director and founder of the modern hospice movement, Dr Cicely Saunders. St Christopher's was the first institution to take an academic approach in confronting the needs of this population, that is to say, giving equal priority to clinical care, research, and teaching. A full report of our findings was to be tabled to the RVH Medical Board.

Our plans were clear. Yet, while interesting, they remained no more than a personal footnote addendum to the existing demands related to my daily clinical, teaching, and research commitments. *This Death and Dying project shouldn't be too great a distraction*, I concluded, *once we get all the wheels in motion.*

But another crossroad event was upon us to dilute my preoccupation with issues academic. It was Tuesday, 10 April, 1973. Faye reached me by phone. "Social Service called. They'll be here just after lunch, depending on the driving."

"I'll be right home." We were excited. Wren and Chris, now six and almost nine, had stayed home from school in anticipation that this might happen. This crossroad would change everything.

Months earlier, Faye and I had taken stock and concluded that we should share our family with one more person. We would adopt a First Nations brother for Chris and Wren. He was coming to us from Great Slave Lake. Our new son was a member of the Dene Nation in the Northwest Territories. Exciting stuff! I assumed that my Meds '63 classmate, Earl Covert, who worked in Hay River, probably knew him and may even have delivered him.

James Edward Mount, who would be three on 29 July, strode through the doorway trailing two beaming social workers and a reinforced cardboard suitcase roughly the same size as he was. Tongue-tied, we stood agape at this bundle of outgoing ebullience. "Jamie," as he instantly became known, marched straight toward Faye standing in the foyer, threw his arms around her with a simultaneous hug and a kiss, and exclaimed, "Hi Mummy!" Then, turning to me, "Hi Daddy!"

A few strides later, he had picked up a wooden mallet from the pile of toys awaiting his arrival and made his way with evident determination into the living room to take a mighty swing at "Tristesse," the marble statue gracing our rosewood coffee table. Four pairs of adult hands intercepted him in mid-swing. "Hi, Jamie dear, welcome home!" He had arrived and, as the announcement to family and friends proudly proclaimed, "Now we are five!"

A letter written a week later provides a progress report: "He is robust, good natured, affectionate, handsome and totally captivating for all family members save [our Samoyed] Nicky who has shown considerable jealousy to the point of biting him once and growling repeatedly. Faye has noticed a tremendous change in her life, of course; one forgets how time-consuming and demanding the care of such a little fellow is."

In June, Chris and I flew to Vancouver to participate in the Canadian Urologic Association meeting where I presented papers on "Urine Cytology with Renal Cell Carcinoma" and "The Impact of Chemotherapy on Germinal Testis Tumours Using the Stevens Model in Mice" as a precursor to horseback riding and a drive across the Rockies to Calgary for the flight home.

THE 1973 ROYAL VICTORIA HOSPITAL STUDY

McGill medical student and summer research assistant Allan Jones stuck his head through my office door. "Got a moment?"

"Sure, Allan, come in."

He looked concerned. Allan was as likely to be dressed in a checkered lumberjack shirt and Kodiak boots as anything else. I cautioned colleagues not to be misled by his informal attire. He was thoughtful, discerning, and highly observant.

"What is it, Allan? Sit down." ˙

As it happened, in addition to being a member of our end-of-life study team that summer, Allan was a "blood man" on Seven West Surgical and other wards. The latter job description entailed arriving at the surgical nursing stations before 7 a.m. to collect the blood-test requisitions, set up the required tubes, labels, and syringes, and draw the necessary blood samples, all of that before the usual frenetic daily busyness overtook the wards.

As destiny would have it, Miss R, one of his blood-test patients that day, was also on our list for inclusion in our study on end-of-life care and that confluence of circumstances had proven to be devastating for

Allan, who suddenly found himself one of the hospital caregivers whose deficient actions we were attempting to document.

As Allan continued his account of Miss R's experiences as a surgical patient, it was my turn to be concerned. "Who is her doctor?" I asked. "I'll speak to him. They're a first-rate group of men on Seven West." I couldn't, however, imagine who among my colleagues might be as insensitive as Allan's tale suggested. Allan's answer surprised me.

"But he's a very fine fellow ... and a good surgeon. He cares about his patients. He would want the very best for them ... always."

With Miss R's tale fully discussed, I suggested to Allan that he go home and write down what he had just told me. Miss R.'s story became the first of nine case studies included in our final report.

Case 1: Miss R, an 80 year old lady, was admitted to a surgical ward eight years [ago] following an anterior resection for carcinoma of the sigmoid colon. On admission she was considered "terminal." The following quotes were extracted from the initial history and physical recorded in her chart. *She appears an independent person who complains very little, but she is not able to give a good history ... Independent but nervous and anxious ... Jovial type, did not treat the examination seriously ... Since admission her condition has deteriorated ... Presence of metastases is clinically apparent. Patient progressively anorexic and losing weight ... Can take small amounts of fluids by mouth, but needs more intensive nursing care ... Patient is terminal and could benefit greatly from being placed in a convalescent home.* Miss R, a graduate nurse without living relatives, remained in hospital thirty-five days before she died.

The interviewer first encountered her prior to my involvement with the Thanatology Committee when I entered her room early one morning to draw a blood sample. As I approached, the bed curtains were drawn. However, I called her name and slipped in. She seemed distressed and in obvious discomfort. A nurse was taking her blood pressure on the right arm and when I expressed my mission to Miss R, she answered raggedly that she was on the bed pan. My response was, "This will only take a moment Miss R, would you mind if I take the blood sample now?" Without waiting for a reply, I applied the tourniquet and began looking for a vein. Dejectedly, she turned her head from me to the nurse saying in a broken voice. "I don't care anymore. Do what you want to me. I don't care anymore! You'll do what you want anyway."

When I next saw Miss R as an interviewer for the Committee, she was unsuccessfully calling for a nurse to help her to the bathroom.

She refused my help but expressed a desire for me to stay. I asked if I
might return later to talk with her. Her eyes filled with tears and she
pleaded, "Yes, yes, please come to talk with me. Please ... please."

I visited Miss R every day from that point until her death on
August 8, 1973. In these visits she expressed her feelings of loneliness, isolation and abandonment. Each day she expressed fear of
being alone. She would beg me, even offered to pay me, to stay longer on each visit and occasionally she asked me to find someone else
she could hire to stay with her. In her loneliness she constantly rang
the bell for the nurses and would make demands, for example, to
go to the bathroom or sit in a chair. These continuous requests were
unsettling to her nurses, resulting in less frequent visits to her room
and increasing delay before answering her calls.

In Miss R's thirty-five day hospital stay she was cared for by thirty-
eight nurses. Only once was she followed by the same nurse on the
same shift for three consecutive days. On only four other occasions
was she cared for during two consecutive days by the same nurse, yet
she cried constantly for a friend to be near her.

The nursing notes in her chart were reviewed as an indicator of a
nursing visit to her bedside during that shift. Of the one hundred and
five nursing shifts during her admission, nursing notes recorded her
status for only sixty-six shifts and only nine included information
regarding Miss R's psychological problems. These notes included,
*crying most of the day, very lonely ... depressed ... asked to die ...
afraid of everything, does not want to be alone.* The majority of
nursing notes included statements such as, *quiet day, not as noisy as
yesterday ... IV running, foley draining ... up in chair today, diet still
poor ... incontinent of stool, intake-output balanced.*

Because Miss R was constantly calling for a nurse and continually
asking those who entered her four-bed room for help, she was moved
to a single room. Miss R feared this move and her new surroundings
and stated, "now they can close the door on me and never visit. She
cried that she would never see anyone again. She mentioned over
and over again that when she was a nurse she "loved everyone and
helped everyone, but now no one helps me." Miss R would not allow
me to help her sit up in bed, go to the bathroom, or feed herself. She
would say, "you can't help me with these things ... a nurse can do
them better."

When a nurse entered the room, her face would brighten considerably and she would plead, "Please, please, talk to me. Stay with
me for a while." The nurse would stay for a short time (when I was

present) and promise to return. Miss R would then turn to me and express her doubts.

The nursing problems were multiple and trying. When she was placed in a chair, she would want to go back to bed minutes later. When offered food, she refused, yet when it was removed she became hungry. She was incontinent of stool and urine. With foley catheter inserted she would demand to get up to urinate. The demands were constant and all were directed at the nurses. On one occasion a nurse whom I approached for assistance angrily stated, "Why doesn't she just die and leave us alone!"

Miss R spoke very little about her medical care, especially concerning her doctors. She said she saw very little of them and assumed they were too busy to care for her. She not infrequently heard them, while on rounds, mutter about a convalescent home and this frightened her very much. She felt she had a few friends at the Royal Victoria Hospital and knew that when she was moved elsewhere she would be completely alone again. Miss R pleaded with me to stop them from moving her, expressing her desire to die rather than move.

The residents on ward rounds spent an average of one minute in Miss R's room. No one would go close enough to touch her and only rarely did someone speak to her. The main theme of discussion after the visit was, "When can we get her into a convalescent home?" There were a few nervous laughs after one visit when Miss R had tried to call the police for help.

During Miss R's thirty-five day stay, there were only eleven doctor's notes recorded in her chart. Only one of the eleven contained some mention of her psychological state – *seems in better spirits ... intake unchanged.*

No clergy ever visited Miss R. When asked if she would like to speak to a minister (she was Protestant) she agreed, adding that when she wanted him she would call, but noting, "the time is not now."

A hospital volunteer visited several times but Miss R's anger, demands and lack of interest in idle conversation seemed to frighten her and these visits soon stopped.

Although Miss R continually acted with anger and aggression during our first encounters, she soon realized that I would continue to visit her on a regular basis. She began to brighten as I entered the room, exclaiming how happy she was to see me, but always asked immediately if I could stay for a long time. Our visits ranged from a half-hour to one hour and consisted mainly of my holding her hand, giving her water and listening. She was aware that I was not a doctor but a medical student who wanted to learn from, as well as help, the very sick people in the hospital. Repeatedly she would plead, "Help me, you are not like the others, help me."

She would beg God to take her. "Ah, God, I don't want to live like this anymore. I want to be with my family. Please take me to my family." When asked about her family, she explained that all were dead: two brothers in the war, her father and mother of old age. She now had no one and her native Nova Scotia was far away. She often commented, "What's the point of living when no one cares."

As she approached her death, Miss R expressed suicidal thoughts of jumping out the window with increasing frequency. "If only I could get out of this bed, I would do it. I would do it. What is the point of living like this? No one cares if I live or die. Help me. Help me."

Because I was not sure what to say, many times I simply held her hand and listened without answering her questions. It seemed that she did not expect an answer because seconds later she would turn to another topic. She did, however, grasp my hand tightly throughout each session and occasionally she would fall asleep holding it.

Three days before her death, I saw her on a Saturday morning. She seemed to be disoriented and slightly sedated. While grasping my hand she said, "You will not see me tomorrow, tonight I am going to die. I am not going to make it through tonight." On Sunday and Monday Miss R was comatose: on Tuesday, Miss R died.

Allan was an invaluable asset for our study. While death anxiety is universal, lack of familiarity with death is often particularly daunting for medical students who haven't yet incorporated the professional escape tactics that enable health-care professionals to distance themselves: the avoidance responses, the conscious and unconscious rationalizations that protect seasoned professionals through selective hearing, patient isolation, and funnelling patient needs through a medicalized observational filter.

In addition, Allan had a second advantage that sharpened his perception of patient needs. As a medical student, he was largely invisible on the ward. Nurses tend to ignore medical students as long as they keep out of their way. Thus, Allan's near-transparent presence was accepted at the nursing station where he could read the patient's chart, make notes, and listen to the nurses' comments about the patients without disturbing anyone. Similarly, he could join the residents on their daily rounds and listen to their comments about the patients he was following.

His approach generally involved the enquiry, "Mind if I join you for rounds?" to which the rejoinder was usually a variation on the theme, "Not at all, tag along, son, and watch how we do it." We had stumbled onto the perfect interviewer, observer, and monitor of hospital practice.

Over the summer, Allan would bring his perceptive observations of hospital staff, patients, and family members to a wide range of inpatient and outpatient settings. The nine case summaries we selected for inclusion in the Final Committee Report would prove to be foundational in convincing the Royal Victoria Hospital Board that we had a serious problem that needed to be addressed.

Administrators Ken MacKinnon and Anne Morgan were key strategists in achieving high-profile, hospital-wide recognition and ownership of the study. It could no longer be viewed as the project of a single investigator. Thus, on 20 March, a letter requesting the support of all physicians was sent to the attending staff by RVH Medical Director Ashton Kerr and Thanatology Committee consultants were recruited from each department. On 11 May an expanded thirty-eight-member committee with representatives from all clinical and administrative arenas met for a detailed review of the issues involved.[3] Open discussion followed. There was now general agreement that this was a problem that required attention.

On 1 June 1973 the Royal Victoria Hospital "Questionnaire on Death and Dying" was distributed to all hospital staff. An accompanying letter requesting participation was signed by Director of Nursing Margaret Clark, Medical Director Ashton Kerr, and Chairman of the Medical Board Jonathan Meakins. As a result, 638 multiple-choice questionnaires on attitudes toward death and dying were completed by the medical and paramedical staff and selected critically ill patients.

The data obtained suggested a variety of patient-care deficiencies. They indicated the patient's desire for openness and honesty in discussions relating to diagnosis and prognosis, the physicians' reluctance to be that candid, the residents' relative lack of concern for patients' emotional needs, and the social workers' tendency to minimize the problem. In addition, there was a consistent tendency to see colleagues' shortcomings more easily than our own.

The primary sources of support in the face of critical illness were the family (50 per cent) and personal faith (25 per cent).[4] Minor variations in attitude were related to the age and religion of the respondent. Comparing the responses of "committed Christian physicians" to those of their "agnostic" colleagues, however, revealed that the two groups held attitudes that were strikingly similar, and widely divergent from those of their patients regarding discussing diagnosis and prognosis.

Both groups demonstrated a similar tendency to judge themselves as being more open than their colleagues were.[5] Two hundred respondents identified more than twenty-six deficiencies they had observed in our care of the critically ill and offered thirty-one suggestions for correcting these deficits.

The Royal Vic study concluded that, like Robert Frost, we had "promises to keep and miles to go before we sleep." We now knew that at our McGill teaching hospital, when cure and prolongation of life were no longer relevant goals, inadequate care ensued. Although these were the sickest and most needy people coming to us for care, we failed them on a daily basis. In addition, we were generally not aware of our failings, largely, it would seem, because of our exclusive focus on investigating, diagnosing, prolonging life, and curing the pathophysiology of disease. Our patients' complex needs consistently fell beyond that skill set, and thus their suffering persisted.

It was clear that, prior to our study, deficiencies in care might be excused on the grounds that we were unaware of their presence. Now, however, with our shortcomings evident, to do nothing would no longer be morally acceptable. By early August, the dimensions of our problem had largely been clarified. The solution remained less clear.

Eighteen months had passed since Dr Kübler-Ross's Palmer Howard amphitheatre presentation. On 8 August I telephoned her to chat about the activities that session had generated. A flurry of letters between us followed. She would be giving a lecture in Ottawa on 11 October and could visit us the next day. Better yet, I could drive to Ottawa to attend her talk and we would then return to Montreal together, thus affording the opportunity for a detailed review of the options before us. She was not surprised by our findings. "Nah... turlee," she affirmed repeatedly.

WHERE TO GO FROM HERE?

I first came across a reference to Cicely Saunders and her work at St Christopher's Hospice in London, England, on reading Elisabeth's book *On Death and Dying*. Intrigued, I had flipped to the bibliography at the back and found seven references attributed to Saunders dating from 1959. They included publications in the *Proceedings of the Royal Society of Medicine* and *Nursing Times*. Interesting! A trip to London seemed to be called for.

"St Christopher's Hospice." The warm response at the first or second ring of the telephone impressed me. It managed to convey an atmosphere of welcoming efficiency.

"Dr Saunders, please. I am calling from McGill University in Montreal."

"One moment please. I shall see if she is available."

"Dr Saunders." Her tone was all business. I offered a brief summary of the RVH study, its findings, and my interest in visiting St Christopher's.

"I see. When do you want to come?"

"Well, I hate to sound so American, but I was wondering about next week. My wife will be coming with me."

"I see. Well, I can't think of such things right now! I am on my way to lunch. Call me back in an hour." *Click.*

An hour later, Dr Saunders was ready for the call.

"Dr Mount ... yes, well, I know you!" (*How odd! ... You do?*). "You want to visit London with your wife, see a few plays, have a quick look 'round the house to see what we're up to, then go home. Well, I won't have it! I'll tell you what, *leave* your wife at home, *plan* to stay for a week, *be prepared to roll up your sleeves and get to work*, and I'll have you." She was, of course, completely accurate in her assessment of my intentions. Faye would have to stay at home; our London theatre dreams must be put on hold. What could I say? "All right, it's a deal."

I was packed and ready to go. Faye was about to drive me to the airport. Only *then* did I think of it! Why hadn't I thought of it earlier? My mind was churning. *Drat! Mount, you twit! If this place is all it's cracked up to be, I'll have to have pictures to prove it. Where in heaven's name can I borrow a camera at this eleventh hour?* With a remarkable leap of faith, Ken Taguchi, a colleague but veritable stranger, handed me his prized camera as Faye waited in our airport-bound car, motor running.

"By the way, you are familiar with SLR cameras, I assume?" Ken asked as I headed down the steps from his door. "No?" He swallowed and blanched. "Well, let me show you a couple of things. First of all ..." Four hours later, over mid-Atlantic, I asked myself what in the world I was doing with this sophisticated Nikon cradled on my knees.

London. Long-established middle-class homes, scattered mature trees, and modest gardens lent a comfortably worn, lived-in ambience to Lawrie Park Road, a quiet residential lane in Sydenham, Bromley. For all of that, Number 51, located on the east side a few blocks north of Crystal Palace Park, fit in curiously well. If somewhat more lustrous than its neighbours, St Christopher's Hospice, with its evident newness and handsome brick, slate, and glass four-storey construction, managed to add understated elegance to its surroundings. A tastefully modern rendering of St Christopher striding across impressionistic waves, his precious bundle perched on one shoulder, occupied a place of prominence over the front door. Shrubbery and a prominent sign marking the entrance offered reassurance and the promise of predictability and order at hand. The first modern, academic hospice was six years old and its skilled caregiving team had settled comfortably into their pioneering vocation with commitment and enthusiasm.

I glanced around the reception area. There, under the front window, was a plaque recalling David Tasma, a young Polish patient Cicely Saunders had fallen in love with as he was dying. It was 1947; she was his social worker, he, an inspiration in formulating her concept of a home for the dying. He had said, "I shall be a window in your home." Now, a quarter-century later, I was standing before that window.

The courteous, neatly attired gentleman behind the nearby desk greeted me with an easy mix of reserve and respect. Could he be of assistance? Indeed, he could; I was here to see Dr Saunders.

"Ah yes, Dr Mount. You will be staying at Wolfson House, I believe. Why don't you leave your suitcase with me, I'll have Miss Reynolds here show you to Dr Saunders's office. She is expecting you."

Dr Saunders's greeting was warm. Taller than I had expected, even stately, she radiated an aura of comfortable authority. Her angular, handsome face bore a lively expression that invited engagement, dialogue, or perhaps a friendly joust in the settlement of any differences that might arise, as she enquired about my flight and confirmed my accommodations in the adjacent, newly opened, Wolfson House.

She waved me into the chair on the other side of her orderly but heavily ladened desk. Her second-floor office was bright and spacious; the windows overlooked the front entrance and tidy parking lot that lay between the hospice and the road. Crowded bookshelves spreading wall to wall behind her suggested the inquisitive mind that I sensed was currently sizing me up as, she would have said, "with a beady eye."

She outlined my schedule for the week. Under the tutelage of the "ward sister," I was to act as an observer on Nuffield, one of the three wards, attend the regular "Mail and Admissions Meetings" with senior staff, and take part in chapel services as well as other activities, as desired. I was welcome to enter fully into ward life, with access to patients, their families, their charts, and the hospice team. Dr Mary Baines was the attending physician on Nuffield and would be available to chat about clinical issues. In addition, Dr Thérèse Vanier would be in the house later that day and was looking forward to saying hello. "You being from Canada and all." Was she the sister of Jean and Father Benedict Vanier? She was. I had met Benedict a year or two earlier when he had agreed to show a dozen or so "Teens Club" members (the club was run by Faye, Phyllis Smyth, and me) around his stately and, to the uninitiated, somewhat austere monastery and explain to our motley group of Protestant teenagers why *anyone* in their right mind would choose a cloistered life. Benedict and I had become close friends.

"Oh, and Dr Mount," Dr. Saunders added, "why don't you plan to join me here for tea at 4:00 P.M. and we can review how the day has gone?"

Dr Baines came by on cue and took me under her wing. She was perhaps a decade my senior. "Let me show you around on our way up to the ward. It will help you get your bearings."

Mary Baines was dark-haired with a gentle openness indicative of her considerable listening skills. Her smile was tentative, as if ready to respond to *your* mood. In contrast, however, she moved right along. I found I had to quicken my pace to have any hope of keeping up with her, physically or intellectually. She and Deputy Medical Director Tom West had been Dr Saunders's medical-school classmates at St Thomas's, though Cicely was considerably older than her peers, having already trained first as a nurse and then as an almoner (social worker) prior to deciding to "swat up Med'sn" as a prelude to starting her home for the dying. Mary had joined St Christopher's soon after it opened, a move considered at the time to be tantamount to professional suicide in the opinion of her medical colleagues.

As we moved through the hospice, I was struck by the exquisite attention to detail in architecture and decor: the sense of space and light throughout, the lack of clutter, the bold, bright, impressionistic paintings displayed on the walls – clearly all the work of one artist. Dr Baines informed me that he was Marian Bohusz-Szyszko, a Polish man Dr Saunders had met a decade earlier and now her close friend (they were to marry in 1980). The centrally placed chapel on the ground floor, with its spacious access for beds and wheelchairs, was an open, airy, sunlit room featuring a prominent Bohusz-Szyszko triptych depicting nativity, crucifixion, and resurrection, executed in bold splashes of blue, white, yellow, and orange.

The tour continued: bay windows, plants, an exquisite sculpture of a kneeling figure; a daycare nursery bubbling with ruddy-faced toddlers, each preoccupied by his/her own delightfully busy presence; the glass-walled dining room overlooking the gardens behind the hospice, which still boasted a degree of end-of-summer exuberance; and, along one side of the garden, the Draper's Wing for the frail elderly, each with its own "bed-sit." The broad, gently rising staircase caught my attention. Each step was only a few inches above its lower neighbour, a thoughtful tip of the hat to weary limbs and spent reserves.

We made our way to the ward where I would be resident observer. Once again, light bathed the scene. It was arranged in bays of four and six beds, each bed positioned parallel to the roadside windows so that the outside world seemed close at hand yet could be viewed without troublesome glare or a sense of its intrusiveness on St Christopher's calm. An open space between beds and the windows overlooking Sydenham Road extended the length of the ward, providing an indoor "balcony" that facilitated a view of passersby, the tennis court across the road, and the changing seasons on the other side of the large windows. Dr Baines introduced me to the ward sister and her team. We were off to a good start.

Following a brief look around at the nursing station, charts, and ward layout, Sister whisked me off to meet Mrs Trenholm, a perky grey-haired woman in her late-fifties. She was ensconced in the six-bed bay nearest the stairs. Introductions were animated. I was said to be a visiting professor from Montreal, she, an adept gardener, retired teacher, and mother of three, her eldest daughter now living in Toronto.

Sister informed me, "Mrs T. has been with us several weeks now and likes to keep a close eye on the ward. She can tell you everything you want to know, and then some." While she had been "poorly" on admission, her uncontrolled pain, nausea, breathlessness, weakness, and depression had responded well to Nuffield care and the medication regimen that had been carefully adjusted by Dr Baines. She was now said to be "blooming" – all this noted with proud satisfaction on the part of Sister and an acknowledging "Hmmmm, yes, quite," from Mrs T.

As I obediently descended into the proffered bedside chair, I was struck by her vigour. Indeed, Mrs T. quickly engaged me in topics ranging from weather, to politics, to my family in Canada, and, finally, to her recent illness. Our dynamic interaction seemed all the more surprising given Sister's report detailing her extensive breast cancer, poor prognosis, and recent considerable distress. At the moment, she did not resemble any imminently dying patient I had ever seen. It didn't add up. Before long we were discussing the murder mystery lying on the bed beside her.

Lunch in the dining room with Dr Thérèse Vanier provided a further infusion of up-beat peace St Christopher's-style. Like her brothers, Jean and Benedict, and their storied mother, Mme Pauline, Thérèse was tall, slender, and moved with grace. Her hair was grey, her patrician face hauntingly lovely, conveying both wisdom and a hint of quiet sadness. In conversation, she deferred to others, but her contributions were always thoughtful and often accompanied by quiet humour and a sparkle in her eye. She was a hematologist at Thomas's Hospital where she had been their first female consultant. Cicely had sought her out as plans for St Christopher's took shape and was delighted to have her join the team on a part-time basis.

A chat around two or three patients with Dr Baines filled the early afternoon. I was impressed by the level of her discussions with the nurses and the depth of their probing considerations as they carefully reviewed the subtle psychosocial and physiologic factors colouring each patient's day. It was highly instructive.

Thérèse came by on her way to see a patient Mary had asked her to review.

"Would it be alright if I tagged along?" I mumbled to Thérèse as I fell in beside her. It hadn't occurred to me that she might say no. She stopped, her face draining somewhat. She clearly felt awkward. "Well ... actually, I would prefer if you didn't. I'm sorry." She flushed, looking down evasively. "You see, I wouldn't know what to say if you were present. For me, talking to a patient is an intimate matter." I was stunned, embarrassed. "Oh, certainly ... of course. I understand." But I didn't.

Later, I passed the patient's bed. The surrounding curtains had been closed, but as I passed I caught a brief glimpse of patient and consultant. Thérèse was sitting hunched on a bedside chair, leaning forward, her face perhaps eighteen inches from the patient's. She was intent, "listening," as I subsequently heard Cicely describe it in reference to one of her nurses, "with every fibre of her being." To my astonishment, I found my eyes welling up with tears. This was "active listening" at the bedside as I had never seen it. Here was radical presence personified. This was how each of my St Christopher's colleagues listened – Mary, Cicely, Thérèse, Tom, the nurses, all of them. Thérèse's comment was suddenly understandable. I felt like a voyeur. For Thérèse, a private discussion with her patient was a moment of union, a time of profound, near-sacred sharing. I had just witnessed a remarkable fusion of the science and the art of medicine.

At 4:00 P.M. I knocked on the director's door. "Come!" With a welcoming nod, she turned to the bookshelf behind her and opened the small cabinet that stood between the *Oxford English Dictionary* and what appeared to be a treasured leather-bound volume of English verse.

"Now then, what will you have? I have sherry and scotch. I am having scotch!" I had sherry.

What a day it had been! Eye opening; transforming; enlightening; wonderful! I had felt unexpectedly engaged and comfortable. I had a sense of peace but also excitement. Who would have thought that a visit to a centre focused on care of the dying could inspire such a reaction? There was much to discuss! Where to start? The Royal Vic study design, our findings, my professional background, her personal journey and professional pilgrimage as nurse, social worker, then physician, and the story behind St Christopher's.

She handed me a sheet of paper, "Drugs most commonly used at St Christopher's Hospice." This single page contained the full St Christopher's pharmacopoeia. Amazing. This first day had suggested what would subsequently be confirmed during the remainder of my visit. In *their* hands, this meagre armamentarium rarely failed! I was astonished by the apparent simplicity of the list. "You mean, this is it?" I asked, looking once again at the humble document. Dr Saunders smiled.

"Well, not exactly. These are our drugs of choice, but pain is more than that, it comes from the depths of a person's being. I think what we are dealing with could more accurately be viewed as 'Total Pain.' The individual's experience of the nociceptive stimuli is always modified by emotional, psychosocial, and spiritual or existential factors. That came to me from a woman I cared for ten years ago. As we talked she actually implicated each of those domains in describing her pain. So, in fact, we have to consider all of that … and also," she paused thoughtfully, "we must keep in mind that the *way* care is given can reach the most hidden places and give space for unexpected development."

I suspect that I did not fully comprehend the implications of what she had just said. Her words were revealing at several levels, but I would fully realize the depth of her wisdom only as it was clarified over the passing decades, through exposure at the bedside to many hundreds of vulnerable fellow travellers.

We were now well past tea time. I was relaxed, brimming over with enthusiasm. It seemed like I had known her for ages.

"What … er … what do, uh … people call you?"

She stiffened and fixed me with her unique "beady eye" scrutiny. She paused.

"My *friends* call me Cicely. Others call me Dr Saunders!" She clearly could read my questioning mind and was not amused. One eyebrow raised heavenward and she added icily, "*Steady* boy! I said my *friends* call me Cicely!!"

That was good enough for me.

I was almost out the door when I remembered. "By the way, Dr Saunders, do you feel it would be alright for me to take some photographs of the patients? The powers that be back home will have to *see* St Christopher's to believe it." She smiled. I didn't know until later that she had already spoken to Sister to get a detailed report on my day.

"I would wait for a day or two, then, as they come to know you, I'm sure that will be fine."

"Will I need a consent form?"

"That shan't be necessary. Simply ask their permission. I should think the photograph itself will make their consent obvious."

I had just come away more or less intact from our first joust. It was 1973. St Christopher's had been open six years. No one yet realized the impact this visionary crusader would have on human suffering and global health care. How did it happen? Who was this larger-than-life woman who would change my life and the lives of countless others?[6]

CICELY MARY SAUNDERS

Cicely Mary Strode Saunders, born 22 June 1918, was the eldest of the three children of Gordon Saunders, a dynamic, highly successful estate agent, and his wife, Chrissie. While father was a conservative extrovert, daughter was a shy, liberal, introvert; both were strong-willed. Childhood challenges were compounded for Cicely by her unpopularity and loneliness at day school and subsequently at Roedean School in East Sussex, where her difficulties were undoubtedly enhanced by being altogether too tall, too bright, and too shy to foster easy relationships with her peers. By the age of sixteen or seventeen, however, she had begun to come into her own, and she emerged an independent, determined young woman with a need for constant activity.[7]

She was accepted by the Society for Home Students (St Anne's College), Oxford, but the outbreak of war in 1939 interrupted her studies and she opted instead to pursue a career in nursing, thus entering the Nightingale School of Nursing at St Thomas's Hospital, with all its pride of tradition, high standards, and considerable esprit de corps. At St Thomas's, she first experienced a deep awareness that in nursing she had "come home." It was there, too, that she would later read medicine. Six decades on, in March 2002, a bronze bust of Dame Cicely would be unveiled in the Central Hall next to the statue of Florence Nightingale, who had been the first woman to receive the Order of Merit (1907), Great Britain's highest honour; Cicely would receive the same high recognition in 1989.

Her nursing career was, however, to be cut short by a chronic back complaint and she was compelled to seek a less physically demanding profession. By 1945, she had completed a degree with distinction in political theory and a diploma of public and social administration at St Anne's College, and in September 1947, at age twenty-nine, she was appointed assistant almoner at St Thomas's Hospital.

Shortly after completing her studies, Cicely converted from atheism to an evangelical understanding of Christianity that over time softened from a need for assertive dogmatism to an acceptance that the Lord had accomplished all that was needed; she observed, "It was for all the world like suddenly finding the wind at your back instead of battling against it all the time." Indeed, she was known for her brilliant linear, logical thinking *and* for her experience of both the imminence and transcendence of the spiritual domain. She commented, "I have always been very lucky in having very definite guidance," and again, "All I know is the way the Spirit has been leading me so far."

I found Cicely's combination of no-nonsense professional practicality and mystical awareness somewhat confusing. Until meeting her, I had heard her style of religious expression only from theologically exclusive Christian evangelicals, yet it became clear to me during our first meeting, as she examined me with her practised and assessing lens, that she had a niggling distrust of such a stance. It was evident that, while she experienced and expressed her faith in down-to-earth concrete terms, and longed for others to have a similar relationship with her Lord, she felt most comfortable when she was simply "getting on with it." She had decided that compassion and a shared will-to-service must trump creed in the community she wished to create at St Christopher's.

David Tasma, a forty-year-old agnostic Polish Jew from the Warsaw ghetto, was dying with advanced cancer on the first St Thomas's ward Cicely was assigned to as a medical social worker. It was her first experience of reciprocal love and its impact was profound. It was in their discussions that her concept of a home for the dying began to crystallize. He provided her fertile mind with the quintessential formulation of "hospice care" in his pithy phrase, "I only want what is in your mind and in your heart." Suffering, she noted, must be addressed with the skills of the mind that are offered by modern medicine, but there must be more. There must also be person-to-person presence, soul-to-soul, Self-to-Self, heart-to-heart.

Here we find a glimpse into how Cicely's mind operated. She intuitively transformed information into insight, then into iconic truth. Cicely was a synthesizer. She heard or saw the pearl, extracted it, integrated it, refined it as required, and then passed it on to others. This happened repeatedly.

Cicely, like all great teachers, had an ear (and eye) for the teachable moment, the lesson, the *nugget* to be integrated and passed on. She rendered insight memorable through articulate expression. A classic example is seen in her observation regarding the importance of clinical presence that she had crystallized for me at our first meeting: *the way care is given can reach the most hidden places and give space for unexpected development.* Similarly, during her personal viewing of the ruins of the bombed-out Warsaw Cathedral, she recalled a theologian's comment that *the hands that hold us in existence are pierced by unimaginable nails*; and the Irish Sisters of Charity's capacity to honour patient individuality led her to adopt their insightful acknowledgment regarding a patient, *Oh, he's himself.* She was learning her craft and storing the recovered wisdom in useable aliquots that would teach the world.

The evening after David's death, a desolate Cicely found the words of the hymn "How Sweet the Name of Jesus Sounds" particularly offensive, since she recognized that, as a Jew, "His name had certainly never sounded sweet to David." "Then," she recounted to me during one of our early discussions, "I had one of those very firm statements I get from time to time saying, *But he knows Him far better than you do already*, and as a result, I never felt I could worry about David ever again, nor indeed about anyone else who dies without apparently any knowledge of Christ." She had recognized within herself a move from an exclusive to an inclusive theology.

This capacity for growth marked her throughout life. In a transatlantic telephone chat on 13 March 1995, she informed me with considerable excitement about a St Christopher's spiritual-care working-group meeting that she had attended that afternoon. She exuded enthusiasm. It was, she exclaimed, one of the most stimulating and stretching meetings she could recall. Cicely was then seventy-six years old. Her excitement led her to admonish, "Bal, one must stay curious. Stay on the learning curve!" She went on to speak in a reassuring tone about finding the pattern we are personally meant to follow. With that cornerstone secure, she noted, a sense of equilibrium may be found and all else may then fall into place.

While continuing her work as an almoner at St Thomas's following David's death, Cicely became a volunteer at St Luke's, a home for the dying. There, she noted that the patients were consistently free of physical pain and anguish yet alert, apparently owing to the novel St Luke's practice of administering oral-pain medication at regular intervals, in doses adjusted to individual need. In spite of their impressive results, this practice appeared to be unknown beyond St Luke's where it had been standard procedure for decades.

Her desire to care for the dying grew and she was advised that to have greatest impact she would have to be a doctor. "So," as Cicely blithely commented to me, brushing aside this epic decision, "I swotted up Med'sn." In fact, it was a bold undertaking. To succeed would amount to a considerable triumph. She was thirty-three years old and had not read science at school. She described her medical training at St Thomas's with customary bluntness: "It was hell." She qualified as a physician in April 1957 at the age of thirty-nine, just as I was beginning my pre-medical studies at Queen's. In 1958 Cicely was awarded a research scholarship to study pain in dying cancer patients.

While still a medical student, she had visited St Joseph's Hospice in Hackney, a 150-bed facility founded in 1905 by the Irish Sisters of Charity to care for the frail elderly and patients with terminal malignant disease. As a student observer, Cicely visited St Joseph's three days a week. Once qualified, she became their first full-time physician. Her goal was to introduce St Luke's oral-analgesic regimen at St Joseph's. Her results demonstrated the potential of this management protocol in achieving an absence of pain accompanied by alertness and increased patient liveliness as well as peacefulness, lessened anxiety, and an enhanced sense of acceptance of death. She also noted a newfound integration in the patient-staff-family triad as complementary equals in this heretofore anxiety-prone setting, and an enhanced respect for the unique individuality of each patient. In the end, Cicely carefully documented more than one thousand cases, thus providing the foundational data that would underpin a revolution in the management of chronic cancer pain and end-of-life care. It was a study of historic significance. Cicely's results demonstrated that the final phase of life may be one of reconciliation and fulfillment, an achievement that relatives may find of great comfort during bereavement.

In this period, a Polish widower, Antoni Michniewicz, was admitted to St Joseph's with advanced cancer. His gentleness and dignity in the face of a poor prognosis impressed the hospice staff. Antoni and Cicely fell in love. She was to describe it as "the hardest, the most peaceful, the most inhibited and the most liberating experience I have ever had." He had only three weeks to live.

With Antoni's death, Cicely's bereavement was intense beyond her imagining. It was a grief that she later felt had been pathological. She was consumed by loss as she attempted to construct a context for the life together that had been denied them. Yet, in their shared faith, there had been support through the sense of a presence that surrounded them. Hereafter she would relate to all who suffer and grieve with new understanding. In true Cicely fashion, she distilled two potent lessons from this terrible but blessed passage: first, that *time is a matter of depth not length*, and second, that *there is something stronger behind it all – not an answer, but a presence.*

This understanding of the nature of time found memorable expression later during a lecture she gave at Whipps Cross University Hospital in which she spoke of the potential impact on the sufferer when caregivers give them time and attention. In response, a rather pompous consultant in the audience remarked that it was fine for her to hold such a view with all the time she had on her hands, *but* as a busy consultant, *he* ...! To this, Cicely responded icily, "Oh, no Doctor, time isn't a question of length, it's a question of depth, isn't it?" Indeed, the consultant had the help of registrars and housemen to cover far fewer beds than Cicely was covering virtually alone.

Perhaps Cicely's most eloquent expression of the "something stronger behind it all" that she had gleaned from Antoni's death is recorded in her book *Beyond the Horizon: A Search for Meaning in Suffering* (1990), a slim volume comprising a collection of readings she had found helpful in her search for meaning in suffering. She states: "Life is about learning to love and most of us have merely begun when we die. This is the main reason why many of us long for and expect another life. But there are other considerations too. Even those who have no faith in the promises of religion know that continuity in change is a consistent pattern in this world. Dying followed by rebirth in a different form happens in many ways: matter and energy are transformed, not destroyed. It would surely be strange if our life of reasoning and loving should be the only form of existence to end abruptly, the amazingly subtle energies of our minds the only thing to leave no trace."[8]

St Christopher's Hospice came into being with all the assorted birth pains and calls on faith one might expect. Simultaneously, Cicely's losses continued. Antoni died in August 1960, her close friend Barbara Galton then died early in 1961, followed by Cicely's father in June 1961. St Christopher's was registered as a company that same year. The Lawrie Park Road site was purchased in February 1963, and the ground was first broken in March 1965. The official opening of St Christopher's Hospice was on 24 July 1967.

THE IMPACT OF THAT WEEK IN SEPTEMBER 1973

Roll up your sleeves and get to work, and I'll have you! Did I adequately "roll up my sleeves"? I can't be sure. Did they "have me"? Absolutely! I found my first day at St Christopher's riveting. The remainder of that September 1973 visit flowed on with a richness I could not have anticipated. The atmosphere of calm that permeated the wards was generated through a sense of confidence, order, and security that was the product of attention to detail. There was a clear sense that knowing hands were running the ship and that all was quietly under control. The shibboleth of fighting disease had given way to a focus on enabling quality of life. *Efficiency is very comforting* was the accepted maxim, the *patient and family* the unit of care. Hospice wasn't a "soft option"; instead, it demanded that each step in the journey be met with discernment. Scrupulous pain and symptom control depended on an individually tailored management program that was finely tuned to hour-by-hour variations in need.

Nursing was the core component of this team-dependent response and, although distinctly hierarchical, in the sense that state-enrolled nurses and staff (state-registered) nurses reported to the ward sister, who, in turn, answered to matron, the observations of *all* were given equal consideration.

The caregiving team was recognized as including patient, family, and *all* other contributors to patient-family well-being. Skilled listening was viewed as being critical for success. "Micro-managing" was foundational, not a derogatory concept. Where else could the Saunders axiom *Nothing matters more than the bowels* be considered sacrosanct and sitting with a patient a higher priority than charting and busyness?

In addition, underlying the high standard of care was the shrewd recognition that optimal medical management depends on continuing concern for the existential, psychosocial, and spiritual issues that are inevitably present throughout life and of universal relevance as life's horizon draws near. At St Christopher's, "spiritual" was taken not to imply religious, though that frequently was central to its expression, but, more broadly, to refer to the search for connection and meaning and to the quest that challenges us all as we face the end of life. Finally, there was a quiet joy and openness to be found in shared celebration, as Cicely emphasized with no-nonsense seriousness over scotch and sherry during that first tea.

I concluded that the essence of the message conveyed to those St Christopher's served was best expressed in her oft-repeated assertion, *You matter because you are you, and you matter to the last moment of your life.* That message was not announced, it was lived out. It was evident when Matron Helen Willans greeted the new patient by name at the hospice door with a warmed bed and turned-down sheets. It was evident in the personalized welcoming card and flower on the bedside table, the tireless pursuit of symptoms, and the attention given to the psychosocial and spiritual gremlins that appear in endless procession. Finally, it was made evident in the lived-out commitment, *You will not be alone at the end.*

Lest a sense of unworldly omniscient tranquility comes to mind with these images of St Christopher's, the full-bore, unromantic human struggle that allowed these hospice benchmarks to be met showed its face reassuringly during the mid-week "Mail and Admissions" meeting on my second or third day at St Christopher's.

It was early morning as Dr Saunders, Matron Helen Willans, Tom West, Mary Baines, Thérèse Vanier, and I gathered to examine the needs of the day ahead. I don't recall the details of the event that triggered the reaction that dominated our meeting, but an absent esteemed colleague, Richard Lamerton, had, a month or two earlier, ruffled the collective feathers of those now present and Mary had been faced with picking up the pieces. During our meeting, Richard was held responsible in no uncertain terms, but the criticism was quickly cut short by Cicely.

"*That* is enough!! I will have *none* of it!! If the rest of you were half as productive as Richard we would be much farther ahead!!" The director had spoken! There was complete silence, heads hung, teeth clenched, as the meeting continued.

What always comes to mind in recalling that incident is the matching story later told to me by Richard himself. With a smile, he recalled the day he found himself trailing behind Cicely as they ascended the St Christopher's stairs to see their respective patients. Suddenly, without warning, Dame Cicely (as she would later be known) stopped and spun around to face him, and Richard, in colliding with her august presence, found himself peering heavenward past her abundant bosom to meet her piercing gaze, as she declared imperiously, "I had forgotten the full horror of you!" She then spun on her heels and continued up the stairs. She was more than ready to stick up for him in his absence, but, in person, that was another matter. And Richard was delightfully ready to acknowledge his feet of clay in sharing this tale with me.

I was fascinated by these compassionate warriors whom I would come to admire as teachers, and so much more, as I discovered, in those full to overflowing September days, my life-defining crossroad. In addition to my discussions with Cicely, Mary, and Thérèse, I encountered a wide range of beachheads through which my St Christopher's colleagues were establishing new clarity of understanding. There were conversations with Tom West, who proved to be both an insightful observer of St Christopher's practices and a probing examiner of our Royal Vic study data. Psychiatrist Colin Murray Parkes (who had worked with the grieving survivors following the 1966 mining disaster in the Welsh village of Aberfan) discussed his work with bereaved families and the complexities of individual grief. Robert Twycross, who had recently been hired as a research assistant, shared his plans to compare morphine and heroin in pain control. And

John Hinton, author of the recent United Kingdom study examining the needs of the dying, discussed his findings. In referring to the efforts of nurses, Hinton had shrewdly observed, "The nurses battled on heroically. They emerge with far greater credit than we, who are still capable of ignoring the conditions which make muted people suffer. The dissatisfied dead cannot noise abroad the negligence they have experienced."[9] Both his study and ours underscored that chilling truth.

Nevertheless, it seemed to me that there was a problem that lay beyond the magnificence of the St Christopher's solution. The large map of London on the wall of the St Christopher's Administration Office indicated, with the help of multicoloured pins, the homes of their patients. The region St Christopher's was serving had a radius of only six miles, with the hospice at its centre. I found that sobering. If at least 70 seventy per cent of us now die in institutions, how could there be a sufficient number of hospices to meet the need? Was there a more cost-effective solution?

Someone, it seemed to me, should carry out a study to see if a St Christopher's-style program could operate effectively within, and as an integrated component of, the existing health-care system, indeed, within a general hospital setting with an associated home-care program, outpatient clinic, and bereavement-support program. That sort of hospice-general hospital (let alone *teaching* hospital) integration had never been attempted in the United Kingdom, or anywhere else for that matter. Would the Vic consider such a program? I mentioned the idea to Dr Saunders.

"It will never happen," she responded.

"Why do you say that?"

"Because hospice goals are antithetical to those of the general hospital, and certainly those of a teaching hospital. The first time there is a shortage of beds, or dollars for nursing staff, the hospice unit would lose out. When the choice is between an urgent medical or surgical admission and a terminally ill patient, who would win out?"

"I'm not so sure," I responded. "You don't know the Royal Victoria Hospital."

During our final afternoon "tea" prior to catching a train to Cambridge for a short family visit with Alice, Peter, Margery, and Wilf, Dr Saunders asked if I would consider returning with my family to work at St Christopher's during the following summer. She and Tom "wished to go birding in Switzerland" and I would be a useful addition to the team in their absence. Without hesitation I agreed.

As I headed out the door, she called after me, "Oh, Bal, incidentally, there is one more thing. You may call me Cicely."

Hospice Care: To Be or Not to Be

Let me see in the sufferer the man alone.

Maimonides

Will you turn me out if I can't get better?

Patient, to Cicely Saunders

*To face death is to face life and to come to terms
with one is to learn much about the other.*

Cicely Saunders

Mid-flight, over the Atlantic en route home to Montreal, my mind was filled with high esteem for Cicely as well as profound respect for St Christopher's and the team who had been my teachers during that eye-opening week.

Our committee's recommendation that the Vic consider developing a hospice had provoked mild interest. *But,* I asked myself, *who in the world could we get to be the lead physician for such an experiment? I can't be the one to take that on, in addition to my practice, surgery, chemotherapy clinic, research, teaching, not to mention family ... We would need a special person ... but who?* Oddly, the question had no sooner occurred to me than a name came to mind. Ina Ajemian.

That was strange indeed! I did not really know Ina. Her husband, George, had been an occasional Royal Vic dentist-on-call roommate during our internship year a decade earlier. I had seen him only once or twice over the intervening years and had briefly met his wife, a family physician, on only one occasion. Why would *she* come to mind?

With a degree of impulsiveness that those I live with might claim was not unique to that occasion, I phoned Ina the next morning and reminded her of our brief encounter. Oh yes, she remembered our having met. I then explained that, "as off the wall as this might sound," I was calling to ask her a hypothetical question. I told her about the Vic study and my visit to St Christopher's. "Now," I wound up my long-shot pitch, feeling more than a little awkward, "*if* the hospital were to agree to such a pilot project, and *if* funding can be located, would you, by any chance, consider taking part? Because, if you would, we should get together for a more detailed chat."

Her answer was immediate and completely unexpected. "It is very strange you should call just now. I have had the strongest feeling lately that I should consider a change in career. I will have to take this call seriously. I would like to hear more."

As we hung up, I realized the hair on the back of my neck was standing up. *That was beyond weird!* The sudden, profoundly mute stillness that, at times, accompanies an unexpected benevolence, that sense of being engulfed in stop-time otherness, confronted and mystified me. *Weird* hardly described it. At a deeper level, I experienced other shadings of response. Shadings that are difficult to express, but no less real for their elusiveness – an undertone of something like anticipated familiarity, an unexpected experience of connectedness, the essence that Cicely referred to as "something stronger, behind it all – not an answer, not an explanation, but a presence," a profound awareness of what the Tibetan Buddhists refer to as an awareness of *the suchness of things*, a sense of newness related somehow to an unanticipated sense of being on prepared ground. The fact is that even now, all these decades later, *this* long-deferred attempt to put into words my reaction to Ina's response is intrusive and I am reminded of Thérèse Vanier's reply to my request to tag along as she made rounds – her sense of hesitation in fostering an exposure of sacredness.

Simply a case of synchronicity, I rationalized (both then and now) in pondering that unlikely phone call and the extreme odds against Ina and me being in contact. But what are the origins of synchronicity when the extremes of probability are stretched as in this case? Is the explanation always simply random chance?

Ina had clearly been pondering the same questions. Ten months later, on 26 July 1974, on the eve of her potentially career-changing first visit to St Christopher's, she wrote me to say, "I have felt very strongly ever since you first approached me that I was being led by the Holy Spirit to get involved. What this means I cannot see, but I pray that we will both be open to the Spirit, if this is to be of God."

"YOU WANT TO START A *WHAT?*"

What was the likelihood that the directors and chiefs of service of McGill's Royal Victoria Hospital would agree to support a new clinical program that addressed a mandate deemed antithetical to teaching-hospital goals, a program that would lead to an increased strain on beds, budget, and administrative structure?

The odds against that *ever* happening were overwhelming! Over the preceding two decades, the Vic had undergone enormous growth. The building projects of 1951–63 had included construction of new medical and surgical wings, extensive renovations to the private wards of the Ross Pavilion, and a new $20,000,000 psychiatric research and training centre. Furthermore, as the 1960s wore on, Quebec adopted the federal plan for state-sponsored health insurance. This had resulted in an increase in the number of patients, required beds, laboratory demands, length of stay, staff, and drug costs. By 1967, the RVH activities, compared to 1960 levels, had risen significantly: days of treatment (117 per cent), surgical procedures (117 per cent), admissions (121 per cent), number of interns and residents (126 per cent), number of honorary and attending staff physicians (132 per cent), number of nursing staff (160 per cent), outpatient visits (160 per cent). In the same period, there was a near doubling in the number of radiologic examinations and radiation-therapy treatments, and a near tripling in the number of electrocardiograms (ECGs) performed, emergency visits, and total staff wages. Over that same interval, total hospital expenses had increased two and a half times. In his 1968 annual report, Executive Director Gilbert Turner noted: "We spent $22,000,000 last year, almost as much every twenty-four hours ($61,000) as it took to operate the Hospital for the whole of 1894 [its opening year]. The suppliers of the funds thought that it was too much; many of the departmental heads thought it was not enough."

The 1970s brought continuing challenges under the new executive director, Douglas MacDonald. There had been a significant infiltration of provincial bureaucracy into daily hospital affairs without apparent enhanced productivity. Also, the venerable and venerated Royal Victoria Hospital Nurses Training School was closed with the opening in 1970 of the junior college (CEGEP) training schools for Quebec nursing education. The Vic would thus no longer be able to recruit, select, and train nurses to its own standard of excellence.

With a determined emphasis on staff initiative during 1973 and 1974, morale remained high and there was an increase in volume of activity as well as a reduction in the length of patient stay. Nevertheless, the rising costs associated with universal health care meant that financial support for hospitals was progressively falling behind inflation and bargained wages, let alone keeping up with the costs associated with improving health-care standards. By 1978, the accumulated deficit of Quebec hospitals would reach $150,000,000 and it was estimated that figure would double in the subsequent few years. During the four-year interval 1975–79, the *annual* Royal Vic budget deficit amounted to nearly $5.8 million.[1]

Protecting one's turf was the order of the day. Service chiefs were concerned with maintaining staff, morale, and their number of beds. The clouds on the fiscal horizon were indeed ominous during the final months of 1973 when the final decision concerning the proposed "end-of-life care" service was to come to a vote.

Among the many correctives introduced by the Royal Vic Board of Governors in an attempt to counter this grim confluence of circumstances was the appointment of Ken MacKinnon as director of professional services (DPS). He would continue as chief of urology, but it was clear to the hospital power-brokers that his thoughtful, calm, conciliatory approach was needed if the Vic was to continue to flourish.

Surprisingly, new provincial programs appeared to have relevance. A notice from Jacques Brunet, deputy minister in the Quebec Ministry of Social Affairs, arrived at the Vic on 15 October 1973. It announced short-term funding for "new job-creating, innovative programs." Ken and his administrative colleague Anne Morgan felt that my proposed program might meet the criteria.

A CONSULTATION REQUEST

The consultation request from the Women's Pavilion read: "Twenty year-old white female with ovarian carcinoma, seizures, hypertension and hypercalcuria. Pyelography demonstrates non-visualization of left kidney and poor visualization of right kidney. Do you recommend further urologic evaluation or intervention?"

The consult had arrived a day or two earlier. I had intended to see the patient immediately but was rushing through a backlog of patients and paperwork prior to hurrying to the airport to pick up EKR. Our schedule in the next couple of days would be full, what with lectures to medical students and discussions involving Elisabeth and our planning group regarding the proposed "Royal Vic hospice program."

There would be just enough time to see either the x-rays or the patient before going to the airport – clearly there wasn't sufficient time to do both. I dashed down to radiology and reviewed the intravenous pyelogram and concluded there was nothing to be gained by further urologic assessment. On calling the ward to let them know that it would be a couple of days before I could get there, the nurse informed me that Carol, the patient, was a student nurse. *A student nurse ... I wonder if she has heard of Elisabeth ... it could be a mountaintop experience for Carol to meet her ... but I can hardly bring Elisabeth to see this young woman without finding out how much she knows about her illness – and about Elisabeth's work, for that matter ... I mean, I can't just wander in with EKR without knowing how all that stands!*

Elisabeth's visit was profitable, the lectures and meetings a great success.[2] I mentioned Carol's consult to her in passing and she was more than agreeable to dropping in to see her – but the timing just didn't work out. *Simply too many people for Elisabeth to meet if we are going to make as much political mileage as we can out of her visit! So much riding on it!*

Returning from the airport after dropping Elisabeth off, I went to Carol's room in the Woman's Pavilion. Her face was slim and somewhat wan, her hair fair. She forced a thin smile as I introduced myself.

"I'm glad to meet you," she offered, "I've been expecting you for several days." Here was a chance both to apologize for my tardiness and to open the door to a meaningful discussion. "I'm sorry I was delayed. Does the name Elisabeth Kübler-Ross mean anything to you?"

"It does," she nodded. "I heard her speak a year and a half ago when she was in Montreal. She has taken all the fear out of dying."

I felt sick – as if I had been kicked! Elisabeth's oft-repeated axiom "The best teachers are the dying patients themselves" came to mind. *Lesson One: Never postpone anything you want to say to, or do for, a dying patient!* It was to be the first of several lessons from Carol. Irony of ironies! I had taken the time to see her films though there was little chance of anything being gained by doing so, but I had missed the chance to explore her emotional needs, where perhaps much could have been done! Mountaintop missed! *Lesson two: Had I cared about the person as much as the x-ray, this wouldn't have happened!*

We chatted. It seemed to her an eternity since her sister's weddings eight weeks earlier. There had been a month of nagging abdominal aches before that and since, an endless stream of investigations, then surgery. Then the hammer fell. It was an aggressive carcinoma of the ovary. Twenty years old. A student nurse. How should she – how *could* she respond?

"Carol, who, or what, has helped you most in dealing with all this?"

"One of the residents. He took the time to sit down with me one morning after the entourage had left the room. He said, 'Hey, I hear you didn't sleep very well last night. How come?' So we talked and I felt so much better." *Lesson three: It takes so little to make a world of difference!'*

On a later visit to Carol, her parents were in the room. A terrible tension was evident as I joined them. Forced smiles. A pressure cooker of awkwardness. The three of us stood stiff and stilted. An electric charge reverberated in the air. They were talking – about the weather, the radio program, her music, the flowers and greeting cards on the bedside table – about *anything* except what was on everyone's mind.

Her father followed me into the hall. He spoke of how tough it was, how he frequently had to leave the room to avoid "breaking down" in front of her. We discussed the alternatives.

"But I don't think she really knows the situation," he said hesitantly. I told him that earlier that day she had squeezed my hand with urgency and asked, "Do you think there is life after death?" Then, with her eyes welling up, she had added with a wistful smile, "I sure hope so! I'm not afraid of dying, but I'm afraid of hurting my family and my boyfriend. I don't want them to suffer."

Her father looked at me in silence, and then, squaring his shoulders, he went into her room. In the flood of openness that followed, the conspiracy of silence was replaced by shared love and mutual support. *Lesson four: Support and growth may flow from healing connections.* The rich flow of lessons from Carol revealed all too clearly how much I had to learn.

To the end, Carol demonstrated courage and strength. While there was acceptance at one level, she carried a protective shield of denial at another, a sense of hope that she needed less and less as the days passed, until the day when, with her father and me beside her, she commented, looking at him and holding tightly to both our hands, "This can't go on. I want to die. I'm sorry to say that, Daddy. I love you so much ..."

In her final days she left us further lessons. *Lesson five: It is the whole health-care team that fails to meet the patient's needs!* There was the nurse who thought that doctors were not supposed to be left alone with Carol because they might say something to upset her; there was the clergyman who attended her at the end but couldn't speak to her needs because he wasn't aware of her faith; there was the doctor who ordered her second electroencephalogram (EEG) that week on the day Carol died.

The lessons from Carol didn't end there. *Lesson six: Openness makes a difference!'* Elisabeth's openness had made a difference to both Carol and me when we heard her speak for the first time eighteen months earlier. It had struck a chord in us, and in many others, a chord that statistically significant data, no matter what the p value, could not have achieved. Later, it was the resident's openness, then her father's, that transformed isolation to accompaniment.

Elisabeth asked me to write a chapter for her upcoming book, *Death: The Final Stage of Growth*. I sent her "Letter to Elisabeth: Dedicated to Carol."[3]

Carol died peacefully on 19 October.

REPORT OF THE RVH COMMITTEE ON THANATOLOGY, OCTOBER 1973

The fifty-page report commenced with the admonition by Maimonides, *Let me see in the sufferer the man alone.* It was sent to each member of the RVH Board of Directors. To ensure that we captured the reader's attention, each copy was individually stamped in red "SENSITIVE & CONFIDENTIAL" on the first page. Once again, the focus of concern was defined as "patients for whom active treatment aimed at cure or prolonging survival is no longer relevant: they may or may not be imminently terminally ill." The document included the history of our research committee, Allan Jones's nine case summaries highlighting deficient Royal Vic care, the findings generated by staff responses to the "RVH Questionnaire on Death and Dying," staff observations regarding existing RVH deficiencies in care, and, finally, the recommendation that the RVH develop a hospice program. The suggested patient population would include those with advanced malignant disease and selected patients with chronic neurologic disorders such as motor-neurone disease. The proposed program would include five clinical arms: a forty-bed inpatient ward, a home-care service, an out-patient clinic, a consultation program to serve the Royal Vic active-treatment wards, and a bereavement follow-up service. The recommended multidisciplinary team would include nurses, physicians, a psychiatrist, physical and occupational therapists, social workers, clergy, and trained volunteers.

The photographs I had taken at St Christopher's had been shot using Kodachrome 64 film. Given my inexperience, I feared the worst. To my astonishment, *all* the images captured during those memorable St Christopher's moments had perfect exposure, focus, and composition. A record of photographic success I have not subsequently come close to equalling! They proved to be an invaluable asset. When combined with the Royal Vic study data, they became a powerful tool in selling the proposal. Cicely had exhorted, "Let the patients do the talking." We did.

I was invited to give Grand Rounds by five of the major Royal Vic services – Surgery, Medicine, Psychiatry, Obstetrics/Gynacology, and

Urology – as well as two research seminars at the Allan Memorial Institute, a multidisciplinary seminar for all staff, and, finally, a seminar for hospital volunteers. In addition, undergraduate training was pursued through lectures to first- and second-year McGill medical students.

The response was gratifying. At the Surgical Grand Rounds presentation, Chief of Surgery Lloyd Maclean summed up the feeling of many present when, on seeing the St Christopher's slides, he commented appreciatively, "Well, I'll tell you one thing, I have never seen a dying patient who looked like that."

I was most uneasy about Psychiatry Grand Rounds. I could all too easily imagine the question period taking me out of my depth in short order. The response of my psychiatrist colleagues was, however, both unexpected and touching. In 1971 Maurice Dongier, a native of France who had trained in psychiatry at the Allan Memorial Institute, returned to McGill as psychiatrist-in-chief following seventeen years of practice and teaching at university hospitals in Marseilles and Liège. His comments during Grand Rounds were strongly supportive. He offered enthusiastic collaboration, noting with a telltale smile, "It is the first time I can recall looking to a urologist for insights regarding my end of the body." He went on to support financially a part-time psychiatrist for our team.

The only negative response in the many Grand Rounds and teaching sessions occurred during the Urology Rounds when a Royal Vic urology colleague – the same man who had opposed my recruitment to the Vic – got to his feet to object to what he considered "all this namby-pamby giving up attitude." In his opinion, such care was "total nonsense!" He argued that he, like Dylan Thomas's father, would choose to "not go gently into that good night, but rage, rage against the dying of the light."

His objections provided the opportunity to consider the cost of denial, the potential that may be gained in actively addressing an unavoidable reality, and his right to die as he chose. He had, I suggested, "a perfect right to rage away, if that is what he preferred to do," but his patients also had the right to something more.

On 18 October our report was presented to the RVH Executive Committee. It was their unanimous opinion that it deserved further consideration by the Medical Advisory Committee. Their support, in turn, was secured on 30 November. During the detailed discussion of the proposal at that meeting, Dr Dongier urged that, in addition to ratifying the program, the chiefs of service commit tangible support in terms of beds, personnel, and financial assistance. As a result, Administrator Anne

Morgan and I were asked to undertake a review of the economic aspects of the proposal, with detailed analysis of those requiring government and private funding.

A MEETING OF THE COUNCIL OF PHYSICIANS
AND DENTISTS AND BEYOND

Since support by the medical staff was considered critical for the proposal to move forward, the full Royal Victoria Hospital Council of Physicians and Dentists was convened to vote on the matter. Ken MacKinnon warned that, while failure to make it over this hurdle wouldn't completely prevent long-term success, it would make it much less likely. While most colleagues might be reluctant to publicly oppose improved care for the dying, if a groundswell of opposition began at the Council meeting, it might be difficult to stop. "It isn't easy to oppose hospice care, it's like coming out against milk and motherhood; nevertheless, most would add I don't want it in my backyard!" Beds were scarce, budget pressures enormous. The stakes were extremely high!

The J.S.L. Browne amphitheatre was as full as I had ever seen it for such a gathering. Ken MacKinnon was in the chair as director of professional services. I had planted one or two colleagues with supportive comments to get us off to a good start. The momentum seemed to be in our favour early on, but after fifteen minutes or so of discussion, a senior oncologist got to his feet to declare his opposition. Such a program, he noted dismissively, was unnecessary. He and his colleagues knew how to care for their patients. Besides, *most* of their patients would at some point die. Such a service would have a devastating impact on their practices. I listened with concern. Did I detect a degree of supportive restlessness among the silent majority in the room? It appeared that way from my vantage point near the back of the auditorium.

I then realized that, among the nine case reports that had been included in the report, three of the most egregious were patients cared for by this particular colleague. No one else would have recognized them as his, but *he* would have had he given the report even a cursory reading. Surely, if he *had* read the report, he would not have had the nerve to speak out. I was certain he had not read it.

The room had grown silent. The level of tension had increased. I motioned to the chairman that I would like to respond. Permission was granted. Turning to my colleague who was sitting across the amphitheatre to my right, I queried, "May I ask if you have had the chance to read the report?" He had not.

"Well, given the seriousness of the findings, I'm amazed that you would feel free to comment on the recommendations." He sat down and the vote in favour was unanimous. The path was clear for a two-year pilot-project trial.

The Royal Victoria Hospital hospice program, should it come into being, would be a first. While other centres had started an in-hospital ward for the dying (St Boniface, Winnipeg) or a home-care program (New Haven, Connecticut), no one in Canada, the United States, or anywhere else had attempted the full-range of clinical services as an integrated system of care offered by a teaching hospital, coupled with undergraduate and graduate multidisciplinary teaching programs and a robust research initiative.

Could it be done? In two years? Cicely thought not, and she was rarely wrong. We would have twenty-four months to obtain ongoing financial support, design and develop the programs, attract a competent whole-person care team (*What disciplines are absolutely necessary? A music therapist, for example?! What if we didn't have one and we later learned of the therapeutic efficacy of music?*), document relevant interventions, obtain objective data reflecting outcomes, and prepare a detailed report! Twenty-four months!

A RVH HOSPICE? HOW? WHAT? WHEN? WHERE?

"A *Hospice* at the Royal Victoria Hospital? Mais non, mon ami, ce n'est pas possbile au Québec!" My friend went on to explain that, while in England, the term *hospice* may evoke images of "hospitality" and "a resting place for travellers," among Quebec francophones the term brought to mind neglect and the warehouse-style nursing-home shabbiness of *les Hospices* in France.

How disappointing! I had liked the idea of the Vic having a "Hospice." The term, I believed, would have the advantage of ambiguity in a culture in which end-of-life care had meant hopelessness rather than excellence of care and quality of life. In 1973 few in North America had ever heard the word "hospice." "Hospice Inc." (later called "Hospice New Haven"), which would be known as the "first American Hospice," was still only a glint in the eye of Florence Wald, dean of nursing at Yale University.[4] The term *hospice* would not bring connotations of death and despair to mind in English-speaking Canada, or any connotations at all, for that matter. I thought the name would be perfect. Apparently not! The implications of the word for our francophone colleagues would be disastrous. But what can we call it? "Critical Care Service"? "End-of-Life Care"? *Hardly!* ... I was drawing a blank.

As I showered the next morning, my name-chasing continued. *What exactly is the goal of our proposed program? Clearly, it is to improve quality of life; to mitigate ... "to improve the quality of"... What about "palliative care"? But what is the etymology of the word palliate?*

The term, as used in 1973, had come to imply "non-curative" as in "palliative radiation therapy" but the etymology of the word was interesting. "Palliate," it turned out, was derived from the Latin word "pallium," meaning a cloak. The pallium was a short outer garment of Greek origin but common among Romans and Jews as well. It was worn by both men and women and was rectangular in shape. Held by a brooch over one shoulder, the pallium descended to just above the knees, and thus it hid or concealed those areas that might be covered by an undergarment and any weapon the person might be carrying. Thus, "to palliate" initially meant to conceal or hide, but by the sixteenth century it had come to mean *to mitigate* or *to make less severe.*[5]

Problem solved! To palliate is to mitigate, thus to improve the quality of! Our program would be the *Royal Victoria Hospital Palliative Care Service* (RVH-PCS).

I wrote both Cicely and Robert Twycross to run the term past them. Both felt it was not suitable and expressed that opinion in no uncertain terms. We used it anyway and when, in 1987, the Royal Colleges of London and Edinburgh officially recognized their new UK discipline as *palliative medicine*, I was delighted!

Where could the proposed Palliative Care Unit (PCU) be located? A long-range possibility existed in the Women's Pavilion but that would be at least three years off. All agreed that an interim location was required to capitalize on the momentum created by recent discussions. "Four Medical" was being considered. It had housed the flagship Endocrine Investigative Unit, but with a decrease in recent activity, hospital planners felt it might be converted to a twelve-bed palliative care ward. A start-up date of December 1974 was thought to be possible.

Meanwhile, many questions needed to be addressed. Hospital deaths over the previous year were shared equally by Medicine, Surgery, and a grouping of other services. As a result, a single department could not be asked to forfeit the total number of beds required. Furthermore, to whom should the administration of the program report? A critical question! "He who holds the cards, calls the shots," I was reminded. There were three clinical budget centres at the RVH: Medicine, Surgery, and Obstetrics-Gynacology. The new Palliative Care Service would be serving the needs of all three. Should Palliative Care report to a triumvirate with representation from all three centres? That formula had been problematic when recently utilized in managing the Vic's new organ-transplantation program.

In addition, there was the question Cicely had raised. Whichever cost centre the PCS answered to, who would make the admission decision when the only available bed in the hospital was on the Palliative Care Unit? Similarly, if an acute-care ward had an unexpected shortage of nurses on a given nursing shift, and the PCU was better staffed, would PCU nurses be expected to meet the need on the acute-care ward?

Dr Sylvia Cruess, an attending physician in the Department of Medicine, became RVH Director of Professional Services in 1978. She later commented on those early days of decision:

> It was a turf war. Basically everyone felt, *What you are doing is*
> *absolutely marvellous! But, not in my space!* Surgery was the most
> vociferous, but then they were more likely to say what was on their
> minds. You didn't know how big a fight you were getting into. What
> saved the PCS was that you were planning an academic program
> and would critically assess outcomes. Otherwise it would have died
> on the spot. The fact that you were a surgical oncologist wasn't
> a factor of particular significance. Physicians listen to physicians.
> The fact that you were a surgeon got the surgeons to listen – they
> wouldn't have believed a medical person. *But,* starting the PCS at
> a time of deficit budgeting *was*, a critical issue! Particularly since
> Palliative Care seemed so aberrant to the main mission of the insti-
> tution. I think Anne Morgan and Ken MacKinnon were probably
> factors arguing for you, but I wasn't DPS at the very first, so I can't
> say for sure who the movers and shakers were. Maurice McGregor
> [chief of medicine at the time of the critical decisions] was always
> thoughtful. He responded to each question with another question,
> and to an assertion with yet another question – very much a Socratic
> approach. He *had* to have been supportive in giving up those beds,
> or it wouldn't have happened, and he wouldn't have agreed unless he
> thought it was worthwhile.

TEACHABLE MOMENTS

My photographs of comfortable, alert, St Christopher's patients led to a flurry of pain-control consultation requests throughout the hospital. With the assistance of Pharmacist-in-Chief Gordon Brooks, we created standardized solutions containing varying doses of morphine together with the other components of the time-honoured "Brompton Mixture"[6] and developed detailed instructions for prescribing this solution, given by mouth in doses carefully adjusted to each patient's individual need.

In our Royal Vic Brompton Mixture, each 20cc. "dose" provided one of four escalating strengths of morphine – the "standard" 10 mg. of morphine, or the increasing concentrations of 20, 30, and 40 mg. of morphine per dose. We knew from Cicely's experience that, when given regularly by mouth every four hours around the clock, the dose required to *consistently prevent* cancer-related pain is often very low.[7] Cicely found that too often painkillers were given by injection in doses that were too high, when they could have been effective by mouth in significantly lower doses. Her message was: *Start by mouth* (rather than injection), *with a low dose,* at *regular intervals to consistently just prevent* pain, rather than letting it crop up again between doses.[8]

The protocol was tested at the Vic during the closing months of 1973 and duplicated Cicely's results. Thus, on 28 January 1974, the Royal Vic medical director, Dr Ashton Kerr, sent an official hospital memorandum, "Brompton's Mixture for Relief of Pain in Terminal Cancer," to all attending staff, house staff, nurses, and pharmacy staff. Vastly improved pain control resulted with the new policy in place. In the three-month period from November 1973 to January 1974, forty patients received the RVH Brompton's Mixture with excellent results.

Sometime later, in Cicely's presence, I mindlessly referred to this type of meticulous St Christopher's-style assessment and management planning as the "Gospel according to St Cicely." When the session ended and the participants had departed, an unamused Dr Saunders turned to me and, looking down from on high, proclaimed, "Oh incidentally, if you ever refer to me as St Cicely again in public, I shall kill you!"

Each new palliative-care consultation request provided the opportunity to introduce yet another group of nurses, medical students, residents, and attending staff to the St Christopher's model of pain relief, detailed patient and family whole-person needs assessment, and the concept of a personalized-care response. Cicely's practice of seizing the "teachable moment" was bearing fruit even before agreement to establish a Palliative Care Service had been finalized. The word was spreading, and the process was accelerated on a vastly wider stage thanks to EKR, who distributed the RVH Brompton Mixture memorandum from country to country at her lectures and seminars.

Two grace-filled reminders of the potential for shared gain through loss rounded out this remarkably eventful pre-PCS year. Our first letter expressing gratitude for bereavement support was received from a nursing colleague following the death of her lovely seventeen-year-old daughter, and the first donations to our Royal Vic Thanatology Fund arrived in memory of Bernard Robert de Massy, sent by his loving, international francophone family. All that the future RVH palliative-care programs would offer might be seen as taking root in and flowing from the template symbolized by these first enabling gifts. Such return to our as yet non-existent service from the appreciative community around us signalled the gratitude that would flow in abundance to the Vic as the years passed. It was a reminder of the wisdom of the would-be peasant of Assisi who observed that it is in giving that we receive.

BES

Lorine Besel was named Royal Victoria Hospital director of nursing and vice-president for nursing services in 1974, a development that directly influenced all subsequent decisions regarding the Palliative Care Service.

It was evident to all that she was gifted with shrewd insight and unswerving determination. She was a woman on a mission that was equally focused on both quality patient care and the role of nursing. She deferred to no one. "Bes," as she was known throughout the hospital, creatively shaped everything she touched. Significant among her many contributions was her edict that Nursing must be involved as an *equal* partner in *all* Royal Vic senior administrative deliberations, a major departure from earlier practices. A graduate of Winnipeg's St Boniface Hospital, McGill University, and Boston University, she was director of nursing at the Allan Memorial Institute prior to assuming her nursing-leadership role in the Vic at large.

As Bes assumed office, the province of Quebec had the most severe nursing shortage in Canada and the lowest ratio of graduate nurses per 100,000 population. Quebec nursing wages were the lowest in the country; the starting salary was 20 per cent less than the national average. The nursing-salary disparity between Quebec and Ontario next door was more than $4,000 per year. Salaries and benefits were higher still in the United States. In addition, following closure of the Royal Vic's Nurses Training School, applicants had widely varying qualifications, thus complicating attempts to develop a cohesive recruitment team. Nursing in Quebec in general, and at the Vic in particular, was in trouble.

With nursing costs accounting for more than one-third of the total hospital budget, and given the financial realities facing Quebec health care in 1974, the pressure to economize was oppressive if not staggering as Bes took office. In response, she presented to the hospital's Board of

Directors a comprehensive analysis documenting external and internal factors adversely affecting nursing, as a means of "helping the whole of the Royal Vic community [and others] to understand nursing problems within their broader context." She also proposed remedies and further studies to be undertaken. Among the latter was a 1975 systems analysis to study the nursing-care needs in each clinical unit, expressed as the mean number of required nursing hours per-patient day. This data enabled a precise needs-based defence of nursing budgets. Through such initiatives, she sought and achieved increased nursing recruitment and retention as well as improved standards and morale. During Bes's watch as director of nursing, the staff-turnover rate would drop from more than 40 per cent per annum to 8–12 per cent.[9]

Reflecting on those turbulent times, Bes would later observe:

I was aware that I was bringing the perspective of a psychiatric nurse to the Director's position and knew I would need to be careful about how I promulgated my views. My central goal was to promote patient-centred care, care of the whole person. I saw that as the nursing mandate throughout the hospital. But in pursuing that end, I realized that there was a risk that I might be considered just another psychiatric wingbat.

I had read Kübler-Ross's book; my own mother had died during that period and I found her work helpful in dealing with my family. I continued to use her insights in teaching on the wards and in the classroom.

I saw the proposed PCS as a model for care of the whole person, but there needed to be no appearance of favouritism. Fortunately, reality was on my side. I simply needed to focus on the everyday occurrences documented in the "Untoward Incidents" reports. They are the medical errors – falls, anything that has gone awry ... all kinds of things. Each morning the reports for all such events during the previous 24-hours were placed on my desk for review. I simply used those incidents to make my case.

Statistics are one thing, but when you're the only female at the Council of Physicians Meeting and a surgeon makes a generalization, you need to respond with relevant fact. I would say, "Just a minute! I have an example of the problem I'm speaking of, and it happened *last night*, on *your ward*! The Untoward Incidents gave me *concrete* examples with *real people* under *their* care! They were personal and relevant in a way that statistics can never be. The Incident Reports were invaluable in making the case for the PCU.

We could be specific about things that were occurring on a daily basis.

For example, we were admitting dying patients to the wards after shoving them through the ER, even when there was no room for them. They would be admitted simply to line the halls on the ward! Without even a call bell! The nurses didn't know what was going on and didn't have time to look. For me it was unacceptable for nursing to accept, without thought, responsibilities they could not deal with, simply on the order of the doctor. So, my question was, "Why are you accepting these patients?! You know you have no one available to give adequate care; there isn't even a call bell! Why don't we simply park them on the corner of St Catherine and Peel streets?!" To me it was just common sense. *Just say no!!* You can, you know. You don't have the staff to give proper care; to accept the patient is dangerous.

In addition, the Untoward Incident Reports were useful in working with the nurses, because the nursing group as a whole did not see the need for a PCS. They would protest, "We just follow the doctors' orders, and besides, we don't have time to give psychosocial support and care for the family; we don't have the staff for that!" They also found it hard to imagine working with the doctors at a collegial rather than subordinate level, or alongside volunteers, or, for that matter, as part of a multidisciplinary team.

When I became Director, there was a need to make nursing respectable, to support the nurses' self-esteem. Up until then, the Head Nurse of each ward was appointed – *anointed actually!* – by the Service Chief. He simply put in whomever he liked. I stopped that! The decision had to be made by the Director of Nursing based on her personal criteria. The Service Chief could be on the selection committee, but *I make the decision*! Nursing needed to be seen as a profession in partnership with the doctors – *partners*, not hand-maidens! But *I* didn't achieve that, *the nurses* did, once given the opportunity!

We saw Four Medical as a temporary site for the PCU, pure and simple. I still had a certain amount of play in terms of budget-ing there, but when dying patients are on the general medical or surgical wards, costing is a problem. I don't know if people really understand how budget discussions go. *Nursing services* is a single budget line, like medical or surgical supplies, or dietary costs, or whatever. Nursing? When you are over-budget there is absolutely murderous questioning. Why is this?! What about that? Why that

other thing?! When that process starts, the discussion of the validity of each contributing item and every minuscule question to do
with Palliative Care that you thought had been settled and agreed
upon long ago, can surface again years later! However, once we had
a separate PCU, it had its *own* budget which gave us more freedom. The heavy nursing care needs of the Palliative Care patients
– higher than any other patient group [as shown by Bes's "nursing
care needs index" data] – meant we could justify the higher nursing
coverage based on documented patient need, but, the higher nurse-
to-patient ratio also made the PCU much more vulnerable. It stood
out in budget terms. Budgets and money ruled *every* question over
those years!

Special nursing disbursements related to Palliative Care required
individual strategies. The Consultation Nurse – and eventually two
consult nurses and the four senior Home Care Nurses, paid for from
the *inpatient* nursing budget, are an example. [All six of these senior
positions were later added to the PCS nursing budget as being critical
for optimum patient care.]

As Director of Nursing you have to think through what is needed
to give the best chance of impacting on the overall goal of the hospital, then make it happen. You look around and ferret your way
through the maze. The detailed rationale underlying each disburse-
ment in the nursing budget is the Director of Nursing's responsibility.
The rationale may be shared with one or two others, but it is up
to the Director to carry forward that priority and make it happen.
There are manoeuvres in relation to *any* war! It's a game – but it's
a tough game! The Service Chief and Head Nurse of the unit under
discussion have to be onside, but these budget meetings are brutal!!
I don't think many people understand the difficulty of trying to provide optimal care under the financial conditions imposed on us. And
it's doubly difficult for nursing – we have to be SO pure! You need a
pit bull and I was a good pit bull.

I didn't consciously set out to be empowering of my nurses, though
that happened. The real goal was to improve patient care. The steps
I took were simply to give nursing a push in the direction in which
nursing and patient care should develop. Nursing had to reconfigure
its self-image, to recognize that nurses are not the only providers
of care, but instead, the *central* members of a team that involves all
disciplines and family members and volunteers … and everyone in the
hospital community, including the cleaners.

PLANNING, PLANNING, PLANNING

What is needed to achieve the metamorphosis from community-based hospice in London, England, to a Palliative Care Service in a McGill teaching hospital? The two models had shared challenges: the needs of patients and families facing life-limiting illness; attention to detail in diagnosis and therapeutics by an experienced multidisciplinary team; and commitment to evaluation and teaching. But there were also myriad issues unique to the demands imposed by our differences in timing, place, and health-care system.

Initially, the Royal Vic service chiefs agreed to commit to a pilot project of only one year's duration, but in due course, influenced by the invaluable high levels of public interest, glowing press coverage, and its own liberal values, the Quebec government upped the ante. It would support us for *two* years! Furthermore, its initial demand that we ask for federal as well as provincial funding was amended to state that *only* provincial finding (that is, from Quebec) should be sought. The chiefs couldn't turn that down.

Two years! *What* we planned to do, *how*, *where*, and *with whom* we would achieve our goals, how to *evaluate* the project, the *writing up*, *presentation of results*, and the final *decision from on high* regarding our future, all of that had to be complete within the two-year pilot-project time span.

We felt deeply privileged. It was a pioneering task in a hospital with a proud tradition. From my first 1963 walk down the marble hall to Queen Victoria's statue while listening to the authors of my medical school *Textbook of Surgery* being paged, the Royal Vic garnered my emotional allegiance like no other institution. To oversimplify, I loved the place and what it stood for! To be sure, we were undertaking the pilot project out of a sense of moral obligation to correct a serious health-care problem, but also, and increasingly, we were acting out of pride of institution and province. It was a pride that would grow as the months and years passed and others failed to follow. Under adverse circumstances, the Vic had stepped up to the plate! Quebec had stepped up! *Other* teaching hospitals and provinces failed to do so, both in Canada and elsewhere. Shame! We were "damn proud" of the Royal Vic and the province that enabled the experiment. We didn't want to let down our patients and their families; we didn't want to let down the Vic or the provincial funders that had supported this unique health-care experiment in tough times.

Could St Christopher's level of excellence be duplicated within the existing institutions of the Canadian health-care system? We would soon know. If we failed, the results would be widely known and the chances of the hypothesis being tested again would be greatly diminished. On the other hand, if we succeeded, that would challenge others in the international community. The stakes continued to be high; if anything, they were getting higher. A sense of pressure was with us daily.

Throughout 1974, regular PCS Core Group meetings[10] were convened to develop policies that would safeguard PCS goals while serving the dynamic, ever-changing Royal Vic environment. RVH patient-care need was estimated by reviewing the inpatient cancer deaths for 1971, 1972, and 1973, accounting for 7,986, 8,234, and 5,165 hospitalization days respectively, with mean lengths of stay being thirty, thirty-two, and thirty-four days. In addition, approximately one hundred additional RVH patients per year were referred for end-of-life placement at other centres. The best estimate of the need for PCU beds was thirty-six to forty beds. The proposed pilot project would be carried out with a twelve-bed PCU. This would involve a reallocation of services rather than an addition of new RVH beds.

Our PCS guidelines were drawn up based on St Christopher's norms of practice. They included:

- PCU decor will be designed to create a therapeutic environment promoting calm, confidence, efficiency, security, and a feeling of welcome that celebrates the individuality of each patient and family. Through traffic to other hospital areas and the traditional busyness and clutter of active treatment wards must be avoided.
- PCS patients at home or admitted to an active treatment ward will be followed by a physician on the PCS Home Care or Consult service, respectively.
- PCU admission decisions and subsequent orders will be written by a PCS doctor rather than the Emergency Room gatekeeper or referring doctor. Continuing involvement by the referring doctor will, however, be encouraged. Patients waiting for PCU admission from the ER or inpatient wards will be prioritized on the basis of need. On PCU admission, the Head Nurse will greet the patient and family by name, see to their comfort and notify the PCS MD.
- Pulse, temperature and blood pressure will *not* be routinely monitored, nor will there be routine laboratory testing. *Any* lab tests ordered must be justified in the patient's chart.
- Problem-oriented charting will be used.

- Volunteers will not have access to patient charts.
- Open, around-the-clock visiting by "family" of all ages will be permitted, with Monday "visitor's day off," thus validating the family's need for respite. Non-family and overnight visiting will be welcomed and monitored by the PCU Head Nurse.
- At death: the bedside curtains may be closed if the family wishes, or if there is a special reason, otherwise they will be left open unless specifically objected to by the family; PCU staff will gather with family and friends to read together at the bedside an inclusive, nonsectarian universal prayer in recognition of the shared significance of this crossroad. Standard RVH nursing procedures with the body will be carried out. The PCU MD, or at night, the ICU Resident on call, will declare the patient dead.
- Weekly meetings will include: the Patient Management Conference with the full multidisciplinary team, the Doctors' Review and Support Meeting, and the Nurses Bull and Beef Session, a staff support session led by the psychiatrist.
- Ongoing PCS Team Evaluation will be carried out by the Clarke Institute of Psychiatry, Toronto.
- Bereavement Follow-Up [BFU] support offered to the family will include, at a minimum, contact at two weeks, a card sent on the anniversary of the death and an invitation to the PCU monthly memorial service at the 3 months and 1 year anniversaries of the death. A standard bereavement risk assessment of all families will be undertaken as an ongoing process during their PCU stay, thus enabling adjusted interventions as indicated.
- A Volunteer Director will be selected by the PCS Director and an appointed committee. Selection criteria for PCU, BFU and Administrative volunteers will be established. PCU volunteers may participate in hands-on patient care under the direct supervision of a PCU nursing colleague. A rigorous volunteer training program, ongoing evaluation norms, opportunities for continuing education, and criteria for dismissal will be established.

As we prepared for our clinical-care programs, it was important to continue our research, teaching, and outreach initiatives. On 31 January 1974 EKR returned to McGill to participate in the medical student Basic Concepts in Oncology lecture series. Once again, her presence brought wide attention to the needs of the terminally ill and the Royal Vic plans for a Palliative Care Service. The *Montreal Star* covered EKR's lecture, as did the *McGill Daily*, and on 14 February the *Montreal Gazette* carried

"A Plan to Humanize Dying," a major two-page article detailing the Royal Vic's PCS plans and an account of Carol's illness. On 15 February the *Gazette* ran an editorial, "In the Midst of Life," thanking the Vic for our "efforts to humanize dying." At the same time, the *Hamilton Spectator* article "Doctors Shun Telling Patients of Death" by Charles Wilkinson reviewed the results of the Vic study and discussed the "conspiracy of silence."

Similar anglophone and francophone press and radio coverage continued through 1974, helping to build and sustain support for the Vic's PCS initiative. In the spring of 1974 the Toronto Christian Fellowship journal *CRUX* published a special edition "On Death and Dying." It brought together compelling photography, quotes to ponder, and original articles by Cicely Saunders, Elisabeth Kübler-Ross, Merville Vincent (psychiatrist), Arthur Boorman (McGill theologian), and myself. This generous contribution by busy colleagues resulted in a document that was useful in reaching potential donors. At the same time, my "A Letter to Elisabeth: Dedicated to Carol" chapter in EKR's book *Death: The Final Stage of Growth* generated further greatly needed support. Public interest was also fostered by a continuing series of presentations, seminars, and discussion groups throughout the province and beyond.

TEAM BUILDING

Over the ten months following the early-morning telephone call when we first spoke, Ina Ajemian remained committed in principle to leaving her family-medicine practice and joining the PCS as physician and PCU clinical director, while I would remain director of the five RVH and community-based PCS programs as well as our research and teaching activities. Her final decision would depend on a plan I had developed with Cicely for Ina to spend one month at St Christopher's during August 1974. In undertaking these activities, Ina would become a full-time member of the RVH attending staff with admitting privileges in the Department of Medicine. Since she was a family physician rather than an internal-medicine fellow of the Royal College, this position would establish a precedent. More prickly still, the Department of Medicine would be expected to contribute funding to sweeten her salary. While the Department of Surgery had moved quickly to support the project and to contribute four beds, the Department of Medicine's deliberations were painfully drawn out, but at the eleventh hour it finally agreed.

Ina enjoyed her month at St Christopher's immensely and on 3 September 1974 Cicely sent me *her* assessment: "We much enjoyed Ina, who is a super person and I do hope that you will get her." We did! Ina opted to leave her thriving private practice and accept the position with an uncertain future at a fraction of the income. For her, it was a calling.

The pilot-project budget was drawn up by Anne Morgan, Bes, and members of the Royal Vic administration. It would call for tough slogging in cash-strapped times. In March 1974 letters were sent to Dr D. Kinloch at Quebec's Ministry of Social Affairs documenting hospital support for the PCS and requesting research and development funding. On 22 July he responded that the minister of health would support our demonstration project for at least two years, with financial implications "to be discussed further."

Then, also in July, there was a game-changer. A grant of $100,000 was received from the J.W. McConnell Family Foundation. In keeping with its wishes, the source of this superb support was not made public. This grant was the catalyst that made further team building and project planning possible and was joyfully received and deeply appreciated. With the McConnell funding in place, all systems were go! It was the vote of confidence that would soon enable reduced suffering at the hospital bedside and throughout the greater Montreal community. In short, as more than one observer commented, "it was a God-send!" In the weeks that followed, a $5,000 donation from the McGill Faculty of Graduate Studies and Research was matched by $5,000 from the Faculty of Medicine. Our clinical care and research initiatives could now take shape without further delay.

The Summer of 1974: Birding Coverage at St C.

This blessed plot, this earth, this realm, this England.

William Shakespeare

The 23 June 1974 Air Canada, Montreal-to-Heathrow flight was a prelude to a forty-five-day Mount family adventure. This time, I arrived at St Christopher's with Faye, the children, and a temporary licence to practise medicine in the United Kingdom. We would become, for a time, part of the southeast London community, Faye, a St Christopher's volunteer, Chris and Wren, students (at their request) at Malcolm School, a few blocks down Lawrie Park Road, and Jamie, a member of the flock at St Christopher's daycare facility. June to August in England; how splendid!

Malcolm School welcomed Chris and Wren as objects of interest, if not minor celebrities, Chris's grade three class having just read "Paddle to the Sea." He was soon immersed in cricket and "proper soccer" while learning to say "'Ello maite'" and "shot yer maoth" under the tutelage of his "best friend," Paul Black. Wren was in the "infants section." Both soon knew how to cross busy Crystal Palace Park Road with the crossing guard. Jamie was homesick and filled with a legion of new fears: the Tower of London ("where they chop your head off"), any building more than ten years old, windy staircases, and all unexpected London street sounds, not to mention Mme Tussaud's ("where people are turned into wax"). He was delighted, however, with daycare, where he quickly developed a happy addiction to "Bobby hats" and was thrilled to learn that puzzle pieces can become a big picture.

Mary Baines and Thérèse Vanier would be covering the hospice while Cicely and Tom were "birding in Switzerland." Robert Twycross was carrying out his morphine/ heroin comparison study and consultant psychiatrist Colin Murray Parkes would be calling in regularly.

It was perhaps the afternoon of my first or second day when the Nuffield ward sister asked me to see Mr S., who was having considerable pain – most unusual for him – and the nurses were concerned. He was a retired (and retiring) solicitor with grown children and wife who was likely to be in for a visit that evening. "Middle bed on your right, in the bay just at hand."

He brightened as he saw me coming, courteously extended his hand, and offered me the bedside chair. "Well then, I understand that you are here from Canada with your family. Splendid!" he beamed. *(Pain?! I thought they said pain. Perhaps I have the wrong bed.)* I glanced around. This *was* the middle bed on the right; it *was* the six-bed bay closest to the nursing station. He continued. "Now then, how many young ones are here with you and how old are they? *(Clearly, the nurses are mistaken.)*

I happily nattered on about the children for far too long before interrupting myself to ask, "I'm sorry ... Mr S., the nurses mentioned you had been having some pain?"

"Hmmm," he affirmed.

"Well, how bad is the pain just now?"

"Excruciating, actually," he observed, quietly.

Caught out again! Several thoughts went through my mind simultaneously. *Welcome to "Good Olde England" – this is the fibre that brought them through the Blitz; Always trust the nurse's judgment!*; and, finally, *When with a patient, the yield is likely to be higher if you* LISTEN *first!*

Each patient on Nuffield was assigned a primary-care nurse whose responsibility it was to tease out and document, with input from her colleagues of all disciplines, the physical, psychosocial, and spiritual/existential issues relevant to their patient's quality of life. The nurses' skill in achieving this through informal, almost casual, chats was striking, as was the depth of their insight and their ability to intuit with astonishing regularity where the next problem might arise.

Among the Nuffield patients, Frances stood out. The nurses held her in particularly high regard. A librarian with ovarian cancer, she had no family, few visitors, and even fewer complaints. Frances carried herself with understated confidence. She had clear opinions and enjoyed discussing the international issues of the day. She could frequently be found walking in St Christopher's garden. Indeed, it was while on one such sojourn in her trademark long pink dressing gown that she first encountered Lauren, to the delight of them both. With all of this in mind, I was astonished when a staff nurse made reference to her "bowel obstruction." *Bowel Obstruction? What bowel obstruction?!* Until then, there had been no reason to examine her. Bowel obstruction? I needed to examine her.

Frances was ensconced on the side of her bed, legs dangling, engrossed in a book while eating a bowl of cherries and organizing the pits into a tidy little pile. We chatted about her book, and then she redirected our conversation to the chapel service that evening. "The new St Christopher's choir is really very good. The director is a volunteer. His wife died here not long ago and it is his way of saying thank you ... The rumour is out that the only doctors they will appoint now are those who can both sing in the choir with Dr Saunders and play squash with Dr West!"

Examination of her abdomen suggested a large bowel obstruction. I was amazed. In Montreal, I might have considered placing a tube through her nose down to her stomach, starting intravenous fluids, and ordering no intake of food or fluids by mouth while reviewing the need for surgery to enable optimal quality of life. Yet here she was! I questioned Cicely, who was on her way out the door for her birding trek. She explained the rationale behind her approach. Her observations were shrewd, her treatment plan insightful and rather clever. Once again, attention to detail had led to a significant improvement in managing advanced disease. I expressed my admiration for their ingenuity and in due course a detailed study of their technique was carried out by Mary Baines, a study that would become part of the medical literature.[1]

Over the ensuing weeks, Frances continued to impress me with her grace and calm. She readily agreed when I asked if I might take her photograph so that she could "accompany me over the years in teaching medical students and telling others about St Christopher's." Her unflappable demeanour in that photo always brings to mind an observation of Cicely's. A colleague had remarked that St Christopher's patients appeared to feel "safe." "I believe the word you are looking for is 'secure,'" commented a psychiatrist friend, adding, "During the Blitz, a baby felt secure when its mother picked it up. In fact, when in its mother's arms it was no safer, but it felt *secure* and that is what counts." Frances personified the security of St Christopher's and the impact of her presence on others led me to conclude that it might well be contagious.

One sunny Sunday afternoon, with nurses busy and visitors trickling onto the ward to visit loved ones, the Italian woman whose bed was directly opposite Frances was alone. She was dying. Her still-black hair suggested that she might be in her early forties, though she looked very much older. Like Frances, the woman had ovarian cancer. She was comfortable but wasted, her gaze poorly focused; she had been somewhat anxious earlier that morning. Clearly, she was nearing the end of her journey, and so the nurses had drawn the curtains around her bed to afford a degree of privacy and asked me if I would sit with her a while.

As I approached, I hesitated on seeing Frances close her book, don her trademark pink robe, and cross to her neighbour's bed, gently pulling the curtain back just enough to slip inside. She then perched on the bed beside her fellow traveller and without a word gently took her hand. The curtains closed around them and around the sense of shared security she had just created. As I recall, Frances stayed with her to the end.

"What helps to diffuse the emotional load when one accompanies the dying, day in and day out?" I queried. My question brought thoughtful comments from my St Christopher's colleagues: the "sense of team" that says we're all in this together; "quiet efficiency," conveying to all involved that things are under control; the "daycare and the ever-present stir of small children" in the house, under the soft-spoken guidance of caring supervision; the regular "Patient Discussion Groups," run by psychiatrist Colin Murray Parkes (one of which Faye and I were privileged to attend at the invitation of the patients, as they exchanged thoughts about being so ill); the "Staff Support Discussions"; the "Case Management Conferences," which foster an airing of feelings; the lighthearted banter that speaks of the "trust and mutual affection" found through common effort; the atmosphere of "shared inclusive faith" nurtured by Tom's wit and Cicely's insights at the Friday afternoon Bible study group; and, finally, the sharing in celebration at "many parties." "There must be many celebrations in hospice," Cicely had proclaimed during my first visit, now almost a year earlier.

In those summer months, the weather was perfect for gatherings in the garden: an open bar, music, and Dr Tom West sporting a flowing cape clasped at his neck and a towering straw "topper" boasting a broad wine-red band wreathed in flowers. His smile lit up the world, and that world, just then, was brightened by a passing parade of couples, each comprised of a nurse and her patient. They brought with them the product of hours of special preparation for this joyful event. The nurses were pushing their partners in elaborately decorated wheelchairs. There was the gracious toga-bedecked gentleman – a favourite of the house, a gracious fellow with amyotrophic lateral sclerosis (ALS) and a wistful smile on his patient face. He wore a laurel wreath round his head. His identity was revealed by two proud signs: one proclaimed "Julius Caesar" and, on his lap, a second, "I came. I saw. I conquered." Farther back in the procession was a craggy-faced fellow whose weight loss and hollowed eyes somehow added intensity to his owl-like gaze with its merest suggestion of a smile. He wore a stovepipe hat that was covered in daffodils and that across its front bore a printed sign proclaiming, "Plant one more in '74." As the evening wore on, Lauren, Jamie, and Chris entered joyfully into the fun and in conclusion all agreed, "What a fine hospice celebration that was!"

The weeks were busy, the time fleeting. Days were filled with countless instructive bedside moments. If Francis offered evidence of skilled care, innovation born of attention to detail, courage in adversity, life fully lived until the end, and the capacity to create community, I was to have another teacher about the potential that each of us has for a journey inward.

Miss Vallor was in a bed near the windows overlooking the outside world. During the last week or so, she had been quietly settling into her final anchorage. Her eyes remained clear. As so often depicted by Rembrandt, her gaze appeared to find its origin in an inner place that some might call the soul, others the Deep Centre. She had few visitors but radiated peace. She may have been in her late sixties, perhaps less. I found it instructive to sit holding her hand. When you are a surgeon accustomed to measuring the value of one's activity in terms of demonstrable productivity, concrete achievements, and mountains scaled, it is, at first, not evident that an equally valid sphere – perhaps *more* valid – lies immediately at hand, hidden in the present moment. I needed to learn that, learn to slow down, to discover that the first steps toward presence involve slowing and opening. Difficult to do.

The telephone rang as I was writing up a chart at the nursing station. There was no one else around, so I answered it. The high-pitched, somewhat imperious voice on the other end of the line was elderly, articulate, and accustomed to being taken seriously.

"Would you please take a message for Miss Vallor? Tell her Miss Brown called. I cannot come in today, but tell her that I give her Isaiah 30:15." I was unprepared. *Good grief, how do you spell Isaiah?!* I repeated the message.

"You send her Isaiah 30:15?"

"That is correct. Tell her I shall get in again as soon as I am able."

Assuming that I should deliver the message, not just the reference, I thumbed through the inevitable Bible shelved at the nursing station. Isaiah 30:15: "For thus saith the Lord God, the Holy One of Israel; In returning and rest shall ye be saved; in quietness and in confidence shall be your strength."

She appeared to be asleep as I sat down beside her. When she opened her eyes, I ventured forth. "Miss Brown called." Her face lit, her eyes holding mine attentively. She was listening carefully. "She said she is unable to come in today but gives you Isaiah 30:15. Would you like me to read it to you?"

"Please do. She was my Sunday School teacher when I was a little girl. I shall take her message very seriously." I read the passage to her, and then, in the silence that followed, I mumbled something about "returning and rest."

"Oh no," she corrected. "Not that. That is not what she intended. *In quietness and in confidence shall be your strength* – that is what she wants me to keep in mind. That is the important bit." She drifted off to sleep.

I sat with her two more times in her last days. Again, she seemed asleep or comatose as I took her hand, but soon, on both occasions, she opened her eyes. On the first, she told me in a whisper filled with awe, "I was just with Jesus. He was with his disciples by the Sea of Galilee." On the last occasion, looking up at me, her face shone with delight. "I was with Him again," she said. "This time He was surrounded by children. So many children! And they were laughing." There was no hint of sentimentality in this, she was simply reporting where she had been.

Among the many students toing and froing through St Christopher's that summer was a young Irishman, Michael Kearney. He was twenty-one years old. Michael had been reading medicine at Cork but was disillusioned. It all seemed too analytical, too impersonal. He felt he should change fields – English literature? The Classics? He needed to get away from the cookie-cutter thinking that reduced human suffering to formulaic numbers. At a 1972 Dublin retreat with Jean Vanier, there had been the opportunity to discuss such concerns. Jean had listened to Michael with focused attention and sympathy and then said, "Before finalizing your decision there is a place you should visit. My sister, Thérèse, works there. It is called St Christopher's Hospice. It is a place of healing."

Michael was overcome by what he found. This was precisely what he was looking for. He would become a hospice physician. He would graduate in 1977 and then come straightaway to St Christopher's to work.

"Not so fast!" said Cicely. "First go off and finish your medical studies, complete either internal-medicine or family-medicine residency and then come back to see us." To this, Tom West had added, "Here are two books I have found helpful." They were *Experiment in Depth: A Study of the Work of Jung, Eliot and Toynbee* by P.W. Martin, and *The Man on a Donkey* by H.F.M. Prescott. Tom was many things: a perceptive physician, a loyal friend, an excellent teacher, and a voracious reader. While my brief meeting with Michael that summer may have carried with it an aura foretelling significance, I cannot vouch for that with certainty. Nevertheless, he ultimately would become my teacher, my companion on this earthly journey, and my guide in my uncertain descent into the mysteries of the inner life.

With our last week at St Christopher's approaching, we were off to Cambridge by train to visit my sister, Alice, and her family. It was Cambridge in all its quietly pristine elegance with picnics in the garden, boating on the Cam, exploring Clare College with brother-in-law Peter, evensong with the sublime choristers at King's College Chapel, origami into the evenings, and hours walking through "the Backs," the grounds and gardens of the colleges where I had a passing encounter with Stephen Hawking and long chats with Al.

My sense of anticipated loss in leaving this welcoming circle of St Christopher colleagues was somehow tempered by my delight in the consistency of their personalities. One had to smile in recognizing that, wherever our next reunion might be, it would be enriched by the unmistakable presence of the same deliciously unchanged friends I had come to cherish.

In those final days, I discussed the plan to develop a hospice program in a teaching hospital with my wise St Christopher's friends. All patients and many of the staff had serious doubts that such a venture could succeed.

SCOTLAND

On Saturday, 20 July, we set out on a family odyssey to Scotland. Our creed was simple. Cleave to the ancient, the quaint, the historic and romantic, far from the madding crowd, motorways, and the entangling webs of urban life.

Monday, 29 July, Faye and I awoke to a small voice that quietly announced, "I'm four!" And he was! All instantly agreed that the *only* suitable place for Jamie's birthday party was the two-thousand-year-old Roman cavalry fort at Hadrian's Wall, three miles north of Hexham. Always impressive, on this particular bleak and windy day, the Roman fort was dripping in atmosphere, a threatening storm menacing from above. The cantankerous wind was gusting ominously, the blustering rain was intermittent and unpredictable. We needed a sheltered spot for the presents, candles, lunch, and cake (a Mars bar with candles), all of which we had lugged lightheartedly along for this auspicious occasion. One passing mustachioed Englishman chuckled on encountering our windswept party literally "up against the wall." "And I thought *we* were supposed to be eccentric!!" Another passerby gave us matches and wouldn't accept payment, commenting, "It's for your contribution to WWII," to which Faye responded, "Have we really aged that much on this trip?"

We headed for Loch Lomond, then west to Oban, on the Firth of Lorn, a mainland port for the Isle of Mull and Iona. By late evening, we had found lodgings with delightful hosts who invited us to join them for an evening of Scottish dancing at the Old Parish Church in Oban. We shopped for the proper attire for Wren, a very excited young lady, eventually finding a perfect MacDuff tartan kilt and lovely white, lace-trimmed ruffled blouse, and Faye bound her hair in a stylish single braid. She was skipping with anticipation, her braid flying. It was her night, her party, her first fling. She was glowing. We found ourselves awash in swashbuckling kilted men, women, and children in party dress who, together with an intoxicating music of piano, accordion, and fiddle, carried us onward and upward.

Leaving our friends, we turned inland, heading into the high glens and mist-covered mountains on a small single-lane road that demanded a sharp eye for oncoming cattle and sheep. Then, passing above great valleys far below us, all mauve and muted olive green, the mountains above bald and brooding, half-blurred by the mist and sporadic rain, we found ourselves in our own private universe – no trees, no homes, no cars, and, as far as the eye could see in all directions, no people. On turning the corner, we came on a solitary piper. He was only a few yards away, his back to us. He was standing at cliff edge facing the distant mountains. A chiselled rock of a man, in his late forties or early fifties, he was playing the Great Highland Bagpipes and was resplendent in bearskin bonnet topped with a fine scarlet hackle, a black doublet with gold trim, flowing full plaid and brooch, belt, sporran, kilt, and hose, the latter only partially concealing his trusty *sgian-dubh*, the single-edged knife that is part of traditional Scottish Highland formal attire. The high drone and skirl of his pipes engulfed us, and, as we slowed to pass, he momentarily looked at us and paused before he turned back toward the solitude of those distant peaks and resumed his playing. There was no eye contact. His mind was elsewhere, far away, cloaked in his personal beyond. The wind and rain picked up and we drove on in silence.

THE MALLAIG AND DISTRICT HIGHLAND GAMES

Pulses quickened one sunbaked afternoon as we joined the crowd making its way to the tents, folding chairs, and blankets that ringed the field of competition for the Mallaig and District Highland Games. There were booths selling ices, "squash," and candy floss and, on the periphery, a sprawling cluster of tents and tables along with the obligatory paraphernalia of Highland Games officialdom.

We were a colourful mix: earnest athletes, each preparing for his or her event surrounded by assistants, trainers, family members, equipment carriers, and admirers; vibrant young lasses preening demurely as they busily stretched and chatted in muted readiness for the dancing competition – their hose and flashes just so, their shoes laced and adjusted with care, swords at the ready nearby (the winner of the Scottish sword dance, or *Gillie Callum*, that day would be the lovely raven-haired Satnum Kainth from Arisaig); young pre-teen girls primping, prancing, and practising their carefully rehearsed steps ad infinitum, only to strip down later for headlong entry in the 100-yard dash; a solemn circle of eight kilted pipers facing one another, eyes fixed straight ahead while taking their cue from the bearded, slightly older member of their group who later, with his son, would be awarded first and second prizes in the *locals* piping competition.

The crowd of several hundred in attendance was, with few exceptions, composed of Scots: kilted children; young couples fondling fondly; an attentive cross-section of the local populace who had been awaiting this day with growing anticipation for the past twelve months; two white-haired judges, perhaps in their seventies, walking toward us in deep conversation, oblivious to all else (one sensed they were respected local institutions, settled elders, each comfortable in his own skin, friends of long standing whose mutual bonds had been chiselled through decades of earnest discussion); one solitary gaitered Englishman with a Sherlock Holmes cap; and, finally, the Mounts.

All of us stood for a moment of solemn reflection as the pipers massed to play a memorial salute to two recently departed neighbours.

To recall that day is to bring to mind a collage of images featuring Highland celebration, beauty, and drama, and I experience once again the repeated low-key response accorded the victors. While they were offered the minimal applause consistent with approval of excellence, one sensed that the recognition was intentionally muted, not through indifference – too many hours spent in laborious preparation for that – but out of respect for the feelings of those who did not win. Grace implied and evident.

My highlight of the day was the performance of Jay Ferguson, one of the athletes. I noticed him early in the proceedings since he was the only competitor wearing a kilt. A handsome lad with broad sideburns and a thick crop of dark auburn hair, he was perhaps 5' 10", trim, muscular, and the only athlete who arrived without a retinue of supporters and a goodly supply of backup equipment. He brought with him only a small kitbag, his perpetual smile, and an aura of understated presence as he walked unaccompanied onto the grounds. He was relaxed and self-contained, neither seeking nor avoiding interaction with others. While an apparent stranger in Mallaig, in competition Ferguson participated in a spirit of implied community. His composure and poise never wavered. It seemed, however, that the local folk did not know him, for he had little or no exchange of small talk with his peers. As his incredible day progressed, Ferguson moved calmly from event to event and I followed, camera in hand. Unlike the other athletes, he did not have, as most did, a particular specialty that he excelled in.

The 100-yard dash opened the day, attracting a strong field, as did all subsequent events. It was the only competition for which Ferguson exchanged his trademark kilt for track shorts. He won with an electrifying sprint from behind over the final yards. It was a breathtaking victory. Next, he handily won the high-jump contest. It featured the only kilt-attired western roll I have ever seen.

Then there was the caber toss. Three massive policemen from Glasgow took part in that testosterone-ladened competition. They were huge fellows of impressive girth and strength. Remarkably, the rather diminutive, by comparison, Ferguson once again won.

His next event was wrestling; he came second. Always, there was the same quiet smile. The hammer throw followed. This traditional event claims Highland Games roots that extend back to the fifteenth century. Given his sparse resources, Ferguson had to borrow shoes from an opponent and came third. Unassuming grace and humility marked his remarkable day, leaving me with an image of quiet leadership, grace under pressure, and poise that would be my final gift from Scotland.

Although we did not meet, Jay Ferguson has remained with me over the ensuing decades, suggesting the potential of the realized Self in confronting the inevitable challenges of life.

As the Games ended I wished to shake his hand, but, as I looked for him in the dispersing crowd, he was nowhere to be found; he had quietly slipped away.

First Steps

[The government of Quebec agrees to the establishment of]
un Projet de Mise en Place d'une Unité de Soins Palliatifs
dans Votre Centre Hospitalier
Quebec government of
Premier Robert Bourassa

Love and steel: how kind. Anyone doing hospice work will need plenty of both.
Dame Cicely Saunders, responding to the observation
that her portrait in the National Portrait Gallery,
London, had captured a look of love and steel.

Compassion is the new radicalism.
His Holiness the Dalai Lama

The official letter from the Quebec Ministry of Social Affairs authorizing a palliative-care demonstration project of "at least two years" duration had arrived while we were in England. The agreed target date and place for start-up was early January 1975 at the RVH's Four Medical ward. The intervening weeks promised to be full, if all was to be ready. The PCS planning team[1] set to work in earnest and an Evaluation Committee was formed to establish a controlled trial that would compare outcomes (pain, mood, drug consumption, laboratory tests and costs) generated by a Study Group (PCS patients and families) compared to those of a comparison group (RVH non-PCS patients and families similar to the Study Group in specified domains).[2]

MME PICOTTE

A consult request arrived one busy afternoon in late August 1974. Though we had not previously met, Mme Picotte had for many years been an administrative secretary for a senior Royal Vic colleague; she was now gravely ill. As I entered her four-bed room on Eight Surgery West, her warmth and wisdom were immediately evident. While I had little to offer her as a urologic oncologist, I lingered, suspecting that she had much to teach me. One thing led to another as we chatted. I asked her to comment on her extensive experience of illness, both as care provider and as one who was now ill. She spoke of the inadequacies of our health-care system and described her desire to be considered a person rather than a patient, to be taken seriously and listened to. She expressed her need for gentle honesty and her hope for accompaniment on the path that lay ahead.

I asked if she would help me spread the message about palliative care. She agreed without hesitation. Returning with the hospital photographer the next day, I asked her to think about the advice she had given me. The resulting image captured what I had been privileged to hear and see – our complex needs in the face of suffering, the human spirit at its best, the richness in potential possible when the journey into the unknown is openly shared, and so much more.

Mme Picotte died days later, but over the subsequent decades her photograph has introduced most if not all of my lectures, expressing with remarkable clarity the need to relate to the whole person and not simply to the disease. She has been my co-presenter. While she did not live to take part in our pilot project, Mme Picotte became, along with Cicely and Elisabeth, a most cherished mentor. With her discerning expression, she continues to ask each of us how we are doing in our quest to ease the burden of those we encounter each day and, in particular, those nearing the end of life.

BIRTH OF THE INTERNATIONAL WORK GROUP ON DEATH, DYING AND BEREAVEMENT (IWG)

The genesis of new clinical programs wasn't the only sign of growth in the field during 1974. A letter from someone identifying himself as "the Executive Director of Philadelphia-based ARS MORIENDI" invited recipients to participate in an event referred to as "The Forthcoming International Convocation of Leaders in the Field of Death and Dying, 14–19 November 1974, Being Called by ARS MORIENDI and the Journal OMEGA." It was to be held at the Urban Life Center in Columbia, Maryland. In her enthusiasm, EKR arranged for me to attend the meeting.

My knowledge of the field and its leaders was at that point more or less limited to Elisabeth's *On Death and Dying* and Cicely's "Drugs Used at St Christopher's." I was largely unaware of the sociocultural, historical, religious, philosophical, educational, and other tomes that had contributed to the collective wisdom concerning "dying well" in the wake of the original *Ars Moriendi* (The Art of Dying) texts dating from the fifteenth century.[3] Additional pre-conference mailings were saturated with rambling, lofty-sounding, rather opaque proclamations, including: "Utilizing the teaching-training continuum, each day's work pattern and agenda will evolve within an interactive problem-solving forma ... Participants will be asked to submit beforehand a statement of study, research, teaching and care problems in which they are interested or working upon ..."

My week had started in the operating room, cystoscopy suite, research lab, and office. There was little time to ponder the deeper meanings of such prose. While these missives did suggest that end-of-life issues were largely neglected in health care and society, I had no idea what else was implied and could only hope that this failing wouldn't be too obvious to my fellow registrants.

Mid-week, mid-afternoon, mid-November Columbia, Maryland, was deserted and silent as the taxi dropped me at the Urban Life Center door. It felt like being deposited into a vacuum. An aura of plastic artificiality permeated everything. Foliage, earlier exuberant, was long past its prime. Muted yellows, browns, and greys dominated that sterile late-fall day. The silent scoured streets, spotless buildings, rows of low white-picket fences, and ruler-straight AstroTurf lawns brought Pete Seeger to mind and I found myself humming, *Little boxes made of ticky tacky, Little boxes all the same*, as I registered at the reception desk.

"Has Dr Saunders arrived from London?"

"Yes, she has just arrived. Down the hall on your right, Room 105." I knocked.

"Come."

Cicely was standing at the far end of the dimly lit room, peering out the vacuum-sealed, ceiling-to-floor, wall-to-wall plate-glass window, studying the muted pastel tones of the skeletal trees and meandering stream that ran soundlessly across the back of the property. She turned. "Oh, *Bal*, I'm *so* glad to see you! There is something terribly Ingmar Bergman about all this!!"

There were about fifty of us.[4] We assembled on cue in the Urban Life Center meeting room. It was to be the last predictable occurrence in a six-day meeting.

John Fryer, a psychiatrist at Temple University, was introduced as our chairman. A large, flamboyant man, he invited us to sit in a circle. We did.

Most were now cross-legged on the floor. He then sat (intermittently lay) on the floor at the centre of our circle, a small brass bell in hand. "I shall ring the bell to bring us together," said Fryer, adding, "Now, I would like some discussion about how you would like to structure our time together."

"There should be *no* imposed structure!" offered a rather intense bearded chap to my right. His salt-and-pepper hair was in a single braid; he wore jeans and a great grey, loose-knit sweater and around his neck hung a leather thong from which a circular bone dangled impressively.

Those of us in the "desperate for structure" crowd visibly paled. Dr Fryer had already started to stir the pot by taking us – taking *me* – out of my comfort zone. A smattering of comments about "Goals," "Process," and "Long-range Objectives" followed.

By day's end, there had been sufficient mystifying dialogue concerning "conceptual frameworks," "deconstruction of hypotheses," "hidden internal assumptions," "affective load," "subversion of apparent significance," and other apparently related weighty issues that I had started to make lists of terms I had never heard before. Dr Fryer seemed to relish the lack of order and predictability. As it ended, our first day seemed to me to have been confusing and monumentally unproductive. Many, probably most, wondered if we were in the hands of the most appropriate leader.[5]

Day two. We dutifully assembled on the floor in the requisite circle with our leader ensconced, whale-like, in our midst and were just underway when the door flew open. In marched Herman Feifel and Edwin Shneidman, powered by a determined and all-too-evident head of steam. They were dressed in podium-ready, city-formal attire. As opposed to the rest of us, *they* remained standing!

Poorly informed as I was, I did know Feifel and Shneidman by reputation. These dynamic psychologists were highly respected trailblazers. They carried a certain presence with them; they were great men and not to be trifled with. Their unexpected entry and the ceremonial formality of their bearing cut though the prevalent quicksand of uncertainty like a knife. The meeting froze in mid-sentence.

Feifel and Shneidman? The first meeting of American psychologists dealing with attitudes toward death and dying had been organized and chaired by Herman Feifel in 1956. It resulted in the publication, in 1959, of his classic book *The Meaning of Death*, which brought together contributions by such eminent thinkers as psychiatrist and psychoanalyst Carl Jung, theologian Paul Tillich, and philosopher Herbert Marcuse. Widely acclaimed, *The Meaning of Death* became the foundational catalyst for a heightened academic interest in death, dying, and bereavement and for Feifel's reputation as "the father of the modern death movement."

Shneidman had similar pioneering credentials. In 1958 he and his colleagues founded the Los Angeles Suicide Prevention Center. Then, in 1966, Shneidman headed a National Institutes of Health project to establish suicide-prevention organizations and in 1968 he founded both the American Association of Suicidology and the journal *Suicide and Life Threatening Behavior*. In 1970 he became professor of thanatology at the University of California at Los Angeles. He went on to publish twenty books on suicide and its prevention.[6]

I came to cherish friendships with both these remarkably gifted and ever-stimulating scholars. Herman Feifel was an opera enthusiast who pronounced the field he had given birth to "thana*th*ology." His distinct "Noo Yahk tawk" was yet further evidence that you can take the boy from Brooklyn but you can't take Brooklyn from the boy.

The razor-edged intellect of Ed Shneidman had a habit of continually spilling over, suggesting to me that you can take the wordsmith from the thesaurus but you can't take the thesaurus from the wordsmith. "Suicidology," "psychological autopsy," "psychache," and "pseudocide notes" (notes written by non-suicidal subject) were *all* his inventions. Ed's favourite English-language masterpiece was *Moby Dick*. He read it once each year. I was not surprised, therefore, when years later, as we walked to a restaurant one fall evening in Montreal, I noticed that his tie bore countless images of small white whales. "Ed, I love your tie."

"You like it?" he asked, promptly stopping dead in his tracks. He pulled it off and placed it around my neck, his eyes agleam. "It's yours." It was an Ed Shneidman moment.

Feifel addressed the assembled Urban Life Center throng on day two, Shneidman by his side. "I am speaking for both Ed and myself. We have booked flights to return to Los Angeles this morning but we want you to know why we are leaving. We were *very* disappointed with yesterday! It was a complete waste of time, money and the effort expended in getting here. We were looking forward to learning from colleagues and discussing our work with them. We both brought presentations with us to share with you, but clearly no one is interested in a collegial academic exchange, so we are leaving. This has been a waste of time!"

There was total silence. I felt embarrassed, mortified, guilty. *How dreadful! This is terrible! (Did I have a sudden impulse to suck my thumb? Who knows.)* Feifel and Shneidman turned to leave.

"Go! For God sake, Go! Feifel and Shneidman, you two arrogant bastards! You know what your problem is?! You always need to have a pedestal, a soapbox. You have to have everyone telling you how wonderful you are. Well, *go!*" It was my neighbour with the ponytail and leather thong.

I was dumbfounded. *This is a catastrophe!*

To my astonishment, Feifel and Shneidman sat down, joined the group, and fully participated in the rest of the meeting.

Highlights of the days that followed included detailed discussions of the goals of optimal end-of-life care and a memorable evening on the impact of war and violence that was convened in a small, seat-less, carpeted amphitheatre in the round referred to as "the pit." It featured St Christopher psychiatrist Colin Murray Parkes in dialogue with the American psychiatrist, writer, author, and theorist Robert Jay Lifton. All present felt privileged.

But the substantive outcomes of our days together went beyond that. We had undergone a pressure-cooker-group meld, an enforced shedding of unconscious veneer in deference to acknowledged vulnerability. At least one of us, a young man with chronic illness, had a major psychological collapse and some of us took a few more halting steps on our inner journey. Occupation-related stances guarding the psychologist, sociologist, funeral director, medical clinician, anthropologist, lawyer, educator, historian, writer, and student were stripped away. It was exhausting yet enlivening. The process had evoked community. Was I the only one so touched? It seemed possible at the time, given that I was just a simple surgeon.

As the meeting ended and we began to disperse, there was a spontaneous after-the-fact call for a discussion about how to sustain what had been started. Twenty of us took part in the hurly-burly of that brief but productive meeting. The final product of our deliberations was the International Work Group on Death, Dying and Bereavement; the next meeting, a year hence, was tentatively planned.

That afternoon, four of us, Cicely, Colin Murray Parkes, Sylvia Lack (the superb young British physician at "Hospice Inc." (New Haven's new end-of-life home-care program and the "First American Hospice"), and I made our way to the airport, still processing the kaleidoscopic turmoil of the preceding six days. As our driver threaded his way through the traffic, Sylvia and I were suddenly shaken into alertness by a loud and

emphatic expletive uttered by Cicely a couple of empty, cavernous lim-
ousine rows forward. Sylvia and I were gobsmacked! We stared at each
other, eyes bugging, mouths agape, our expressions silently asking *Did
you hear what I just heard?!* It seemed that we weren't the only ones
affected by the post-Columbia syndrome!

A year later, "IWG II" commenced with an introductory session
reviewing the "Columbia experience" with the aid of slides I had taken
during the first meeting. We were standing informally, sipping cocktails;
the atmosphere was relaxed. How could I convey the impact of that earlier, still graphic, potboiler? I hesitated in mid-presentation groping for
words. "It would be hard for those of you who were not present to fully
appreciate the process we went through. Perhaps it will convey something of the nature of the event if I say that on the way to the airport
following the meeting, Dr Saunders was clearly heard to say to Colin
Murray Parkes ..."

"YOU WOULDN'T 'DAY-AH!!'" came thundering from the shadowy
back row of the gathering. Cicely had spoken!!

"I guess you're right," I responded, quickly regaining my senses. "I
guess I wouldn't!"

THE RVH PCS PILOT-PROJECT PRELUDE

As we worked our way through 1974, the challenges facing us became
increasingly clear. The central question was: "Can a hospice program
function successfully within a general hospital? How about a major
teaching hospital?" Optimal whole-person care would demand state-of-
the-art skills pertaining to each patient and family member – *physical,
psychological, social, and existential/spiritual* – as well as skilled interaction between multidisciplinary caregivers, persons who actually *listen* to
each other and take each other's insights seriously.

To cite an early instructive example, would a consultant neurologist
seeing a PCU patient with complex neuropathic pain feel comfortable
calling on the insights of the PCU floor cleaner who, like the patient,
happened to be Portuguese? And, even if we happened to have such a
neurologist, how likely would it be that the ward cleaner would disclose
what he knew about that patient's sociocultural realities, things that
only someone with a similar background could possibly understand?
Moreover, given the pressures on time, what sort of team meetings would
be necessary to transmit such multilayered information? What about the
problems involved in developing such a team? The funding needed? The
time necessary?

In the case of the consultant neurologist referred to, he *was* ready to listen to the cleaner, who was a thoughtful man highly respected by all. The cleaner was, however, rendered speechless by the unaccustomed attention of the doctors and nurses and his discomfort rendered all communication about sensitive psychosocial matters impossible. And the story didn't end there. When, following our patient's death, the bereavement-support coordinator contacted the grieving family for the first time, she was alarmed to hear from the widow that a PCS visitor had already made several bereavement calls and had been very helpful. Alarming! *What visitor?* There had been a visitor claiming to be from the PCS! A delicate situation. Who could be posing as our representative? Gentle, if anxious, questioning revealed his identity. It was our thoughtful member of housekeeping.

Clearly, a non-hierarchical, egalitarian, or, as Ina described it, matrix-style team was required, one that included the full range of disciplines. In addition, the service must operate in vastly different settings given the five proposed PCS clinical arms: the Hospital Ward (Palliative Care Unit), the Home Care Service, the Consult Service, the Outpatient Clinic, and the Bereavement Follow-Up Program. And, while functioning in synchrony with our colleagues throughout our one-thousand-bed teaching hospital and the multilingual population they serve, the PCS must operate within the constraints of the budgets, union rules, and operational guidelines of the larger institution.

What would be necessary to achieve success on each of the clinical arms? Indeed, what would "success" in each setting look like? How could it be measured? What would be the minimal team requirements for each PCS clinical arm? How could the whole multifaceted program be designed, operationalized, and evaluated within the time and financial constraints of a two-year pilot project?

Complex administrative and interrelated challenges were evident. The need for a Palliative Administration Coordinator (PAC) to interface between the many PCS disciplines, the five PCS clinical arms, the clinical and evaluation teams, and the PCS and the RVH administrations, as well as to deal with a steady stream of students and visitors, was clear to all involved. An experienced person with administrative and health-care experience was required. Dottie Wilson submitted her name as applicant for PAC in a letter dated 7 March 1974. I was delighted beyond words.

Dottie was my cousin by marriage, her husband being my aunt's son, David. More than a decade my senior, Dottie had the needed credentials,[7] possessed a quick, discerning mind, and was a good listener. She was engaging, direct, and at ease in conversations with everyone from the lowest in the pecking order to the most self-assured CEO. I cannot recall a person or situation that fazed her. Radiating professionalism, she generated immediate trust. She was practical and down-to-earth, and she brooked no nonsense.

My relationship with Dottie was like no other I have known. It was marked by unbounded mutual respect and ferocious loyalty, qualities rendered priceless by her withering honesty and forthrightness. When Dottie considered my words or actions below par, she never hesitated to let me have it straight between the eyes at the earliest private opportunity. In short, she was invaluable, a gift beyond measure in the role she was asked to assume.

Dottie was hired in November 1974 over loud protests from all manner of RVH administrative directors. ("What do you mean you need a 'Program Manager'? First of all, there is no such position. Second, not even the Chiefs of Surgery or Medicine have someone in the role you describe!") Finally, however, following endless explaining and a title change to "research assistant," they reluctantly agreed in a "this-better-be-good, you're-out-of-your-mind, *and* out-on-a-limb!" tone. Everyone's credibility – mine, Dottie's, theirs – was clearly at risk!

With the January 1975 start-up rapidly approaching, preparations were full-steam ahead:

- Bes's newspaper advertisement read: "A unique hospital unit for the care of the terminally ill based on concepts of care developed by Dr Elisabeth Kübler-Ross and Dr Cicely Saunders at St Christopher's Hospice, London. Opening early 1975. Applications for Domiciliary Care Nurses, Head Nurses, Staff Nursing Assistants, male and female are invited."
- A late January 1975 seminar with Elisabeth was planned; eighteen team members registered.
- A study of the efficacy and mode of action of the RVH Brompton Mixture in the control of terminal-cancer pain was initiated by McGill researcher Professor Ron Melzack, who, in 1965 at the Massachusetts Institute of Technology (MIT) with his colleague Patrick Wall, developed the gate-control theory of pain which states that pain is "gated" or modulated by past experience. Gate-control theory led to the valuable discovery of endorphins and enkephalins, the body's natural opiates.
- Procedural norms were established for each of the five PCS clinical arms.
- Discussions were held with Anesthesiology and the Montreal

Neurologic Institute (pain consultation), Radiation Therapy (treatment availability), and Oncology (appropriate referral criteria).
· The document "How the PCU Will Work" was distributed to all
Royal Vic clinical departments.
· The potential merits and liabilities of media requests were discussed,
including TV special programs (both French-language Radio Canada
and English-language CBC's *Man Alive*).
· K.J. MacKinnon, as director of professional services, identified
15 January 1975 as the target PCU start-up date, depending on bed
and staff availability.
· A weekly, in-depth PCS Volunteer Training Program was initiated.[8]
· On 26 November 1974 the RVH clinical staff was notified that the
PCS Consult Service was now available.

The year ended on a hopeful note when the RVH executive director
wrote in the hospital's Annual Report:

During the past year or two, the conceptual definition of a Palliative
Care Unit in the Royal Victoria Hospital was produced. The concept
received wide publicity throughout the mass media and was enthusiastically endorsed by the Minister of Social Affairs. While final
budgetary arrangements have not yet been worked out, including
an appropriate home care program, a pilot unit was opened in late
1974 on 4 Medical. I believe sincerely and without reservation that
this unit has generated more awareness and appreciation within the
community than any individual program that the Hospital may have
established in the recent past, with this being particularly true with
respect to the patients and families involved. It should be emphasized
that the unit is interdisciplinary and I believe that it has the general
strong support of most of our institution.

Now all we had to do was live up to the advance billing!

PCS PILOT PROJECT: THE FIRST FOUR MONTHS

A noteworthy feature of the initial Volunteer Training Program was
the fact that attendance was taken at *each* session and the *reason for
absence* (from even a single session) was investigated through a telephone call. PCS volunteer training was, we believed, essential to our
goal of creating an egalitarian team. The volunteers were believed to be
indispensable in optimal patient and family assessment and care; thus,

old teaching hospital norms needed to give way to new patterns of functioning through which that potential could be celebrated. On the ward, volunteers might be involved in psychosocial support and, in addition, they might participate in hands-on patient care under the supervision of a nurse. In the Bereavement Follow-Up program, volunteers were the front-line workers, reporting to the PCS psychiatrist. In all activities our volunteers answered to the PCS director of volunteers, a senior position that was independent of the RVH director of volunteers.

We learned that five factors were needed to ensure optimal volunteer functioning: a skilled screening interview of each applicant, a rigorous training program, a stimulating continuing-education program, regular performance assessment and feedback, and a mechanism for uncomplicated termination ("time to move on").

Kitty Markey became our first volunteer director. When Kitty walked into a room, her bearing and personal appearance suggested that she might well be listed in Burke's Peerage. Within a few minutes over a cup of tea, however, the applicant Kitty was assessing, whether prince or pauper, felt that Kitty was a long-trusted friend. She had both Cicely's "beady eye" and a social ease that was completely disarming. For years, I made a habit of casually asking new volunteers how their initial interview with Kitty had gone. The usual response was a variation of, "Well, it was the oddest thing [laughing] ... I had decided there were things she didn't need to know, but once we got chatting ... well ... I told her everything."

Kitty's assessment was critically important since, unlike St Christopher's, we planned to use volunteers in hands-on bedside care. Later, St Christopher's would follow our lead in this regard, as would other centres, but Cicely had serious misgivings about this decision during the early years.

When well into their rigorous fourteen-week training-program agenda, with its extensive reading list, our volunteers were offered two additional "optional" training sessions as well as notification that they could audit the new March-May 1975 McGill medical-student "Thanatology Options Course." When the PCU beds opened on 22 January 1975, our three dozen shiny new volunteers were impatiently pawing the ground at the starting gate, anxious to put their newly acquired knowledge to use.

Our new nurses, on the other hand, arrived at the PCU totally exhausted, having left their previous posts only hours earlier. They had come from the OR, OB/GYN, Emergency, Surgery, or Medicine and were, at best, just coming up for air as they negotiated this career change into the unknown. They had applied for something called "palliative care" but what exactly was that?

Their challenges were many: new job, new ward, uncertain mandate, untried colleagues, and a head nurse who was a palliative-care novice. And, on top of it all, their life was to be complicated by this bevy of enthusiastic, hyper-dynamic volunteers who knew so much more about "death and dying" than they, we, or almost anyone did. It was surreal, a nightmare! To a person, our new nurses developed an instant allergy to the mere word "volunteer" as their dizzying orientation program was crammed into two days in preparation for the opening of our first beds. Our errors in start-up planning were oh so clear – in retrospect!

Mr Lévesque, a man in his early sixties with advanced cancer, was our first PCU admission. Though weak and in need of oxygen assistance in breathing, he was comfortable. Bushy black eyebrows and a receding hair-line framed his consistently calm expression. He had read about the PCU in the newspaper and smiled as he spoke of his delight at being our first patient. We claimed equal pleasure and asked if we might capture the moment with a picture. As it happened, Barb Carter, a nursing assistant who became an instant team stalwart, was at his bedside, thus rendering that photograph doubly meaningful. Barb, with her short, cropped hair, salty vocabulary, and easygoing ways, drove a motorcycle and wore quarter Wellington boots. She was warmly brusque and had a heart of gold. It soon became clear that there was a sizeable sector of our patient population that Barb alone could help to feel completely at home; the rest of us, too often, made them feel awkward. We were off to an auspicious start.

Mr André was our second admission. A man of swarthy complexion and abundant dark hair, he was drowsy when Ina examined him, his attentive wife at his side. He would be the first to die on the PCU. His widow later returned to join our team as a volunteer.

Our Four Medical location in the hospital was always intended to be temporary. Following the pilot project, if successful, we would move to an as yet unidentified locale. In its previous incarnation, Four Medical had been home for the Royal Vic's highly acclaimed centre of metabolic research under the leadership of Drs Eleanor McGarry and J.C. Beck, the chief of the RVH Endocrinology and Metabolism Service. They had been leaders in use of human pituitary growth hormone and Four Medical had been their internationally renowned clinical laboratory. Its meta-morphosis to a ward for the care of the dying was painful for many in the Department of Medicine and Dr McGarry's frequent visits to check on the status of her old home during our early weeks was a continuing reminder that the stakes were high.

The PCU was a compact twelve-bed unit with four private rooms, two three-bed rooms, and one room with two beds. The nursing station, charting area, utility room, linen closet, and the rest were, to be charitable, compact. There was no doctor's office; the family waiting area was a small cubicle off the main hall.

Four Medical did, however, have several advantages. The PCU main entrance was across a short private hallway from the modest Royal Vic interfaith chapel, and, of equal significance, our location offered privacy. While Four Medical had none of St Christopher's bright, airy spaciousness, it did manage to present a quiet and welcoming calm. One could establish a "therapeutic milieu" free from the intense pressures and pace common to teaching-hospital daily life. We could adjust wall colour (soft, pleasant tones) and lighting (florescent lighting that offered a healthy pink off-white light rather than the cyanotic blue off-white found elsewhere in the hospital), select wallpaper (our most notable mistake!), and so on. We would make it work.

In late May 1975 the Department of Nursing reviewed our first four months. It had been a challenging time for the team. A staffing shortage throughout the hospital had led to widespread bed closures, with the PCU being temporarily cut to seven beds. In addition, significant initial teething pains, particularly evident among our nurses, had persisted. Anne Dubrofsky, our head nurse, had been selected by Bes based on her outstanding personal and professional qualities. In June, a month after the four-month review, Anne resigned to take on other responsibilities, but not before providing an insightful critique of the issues facing us.

We had experienced head-on the challenge death represents. In her book *Watch with Me*, Cicely wisely observed: "To face death means to face the ending of hopes and plans. Pain is not only physical and social, it is also deeply emotional. Indeed, mental pain may be the most intractable of all."[9] Those first months taught us that the sting of transience that Cicely spoke of is a challenge for *each* person in the therapeutic triad, patient, family member, and caregiver alike. While our reactions to death may often be evident at a conscious level, they are frequently more subtle and pass unrecognized. In the early days of hospice care in the United States, there was a trite bit of naivety that glibly pronounced, "One should not work in hospice until you have 'worked through' your own feelings about death." What arrogance, what ingenuous nonsense, to suggest that we can "work through" our response to death as if part of an imagined pre-employment checklist! Cicely's warning was underscored by our departing head nurse's observations: "There's such a huge opportunity to do so much good, [but] it can be overwhelming. You sit and take stock of yourself. All of us cry, all of us do – torrents. It's very difficult and sometimes I go home depressed. There are days when one leaves the unit completely drained, with no energy left to conduct one's personal life and business."[10] And yet the efficacy of palliative care was also noted by Anne. In her resignation report, she observed prophetically: "I believe that the viability of the PCU has been established. The care that patients and their families receive is of the highest quality; patients die comfortably for the most part. Their families maintain contact with [the PCU following their loved one's death], the initiative for contact [coming from them] in many instances. Preliminary investigations indicate significant savings in hospitalization costs as an effect of PCS Domiciliary Care."

We needed an additional objective assessment. With customary generosity, St Christopher's offered Dr Tom West as a visiting consultant to assist with both PCU evaluation and a team retreat. His subsequent assessment report read:

Information: Big city hospital that has now had open, for two months, their PCU which is a ward situated in the middle of the hospital.
Assets: 1) A real live base that is functioning; 2) Eight patients with terminal disease whose degree of care St Christopher's would have been proud of; 3) Dr Bal Mount who has worked at St Christopher's twice but is a very busy surgeon in his own right; 4) Dr Ina Ajemian who has worked at St Christopher's once and visited again this year but is also a housewife; 5) a very well prepared and organized volunteer group.

Problems / Suggestions:
1) Need for 24-hour medical coverage;
2) Nursing meetings, planning sessions and discussions (similar to those given volunteers) needed;
3) Increased team discussion and teaching regarding i] medical management issues, ii] the need to continually practice the art of *not* being busy, iii] you *will* be upset by death;
4) Head Nurse and Volunteer co-ordinator to meet daily;
5) Whenever things seem to be going badly, staff should be encouraged to do what we have to do here at St Christopher's – stop looking at the problems, stop looking at each other, stop looking at themselves and go and sit with the patients. But *then* we have to go back and look at each other! [that last phrase added by Dr Saunders, who had signed this brief addendum].

In a follow-up letter, Tom wrote: "[Cicely] and I mourn with you that your nursing staff are still bothered and bewildered. There sometimes comes a time when someone does have to lose their temper but I doubt this can be planned and one should only lose one's temper if one is prepared to apologize afterwards!! // I hope you now have some patients back again [post-retreat and RVH bed closures]. I think you have a greater chance of clearing things up with patients, albeit limited in number, in the background rather than letting the histrionics reverberate through an empty ward. // love to all of you. Tom."

It was 2:00 A.M. While I had been deeply asleep, I suddenly found myself sitting bolt upright, wide awake, completely focused, and feeling distinctly anxious. Why? The Consult Service had been in operation for eight weeks, the PCU for five weeks, and Home Care for one week; my surgical practice was busier than ever; my medical-student and residency teaching and research obligations were keeping me off the streets. In addition, there were the presentations, talks, interviews.[11] I wasn't spending enough time with Miriam in our mouse-research lab, and I had a gaping deficit in our family time! The issue that had awakened me was clear! *The PCS is gathering steam! If anything happens to Ina this house of cards will collapse. It would be a disaster. We have an urgent need for another PCS doc. But who?*

Oddly, as in my mid-Atlantic-flight awakening that came up with Ina's name, the answer was there the moment the question had formed in my mind. *John Scott.* Now that *really was* weird! I did not know John but had almost met him once, a year earlier. Ina had started to introduce us just as an evening community-based meeting we all were attending was getting underway. We never did get beyond names. I rummaged through my memory. *I think Ina mentioned that he planned to start a family practice on the West Island. I'll call him in the morning.* Getting his phone number from Ina, I gave him a call. It was not yet 8:00 A.M.

Reminding him of our brief contact a year earlier, I apologized for the early hour and told him in a sentence or two about the PCS and our need for a physician. Apologizing once again, I said that I was calling to see if there was any possibility that he might be interested in joining us. If not, I would certainly understand, but if so, we should get together for a longer chat. I paused, feeling rather embarrassed. His response left me speechless.

"It's a funny thing that you should call just now. I am sitting here reading about the calling of Abraham. I shall have to take this call seriously." The parallel to Ina's response a year earlier was stunning. That sense of "deeper meaning" that Cicely spoke of came to mind. We arranged to meet.

I was booked to do a cystoscopy the next morning. Had John ever seen a cysto? No. Would he find that interesting? Well, he supposed so.

We met in my office at 10:00 A.M. and that day John observed his first cystoscopy, learned about St Christopher's, and heard an account of the Royal Vic study and our PCS plans.

John Fraser Scott proved to be an interesting young man. A 1973 medical graduate of the University of Toronto, he had chosen student electives in rural India, St Bartholomew's Hospital, London, and the Royal Infirmary, Edinburgh. Then, because he felt obliged as a unilingual anglophone Canadian to learn French, he had chosen to do his internship *en français* at the Université de Montréal's Hôpital Notre Dame. Remarkable! *Not* your average medical student, intern, or, for that matter, Canadian! Letters of reference described him as "sensitive and responsible" and his undergraduate clinical work as "excellent," and noted that his particular "strength [was] in medicine, community medicine and therapeutic radiology, where he excelled." Rapport with nurses and patients was described as "extremely good, far above average."

A short time before my telephone call, John had taken out a loan to purchase a building in a Montreal's West Island suburb where he would live, establish a Christian community, and set up a private family practice. Following our discussions, he cancelled those commitments and moved to a small downtown apartment in preparation for training as a palliative-care physician.

With the agreement of Lloyd MacLean, chief of surgery, Peter Mansell, director of oncology, and Dr MacKinnon as director of professional services, John joined the Royal Vic staff as an oncology fellow for a period of two years, with the agreement that this would lead to a subsequent RVH staff appointment in palliative care, assuming two things: first, that the PCS survived the pilot-project phase, and second, that I could find funding to support his two-year fellowship.

On 3 April the Cedars Cancer Fund agreed to meet John's two-year funding requirements. It was support that I found personally meaningful. Years earlier as a resident in surgery, I had assisted Dr Edward Tabah as he operated on a young man named Harley Chamandy. Harley subsequently died of his cancer, but he lived on in my memory, and also in name, through a memorial fund created by the Montreal Lebanese community, known today as the Cedars Cancer Foundation. In 1975 that fund helped secure the program and the training of John, a future leader in this new field. (John, like Ina, would leave a lucrative family practice for an annual income of less than $30,000.)

In mid-April, John left for Connecticut to spend two weeks with Dr Sylvia Lack and her team offering community-based care at Hospice New Haven, prior to a six-week training period at St Christopher's.

John's official Royal Vic fellowship commenced on 1 April 1975, twenty-nine days after our first early-morning phone call.

Our first real glimpse of John's quality came in his detailed handwritten report following his New Haven visit. It was forthright, bordering on blunt, in assessing the areas we needed to work on. His tightly organized insights regarding our deficiencies became for us a sobering cautionary tale. In summary, his comments included:

> *Limit Goals*: Our instant start-up of all five PCS clinical services – PCU, Consult, Home Care, Clinic, and Bereavement – had raised eyebrows in New Haven and London.

> *Staff*: John had considered his first priority while in New Haven to be examination of their staff recruitment, screening, communication, support, authority structure, and relationships between the various professional groups. He concluded that New Haven had a great deal to teach us. In contrast to our PCS, New Haven was noteworthy for the excellent communication among its staff and its genuine team approach, with very little interpersonal friction, and this was reflected in its efficiency and excellence in patient care.

> *Staff Selection*: Here John included a detailed analysis of the highly evolved New Haven screening-and-selection process, which was far superior to ours in the areas of leadership, team communication, staff support, volunteers, and space. He followed with a detailed analysis of New Haven's program and of services at St Luke's, New York, and the Marin County Hospice in northern California.

He closed his report with: "Despite all the attention to staff, probably one large factor in the stress problem [we have] is not having the right persons." John therefore enclosed the criteria for hospice-nurse selection suggested by New Haven's Sister Mary Kaye, who suggested: "*Look for*: a loving, open person who does well in interpersonal relationships; good general nursing skills with wide knowledge and experience; inner strength, personal emotional and spiritual wholeness; personal faith; support system outside hospice – family, friends, interests; experience in working as a team player. *Be Leery of*: the academic nurse, the psychiatric nurse who specializes in 'communication,' nurses who consider terminal care to be her/his 'specialty' and goes from one death and dying seminar to another, as well as those in it to solve their own personal problems."

It was clear from the outset that in John Scott we had struck gold. He brought us organizational and problem-solving skills; he was an adept clinician; he was outspoken and liked by his peers; and, as soon became apparent, he gave teammates memorable backrubs.

GAINING AN ALLY

It had been a busy morning: a long but satisfying eight o'clock case in the OR, then rounds in the Ross Pavilion to check on my surgical patients (*Mme L. isn't picking up as quickly as I would have liked, but the rest are on track*). I was now on my way to the hospital cafeteria to catch a quick lunch before what promised to be a long afternoon.

Passing along the corridor from "the Ross" to "the Main," I was deep in thoughts of soup and a sandwich when it registered that the figure that had just swept past me, en route to the Ross, was "L.D.," our dynamic chief of surgery, Lloyd MacLean. At that same moment, his voice broke my reverie. "BAL," he coughed absentmindedly in a manner suggesting that he too had been lost in thought.

"*BAL* ..." We both stopped abruptly in our tracks, and a couple of anonymous figures had to steer around us or risk running amok in our wake. "By the way," he continued, reaching for words, "*That girl* ... She's VERY good!" He was speaking in that high-pitched semi-yell that reflected "LD enthusiasm in living.

Love that man! But what in God's green earth is he talking about? When I turned, he had already moved on and was now lost in the bustling crowd. *That girl?* Then I remembered: Ina had done a consult on one of L.D.'s patients a couple of days earlier. *That girl? He's talking about Ina; his assessment was based on her consult!*

I asked her about it when I finally got to the PCU at the end of the day. The pieces fell into place. L.D.'s patient had cancer of the pancreas with intractable back pain. L.D. had been following him as an outpatient for weeks in a futile attempt to obtain consistent pain relief without excessive sedation. He then had admitted him, but to no avail. He sent us a consult. It was his first PCS consult. Ina saw the man. Within forty-eight hours he was consistently pain-free *and* awake. From then on, L.D. was a staunch PCS supporter. He had our backs.

I came to hear from various sources as months merged into years that he aggressively took up our cause in more than one shouting match around the "Table of the Gods" during battles about cutting beds and closing wards in those cash-strapped days. L.D. had unofficially joined the PCS team and I slept more soundly knowing that.

TRACKING PROGRESS

During those early months, team members recorded instructive moments as we learned together about the nature of patient and family needs. Perhaps, we thought, a record of these early experiences might provide useful reminders of our patient and family teachers as we inched toward a deeper understanding of our goals and the process of becoming a team. What follows are a few of these experiences from the period January to May 1975.

Miss B, a fifty-year-old woman with head and neck carcinoma, had refused to look in a mirror for weeks prior to her transfer to the PCU, noting, "I did not want to see how ugly I have become." A week following admission, her transformation was evident and particularly gratifying. She was delighted with the attractive scarf the nurses had found to conceal the mass in her neck and agreed to wear makeup as she began to enter into conversations with other patients and their families. She commented to her nurse with gratitude that "now she once again felt like a person."

Mrs V. had been ill at ease and withdrawn since her husband's PCU admission. When Norma, their nurse, asked if Mrs V. would like to help give her husband his bed bath, Mrs V. looked surprised that this was permitted and responded with delight, "All right, I'll wash and you dry." Norma was impressed by the power of such a simple suggestion aimed at deinstitutionalizing care and was deeply moved by the evident tenderness involved as Mrs V. ministered to her husband of thirty-five years.

Paul-Émile was admitted to the PCU with a history of lung cancer and epilepsy. His greatest problem, however, was his lifelong isolation. He had no visitors, indeed, no family or friends. Throughout life he had been ignored by everyone. A diminutive man in his fifties, he was now bedbound and profoundly withdrawn. As he settled into his new environment, however, the PCU became his home and the staff his family. He responded as a plant to sun and rain. For the first time, he experienced being valued by others. Day after day he continued to respond, in time leaving his room, helping the nurses make his bed, returning his meal tray to the transport cart, and starting to socialize in the lounge. As time passed, he increasingly engaged others in conversation. Toward the end, the PCU team saw to it that he was presented with a framed RVH Meritorious Service Award "in grateful recognition of your many hours of devoted service to the patients and families of the PCU." We were delighted; so was he. But it proved to be too much. The attention overwhelmed him and his newfound pleasure in daily life and heightened activity gave way to catatonic withdrawal. The team backed off; he recovered, and in his final weeks, he remained quietly happy with his PCU "family" close by. In dying, he left the team a note: "Memo: Thank you for your affection and devotion to me. After I am dead call to me and I will pray the Lord any time you are troubled."

Our need to err toward being over-inclusive in defining the patient, family, caregiver triad was becoming increasingly clear. And, on the whole, I think we did a pretty good job of it. A few examples: finding one morning two beds pushed together, the patient asleep in one, her twenty-two-year-old son asleep in the other, their hands touching across the beds; the PCU orderly studiously drawing a hot bath for an exhausted visiting grandmother, then tucking her into bed; two teenage daughters, together with their friends, softly playing their guitars while singing to their mother as she died, her tense face relaxing as she enjoyed a new sense of peace and comfort; Mr D. quietly enjoying family time with both his wife and their only "child," their dog Butch.

Mrs C. could not face her dying husband without bursting into tears, so she restricted her visits to brief encounters in the lounge when others would be present. Then one day, following an informal social chat over coffee with Mel, the PCU chaplain, she requested a brief bedside group prayer that included several members of the PCU team as she stood by her husband's head. As Mel concluded, Mrs C. silently bent over her husband for several minutes before straightening to state calmly, "It's going to be all right," and she sat down at his side. Now at ease in his presence, she was able to stay with him to the end, two days later.

When a blind organist offered to play for the PCU, the concert was enjoyed by all. One of the patients present that day was a retired piano teacher who had, since admission, steadfastly refused offers of music, whether recorded or by radio. Now, the day after the recital, she left her bed for the first time, went to the lounge, and started to play the piano. She continued to play during her final days.

C.T. was dying and was depressed. A thoughtful man with an enquiring mind, he seemed haunted by a private darkness. Like Barb Carter, "Magoo," our forty-year-old nursing assistant who referred to himself as "the world's greatest unpublished poet," was known for his ability to relate to patients. As he puttered about C.T.'s bed one afternoon, they gradually fell into an easy, if sparse, conversation. It was *not*, C.T. explained to Magoo, that he was afraid of dying, nor did he fear heaven or hell. He was struggling for words. "It's just that when I think of death, all I see is a void." Magoo straightened pensively. "Well," he replied, "at least a void is better than nothing at all." The two men dissolved into gales of laughter, all the more rollicking for being so unexpected. A bond had been created: C.T. began to relax.[12]

GROWING PAINS AND BUILDING THE "TEAM"

It soon became clear that the "RVH PCS Team" had to include the larger public, the provincial government, the RVH community at large, and then, with these foundational elements in place, a skilled, carefully selected, collegial, interdisciplinary group of professionals and volunteers. *Team building* had to be intentional and inclusive of the broader community, with wide layers of support, for the critical nucleus of day-to-day caregivers to grow synergistically.

On return from his obligatory visit to St Christopher's, John Scott joined us as a RVH fellow in oncology. The extra pair of hands lightened Ina's load significantly. His thoughtful, ordered approach brought a sense of reassurance and calm to the nurses. The patients and families loved him. On 11 September 1975 John was notified that he had been officially appointed to the Royal Victoria Hospital's attending staff, two years ahead of schedule. He was twenty-six years old, hardly the Royal Vic norm. In fact, it was unprecedented.

During the first four months of operation, there were forty-seven PCU admissions. Two patients were admitted from our Home Care Service, having saved a total of five weeks' hospitalization as a result of that program. Seven other patients were discharged to Home Care from the PCU, with the hospitalization time saved due to Home Care totalling thirty-four weeks. In this brief experience with one home-care nurse and only eight PCU beds, the PCS had freed up a total of thirty-nine weeks of hospital-bed utilization.[13] During the same period there were forty-nine consults. Of these, twenty-two patients were admitted to the PCU. Their waiting had blocked a total of 110 days of active-treatment beds for incoming patients. Fifteen additional patients died off-service while waiting for a bed. Clearly, the Vic would benefit from having more PCU beds.

Over these early months, our experience of a baptism by fire arose from many quarters. In addition to the challenges related to bed closures, tight budgets, the skepticism of academic colleagues, and the pressures of PCS program development, there were funding and evaluation complexities, and we also had to deal with requests for media interviews, inquiries about visits to the PCU, and invitations to speak to audiences that ranged from local church groups to international annual meetings of the various health-care disciplines. The more the interest grew, the broader the spectrum of demands became. Soon, every PCS team member had a significant probability of being contacted to tell their story. The RVH administration monitored the situation. The simplest response was to "just say no," but the PCS required financial support from the private sector, and, furthermore, the scarcity of community-based resources for palliative-care patients throughout Quebec and beyond and the resultant thirst for further information about palliative care presented a golden opportunity to disseminate our message. In these tough times, health-care news was generally bad. There was an appetite in the community for something positive, something new, something that was patient and family-centred. It was clear that we should make the most of this opportunity.

In March 1975, following less than three months of PCS operation, the hospital's director of public relations wrote, "I would like to congratulate you on the lustre you have brought to the RVH through your service and not being backward in coming forward when in the interest of those suffering." Similarly, a month later, a letter from the director of professional services stated: "In a period when our newspapers are filled with reports of turbulent events and the hospital is beset with numerous problems, it is gratifying to note the outstanding success of your unit. Many favourable reports have come to our attention and we are well aware of the outstanding public relations which you have developed. The 'feedback' has been most favourable."

We attempted to review each media request with care, but it wasn't until the airing of the CBC film *Death Shall Have No Dominion* that we fully recognized the risks involved. We had worked painstakingly with the producers in discussing the scenes to be included and had suggested that, rather than dramatizing the anxiety generally associated with death, the emphasis should be on compassionate, comprehensive care, a focus that would highlight the opportunity for comfort, peace, and reconciliation, even growth, at the end of life. The objective, we suggested, should be reassurance through recognition of what is possible. Watching the completed film on TV at home, I became apoplectic! How *could* they? The scenes were as we had planned, but the whole closing segment was presented over a low continuo that featured the *lub dub, lub dub, lub dub* of a beating heart. It was completely terrifying! Following discussion with the RVH administration, a memo was sent to PCS team members and associated Royal Vic colleagues requesting that *all* media requests be referred to our PCS administrator, Dottie. It was a directive that incensed three senior oncology colleagues – I mean, the very idea that *they* must seek permission! What were things coming to?

A month later, the RVH received a letter from a man in Ontario; he was responding to a Toronto *Globe and Mail* article on the PCS. His donation of $8,000 in support of our urgent financial needs followed.

How did the PCS evolve over these initial pilot-project months? By September 1975, we had added a second full-time physician and a full-time social worker (50 per cent, research; 50 per cent, clinical). All twelve beds were now open under the leadership of Head Nurse Sue Britton, who had a keen, assessing eye, a catalytic sense of humour, and a take-charge presence. The home-care team now consisted of three full-time nurses, a dedicated physician, and a consultant social worker offering care to Royal Vic cancer patients living on the roughly 200-square-mile Island of Montreal. Our revised five-page document "Drugs Useful in Palliative Care" (adapted from Cicely's original "Drugs Most Commonly Used" sheet), with its list of medications and comments on the management of frequently encountered symptoms,[14] had been made widely available.

As time passed, we were developing a more sensitive awareness of the full spectrum of physical, psychosocial, and existential/spiritual variables that predictably influence the quality of life of our patients and families. We were getting better at round-the-clock pre-emptive dosing to enable consistent minimal-dose prevention of, rather than repeated treatment for, troublesome symptoms, and we were recognizing more quickly the subtle indicators of need for diurnal variations in medication doses.

Optimal care is always person-specific, thus requiring shrewd awareness of the potential contributors to each individual's suffering. A woman on home care demonstrated the point. Her records documented a daily late-afternoon spike in morphine requirements that was difficult to explain until it was recognized that her increased distress was related to her husband's return home from work. Optimal-care plans require accurate diagnosis. As the months passed, discussions at the bedside and weekly rounds were becoming infinitely more nuanced and our listening to each other across disciplines more attentive.

As our awareness deepened regarding the complex mix of influences shaping patient experience, we noted that the same issues held true for family members and for ourselves as caregivers. Finally, as our shared personhood came into clearer focus, hierarchical distinctions between caregiver and care receiver blurred. We became increasingly ready to lower our defences and recognize that, in truth, we are all in the same boat – exactly the same boat! Once "the other" is seen in the uncompromising brilliance of that light, accompaniment that is different in quality and quantity follows. Patients, family members, and caregivers come to experience that we are all fellow travellers on the voyage and, at best, wounded healers.

As these changes in perception evolved, team effectiveness increased, friction decreased, and staff stress became more manageable. It didn't disappear. It never does. But when the inevitable anxieties surfaced we were becoming more able to mobilize support systems and assist each other.

The PCS team was now functioning with confidence and optimism as we moved forward with the assistance of periodic team potluck suppers in one of our homes for upwards of sixty staff members, volunteers, spouses, and friends to eat, drink, sing, and become better acquainted.[15] And so, into the second year.

BARRY

The Ross elevator was in "slo-mo" and I was running late! On every floor the doors opened, paused, seemed to look around, then finally, gradually, closed – on *evvverryy* floor! We were about to ascend to the next floor when a voice that, if half an octave higher, would have shattered glass, froze us in place. *Stella* had just glanced up from her Ross 3 Department of Medicine nursing-station control tower, directly across from the elevator.

"DR MOUNT!" Stella was gritty, with a veritable-carnival barker presence; she was also warm, open, and undaunted by life or anything else. Her gene pool was Mediterranean, but her flair Aussie in character. She ran a tight ship. "Got a minute? I need to speak to you about something." She looked determined. You didn't say no to that look! "I've got this young man I want you to see – twenty-one years old. It's serious. He's dying, actually. We don't know what's wrong with him. Would you take a look?"

"Stella ... hold it! Stella, just a moment." I had left the elevator and she now had enclosed my head in the young man's chart. "Who's he under? Who's his doctor?" She mentioned a highly respected senior internist. "Stella! Hold it!" But she was in full flight.

"He has an abdominal mass; the biopsy showed undifferentiated CA [cancer]. He has a high fever. I wondered if it might be a testis tumour, what with his age and all. Thought you should see him."

"Stella. Hold it! Is there a consult? Have I been asked to see him?"

"No, but he won't mind. He will agree. The patient's name is Barry." At this point she had linked our arms and I was struggling to keep up as she marched down the hall to the patient's room.

The patient lay in a swirl of twisted, damp sheets, barely awake. There had been significant weight loss and a spiking fever. It was now too late either to either back out or to shoot Stella – the two options that came to mind. We were at the bedside.

He was curled into a fetal position, pillowed onto his right side. I pulled up a chair. "Hello, Barry." He moaned. "I'm Dr Mount. Let me have a look at you." His pulse was fast, his abdomen tense, the right lower quadrant full; there was guarding, perhaps moderate rebound tenderness. I finished my brief physical examination.

Back at the desk, I phoned the pathologist who had studied the slides resulting from the biopsy done earlier in his admission.

"Well," he mulled thoughtfully in response to my query whether this could be a germ-cell tumour, "It's pretty undifferentiated; could be a number of things. Let me have another look at the slides and pass them around the department to see what the others have to say. I'll call you back." The conclusion was that they couldn't rule it out, but there was nothing specific to hang your hat on. He listed several other possibilities.

When I hung up following my second chat with the pathologist, Stella had already spoken to the attending physician about my participation. He would be most grateful for anything I might suggest.

I reviewed his chart. Barry had been admitted on 11 September with a two-month history of right abdominal and flank pain, nausea, vomiting, chills, and fever. Tests had revealed an obstructed right kidney owing to compression of its outflow by a mass, perhaps an abscess. He had been taken to the operating room on 12 September. At surgical exploration, an extensive mass in the right-lower abdomen was seen to be distorting the anatomy, resulting in progressive damage to the right kidney and pressure on the abdominal contents. The pathology was undifferentiated cancer. The post-operative course was tumultuous, with fever, persistent anemia, and troubling nausea and vomiting.

Radiation therapy had been started on 24 September and hyperalimentation feeding on 3 October. On 7 October, Barry had again been taken to the operating room to determine whether there was any evidence of cancer of the right testis. None was found. As the days passed, chemotherapy was started, though the absence of an exact tumour diagnosis made the choice of agents something of a shot in the dark. Things were deteriorating and once again Barry's temperature began to climb. It was clear that his time was limited. It was at that point that Stella and I crossed paths at the elevator.

With his internist's permission, I met with Barry and his mother and explained the situation. Barry had extensive cancer that had damaged his right kidney. While we could not be certain where the cancer had started, we did know that it was an aggressive form and that to date it had not shown any response to treatment.

They listened, motionless, as I continued. In the interest of pursuing every option, I noted, there was one more possibility to consider. Looking at the tumour under the microscope, the pathologists could not rule out it being a testis tumour. As they knew, the doctors had checked the right testis and it appeared to be normal, as did the left. While that seemed to rule out the testis as the source of the cancer, occasionally cells similar to those in the testis lie dormant elsewhere; therefore, we couldn't completely rule out that rare type of tumour. If that was to be the case, it was theoretically – *remotely* – possible that surgery and chemotherapy might cure his cancer. I stressed it was *highly* unlikely that it was that type of tumour and equally unlikely that it could be completely removed given its extensive spread. Following our detailed and gently frank discussion, I asked Barry and his mother if they were in favour of pursuing what was, at best, a long-shot return to the operating room. They wished to proceed.

The 28 October surgical procedure was challenging and extensive, taking fourteen hours. The subsequent chemotherapy was prolonged. Barry was cured. It had indeed been a primary retroperitoneal germ-cell tumour and the resection plus combination chemotherapy designed for testis tumours had worked their wonders.

Why did I feel compelled to speak about Barry in these pages? He has held a particular significance for me. Undoubtedly, I identified with this young man with a life-threatening germ-cell tumour. Perhaps, in mid-PCS pilot project, a result like Barry's offered me a welcome (needed?) "victory" over death. But there was something more. It seemed to me that it was more difficult for my academic colleagues to dismiss the PCS experiment as a mere exercise in sentimentality and handholding given results like Barry's at the hands of the same responsible investigator. Had I been a psychologist or pastoral-care person, instead of one involved in aggressive surgical oncology, the pilot project might not have been viewed in the same light. Our interest in detailed documentation and research was the other key to Royal Vic acceptance. These were tough times and any factor strengthening PCS support was welcome.

An additional reason to recount my encounter with Barry would arise much later. It involves a close friend of Barry's, named Kevin, or, as he himself pronounces it, *Keevin*. That story will be told in the book's concluding chapter.

Of course, it is always more comfortable to speak about our successes than our mistakes and failures, but the latter also remain with one as the years pass. I recall all too clearly a very pleasant gentleman on whom I undertook removal of the bladder (a radical cystectomy and ileal conduit urinary diversion) for cancer. The surgery went well and his early post-operative course was smooth, but after several days, when he should have been on the mend, he began to lose ground. He developed a low-grade fever. Efforts to chase down the cause were leading nowhere, but then an x-ray of the abdomen showed a telltale radiopaque marker near his new "bladder." I was mortified. It meant that a "sponge" used during his surgery had been left inside at the operative site. Who was to blame? What in the world had the nurses been doing? *They* do the counts before closing! That is *their* job! I had been told "the count is correct," thus confirming that the sponge count was correct before closing. That fail-safe guarantee is always a prerequisite to closing. I had been told, "the count is correct. On the other hand, *The buck stops here!* And *here* is always with the surgeon! It is that simple. No passing the buck!

To my relief, the problem was easily rectified. In the OR the sponge was retrieved in moments and my patient was discharged after a trouble-free few days. His hospitalization had not been prolonged on that account. What haunts me, however, is that I never did discuss the source of that transient low-grade fever with my patient or his wife. I rationalized that they didn't need something other than his hoped for cancer-free state to dwell on during their uphill climb back to health. But looking back, I suspect that they deserved a more complete report.

THE HOME STRETCH

Year two of the pilot project – the final year – was upon us, and our detailed report would need to be delivered to the RVH Board of Directors and the Quebec Ministry of Social Affairs on or before 13 October 1976 to enable a timely decision regarding the future of the PCS. Imperative deadlines for data concerning our success or failure were therefore imminent.

How were we to most effectively communicate what had been achieved? Our Evaluation committee opted for a multipronged attack involving the following elements:

1 the RVH PCS *October 1976 Pilot Project Report* documenting all aspects of the project and our findings authored by team members;[16]
2 the RVH *Manual on Palliative/Hospice Care*, a 555-page teaching manual for palliative/hospice-care planners and providers;[17]
3 published reports and articles in peer-reviewed journals;[18]
4 a McGill International Seminar on Care of the Terminally Ill, to be convened in Montreal on 3–5 November 1976;
5 two *presentation volumes*: identical, bilingual, colour, photo-journalistic volumes for rapid perusal containing summaries of the pilot-project philosophy, goals, clinical programs, conclusions, and recommendations; and

6 a participant-observation qualitative study of the lived experience of palliative-care patients and their families, the *Marmalade
   Project*.

THE MARMALADE PROJECT

From the outset, PCS evaluation included studies examining pain management, staff stress, patient attitudes, bereavement follow-up, demographics, and cost analysis. While the data generated by these efforts
would be useful, what if they failed to reflect fully the impact of palliative care on patient and family quality of life, an impact that had been
evident to us on a daily basis? As Einstein is said to have noted, "not
everything that counts can be counted, and not everything that can be
counted counts."

   How could we account for the improved quality of life consistently
claimed by our patients and their loved ones? How might we explore
the root causes of that improvement? Anecdotal accounts such as Allan
Jones's disturbing 1973 case studies and the contrasting 1975 PCS
vignettes collected during the early weeks of the pilot project were compelling, but what research methodology would best capture the lived
experience of patients and families?

   Dr Sylvia Lack and her New Haven Hospice colleague Bob Buckingham
came to meet with Ina and me shortly after the PCU opened. Bob was a
full-time doctoral student at the Yale School of Medicine's Department
of Epidemiology and Public Health. He was teaching a course in anthropology, community development, and public health to graduate and
medical students at Yale. In addition, he had participated in an ethno-
graphic participant-observation study on a Navajo Reservation during
the summer of 1972. Now, Sylvia and Bob were responsible for the evaluation of New Haven's Hospice. They were struggling with the same
issues we were facing. As we chatted, sitting around the kitchen table at
my home, the conversation was relaxed but focused. "Well," Bob sighed.
"I know what *would* position us to observe what is really making the
difference!"

   "What?" I asked. "Participant observation!" Bob elaborated. "A psychologist at Stanford – David Rosenhan – published a study a year or so
ago in the journal *Science*. It was titled, "On Being Sane in Insane Places."
He wanted to examine the efficacy of the techniques involved in diagnosing schizophrenia, and so he and a number of healthy co-investigators
posed as psychiatric patients in order to observe first-hand both the
diagnostic process and the milieu of psychiatric hospitals.[19] In any event,

you won't be able to repeat what they did. It would never pass an ethics committee."

"Why do you say that?"

"Because, they'd argue that all study participants must be aware that they are subjects in a research study."

"I'm not so sure that would be an obstacle," I responded. "Currently at the Vic, it is common knowledge that the quality of life of dying patients and their families is being assessed throughout the hospital. Certainly, everyone working on the PCS is aware that every aspect of their work is being evaluated. If 'participant observation' has something to offer, it seems to me it should be carefully considered. I'd like to see that Rosenhan paper. We can at least run it past the powers that be. If this is the closest we can come to examining the experiences of all concerned, they may feel it is the way to go. *However,* even if we *are* given the green light, where would we get the volunteer patient?"

Bob responded without hesitation. "I would do it. If you can get it through the ethical review, I'll be your patient."

The hypothetical *what if* wheels started to spin more quickly as Sylvia, Bob, Ina, and I dug deeper. Each of our successive queries generated further intriguing possibilities. The number of people aware of the project would have to be kept to a strict minimum. I would need to involve Dr MacKinnon as director of professional services. Bob's Royal Vic admission could be linked to his having come to Montreal for a second opinion. He could be admitted to a surgical ward and then transferred to the PCU – he would thus be able to make observations in both environments. If that was the case, he would have to cancel his planned tour of the PCU on this visit – can't have him bumping into his future caregivers!

There were endless details to be worked out. What cancer and clinical situation would lend themselves to our specific needs? Why would Bob be seeking his "second opinion" in Montreal? Perhaps he could have a family member in town. How could Bob avoid all invasive tests and treatment yet be admitted on the basis of his condition? Why would he be admitted to Surgery, then transferred to the PCU? What observations would Bob be documenting in assessing the impact of care in both settings? We talked well into the night.

Dr MacKinnon listened to my explanation with rapt attention. He would read the Stanford study published in *Science* and the information on participant observation which Bob promised to send, and then consult the hospital lawyers. In a second meeting I met with the senior Royal Vic lawyer, Alex Paterson, and Dr MacKinnon. They promised to get back to us after further consultation.

Mr Paterson's confidential letter to Dr MacKinnon of 16 February 1976 outlined the risks to each party, noting that the recommendation of the World Medical Association and similar bodies that local, provincial, or federal authorities be consulted *prior to* human experimentation would *not* be possible in our study given the need for secrecy. He then stipulated three prerequisites for study acceptability: 1) the aims, methods, anticipated benefits, and potential hazards must be fully explained to Buckingham; 2) he must be able to abstain or withdraw at any time; 3) any examination or treatment judged potentially harmful must be avoided. A four-page legal agreement and a one-page consent form had been drawn up. They would require Buckingham's signature.

In the scenario chosen as being most likely to meet our requirements, it would be necessary to involve Lloyd MacLean, chief of surgery. He listened carefully as I described the research rationale, the *Science* article, the proposed scenario for Bob's medical condition, and Alex Paterson's stipulations. There was a moment of silence, then, "BAl, it's *got* to be done!!" L.D. was on board.

The Ethics Committee included those currently informed along with two outside colleagues experienced in research-protocol review. It was decided to proceed, with the proviso that there be a detailed debriefing of all concerned on both wards immediately following the discharge of the pseudo-patient. The date for Bob to present himself at the Emergency Department was selected.

In a moment of enthusiasm, I commented, "Well, if anthropology isn't the bread of life, it may well be the marmalade on the bread." Sylvia grinned. We suddenly had a code name to facilitate ambiguity in future discussions. The study had just become the *Marmalade Project*.

The scenario: Bob, now "Robert James Murray," was to arrive at the Royal Vic Emergency Department complaining of abdominal pain, nausea, and vomiting on Sunday afternoon, 16 May, 1976, having travelled to Montreal for a second opinion from Dr MacLean. His office appointment (booked with L.D. for Monday, 17 May) had been arranged by Robert's Montreal-based "cousin," Breen Murray, "his only relative." Breen Murray (his real name), an anthropology graduate student at McGill, was not related to Bob. Buckingham was to arrive at the ER equipped with x-rays, pathology slides, and a discharge summary pertaining to a fictitious New Haven hospital admission on 24 March 1976. He was to be admitted from the ER to a surgical bed under Dr MacLean and then transferred to the PCU. He would then be discharged to the care of his "cousin."

Preparations would need to be painstaking. The "discharge summary" from Robert Murray's reported New Haven admission for "epigastric

pain" documented an enlarged lymph node in his neck just above the
left clavicle. It had been subjected to an excisional biopsy that revealed
an adenocarcinoma compatible with cancer of the pancreas. This diagnosis had been confirmed by radiology studies (an arteriogram and a
retrograde pancreatogram). Local radiation therapy was given (3600
rads) to the upper abdomen and chemotherapy initiated prior to Robert
Murray's refusal of all further investigations and treatment.

Each aspect of the story required collaborative evidence: the name
Robert James Murray appearing on all medical records of the case –
discharge summary, pathology slides, arteriogram, and pancreatogram
x-rays; a "post-biopsy" left-lower-neck incision that had healed to a
degree compatible with the seven-week interval since the reported lymph-
node biopsy; skin changes in the abdominal "radiation field"; a shaved
abdominal field, with the desired erythema achieved through exposure
to a sun lamp; bruises up and down both arms compatible with numerous venipunctures. To ensure familiarity with how Robert Murray might
be feeling, during the weeks prior to his Vic admission, Bob arranged
several chats with a man in New Haven who had pancreatic cancer.

During the weeks leading up to the 16 May Emergency Room visit,
Bob experienced increasing stress, loss of appetite, and a twenty-pound
weight loss; he became anxious and somewhat depressed. *What if we're
discovered?* Whether detected or not, this was far more stressful than
he/we had anticipated! He developed psoriasis and plantar warts and
started to lose his hair. He also became impotent, a problem that would
continue for five weeks.

On Sunday afternoon, 16 May, Bob, Breen, Sylvia, Lloyd MacLean,
Dottie, Ken MacKinnon, and I met at my home. An undercurrent of
apprehension cut short any thought of lighthearted banter and bravado.
Bob was unwashed and unshaven, with several days of stubble. He
looked pale. His weight loss was evident.

We reviewed the plans for the umpteenth time, and then L.D. phoned
the ER. "Hello, this is Dr MacLean, who am I speaking to? May I speak to
a nurse? Hello, it's Dr MacLean. I just wanted to let you know that there's
a young man coming in. American, with recently diagnosed cancer of the
pancreas. I am booked to see him in the office tomorrow but his pain is
worse and he has developed nausea and vomiting – may have a degree of
bowel obstruction. You may want to admit him to the Holding Unit."

"Well, no point postponing this any longer, we're off." Bob and Breen
left us. It was agreed that Breen would give us a telephone update as
soon as possible. We settled back for another cup of coffee. The wait
seemed endless; time had slowed to a crawl; we became restless.

Bob and Breen made their way through the shabby ambulance entrance to the old Royal Vic Emergency Room and into the cramped waiting area with its dishevelled mixed-salad aroma of recycled humanity, stale tobacco, beer, and gin.

Bob headed for the two empty chairs in the front row and slumped down. It really didn't require acting at this point. He was exhausted and, to make it worse, he knew – absolutely *knew* – that, in an inevitable *One Flew Over the Cuckoo's Nest* moment, "Nurse Ratched" was about to burst in, see him, and shout "FAKE!" He was certain of it! Breen went to register and then took the seat next to Robert just as an encrusted old-timer with bad breath sitting in the next chair was giving Bob a careful once-over.

"What's the matter with the young fella?" he breathed into Breen's ear.

"Cancer," replied Breen softly, behind a raised forefinger. Now, the old-timer was an ER regular and both Breen and Bob suspected as much. He had become an experienced diagnostician in his own right – and they assumed that as well! His eyes narrowed as he studied Robert once more.

"Ahh, that's a shame," he grunted with reassuring sympathy. And that, Bob later confessed, was when he started to relax a little. If he passed *that* test, chances were that he would get past most others!

They called Robert Murray's number; he made his way through the tight, cramped maze into the back room and clambered onto a vacant stretcher.

"I've been over your New Haven notes, Mr Murray," reported the unsmiling young man blankly, "and we're going to do some blood tests."

"No, you're not," Bob started to blurt, but he quickly thought better of it.

Hour upon hour later, the resident was back. "OK, Mr Murray, the blood tests have just come back and we now know what's wrong with you. You have evidence of pancreatitis – an inflammation of your pancreas. It's common with cancer of the pancreas."

Bob was now wide-eyed! *Pancreatitis! He knows what is wrong? WRONG? What in God's name?!*

"Now we're just going to put a tube down your nose into your stom-ach. It'll help your nausea and vomiting."

"Oh, I don't think that will be necessary, doctor. It's been a little better since coming in," Bob stammered. "I'd like to try going without it for a while." *What is going on?! Dear God! A Cuckoo's Nest moment if there ever was one!* "But, I need to go to the bathroom, if that's OK."

"Just down the hall there, on your left."

Bob called us from the pay phone in the hall. L.D. reassured him and said he would phone and speak to the resident.

The blood-test values had been borderline normal/abnormal. The astute residents had read "pancreatitis" into the results. L.D. suggested they admit Robert Murray to the Holding Unit, and, following a shot of Demerol for his "pain," that is exactly what they did.

The next day Robert Murray was transferred from the Holding Unit to a bed on a surgical ward under Dr MacLean. Oncology and palliative-care consults were obtained. After four days on Surgery, Robert Murray was transferred to Palliative Care, once again for four days. He was then discharged to the care of his "cousin."

During his ten-day hospitalization, Robert attempted to maintain passive, compliant behaviour and a quiet affect. While he rang the bell for assistance when he could have acted on his own behalf, otherwise, the content of his actions, conversations, and expressed philosophies, likes and dislikes were representative of his personal feelings. Throughout his stay he kept detailed records of his observations, explaining that he was writing a book, an activity that drew only one comment from a surgical nurse who said that she hoped he was not writing about the hospital.

It wasn't easy! Heightening Bob's mounting anxiety was the fact that, within forty-eight hours, he began to experience "real" back pain. In an act of defiance, he discarded his pyjamas for slacks and shirt "to preserve accurate observations, feel better and silently remind myself that I'm really not sick!"

On the surgical ward, Bob quickly became bored and frustrated. He felt isolated and attributed that to the absence of meaningful social interactions. In spite of his determination to remain passive, he found himself initiating conversations. After the first forty-eight hours, when asked how he was, he spoke of back pain and weakness, problems he was *actually* experiencing.

Given his reaction to the surgical ward, Bob worried that when he was transferred to the PCU he would probably experience even more isolation. He assumed that he would have an even greater risk of being recognized as a fraud since his fellow patients would be sicker and his relative well-being would be even more evident.

Once on the PCU, however, he identified more closely with the patients and found himself becoming weaker, more anorexic, and increasingly exhausted. He developed a constant ache in his left leg and had increasingly restless nights during which families of other patients commented on his moaning and groaning – a manifestation that he was completely unaware of.

Throughout his admission, Bob observed the frequency, quality, and duration of verbal interactions on each ward among staff, patients, and family members. While the number of patient-staff verbal contacts was virtually the same on the two wards, their mean duration on Surgery was 5.5 minutes and on the PCU 19; for nurses, the difference was even more pronounced: 2.4 minutes (Surgery) compared to 13 (PCU). The quality of contact was also strikingly different. He noted that patients, in general, experienced monotony and loneliness on the surgical ward whereas engagement, kindness, and individual attention were evident, indeed a matter of policy, on the PCU.

In his notes on the surgery ward, Bob wrote: "The only staff who initiate conversations are the student nurses and orderlies. Personal requests made to other staff were frequently ignored or forgotten." The PCU experience was vastly different. On arrival at the PCU, he was greeted by flowers and a bedside card saying, "Welcome Mr Murray." Glynnis, the admitting nurse, introduced herself by name, sat down so that her eyes and his were on the same level, and proceeded to listen. There was no hurry; her questions flowed from Robert's previous answers and there was acknowledgment and acceptance of his expressions of concern. She asked such questions as, "What do you like to eat?" and "Is there anything special you like to do?"

The difference in the ease of discussion with doctors on the two wards also impressed Bob. On surgery, resident doctors travelled in groups, a pattern that fostered professional and social discussion among themselves but prevented conversation with the patients. Patients appeared to be intimidated and were reluctant to question these groups of young surgeons. On the PCU, the patient-doctor contact was one-on-one and private.

Murray observed that the surgical team excelled at pre- and post-operative acute care of the body while neglecting emotional needs and "needs of the spirit." They concealed their personalities, rarely smiled, and frequently gave orders to the patients. In contrast, on the PCU, staff professionalism was balanced by a notable freedom to express individuality; orders were never given to patients. Instead, Bob noted a "happy spirit" and "atmosphere of caring" that patients and family members repeatedly commented on.

Bob felt that relatives suffered from the doctors' inaccessibility on the surgical ward, where queries about medications, diet, and other topics were deferred to "the doctor," whose absence meant they were left unanswered. He concluded that this lack of access to the doctor "contributed to family grief, fear, sense of loss, resentment, anger, guilt and other similar reactions." On the PCU, however, he observed a family member requesting a doctor on five occasions and on each occasion the doctor was reached and spoke to the family in person or over the phone. In addition, on the PCU, the nurses, volunteers, and other staff were more willing and permitted to answer questions. Finally, on the surgical ward, the family was more likely to feel in the way at the bedside, while on the PCU they were encouraged to be active participants in bedside care.

Following Robert Murray's discharge, Ina and I held the planned "full disclosure" meetings first with the staff of the Surgical Holding Unit and then with the PCS team. I had anticipated distinct interest in the Marmalade methodology and an appreciative response for the care and attention to detail we had shown in attempting to evaluate the experience of our patients and families. Surely, there would be great relief on hearing that "Robert Murray" was actually healthy. Would our colleagues resent the fact that they had been misled? I assumed that issue would be quickly resolved through discussion of our need for qualitative data with which to explain our consistently observed palliative-care effectiveness, not to mention the unimpeachable credentials surrounding Rosenhan's *Science* publication.[20]

On meeting with the surgical staff, Ina and I encountered disinterest bordering on boredom; with the PCS team, however, there was disbelief, then *more* disbelief, then anger! They had been *betrayed*! How *could* we? How could they *ever* trust us again? How *could* we justify such dishonesty? How total had been their commitment to and emotional engagement with that appealing young man!

Did we reach a common understanding at the end of that long and painful meeting? Perhaps, to some degree. But, to the extent that common ground *was* achieved, it resulted largely from the desperately earnest willingness of each person present to question, challenge, listen, strive to understand, disagree, and then listen again to each other's point of view rather than from any sense of justification for doing such a study.

Participant observation had successfully laid bare both the compassion and commitment at the heart of effective palliative care and the reductionist depersonalization endemic in many other settings. The critical issue, in my opinion, wasn't that the caregiver subjects "didn't know they were in a study" – the whole two years was a study and everyone knew it! Instead, paradoxically, the problem, and our strength, was the totality of investment offered by our PCU colleagues.

Reaction to the planned research presentations at the RVH Surgical Grand Rounds and the 3–5 November 1976 International Seminar, and also in a *Canadian Medical Association Journal* (*CMAJ*) article, lay ahead. We had been forewarned.

FEEDBACK

By 30 September 1976, after twenty months spent learning our way, there had been 288 PCU admissions with a median length of stay of 11 days, 156 dying men and women had been cared for by the Home Care Service, and 413 PCS consultations were completed concerning patients on the Royal Vic active-treatment wards. In spite of the endemic emotional heaviness related to so much loss and the exacting challenges encountered in symptom control and support, the commonly expressed observation by PCS team members was, "We get more than we give."

In the early months of our second year, Margaret Archibald died on the PCU, thus bringing to a peaceful close an atypically lengthy PCU admission. The next morning, her close friend, Mardee Cork, penned a letter to the RVH's executive director:

> I would like to express my impression of this inspiring exemplification of man's humanity to man. In the paradox that is the Unit, where a general atmosphere of depression might be expected, there is one of warmth and cheerfulness; where death is imminent, there is affirmation of life to its fullest possible capacity; where there is grief and apprehension, there is solace and reassurance; where there is great diversity of individuals, there is fellowship in the shared experience of heartbreak and bereavement; where there is weeping, weariness and discouragement, there is laughter, uplift, overwhelming bravery and faith; where strain and taxed emotions accompany demanding, difficult service, there is the consistent kindness, sensitivity, understanding, ready attention, skilled care, frankness and friendliness of an exceptionally special professional staff, supported by the finest volunteers. The genuine concern and generosity with which all these truly "beautiful people" give of themselves to both patients and visitors are profoundly and inexpressibly appreciated.

In the process, our team experienced once again the feedback loop. Healing begets healing, begets healing, and, as a result, we the caregivers found ourselves the unintended beneficiaries.

OLYMPIAN DAYS AND NIGHTS

The summer of 1976 involved Olympian output with eighteen-hour days as we attempted to keep all the balls in the air while writing the PCS

Pilot Project Final Report, collating and analyzing clinical and research data, and planning the first McGill International Seminar on Care of the Terminally Ill.

John Scott laid it out for us at a physicians' meeting that rounded out yet another gruelling day. "This pace is neither healthy nor sustainable; it has to stop! If the service goes beyond the Pilot Project phase, there must be major changes. We are currently on a collision course with personal and collective disaster. Each of us needs to recalibrate. There must be time for reflection, renewal, personal life, team building and so much more!" All agreed, and we plodded on.

The incoming data from the various studies were compelling:

Pain Study: Ron Melzack and colleagues studied the impact of the liquid medication (our version of the British Brompton Mixture) on pain in cancer patients and found that the RVH version of the time-honoured mix controlled pain in 90 per cent of PCU patients and 75–80 per cent in other RVH settings – a significant difference. Moreover, it produced substantial reductions in all three main dimensions of pain assessed – sensory, affective, and evaluative. Finally, these results were "strikingly more effective" than those observed in an outpatient pain clinic using traditional cancer pain-management strategies.

Staff Stress: Toronto's Clarke Institute of Psychiatry team[21] tracked PCS staff stress using both standardized measures and participant observation at three-monthly intervals during the initial fifteen months of the Pilot Project.[22] Three months into the study, more than half the palliative-care nurses had stress levels (Goldberg questionnaire) similar to those of newly bereaved widows.[23] As the PCS staff changed and team experience grew, stress levels decreased to levels approximating those on another new clinical-care unit in the hospital. Ongoing factors that contributed to episodic palliative-caregiver stress included: inconsistent hierarchical vs. matrix-style team relating; communication confusion around religious vs. standard caregiver terminology; the need experienced by PCS staff to minimize expression of personal reaction to death in the interest of honouring perceived PCS team norms; and my lessening day-to-day involvement as director.[24] While stress levels had decreased to much lower levels by six months, it appeared that the very real administrative and interpersonal difficulties seen with any new unit were magnified by displacement of anxieties about death to these interpersonal topics, giving rise to stereotyping and scapegoating. ("If it wasn't for those x or y group members, things would be just fine around here!") Rather bitter scapegoating up the hierarchical ladder was also seen, particularly regarding the now less-available PCS director. Finally, although stress levels had decreased markedly after the first half year, "it remained high enough to remind us that the needs of staff should remain at the forefront of our minds."

Bereavement Study: British-trained social worker Jean Cameron,[25] in consultation with St Christopher consultant psychiatrist and bereavement researcher Colin Murray Parkes, examined the experience of twenty PCU bereaved "key persons" (KPs) and a "comparison group" of twenty non-PCU KPs one year after bereavement:[26] 75 per cent of the non-PCU KPs claimed they had no advance warning of the death and expressed strong anger about the indifference, neglect, and callous treatment encountered by their dying loved one. Only one PCU KP complained of similar inadequate care and that had occurred prior to transfer to the PCU. Fifty per cent of non-PCU KPs found "the hardest thing to bear in the past year" was the "terrible and unrelieved pain and suffering" of their loved one. There was, however, no mention of their loved one experiencing unrelieved suffering by PCU KPs. Loneliness was a common response to the "hardest thing to bear" question in both groups. Sixty per cent of the non-PCU KPs said they were troubled by not being present when their loved one died, either because the death was unexpected or because they were not permitted to stay "outside visiting hours or overnight." This anguish was often enhanced by the sense that their relative had been neglected and ignored. Only one PCU KP expressed regret at not being present for the death, an event that had occurred because the imminent death had not been anticipated and the KP had chosen to go home. Bereavement follow-up was received by 80 per cent of PCU KPs and their grief factor scores were lower (better) than the more troubled non-PCU KPs. Interestingly, the four PCU KPs who had *not* (for a variety of reasons) received BFU support all had troubled bereavement experiences and scores similar to the non-PCU KPs. The non-PCU KPs had significantly greater manifestations of grief at one year than did the PCU KPs. Those in both groups who had *not* anticipated the deaths had more prolonged and intense grief and they seemed to feel the "presence" of their dead relative more frequently. In both groups, women showed more overt manifestations of grief than men and more women continued to take sleeping pills and tranquilizers, especially in the younger (eighteen to forty-five) age group. Prolonged "pining," depression, solitariness, and sense of health deterioration were more common in the elderly of both groups, yet they remained unwilling to seek medical attention. Parental grief was particularly intense and prolonged in both groups, and in both, the KPs happened to be elderly. Rumination about the past seemed to be more prevalent in the non-PCU group and this troubling problem seemed to be linked to their sense that the loved one's care had been deficient during the final illness.

The Marmalade Project: With the qualitative participant-observation study now behind us, the reading of Bob's endless careful notes and summaries followed, as did the synthesis, analysis, discussion, and review of emerging themes, the preparation of manuscripts, and the critique of findings (with input from Lloyd MacLean). Plans were finalized to present the Marmalade study at RVH Surgical Grand Rounds on 28 October ("Terminal Care: An Anthropologist's Perspective"), then, once again, at the November 1976 McGill International Seminar, and finally through publication in the *CMAJ*. Three days after the Surgical Grand Rounds, on Sunday, 31 October, the *Washington Post* published a feature article on the Marmalade study. Staff writer B.D. Colen's "Ten Bad Days among the Dying" provided a detailed description of Marmalade accompanied by a comment by Dr Robert Veatch of the Hastings Institute of Society, Ethics and the Life Sciences noting that the study, as described to him, would probably not meet the informed-consent guidelines for funding by the Department of Health, Education and Welfare. In the article Bob Buckingham observed that, while he felt the study findings made it worth doing once, he would not do it again based on the stress involved.[27]

Pilot Project Data to 31 December 1976: The multidisciplinary PCS team[28] generated a wealth of data related to the PCU, Home Care, and Consult services.[29]

We weren't the only ones in town experiencing all-out, effort-filled Olympian days during Montreal's summer of 1976. Indeed, the Games of the XXI Olympiad commanded centre stage from 17 July until 1 August as Montreal hosted the world!

Faye and I attended only two events, diving and, on the last full day of competition, track and field. It had been a grim two weeks. Canada was to become the first Olympic host country to fail to win a single gold medal.

On Saturday, 31 July, we were sitting nosebleed high in the stands. Not only had Canada not won a gold medal, we hadn't even won a silver medal. The stadium was sold out with 70,000 in attendance. At a particular moment, all eyes shifted to the high-jump competition directly below our seats – far, far below. We still had a competitor in the running, a twenty-year-old Canadian kid named Greg Joy. The bar was set at 7'4" – that's *seven feet*, four inches!

As Greg said later, "It was more like a hockey game than high jumping. I was amazingly relaxed; I didn't notice the people ... My mind was on jumping and nothing else. I heard the crowd, but they were sort of inanimate. While I did my 'walk through' they were cheering and everything, but when I started walking back they started to chant and my heart started going like crazy. And then I stood back, ready to jump and was totally relaxed. And when I dropped my head the crowd just went *whsshhh* and there wasn't a sound and when that happened I just went ... I got it! I knew I had it right then."

The crowd was still; Greg's head was down; 70,000 of us held our collective breath. He was dancing toward destiny, his long brown-blond hair streaming – a bouncing spring in his step – we're still not breathing – he's obviously relaxed – up, up, up, his back arched gracefully – the kid's flying. Now he is on his feet – the bar is still in place above him – arms extended high about his head, fists punching the air – he knows what has happened – it sinks in for the rest of us – 70,000 of us are cheering now; the whole stadium is pulsating, Greg is prancing toward the stands, coming directly toward Faye and me – arms still pumping over his head, the crowd's screaming. Time is locked in those seconds for all who were there.

I lost my voice in that single delirious moment. We were all on our feet, ecstatic. The roar of the crowd was sustained, on and on and on. You see, it wasn't simply about a high jump, or the silver medal he won. It was about national pride. It was about a kid pulling the iron out of the fire at the last moment; it was an eruption of unity and it was better than all the gold medals put together.[30] Greg Joy was in the zone and we were there with him. Like the Canada-Russia hockey victory, it was, "an iconic Canadian moment for the ages." My celebration of Greg Joy's success was also, unconsciously, my recognition of the completion of a pilot project that would change health care.

THE VERDICT

October 22, 1976

Dear Balfour:

On my recommendation to the Board of Directors at their meeting
of October 22 1976, the Palliative Care Service was confirmed as a
continuing patient care service in this hospital. This takes it out of
the category of a pilot project and assures its future activities.

With reference to the various recommendations included in your
report, steps were initiated to study these recommendations and their
financial implications, at the conclusion of which, decisions will be
taken concerning the proposed expansion of the service.

I would like to add that your report and the function of the
Palliative Care Service received nothing but commendation and
praise from the Board members.

Sincerely yours,
F.J. Tweedie, Chairman,
RVH Executive Committee

I responded: "During the past two years we have had the privilege of seeing a problem give way to an idea, an idea become a plan, a plan develop
into an experiment, and an experiment reap a rich harvest. We have all
grown through the experience! Those of us who have been involved have
received more from our patients than we have given."[31]

THE INTERNATIONAL SEMINAR ON CARE OF THE
TERMINALLY ILL: 3–5 NOVEMBER 1976

From early in the pilot project, a cornerstone outcome of our experience
was to be the McGill International Seminar on Care of the Terminally Ill.
We planned to present three models of care of the dying: St Christopher's
Hospice, London (Cicely); the individual consultant working within a
teaching hospital[32] (Elisabeth); and the RVH teaching hospital and community-based PCS (Bal). We envisioned an interactive format designed
to foster active participation by all registrants sitting at round tables for
ten, each with a trained discussion coordinator.

The 317 seminar registrants (Canada 193; United States 123; Sweden
1) who assembled for the Opening Plenary on 3 November were welcomed by McGill's dean of medicine, Patrick Cronin, and the Royal
Vic's DPS, Ken MacKinnon. The program promised to be rich and

groundbreaking. From the initial introductions at the tables, interactive sessions were lively.[33] Editor Dr David Shephard was present for all three days to prepare a detailed report on the meeting for the *Canadian Medical Association Journal*. We were off to a flying start. The hall was abuzz with enthusiasm and expectation.

The first day's sessions focused on "Total Care" (Cicely, Bal, and colleagues) and "Intractable Pain" (Ron Melzack and Ina); day two, "Symptomatic Care Other Than Pain" (John Scott and multidisciplinary colleagues with comments by Cicely); and "Staff Support Systems" (PCS psychiatrist Akos Beszterczey, the Clarke Institute team, and Sylvia Lack). The third day, devoted to "Emotional Aspects," opened with my presentation of our data on "Attitudes to the Terminally Ill in Present Health Care," followed by Elisabeth's "Psychological Needs of the Patient and Family" and then, closing the morning, Bob Buckingham's participant-observation presentation, listed in the program simply as "Case Study."

I was standing at the back of the room taking the pulse of the audience. The response to the Marmalade Project could perhaps best be described as *charged*. One registrant wrote, "I'm sure you knew there would be plenty of static – but did you realize there would be an electric storm?"

Carol Hancock, a McGill pastoral-care student at the time of the study, had cared for Robert Murray on the PCU and then been posted to a church in western Canada prior to the post-study debriefing of the PCU team. She had not heard! Now she was in the audience. She gave an audible gasp as Bob, her presumed dead patient, bounded onto the stage. Ina and I made eye contact – *Groan!*

As Bob proceeded with the presentation, a collective restlessness became increasingly evident. It appeared to feed on itself. Registrants started to line up at the floor microphones before the table-discussion period had ended. The most memorable comment was the theatrical pronouncement by British psychiatrist Michael Simpson that Marmalade was "the most unethical study since WWII." Several, including Elisabeth, expressed concern that Bob might be at risk for developing cancer as a result of the stress he had experienced.

The lines at the microphones swelled. It was as if the expanding aura of sustained excitement that had been joyously building since the first day had suddenly been lanced to reveal a boil rather than the giddy bouquet that had permeated the proceedings to that point. Suddenly, everyone had a need to voice one concern or another – Bob's stress, a perceived ethical lapse, disillusionment, anger!

From my position at the back of the room, I carefully assessed the situation, came to a measured assessment, and concluded, thoughtfully,

#/@*Z^+! while striding to the nearest floor microphone. Frankly, I found the growing flood of holier-than-thou, "ethical" critiques light-weight at best and irritating as hell!

With my sleeves rolled up, I stridently responded that, in my opinion, there *was* a critical ethical issue before us – our demonstrated ability to ignore the needs of the 70 per cent of our citizens who die in insti-tutions, not to mention the non-quantitative factors that other study methodologies might fail to highlight fully as we attempt to explain the enhanced quality of life that was the consistent experience of our patients and families!

Informed consent, in my view, had been attended to since our "patient," the person actually at risk, had been *thoroughly* informed through the detailed consent form that had been carefully drawn up by the hospital lawyers. Furthermore, he was aware that he could withdraw at any time. As for the caregivers on the two wards not being "informed," I argued that the staff on both wards were aware that *all* Royal Vic end-of-life care was being assessed.

As far as *deception* was concerned, I reminded our critics that full disclosure is *not an invariable and absolute right*. For example, a ques-tioner does not have a "right" to the details of another's intimate life. I argued that deception becomes an ethical concern under two circum-stances: *first*, when you deny the truth to someone who has a right to information critical to his or her personal well-being, which was not the case here; and *second*, when you deny the truth for the purpose of elic-iting behaviour from an individual that would not otherwise have been elicited, and that also was *not* the case in this instance.[34]

Finally, I suggested that the ethical standards of the model we had followed, set out in the Rosenhan study published in the journal *Science*, could not be dismissed as casually as some seemed to have done. The journal *Science* is a universally respected publication and Rosenhan is a well-credentialled Stanford Law School faculty "expert on psychology and the law." Out-of-hand condemnations of disregard for ethics, while interesting, were in my view facile. Should the PCS pilot project have failed for lack of qualitative evidence, hollow ethical arguments would now seem shameful and anemic indeed!

Cicely's comment from the floor noted Marmalade's significant find-ings but suggested that such a study should not be repeated. Elisabeth's comments – delivered with literally one foot out the door as a result of conference-scheduling chaos in the wake of the Marmalade uproar – were variously recalled by those present as: "I don't agree with your hav-ing done the study, but that's OK; the findings are important, and that's

OK; Bob, you're not OK, and we're not OK, but that's OK." Then she was
gone, to a chorus of laughter and a burst of applause.

Postscripts from three psychiatrist colleagues seem relevant. Bill
Lamers, who in 1974 had pioneered the Hospice of Marin home-care
program in northern California, commented, "We all have a lot to learn
from the way we reacted to Operation Marmalade." John Fryer suggested, "Please take some advice from us affective *nuts* about how to
deal with the inevitable expression of feelings – There are ways of planning for them. Please, no more big surprises!" The third psychiatric postscript arrived that evening. The telephone rang. It was Elisabeth, now
home in Chicago. "Bal," she intoned in that reassuring Switzerdeutsch
voice of hers, "I just vant to say two things. First, it vas a *loovely* conference! And second, give up your insecurity, you don't need it." ... *Click*.

Of my many personal reactions to what would become the first in a
continuing, decades-long, unbroken chain of biennial McGill international conferences on palliative care, the response that took root most
deeply as the November 1976 dust began to settle was the realization
that at some point my crossroad decision must be faced: Which path
would I follow? Surgical oncology or palliative care?

TAKING STOCK

On 15 November 1976, ten days after the McGill International Seminar,
the Parti Québécois, which had been formed in 1968 to promote Quebec
independence, swept to victory in a Quebec provincial election. The PQ's
first priority was to pass the Charter of the French Language (Bill 101).[35]
The country took a deep breath. The future once again looked uncertain.
It was time to take stock.

It had been a highly focused year – make that *three* years! Being unrelated to our all-consuming pilot project, the parade of events – family,
local, national, and world – had largely passed me by unnoticed. Some,
however, had, gained a foothold in my unconscious and now, as Faye and
I paused with the children for a year-end celebration in front of the fireplace, those events may have, could have, should have, drifted to the fore.

Chris was twelve, determined, a dynamic force, interested in music.
Not long before our evening of taking stock, he had proudly brought
home a recently acquired record album – Elton John's *Goodbye Yellow
Brick Road*. One glance at the back cover, where the band members
looked distinctly gay, and several suspicious song titles led me to declare
the album forbidden fruit without bothering to take the time to listen to
a single song. Did I know that my son needed a father with a supportive,

listening ear? Apparently not. Did I know what "homophobic" meant? Did I realize that many of my closest colleagues and friends were gay? Was I aware of the wounding that attitudes like mine had caused them? Did I know it was *my* problem not theirs? Apparently not. Did I know what perennial joy would have been kindled in my heart and soul if I had let Chris introduce me to Elton that afternoon? Obviously not. Did I recall this incident as we reflected during that 1976–77 New Year's Eve stock taking? I'm not certain, but it has haunted me ever since.

Lauren – to me, always *Wrennie* – was nine. Inquisitive, thoughtful, reflective, and perceptive from her earliest days, she quietly carved her own path. Did I protect her enough from the predicament of being the middle child that had burdened her Aunt Alice? Was it even an issue? While she was vigorously independent, her participation in family play, outings, and story time was joyful and full. Images of her burrowing her face and hands in Samoyed Nicky's thick white coat as they lay wrapped in a mutual hug come to mind. She also had a private side that had to do with books and papers and secret notes that were inevitably balled up and squirrelled away in drawers. She repeatedly surprised me with her willingness as she took on, with quiet enthusiasm, cycling, skiing, water skiing, horseback riding, and cooking lessons.

Jamie was six, outgoing, fun, ever-ebullient, the entertainer! Did I realize how he was being bullied at school, called "stupid Indian," "redskin," "savage"? Come to think of it, what did I say to him when the man passing us on Sherbrooke Street said to his son, "Now there's a *real* Kung Fu!?" His buoyant demeanour seemed to carry him through, but abuse continued. Why didn't I know that? Mother, *Nana Maude*, was holding the fort on the day, a few years later, when he came home from school in tears with a bloody nose and battle scars in the wake of an obvious dust-up. After giving him a greatly needed hug and a drink of hot cocoa, and cleaning up the blood, Nana extracted the details of his after-school encounter with three classmates – Justin, Adam, and Allan. A flurry of racial slurs had informed him that he was Indian trash, then, that his parents must be very embarrassed to have him as a son. A beating followed. It was when Justin was kicking Jamie in the head that he became enraged and fought back. After he had sailed into two of his surprised assailants, the third ran off. "Did you hit them in the snout?" asked Nana, going for a laugh. "Yes, I did," Jamie confessed between sobs and a grin. She nodded with sympathetic understanding. Then, after a reassuring pause, more nods, and a backrub, she offered a word of advice. "You did exactly the right thing! You should always try to make friends, but when bullies beat you up, you must stand up for yourself and let them have it." His anxiety that he would be punished for fighting dissolved. They sat for a long time. She held him tightly. When he returned to class next day, it seemed that word had gotten out. He was never bullied at school again.

Mother's support for each of us was ever ready. On a subsequent early-fall occasion, she and Dad were watching the home-based flock when she wakened, feeling thirsty, during the night. It had been uncomfortably warm. Going downstairs without bothering to turn on the lights, she settled on a stool against the kitchen wall to sip her water and enjoy the slight breeze from the partially open window beside her. It had been left ajar when they went to bed. To her amazement, two hands silently appeared out of the moonless night and started to slide the window open. Without a word, she stood up, placed her glass on the nearby counter, and slammed the window down with all the strength she could muster. There was a muffled groan. Neither spoke. She caught both the intruder's hands with a ferocious force, doubly effective since totally unexpected. In a moment he had vanished. They had not had even a glimpse of each other. Apart from the slight whimper, the silence had remained unbroken. When the police arrived, there was nothing much to record. Mother took it all in stride. Her only comment later was that the whole thing had seemed surreal.

Faye was keeping the ship afloat at home. A master tactician, she approached every facet of life as a problem to be solved. Was the challenge how to get from A to B? She would calculate the three or four best strategies and then weigh each option against the others – their merits and disadvantages, their costs and potential benefits, their ethical, moral, psychological, and cultural strengths and weaknesses. Tackling life this way was, at the same time, both her particular skill and her evident delight, a never-ending chess game, a jousting match with reality, an exercise in thoughtful living. Not surprisingly, her talents as a debater were legendary. We were proud of her. She was tireless.

But where were our detailed discussions about her dreams? She kept such matters to herself. Indeed, her first comment about seeking a career change had been made without discussion, as we sat on the Point at the Island. She had been drawing. She simply glanced up from the drawing and announced her decision. She would return to university and be a candidate for ordination in the United Church. It was a fait accompli. That was, as I recall, in 1973. I was surprised and proud. I mentioned my support, but that, she informed me, was irrelevant at best and had been heard as inappropriate paternalism. The rudiment of a wall between us that neither of us wanted was already apparent, but ignored, even denied. It brought to mind the moment years earlier in New York when the Medins, our Central Presbyterian friends, had observed that we continually undermined each other in feigned jesting. We were stunned; we had been unaware.

Beyond family affairs, those twenty-four PCS pilot-project months had witnessed the usual mosaic of events, from trivial to historic, some to become part of my tapestry of memories of those years: the discovery in northwest China of the life-size Terra Cotta Army, estimated to include over eight thousand warriors; Robert De Niro in *Taxi Driver*; Jack Nicholson in *One Flew Over the Cuckoo's Nest*; Jimmy Hoffa, of organized-crime fame, disappearing – permanently; spacecrafts Viking I and II landing safely on Mars and sending back the first close-up photographs; the Habs winning the Stanley Cup; recurrent reminders of transience with the news of particular deaths – Field Marshall "Monty" Montgomery, composers Leroy Anderson and Benjamin Britten, and singers Richard Tucker and Paul Robson.

But for all of that, my most indelible stock-taking moment came during a meeting with Dr Michael Strobel that fall. Michael was a statistician at the Université de Montréal. A colleague had put me in touch with him when I needed assistance in sorting out the statistical significance of some research data.

We met around the small desk in his tiny book-lined office. He presented a sober, Germanic demeanour. Serious, square-jawed, black-haired, Michael was a lover of music, that is to say, the German composers. It took him not more than three or four minutes to sort out my data issues. Then, rather than ending our encounter, we settled into a chat. He was quietly welcoming but looked distinctly sad and preoccupied.

"Michael, you look like you have something on your mind." He turned his head to peer at me, his gaze unwavering. Pulling out one of those long pads of lined yellow paper that are so beloved of statisticians, he picked up a pencil. "How much have you heard about the 'The Limits to Growth' work of the MIT scientists Donella and Dennis Meadows?"[36]

"I have not the faintest idea what you are referring to."

"Take a look at this." He quickly sketched a graph with "Time" in centuries on the "x axis," leaving the "y axis" unlabelled. "Now, let me draw you three curves."

Michael commented as he drew. The first line extended horizontally across the bottom of the graph from left to right, then suddenly sloped north. "This shows the population for the planet. It has been plotted since way back: for example, it took over 500,000 years to reach a population of 5 million in 5000 BCE; at the time of Jesus, there were only 200 million of us, worldwide." He continued the slightly sloped line as it moved to the right on the page as centuries passed. "In 1900 there were 1.6 billion. Bal, it took *half a million years* to reach 1.6 billion! That was in *1900!* But *now*, in 1970, there are *3.7 billion*, only seventy years later." The curve was now climbing steeply. I didn't need further explanation to feel my temples warm and a heaviness in the pit of my stomach. "By 2000, there will be over 6 billion! By 2011, 7 billion. By 2045, 9 billion and by 2050, 10.5 billion. In that last *five-year* span world population will increase by a number that initially it took us *500,000 years* to achieve!" Michael was pale, his face drawn, his expression intense.

"And here's another thing! We in the West won't be the ones calling the shots! You can count on that! By 2050 the population distribution will have shifted. Here are the 2050 population projections: Asia 62.0 per cent, Africa 20.8 per cent, North America 7.3 per cent, South Africa 4.8 per cent, Europe 4.6 per cent, and OceanaAustralia 0.4 per cent!"

He returned to the page in front of us, pencil poised. "Now, Bal, let's look at two more graphs, dealing with *non-renewable resources* and the *cost of food and industrial production*." The former, plotting non-renewable resources, featured a horizontal line near the top of the graph, and then, as it reached the right side of the page, the planet's non-renewable resources line plummeted southward, reflecting the disappearance of fossil fuels and other non-renewable variables. In contrast, the final graph, representing the cost of food and industrial production, became a horizontal line near the bottom of the graph, and then, toward the right side of the page, it swept north as costs soared and resources became inadequate to sustain the system. The result was an ominous crossing of the three lines toward the right side of the page. "This point of crossing, when human demand outstrips earth's resources, will occur sometime in the 21st century!"

"What happens then?" I asked.

"Catastrophe! The mix of inevitable consequences will be devastating." Michael went on to list the predicted disasters before adding: "The MIT group felt hopeful that their data would sound an international alarm bell, but so far that doesn't seem to be the case. Unless we come to our senses quickly and work together, we will be finished as a species."

We sat in silence for several minutes before I pushed back my chair. There was little to say. I mumbled my thanks for his help, got in the car, and drove home. I couldn't muster the energy to return to the Vic that afternoon.

Moving on, 1977–80

Ask not what disease the person has,
but rather what person the disease has.

William Osler

To be not the servants of science, nature, nations, personal beliefs
or even our desire to preserve life
Understanding the reality of our own mortality,
we endeavour, instead,
to heal our fellow human beings
and free them from constraint, so that they may flourish.

Pledge of the McGill
Medical Class of 2012

Dying makes a room a sanctuary and holy soil of dirty sheets.

Laurence Freeman, OSB

At the completion of the pilot project in December 1976, a forty-item questionnaire was distributed to our PCS colleagues. The covering letter from Ina as PCU clinical director stated: "The challenge now is to convert an explosive Pilot Project into a smoothly running on-going permanent hospital service. We are now entering a phase of consolidation and re-definition, as a prelude to a move in location and future growth."

At the same time, Ina, Dottie, the physicians, three head nurses (Sue Britton, Cathy Macaulay, Pierrette Lambert),[1] social worker Anne Chant, and Volunteer Director Kitty Markey prepared for an intensive two-day January retreat to review standards, policies and procedures, team functioning, staff support, data management, administrative functions, and PCS integration with other RVH services.

The river of visitors wishing to examine the minutiae of our programs continued to astonish us. Our *daily* number of two to twenty visitors on fact-finding missions had become seriously taxing for our already over-burdened team. In general, these visits varied from half a day to several days, but longer visits could last weeks or months and up to a year. We were painfully aware that each visitor came at personal hardship and cost. Each was armed with a long list of highly specific questions; each sought a personal response tailored to their needs. We offered visits that varied from a brief PCU group tour followed by a question-and-answer period to an individually tailored training program. Jocelyne Tanguay was hired as a full-time "Education Co-ordinator" for visitors and student and graduate trainees.

Many of the questions asked were similar from visitor to visitor. How did we define our patient population? How did we fit into the hospital administration? What were our problems in attempting to meet Royal Vic needs? Did a ward for the dying frighten prospective patients? What should the nurse-to-patient ratio be, and why?

As our responses evolved, they led to further clarification and in due course a document took shape that became the first detailed description of a hospital-based palliative-care program. It would continue to mature, but as the 1970s drew to a close we had a detailed snapshot of where things stood, "The Royal Victoria Hospital Palliative Care Service Answers to Most Commonly Asked Questions."[2]

Our already high regard and boundless gratitude for the generous response shown by Cicely and her St Christopher colleagues as the world came knocking on *their* door reached reverential levels. Year after year, St Christopher's acted as a gracious benefactor, without charge – truly a "hospice" in the medieval sense, a place of succour that hosts those on a quest, a resting place for travellers.

CHIP

It had been a typically busy morning as I multi-tasked my way toward the heavily booked afternoon office: two or three cystoscopies; a transurethral prostatic resection under the supervising eye of Endoscopy Head Nurse Miss Stewart, who consistently brought a mixed presence suggestive of both a circling hawk and an ever-caring mother hen; dictating case notes; discussing results with patients and family members; reviewing current clinical problems on Six West with the urology residents; noting that a family was waiting to see me on Ross V; pausing to talk with Miriam Husk about an impending order for more mice from the Jackson Laboratory. *Dear Miriam! What would I do without her?* All of this under the observant eye of Executive Secretary Joanne McPhail, who rode shotgun for K.J. and me from her desk stationed by our office doors.

Ken's door remained ajar these days, the room mostly vacant. Contact dermatitis caused by latex OR gloves had sidelined him to administrative tasks as RVH director of professional services – a great blessing for the hospital at large and for the process of initiating the Palliative Care Service, but not for his patients. Always an exemplar of the thoughtful life graciously lived, he never complained.

Joanne called through with a message: "There's a doctor on the line – didn't catch his name. He'd like to have a brief word with you. Seems insistent." I picked up the phone. "Hello, Dr Mount, *X Y* here." Like Joanne, I didn't catch his name. He went on to identify himself. "Oh, hello," I responded, rather vaguely, now fully focused on attempting to understand the reason for this call. He continued, "I believe you will be seeing a new patient this afternoon, Chip Drury. A rather special young man. I just wanted you to know that if there is anything I can do to help in any way I'd be happy to do so. *Anything!*" ... "How good of you to call. Thank you so much. I appreciate it." We hung up. *Odd. What was that all about?*

It may have been thirty or forty minutes later when a second call was put through by Joanne. Another medical colleague with essentially the same message: a special young man; an offer of assistance – "*anything* at all!" My second unknown colleague had further focused my attention. *What is this all about?* I returned to swimming upstream against the rising tide of issues needing attention before the first office patient arrived at 1:00 P.M.

It was mid-afternoon; I was finishing up my notes on the previous patient when the door opened. I glanced up. Instant understanding. *This has to be the young man in question. Now I get it!* In his late twenties, maybe thirty. He had a commanding presence and a relaxed smile as he extended his hand.

"Hello, Dr Mount, Chip Drury."

He slid into the chair across from me and handed me the empty file from Joanne with his name and basic identifiers neatly in place.

Here was one of those rare individuals who emits grace, warmth, calm, and openness while at the same time conveying a down-to-earth self-confidence that does not require bolstering by a needy ego. Here was a sense of energy, enthusiasm, and grounded joy.[3] Here was *man fully alive*, as Irenaeus might have phrased it. I noted my sense of bonding with this complete stranger. How could it not be so? I thought once again of Cicely's dictum – *Healing begets healing, begets healing, even as wounding begets wounding, begets wounding.* The essential wholeness of this young man was contagious. *Like Whit,* I thought.

The story was all too familiar: an aggressive testicular cancer; evidence of extensive spread to the abdomen; chest x-ray clear; referral for retroperitoneal lymph-node dissection and post-operative chemotherapy. I issued Chip into the examining room and he slid onto the table. No supraclavicular nodes. His abdomen, however, stopped me in my tracks, not because of apparent disease, but because of the prominent bands of clearly defined muscle across his anterior abdominal wall that caused me to blurt out without forethought, "Why don't I look like that? Are you on steroids?" He laughed.

"No, I ski." Chip was a member of the National Ski Team fraternity. He had been a good student, head boy at Montreal's Lower Canada College, and now he was heading into a career in business. He was the son of Chipman Drury and his dynamic wife, Janet, and nephew of politician Bud Drury.[4] He and his delightful, high-functioning siblings and extended family were representatives of a storied clan.

The surgery was long and challenging, the tumour extensive. Nevertheless, I was guardedly optimistic. Testicular tumours of that particular type and degree of spread were potentially curable with radical surgery and chemotherapy.

A 6 August 1977 letter of thanks from Chip and his fiancée spoke of their gratitude, our close ties, and a sense of travelling this road together as his chemotherapy continued. Chip remained fit for month after month. It appeared that the battle may have been won.

Then the tables turned. He started to lose weight; "muscular and fit" became "slim and asthenic." Further chemotherapy was not helpful. I readmitted him. His wasting was marked and deeply troubling. Visitors were limited to his fiancée and the immediate family. As the days passed, his physical magnificence morphed into a sad caricature.

Through it all he never complained. He met overwhelming weakness with persistent grace. The score card wasn't Cancer 1 / Chip 0, it was Human Spirit 10 / Cancer irrelevant. Yet, with all of that, I knew that my sense of failure would remain. He was my patient, but he had also become a friend and brother.

Chip's hospital bed was in the Ross Pavilion. I considered suggesting a transfer to the PCU but concluded that we could not improve on the care he was receiving. It was now April 1978; the end was nearing. I slipped into his room for what would be our last conversation. Chip was calm and of a philosophical turn of mind as I settled in the chair by his head. He spoke quietly but deliberately.

"You know, Bal, I need to tell you two things. The first is that I love you."

I replied, "And I you, Chip." As he spoke, I heard his words for what they were, acknowledgment of our continuing bond at the finish line. They spoke of the potential for unexpected healing in confronting death, and the possibility that both caregiver and patient may be catalysts in establishing attachment solutions to life's ultimate separation challenge, the significance of which would, in due course, be documented by Harvard neuroscientist and psychiatrist Gregory Fricchione.[5]

Chip exemplified grace. He had run the race and completed each lap with remarkable composure. Now, he was ready to hang up his cleats. He was acknowledging his total acceptance and an experience of multifaceted connectedness. I thought of T.S. Eliot's words: "We shall not cease from exploration / And the end of all our exploring / Will be to arrive where we started / And know the place for the first time."[6]

Though profoundly weak, Chip continued, "The second thing I want to say is that this last year has been the best year of my life."

I was stunned. *This last year?* This *last year, that took you from mountain top to death's door? The best year of* that *life?* I was overcome by a sense of wonderment. "The *best* year? Tell me about that Chip."

"I have had a good life. It has been a *great* life. But all my life I have been directed outward. This last year, for the first time, I have travelled inward and it has been the most exciting journey of my life." We spoke briefly and sat together in silence for a while. A day or two later, Chip married his fiancée, then he died.

Chip's funeral service at St Matthias Anglican Church, Westmount, established something of a milestone in the crowd of youthful attendees it attracted. There was respectful solemnity marked by musical grandeur and liturgical formality, with more than a hint of "old school tie."

At the completion of the service, the Drury clan lined up outside the door, spilling down the stairs onto the street, oblivious to the passing traffic that respectfully detoured past at a snail's pace. As we made our way down the stone steps and into the sunlight, each family member shook hands in gratitude for our presence. There was a touching air of subdued occasion – Chip's last hurrah, as it were.

As I arrived at Janet, Chip's mother, in the reception line, her composure and faint, slightly regal, smile were impeccable. We embraced silently, then she leaned into my ear to comment privately, with the quiet restrained air of one noting a fleck of failure on my cheek, "Bal, cancer is a terrible disease!"

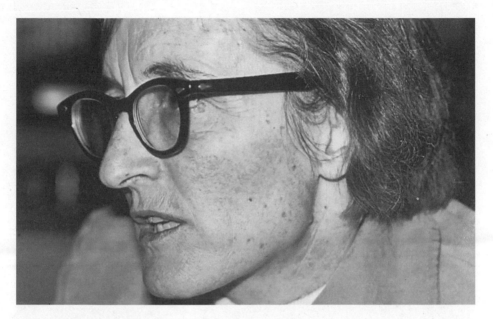

Elisabeth Kübler-Ross ("EKR"): guest lecturer at McGill.

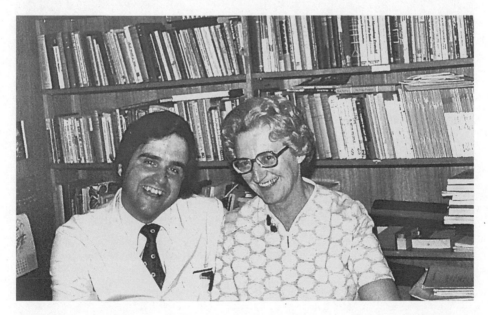

With Dr Cicely Saunders, 1974: "*Steady boy*, I said my *friends* call me Cicely" – "You may call me Cicely."

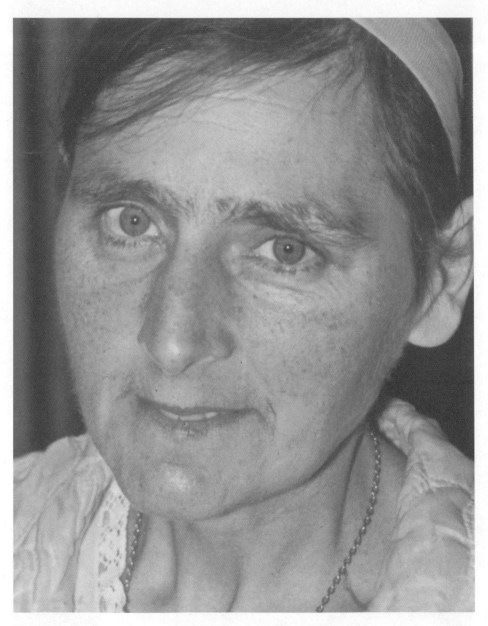

Francis Hickey: exemplar of our potential at the end of life.

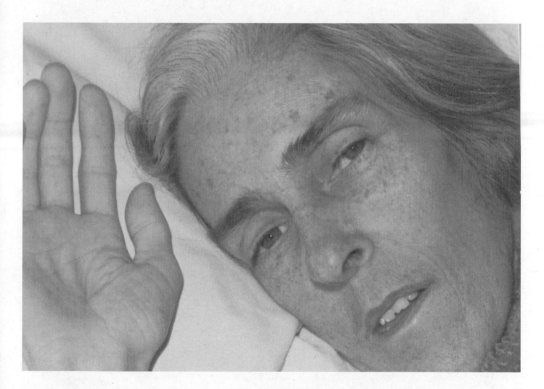

Miss Vallor: wonderment on seeing children with the Nazarene.

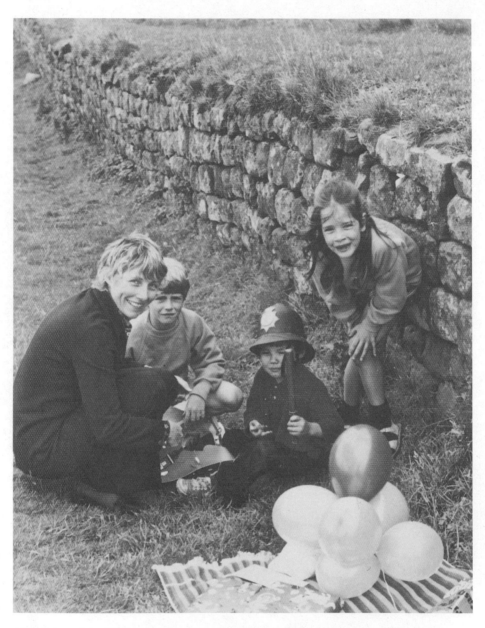

With Faye, Chris, Jamie, and Wrennie at Hadrian's Wall on Jamie's fourth birthday.

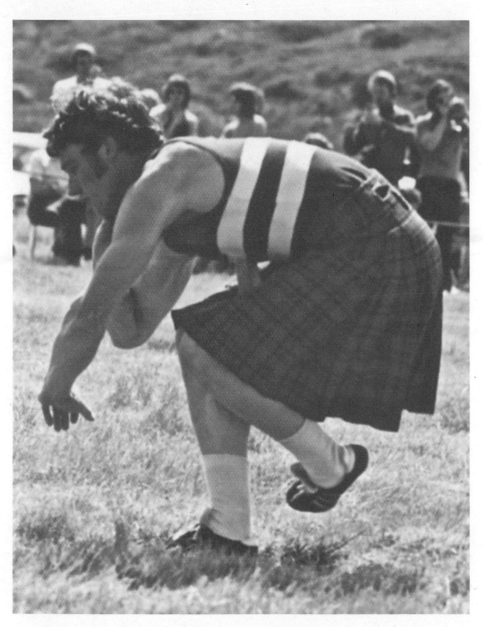

Jay Ferguson at the Mallaig and District Highland Games.

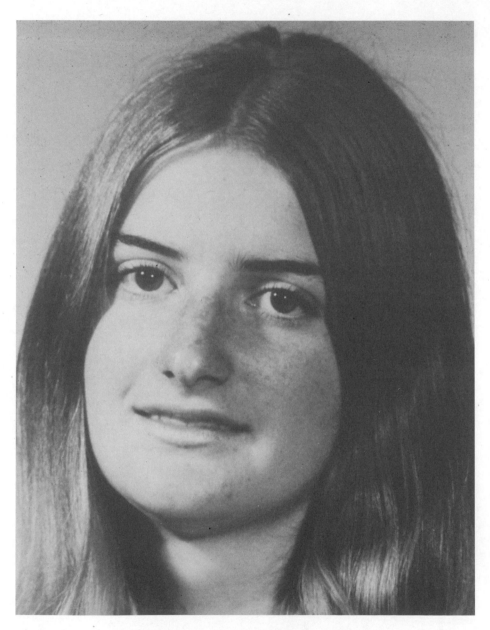

Carol: student nurse and subject of a consult request.

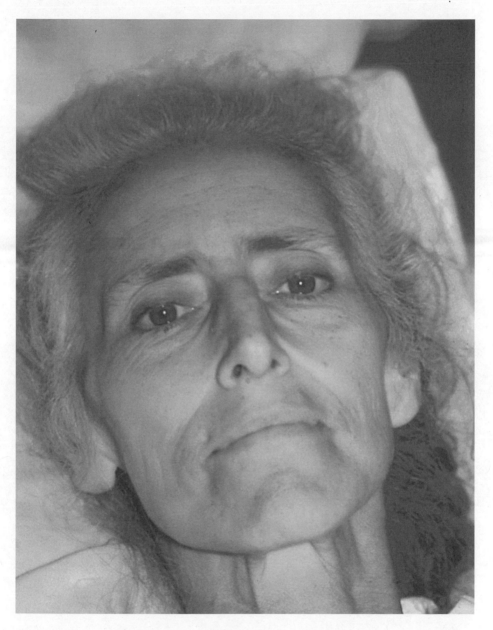

Mme Picotte: my silent teaching partner through decades of lectures.

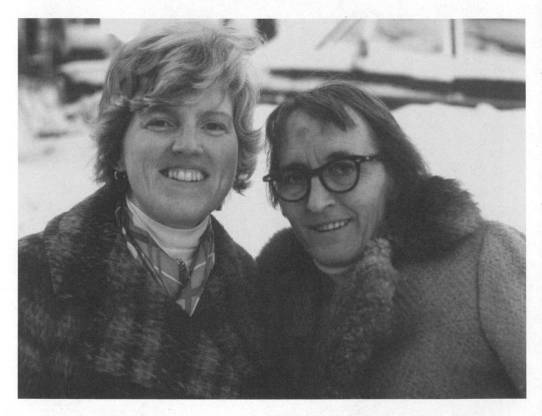

Ina Cummings Ajemian and EKR: world-class listening skills and insight personified.

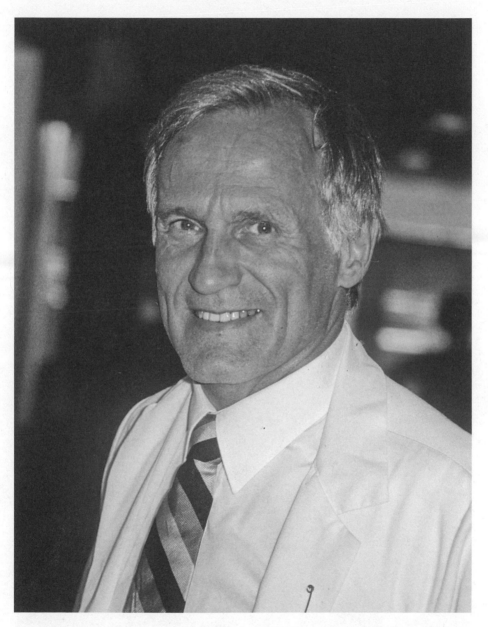

Marcel Boisvert: discerning clinician, musician, linguist, philosopher, healer.

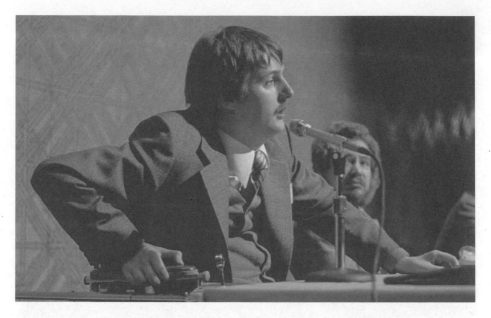

Jacques Voyer: PCS psychiatrist and man of grace in confronting adversity.

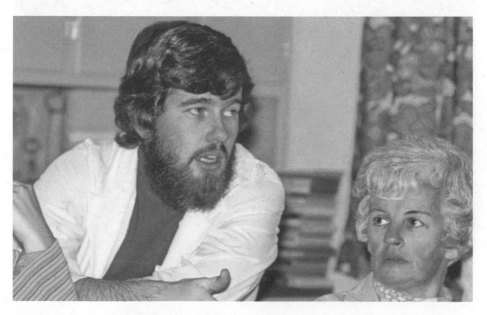

John Scott: student of the depths – medical, psychosocial, and spiritual, with Kitty Markey, pioneering director of RVH PCS volunteers.

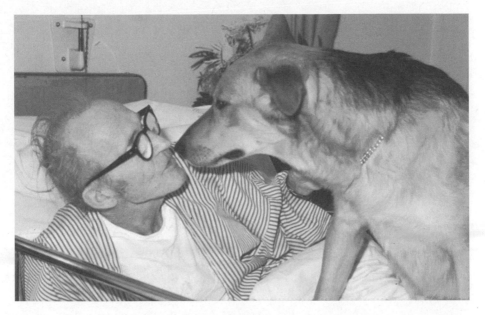

The focus of palliative care: the patient *and* family.

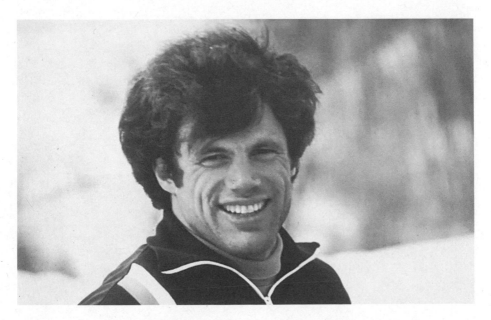

Chip: my patient, teacher, and brother.

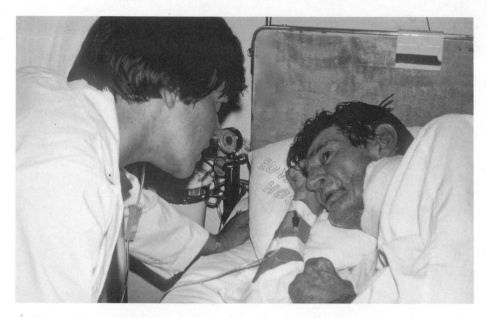

Pierrette Lambert: Consult Service nurse, diagnostician, and systems analyst.

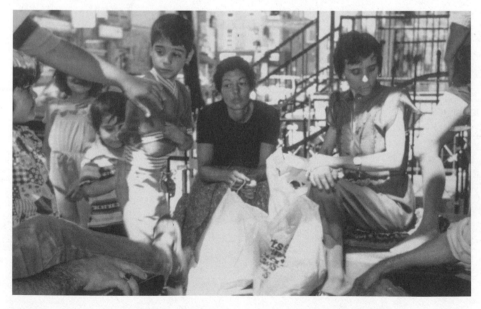

Nelleke Nieuwendijk: Home Care nurse and assessor of community-based needs.

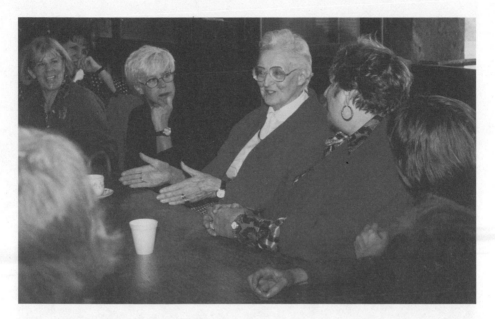

PCS team discussion with Visiting Professor Dame Cicely Saunders.

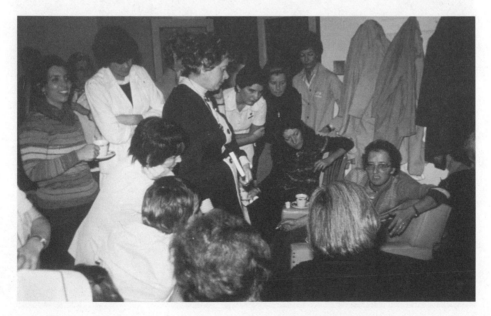

Digging deeper: examining the needs of the therapeutic triad with EKR.

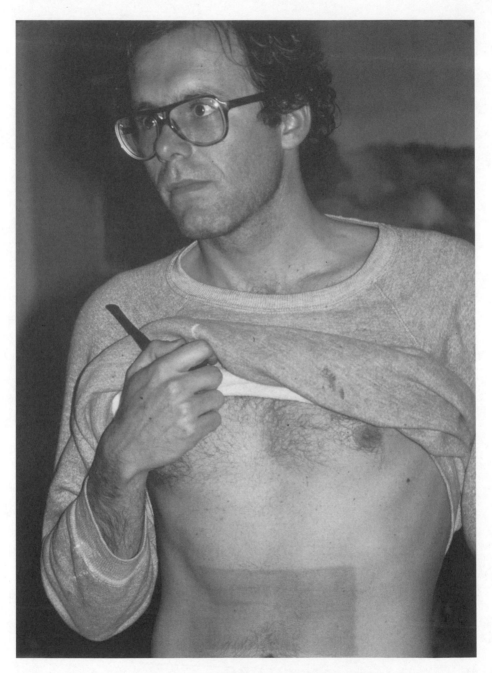

Marmalade Project: Bob Buckingham following (sun lamp) "radiation therapy."

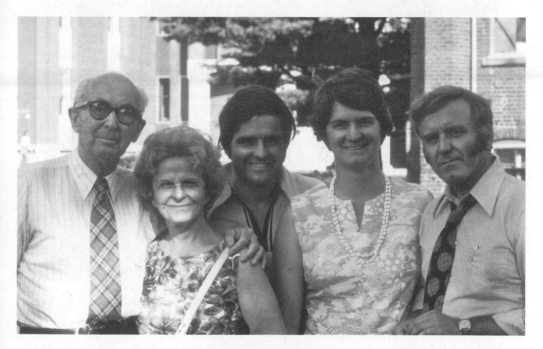

Harry and Maude, 1975, on their fiftieth wedding anniversary, with Bal, Alice, and Jim.

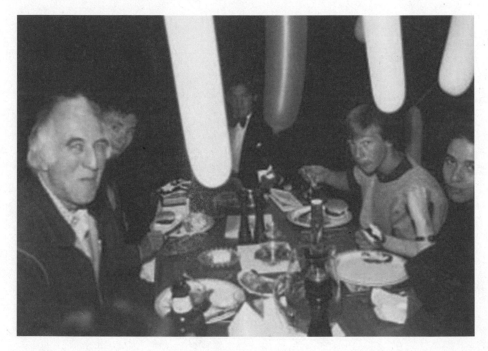

Jean Vanier, having arrived unannounced, joined Jamie (black tie) for his fourteenth birthday with friends and sister Wren.

Chip was to be a linchpin anchoring my two careers, a symbol of ultimate victory in the face of defeat, evidence of the promising potential of
the inner journey when turned to with singular focus.

Decades later, he remains my teacher, friend, and inspiration. It is
with the permission of both Chip and his parents that I identify them
as benefactors, fellow travellers from whom I have received so much,
and I have done so in numerous teaching sessions down the years.
Chip's parents, Janet and Chipman, later joined the RVH PCS Executive
Committee and Advisory Board respectively,[7] living proof that it isn't
the cards you are dealt but the way you play them that defines life's
potential.

THE WALL

The PCU was to move to Eight West in the Surgery wing. At least, that
was the idea. Simple enough! In a memo dated 4 October 1976, Ken
MacKinnon, as DPS, cheerily noted, "It is hoped that we can make the
proposed PCU move to 8 West by mid-November."

There would, of course, need to be a number of renovations and program relocations. That was to be expected. When you move a service
in an already crowded hospital, a domino effect is set in motion: move
one program into another's space and the current occupant must relo-
cate. Moreover, the new home for *that* program must be freed up by
yet another service moving, which entails ... and so on. The chess game
involved the uprooting and relocation of eight major activities.[8] It was
to be a process that would take months, not weeks.

But the critical problem was not the domino effect; the *real*
blood-pressure raiser lay elsewhere! Eight West would certainly be
more spacious and, in general, better suited to our needs, but it was
the major thoroughfare between the Medical Pavilion and three critical
Royal Vic centres of patient care – the Surgical Pavilion, the Women's
Pavilion, (*the Mat*), and "the Ross," with its medical and surgical private accommodations.

Eight West Surgical was high-traffic real estate! It was, among other
things, the route of choice for the Cardiac Arrest Team and their "crash
cart" as they careened from the Medical wards to the ward in crisis. It
was also the preferred route for staff bound for all manner of meetings,
consultations, rounds, and appointments. Taken together, there was a
never-ending stream of travellers making their way through Eight West
en route to countless destinations. It had *always* been that way! Clearly,

this particular highway could *not* be tampered with! Why, tampering with this time-honoured path could lead to war!

My assessment was sympathetic but resolute: we must identify an alternate home for the PCU. Why? Because the two foundational predictors of success in creating a home for the dying are the team and the therapeutic environment. Surroundings that foster a sense of security, peace, and quiet are imperative. The most elementary scrutiny of St Christopher's and our original Four Medical PCU home would clarify that their success was linked to having achieved a carefully crafted ambience characterized by low traffic flow, minimal noise levels, reduced lighting glare, calming decor, and a variety of similar considerations. Attention to such details was absolutely essential! It seemed self-evident. The traffic demands of Eight West meant that it could *not* be used as the PCU!

"What," I was asked by the top brass, "would be needed to ensure the success of the Eight West site?" I replied that it would necessitate erecting a full partition across the hallway connecting Eight Medical and Eight West Surgical. The planners took that notion back to the administrative powers that be and in due course I was informed that a decision had been taken. The Wall would be built! The PCU would move to Eight West!

When it was labelled by some "the Berlin Wall," I observed that "the Berlin Wall it may be, but whereas the East German original was erected to block the most needy from achieving their ends, this namesake will *assist* our most needy in meeting theirs." To a degree, necessity became the mother of invention and a repositioned crash cart nearer the other pavilions solved the medical-emergency issue. But for many colleagues, the PCU-initiated detour in their daily routine remained a chronic bone of contention. While the decision had been made by the RVH administration, some colleagues remained convinced for years to come that I had personally built the wall, hammer and nail.

As fate would have it, the mystique and archetypal significance of the Wall was enhanced by a chance occurrence on the night of its birth. To minimize the blow, it had been agreed that the barrier would be erected at the last possible moment, thus maintaining the traditional traffic flow as long as possible. The long list of Eight West renovations needed for our new PCU would be completed, and *then*, at the eleventh hour (literally), the carpenters and masons would do the dirty deed. Better yet, to avoid any possible confrontations with the irritated multitudes, the Wall would be constructed in the dead of night. And so it was.

Unfortunately, it was precisely in those midnight hours, just as the irritating impertinence was inching its way skyward, that a medical resident was called to the Ross Pavilion. Now, I am quite certain that his clambering up-and-over to make his way through the diminishing gap between the expanding wall and the ceiling was *not* caught on film, but it might just as well have been! The resident's anger and determination, not to mention the workmen's consternation, were preserved in legend within twenty-four hours.

The PCU moved from Four Medical to Eight West Surgical on 18 May 1977 but the controversy raged on for some time.

CHALLENGE, CHANGE, AND LOSS

If the Wall retained archetypal significance for Royal Vic colleagues as a symbol of challenge, change, and loss, a similar spectrum of issues had been smouldering in my personal consciousness. What were my plans for the future?

In a March 1977 letter, Dottie documented my contributions to the PCS but also the cost to the team caused by my frequent absences resulting from my surgical, research, and teaching commitments, not to mention my ever-expanding lecture tours. While I saw the lecture invitations as golden opportunities to spread the palliative-care message, the team saw them as chances to gallivant around the world while *they* soldiered on in the trenches.

The immediate post-pilot-project period was marked by restlessness and staffing changes in the PCS team, as well as in the Royal Vic administrative and oncology departments. Where would palliative care fit in a new RVH structure? What level of financial support could we count on given the Vic's large annual budget deficits?

And there was more. Had I been meeting my family obligations? Should we stay in Quebec with its Parti Québécois government and its separatist aspirations? Should I investigate further the recent out-of-province palliative-care job offers?

A May 1977 note from EKR (written, as usual, "in transit") suggested I seek input from "friends and therapists." Psychotherapy? Elisabeth and I had discussed its potential and the importance of the unconscious and personal "inner work" for those who confront death on a daily basis, noting the validity of Rochefoucauld's maxim 26, *Neither the sun nor death can be looked at with a steady gaze.* How delusional to think that we could *ever* neatly work through, package, and dispense with death anxiety! Death anxiety, we both recognized, may be banished to the unconscious by frantic ego defences, but it still lurks. Insight gained through psychotherapy under the supervision of an experienced guide, Elisabeth noted, has often been a valuable avenue of support at life's crossroads.

In a phone conversation, I admitted that I had no doubt that psycho-therapy would be informative and endlessly interesting. But not now! Another time perhaps. I could hear in her silence, on the other end of the line, a shrug and shake of the head, then a quiet Switzerdeutsch, "Yah, yah, yah ..."

The pace has been horrific. I should cut back? But, where? How? The stream of invitations to spread the word about palliative care had become a flood. Both providential and seductive, no doubt. Nevertheless, the lec-turing wasn't as simple as many supposed. In preparing for each presen-tation, I spent considerable time thinking through who would be in that particular audience. What evidence would speak most clearly to their rel-evant issues? If skeptical, where did their skepticism lie? How could it be addressed? These were the days when there was one, and *only* one, accept-able cancer-treatment goal. Cure. For example, in the spring of 1976, I was invited to give Grand Rounds at Buffalo's Roswell Park Memorial Institute. During my introduction, the director, Dr Gerald P. Murphy, took the trouble to advise the packed auditorium, "This Institute does not sup-port the views of the speaker you are about to hear!"[9]

My list of 1976–80 lectures tell the story.[10] During that interval I had also authored twenty-six publications. What was the personal price paid? Moreover, one might well ask, as many did, "When the Director, clinician, surgeon, investigator, and, oh yes, husband and father is away, what are the consequences? Who *else* has paid a price?" And I heard once again a vocal continuo add, "Who is getting all the glory and fun trips while we are left here holding the bag?"

On one particular Thursday afternoon, I was hurrying from operating room to office, a lab coat pulled on over my OR greens. There hadn't been time for lunch. The morning surgical cases had been delayed and I was now *very* late. While the office throng would undoubtedly be doing their best to be patient, their understanding would be wearing thin.

As I rushed through the surgical ward toward my office and the wait-ing masses, I passed the man in "bed 4" of the nearby room and auto-matically registered: *M.T., late fifties; radical cystectomy on Tuesday; stable; fluid and electrolyte balance OK; the boys are watching his crit; the surgery went well; haven't been to see him since the surgery; he was still in the recovery room until well into the night on Tuesday; just not possible to get in to see him yesterday, but, I have been in close contact with the residents and know his lab values; I know he's fine.*

Just then our eyes met and locked for a split-second. He looked drained. But what I *really* saw in his gaze was his need to hear *me* tell him that things were OK. He needed *me* to pat his arm, call him by name, reassure him. It was an infusion of confidence from his surgeon that he longed for. But there just wasn't time. In that fleeting moment, it occurred to me: *What a paradox! If he was on the* PCU, *I would have found a way to see him, even if only for a minute or two ... That's crazy!*

The pondering was unending: *Surgery or Palliative Care?!* Impending uncertainties loomed everywhere: Quebec health-care funding; impending Royal Vic administration changes; Ken MacKinnon's acceptance of a two-year appointment as director of the Aga Khan University Hospital in Nairobi, Kenya; my uncertain source of funding as a urologist doing palliative care (*and there was no established mechanism for me to be reimbursed as a palliative-care physician in any other Canadian province*); an uncertain political future with René Lévesque and the separatist PQ in power. (*While I admired many of their inclusive left-wing values and respected Lévesque's stance as a committed democrat, I would certainly* not *remain in Quebec if the province were to leave the Canadian confederation.*)

Such issues were fundamental to my career decision, but, at a deeper level, the essence of the two crafts – surgery and palliative care – was also central. A core consideration was the privilege palliative care offered to examine the nature of the whole person – physical, psychosocial, existential/spiritual, in sickness and in health; the determinants of suffering and quality of life; the significance of meaning and how it shapes our sense of well-being; the factors influencing our inner growth; the opportunity to take part in the development of a new field and to work with people of the calibre of Cicely, Elisabeth, Ina, John, and my other remarkable PCS colleagues, both professional and volunteer. Mythologist Joseph Campbell might have called it "following my bliss," Jungian analyst Robert Johnson, "my golden thread," others, a desire to further deepen "right-brain" function, an endeavour that had enriched my life through drawing since childhood.

In July 1977 the Vic hired Steve Herbert as director of patient diagnostic, therapeutic, and support services. My first meeting with Steve occurred as he arrived. Welcoming him aboard, I dropped off a copy of the PCS report. We hit it off. He was, at once, relaxed, pleasant, and shrewd. His questions were to the point, his competence evident. I requested a permanent salary for Dottie. He noted the uniqueness of her position and, while that intrigued him, asked me to send him her CV and a formal job description. He would see what could be done.

Two years later, Steve would become the seventh chief executive officer in the Vic's eighty-five-year history. He would be charged with reining in the hospital deficit. The result? After three traumatic years of belt tightening, he was able to report: "By March 31, 1981 we had success-fully implemented our financial recovery program, which resulted in a reduction of $5 million in expenses to operate the hospital, without reducing beds, closing services, affecting the quality of care, or placing an undue workload on any group of employees." He had pulled the rab-bit out of a hat.

Dr Sylvia Cruess had replaced Ken MacKinnon as director of profes-sional services in 1978. Sylvia was a professor of medicine, an endocri-nologist, and the previous director of the Vic's Metabolic Day Centre. Affable and direct, she quickly demonstrated her warmth, humour, and no-nonsense discernment, a combination that frequently found expres-sion in a memorable offhand bon mot. For example, there was the day I asked how best to deal with a contentious issue. She advised, "Leave her lay where Jesus flung her!" In Sylvia, I had a wise, insightful, and practical mentor. Working with her was a breath of fresh air. The ship was in good hands!

Since the PCS served the patients of all clinical departments – Medicine, Surgery, and Obstetrics/Gynacology – we were concerned that, in responding to the needs of all, we could not afford to be subject to the priorities and demands of any single program. In the end, it was decided that we would answer directly to Steve for operational matters and to Sylvia for matters pertaining to patient care. In addition, Bes, director of nursing, sanctioned the funding of our home-care nurses and consultation nurse (out of the inpatient nursing budget) in the interest of efficiency of bed utilization. We were up and running with an efficient and effective new administrative cadre. Encouraging!

MEANWHILE, HOW WERE THINGS AT HOME?

In my frequent absences Faye was yet again left having to cover the bases at home in addition to her theology studies. Chris, Wren, and Jamie each had their own constellation of needs. Each would have benefited from the full-time undivided attention of both of us. Additional issues facing us were complex, their origins multifaceted. The result was countless late-night deliberations. We sought and found willing help from many quar-ters, but few solutions, as we pursued with determination a wide variety of corrective strategies. If we failed it wouldn't be for lack of effort.

"The more she comes the worse she looks." This old rural saying sum-ming up mounting concerns regarding topics that could be as disparate as the weather or raising a young calf felt relevant. It was a prudent warning. Family stakes were high and anguish-filled, that was clear. I repeatedly thought of Cicely's comments to those under her care: "You matter because you are you, and you matter to the end of your life." The urgent relevance of those words for each member of our family of five was clear and was reflected in my daily diary notes as matters deteriorated. The wisdom of three further maxims came to mind as painful incompatibilities and challenges became achingly obvious: "admit your limitations"; "save what you can while you can"; and "rearranging furniture isn't going to do it when the house is burning down."

These home-front concerns were growing increasingly worrisome when Mother and Dad developed escalating medical problems. Dad was subjected to multiple surgical adventures for cataracts and a retinal detachment; he suffered a laceration to his scalp during a fall at the Island; his asthma attacks and weakness were becoming more marked; chronic lumbar disc disease and back pain flared. Then, on 15 March 1978, Mother was admitted briefly to the Ottawa Civic with "diverticulitis and bowel obstruction," a problem that smouldered on following her return home a few days later.

On 11 August, Dad was admitted to the hospital with encephalitis. With his status stabilizing at a profoundly compromised level of cognitive functioning, he was transferred to the geriatric ward where his touching sense of responsibility and need to be of service to others was creatively supported by the nurses who put him to work cutting up sheets of paper at a desk they had equipped with a stethoscope and set aside for his use at the nursing station. How painful to accompany this beloved pillar of neurosurgery, academic medicine, family, and community as he was reduced to such tasks. How characteristic of him to cut short our conversations with the comment, "I must get back to work." How grateful we were for the respectful, nurturing presence of those attentive nurses, and how profoundly relieved we were when, after some months, his encephalitis gradually cleared. On 13 December he returned home, now completely clear of mind and fascinated by those "several lost months!"

The viral encephalitis was gone, but mother's grumbling abdominal pains persisted. Although the diagnosis would not be clear for another two years, the leiomyosarcoma of the small bowel that would take her life had delivered its first warning shot across our collective bow.

In early 1977 a welcome support system for Faye and me unexpectedly fell into place. Judy and David Bourke were vigorous, dynamic members of their church and community. They were a couple one could always count on to pick up the slack. To the consternation of our circle, Judy had developed cancer and we, among their many friends, were devastated and anxious to help. Out of that desire came an ongoing weekly prayer group – not something that *any* of us United Church stalwarts had previously experienced – ever!

David and Judy agreed to the proposal, on the condition that our gatherings didn't focus solely on them. Instead, they must concern the well-being of all present. We met on Wednesdays at 4:00 P.M. – thus, "Prayer on Wednesday," or "POW. *Lord! How corny, if not embarrassing! Clearly this is something I'll keep to myself as questions about my early departure from the hospital on Wednesdays begin to surface!'*

Each week, a member of the group volunteered to prepare a brief prelude for our next meeting in the form of a reading, musical piece, or poem. An open conversation about our concerns of the week – personal, community, national, or global – followed, then a half-hour or so of shared, informal prayer about the issues raised. *Pray? Out loud? As a group? Horrors!* To my surprise and gratitude, a sense of comfort and atmosphere of relaxed community evolved.

We were a varied group. Men and women from twenty-seven years old to late seventies, we represented a cross-section of the congregation. Each contributed to the prayers according to personality and background – from the few occasional halting self- conscious words (the initial stance of most of us) to the eloquence of Carol, one young participant who was capable of a flowing, articulate cascade of word and thought that invariably summed up all preceding concerns. In awe, I once accused her of having the words typed on the back of her closed eyelids! The weekly attendance varied from fifteen to thirty, generally about twenty. It was on a Wednesday afternoon in August 1979, while we were at POW, that Judy died at home, cared for by the Royal Vic PCS nurses.

The group continued for another year and during that time the husband of one of our circle developed a fatal neurodegenerative disease; another member, a gentle man in his early sixties, was murdered in his apartment; and several others were supported through less dramatic, but serious, crises. We were on a path toward a deepening experience of community and the journey inward toward our existential/spiritual core.

Over that time, Faye and I rarely missed a POW meeting. We welcomed the oasis of shared peace but our personal problems were not diminishing. It was difficult to express our multifaceted challenges in words. Years later, however, the writings of analyst Robert Johnson described one of several core aspects of our dilemma: "Marriage is a sacrament in and of itself, but when we marry seeking our own gold in someone else, then at some point in the marriage each partner has to take his or her gold back. This leads to terrible disillusionment and often results in divorce. The wife says, 'You are not the knight on the white horse like I thought,' and the husband says, 'You are not the princess I married.' The gold comes clattering down, followed by accusations and incriminations."[11]

THE EIGHT WEST PCU AND THE CONCEPT OF TEAM

Settling into our new PCU in the surgical pavilion felt like arriving at the Promised Land. There was a feeling of spacious freshness and calm that was enhanced by muted colours, unobtrusive lighting, and newly installed handrails lining the clutter-free halls. We now had a lounge for patient and family activities, a room for weekly rounds and other team meetings, and more adequate accommodations for charting and for the nursing staff as well as a corner to call home for each of the various part-time team members. Moreover, the northwest end of the new ward opened onto a quiet outdoor patio that overlooked the forested slopes of Mount Royal and the stately stone facade of the Ross Pavilion. While the number of patients remained the same, there was potential for adding to the bed count should future circumstances permit.

It was a time of change. Ursula Rau was named PCU head nurse as Sue Britton moved to Home Care. Ursula, a multi-talented Swiss nurse and alpine skiing instructor, was an experienced leader who brought an easy-going, attentive, and questioning presence to all she did.

At the same time, Akos, our psychiatrist, moved to another department. At our request, prior to his departure, he compiled his observations concerning staff stress,[12] and Director of Psychiatry Maurice Dongier named Jacques Voyer as the new PCS psychiatrist. As a twenty-one-year-old Université de Laval medical student, Jacques had suffered a broken neck on diving into a friend's swimming pool. Instantly, the six-foot athlete and self-proclaimed "ladies man" was rendered quadriplegic. His battles with suicidal depression and staggering physical disability were precursors to what he later described as a sense of "shame at being a doctor in a wheelchair," but, returning to medical school, he went on to train at McGill as a psychiatrist.

Jacques managed his adapted aids for writing, eating, and activities of daily living, including a motorized wheelchair and a modified van, without complaint. He brought to our team a deep understanding of loss and a remarkable capacity to sustain a positive attitude in the face of epic moment-to-moment challenges. When asked how he was doing on any given day, he was likely to reply with a chuckle, "Not bad for a psychiatrist." He enjoyed poking holes in our imperfect pretensions to "whole-person care." "Well, Reverend Bal, how are things going today?"

His professional priorities on the PCS were first the team, then the family members of our patients, and, finally, the patients themselves. Jacques was an enabler. He developed PCS staff-support sessions, was responsible for the weekly meetings of the Bereavement Follow-Up team, and offered short-term counselling, as required, to team members as well as consultations with PCS Home Care staff and clients. His consistently sunny persona was an inspiration to all, as was his advocacy on behalf of the disabled and his autobiography, *Que Freud Me Pardonne* (Freud, forgive me), the title relating to his willingness, contrary to Freud's teaching, to discuss openly his personal experience of disability during therapeutic sessions. In addition to his PCS activities and private practice, Jacques worked at Montreal's Philippe-Pinel Institute for the criminally insane, the only institution of its kind in Canada.[13]

A formal survey of PCS teammates explored our perceived deficits in addressing the various components of whole-person care. Spiritual needs stood out. While generally supportive of the concept of whole-person care, some team members felt ill-at-ease in addressing spiritual issues as part of their job alongside bowel function and matters of family dynamics. This led us to re-examine our need for a full-time chaplain as part of our day-to-day care team – a recommendation that was sure to raise eyebrows in our McGill teaching hospital! During our initial years, Sister Brenda Halton, as a PCS volunteer, had offered pastoral care with patience, gentleness, and great effectiveness. If, however, we were to secure funding from the Faculty of Medicine for a full-time position, the candidate would require academic qualifications commensurate with that salary.

I sought an appointment with McGill Dean of Medicine Sam Freedman. As I discussed the role of chaplain in evaluating whole-person care, Sam asked for clarification of the sort of candidate I had in mind. In that context, I mentioned the Reverend Doctor Phyllis Smyth. His response was immediate. "If you can recruit Dr Smyth, I'll fund the position. She'll have to earn tenure, but I'll fund the position and give her that opportunity."

In 1979 Phyllis had resigned from Montreal's Dominion Douglas United Church to accept a position in the Faculty of Theology at the University of Winnipeg. In early 1980 we recruited her back to Montreal and McGill as an assistant professor in the Faculty of Medicine with a mandate of further developing the pastoral-care role on our multidisciplinary team. She was to be a favourite focus of discussion in our cash-strapped faculty for weeks to come: "Hey, did you hear who the dean just funded to an academic position?"

By early 1979, our need for another full-time physician was urgent. The coordinator of the Royal Vic's Community Clinic at that time was Marcel Boisvert, a skilled and thoughtful clinician who was devoted to patient well-being. I first met with Marcel in June 1979. Would he consider a palliative-care career if I arranged for him to have an introductory month at St Christopher's Hospice that August? Thus began a landmark chapter in the history of palliative care, both in Quebec and in other francophone settings in the international community.

Marcel and I were to be brothers in arms save for four issues. First, he was a card-carrying Quebec separatist. Second, he felt that the *worst* musical instrument in the world, "with rare exceptions," was the human voice. (He preferred Chopin and was himself a competent composer.) Third, he, like the majority of his Quebec countrymen, had unwavering disdain for organized religion, particularly the Catholic Church. Finally, Marcel was an ardent proponent of euthanasia. In this regard, he was given to quoting Cicely: "Dr Saunders frequently reminds us that we need to *meet patients where they are, not where we think they should be*, but all of that is empty rhetoric if your care doesn't respect their wish to have life end!" On these four topics we agreed to disagree.

Marcel and I respected each other's integrity and passion for whole-person care. Through our rich eighteen-year span as colleagues (he left the team in 1997), Marcel tolerated our differences with grace and showed endless patience with my abysmal *franglais* as he translated my thoughts into the scholarly prose that revealed his deep love of French literature. In a word, we shared a strong bond in spite of, or perhaps because of, the distances that separated us. Marcel, my enduring friend, was to be a crucial pioneer of palliative medicine in the francophone world and, on countless occasions, my teacher at the bedside.

MUSIC THERAPY: AN EXPERIMENT IN WHOLE-PERSON CARE

Given the power of music as a determinant of quality of life, its efficacy in end-of-life care under the guidance of a music therapist demanded exploration. Music had been part of the caring environment in the modern hospice movement from the opening of St Christopher's, but to date the impact of a trained music therapist remained untested.[14] Susan Munro, a 1973 music-therapy graduate of London's Guildhall School of Music and Drama, had previous experience working with severely handicapped children and psychiatric patients when I invited her to join our team.

Susan was determined and confident in her craft, but at the same time she could be light and humorous. A skilled listener, she knew when to push and when to pull. Her insight and capacity for focused presence were evident from the first. She had an innate ability to accompany suffering with gentleness while nurturing the path of a sufferer toward an increasingly secure perspective. I watched with delight as her diagnostic and therapeutic skills became a part of our inpatient and home-care programs. In time, her work contributed to growth in both end-of-life care and music therapy. She was soon asked to consult on off-service Royal Vic patients in distress. We published our early experience in the *CMAJ* in 1978 and she followed with her acclaimed book on music therapy in palliative care in 1984.[15] Our early music-therapy successes spoke clearly of the new insights we were gaining:

Anne, thirty-two years old, was admitted to the PCU in great distress six months after a hysterectomy for advanced cancer of the cervix. Her many symptoms included uncontrolled pain, shortness of breath, difficulty swallowing, urinary incontinence, constipation, swelling of her abdomen and legs, and insomnia. Her previous outgoing, dynamic personality had been overtaken by shattering episodes of anxiety during which she lay with body rigid and fists clenched in the air a little off the bed sheets, her grimaces expressing total anguish. She was aware of her prognosis and hoped she would die quickly.

Attentive titration of analgesics, laxatives, urinary-tract catheterization, frequent repositioning with regular turning and massage of her back and legs, elevation of her arms, meticulous mouth and skin care, a liquid diet, and chest physiotherapy provided symptomatic relief. The panic attacks, however, persisted, to the distress of her attentive family and our team. Susan, our music therapist, was consulted. Following an assessment interview, she assembled an audiocassette tape of musical selections aimed at inducing relaxation with their steady reassuring rhythms, low-frequency tones, soothing orchestral effects, and comforting, serene, melodies.

Anne's response was immediate and impressive. Within a few minutes her facial expression softened and her respirations deepened and slowed; her hands relaxed and lowered to rest on the bed as she fell into a deep sleep which continued uninterrupted as family and staff passed quietly in and out of her room. As the tape ended, however, Anne wakened and the profound tension and anxiety returned. An intimate, quiet conversation with Susan ensued in which Anne disclosed that she was afraid to sleep since she was not ready "to let go." This led to a natural chat about Anne's fears and the recognition that she could turn on the relaxation music when she felt the need; it was up to her. She was in control. Relaxation promptly followed each return to her music.

A week or two later, Anne was comatose. The music had worked its miracles consistently thus far. Now, Susan sat by Anne's bed and, for the first time, played soothing selections to her on the flute. While there was no visible response, on awakening the following day, Anne asked Susan to play the flute. When questioned, she could not recall having heard her play it the day before. During Anne's admission, we witnessed once more the wisdom in Cicely's concept of "Total Pain," the power of music to lead us into the full potential of the present moment and the need to treat the unconscious patient as if fully alert.

J.N., a married fifty-three-year-old accountant of central European origin with two teenage children, described himself as a perfectionist and a very private person. Throughout life he had been uncomfortable expressing feelings, preferring to let the high standards he set for himself express his values. When transferred to the PCU, nine months following diagnosis of a very aggressive base of skull cancer of the sphenoid sinus, he was weak, emaciated, had blurred vision, and was intermittently disoriented. Metastases to his cervical spine had rendered him paraplegic with weakness and pain in both arms. A pressure sore over his lower spine was painful; he had little appetite. While on occasion he raised questions about his prognosis, he generally chose to deny the gravity of his situation. He was depressed, anxious, demanding of family and staff, and had a desperate need to control his environment.

Symptom control was pursued with customary attention to detail and frequent review; special effort was given to including J.N. in decisions regarding his daily-care routines which were scheduled according to his wishes. Family counselling focused on the many needs of his wife and children. Carefully planned supportive interactions with J.N. and his family were held over many weeks; they included nurses, physicians, psychiatrist, chaplain, social worker, and volunteers.

The music therapist came to play a key role in our attempts to meet the needs of J.N. and his family. He had, we soon discovered, a strong baritone voice and loved to sing. His carefully constructed intellectualization quickly fell away when he sang his favourite songs. Tears flowed easily as he listened to Stephen Foster's lyrics, "I hear the gentle voices calling, old black Joe." His choice and interpretation of songs revealed a very sensitive man struggling for understanding and acceptance. He deeply appreciated these sessions of musical sharing. Music had been an important part of his life. Now, it became a treasured vehicle for expressing his search for meaning during his final weeks. It also proved to be

effective in relieving his pain. When he sustained a pathologic fracture
of his right arm, his love of music became a welcome distraction during
painful repositioning: muscle spasms decreased and his level of coop-
eration grew as the music dissolved his "Total Pain." Nursing time for
each physical-care procedure decreased and the support of, and bonding
with, staff increased. At the same time, the use of liturgical music helped
the whole family express the strong religious faith that supported them.
Finally, as the end of his courageous journey drew near, he planned and
prepared, with gentle encouragement and assistance from Susan, a tape
of his favourite songs with the dedication, "For my wife on our last
anniversary."

Mme Levkova, an eighty-four-year-old Russian-born matriarch who
spoke few words in French and no English, was admitted to the PCU
three months after refusing all investigations and treatment for an
advanced abdominal cancer thought to be of pancreatic origin. A lessening of her symptomatic distress was achieved with rigorous medical
management but marked anti-social behaviour and refusal of all hospital food persisted. The latter problem was solved by implementing an
ongoing diet of baked or boiled potatoes and black bread brought in
by the family, but her turbulent social interactions continued. A nursing
progress note written following the music-therapy evaluation interview
noted: "She seems to be extremely difficult to handle; language barrier;
hostility; paranoia; apparent confusion; positive interaction with her
almost impossible."

Susan sought out a recording by a Russian choir that came with lyrics
in English and Russian on the cover. She later reported: "As the first
strains of the initial chorus swelled to fill the room the patient's facial
expression changed to an alert, proud look and she seemed to grow in
stature. With dignity and secure intonation she read the Russian text
aloud, her diction perfect. A pause followed, then the patient, in adequate French, told the story of her childhood as a member of an aristocratic Russian family, where music, dance, literature and art were of
great importance. She went on to speak of her bitterness at the loss of
prestige, homeland, beauty and eventually health. In the ensuing days
music became the bridge to otherwise impossible communication."

The striking impact of end-of-life music therapy, as pioneered by Susan,
gave way to years of equally impressive results under the leadership of
other trained music therapists, including the multi-talented Deborah
Salmon, who would become the longest-serving caregiver during the first
four decades of the McGill palliative-care programs.

PERSONNEL SELECTION: SCIENCE OR ART?

It was Dottie's husband, my cousin Dave Wilson, who suggested it.

"Bal, would you like some advice?"

"Sure, Dave."

"The most important lesson I had in setting up my business is that 'team' means as much, if not more, than 'product'! Everything depends on the people working with you. Without a good team you're dead in the water. Taking a course in personnel hiring was critical to our success."

The practices followed in hiring health-care professionals had always seemed notoriously ad hoc in my experience, whether in medical school, residency, or, more recently, during my clinical practice, research, and teaching years. Indeed, we had made important mistakes in PCS team selection early on. It seemed clear that we might benefit by incorporating the tested hiring practices used in the business world. One thing led to another and, before I knew it, Dottie, Ina and I were winging our way to Chicago for a two-day course on "Techniques in Personnel Selection."

The curriculum was an eye-opener. We examined issues that, in retrospect, seemed self-evident: basic principles; writing the job description; recruitment ("Recruit! Recruit! Recruit!"); screening applicants; the patterned interview; getting the facts without wasting time; interpreting the results. Fabulous! We were about to fly home experiencing a definite sense of superiority! Why did no one in health-care hiring know all this?

The course ended with an IQ test which we registrants could choose to take as an optional learning experience, though it was not a legal hiring criterion in most states. Dottie ranked in the 94th percentile, Ina in the 98th, and I, as I recall, fell in somewhere around the 65th percentile. Ah well ...

After diligently applying our new skills for a year or so, I asked Ina whether she thought our personnel-hiring batting average had improved compared to the early days when we simply relied on happenstance and prayer. We agreed that it probably *hadn't*, but that we now understood more clearly where we had gone wrong!

AN EXPERIMENT IN ORGANIZATIONAL DEVELOPMENT

As the pioneering spirit of the pilot-project years and the excitement around our newly accomplished goals waned during 1977 and 1978, so did staff morale. While motivation and concern for our patients remained high, tensions within the team escalated to worrisome levels. Meetings aimed at enhancing staff support resulted in awkward silence or heated comments. There was an absence of trust. The intensity of frustration was illustrated by an outburst from V.J., a nurse generally considered a team leader and enthusiast, when she exclaimed, "We're up to our shoulders in shit and others get all the goodies." While we could identify role-related problems, we knew that other issues lay beyond our capacity for self-analysis. We needed outside help.

The services of organizational-development consultant John Little were sought, resulting in the decision that we would hold a full team retreat under his leadership. We were informed that a five-day event was the norm for situations similar to ours. That was out of the question financially. After much discussion we settled on a one-day "off-campus" seminar. Would it be worth it? Though John Little was clearly experienced and skilled, could an outsider shed light on our problems when we had failed to do so? Could our problems be corrected? Finances were tight. Would it all be worthwhile?

Preparations for what became known as the "Advance Retreat" were many: five of our senior nurses met with the consultant on two occasions; a large meeting hall and five smaller group discussion rooms were donated for the retreat by a local church; John graciously agreed to waive his customary fee; nursing-roster adjustments were made for the day of the meeting as well as the night shifts prior and following, and modifications in reimbursement and off-duty days were arranged so that all nurses could participate without financial penalty; the $1,146 cost for nursing coverage and materials was covered by PCS donated funds.

Symbolic of the ambient anxiety levels, the five selected PCS nursing leaders all resigned from their seminar-leadership roles twenty-four hours prior to the retreat so as to free up their participation *as equals* in the proceedings; and five new "non-PCS" group leaders were hurriedly recruited (two senior PCS volunteers, the new bereavement-program coordinator, and two knowledgeable "outsiders") and given a last-minute briefing.

Approximately seventy nursing staff, volunteers, physicians, and administrative staff, as well as the psychiatrist, chaplain, music therapist, education coordinator, and physiotherapist, attended the retreat. The schedule for the day alternated between full-team meetings in the large hall and break-out sessions in the group-discussion rooms. As the day proceeded, each breakout session worked on the material generated by the preceding meeting.

On arrival, participants were allocated to one of the five discussion groups, with care taken to maintain a multidisciplinary composition in each group. In addition, each was asked to contribute anonymously to a large sheet entitled "Je me souviens" (I remember) that hung on the wall of the main meeting room. The names they added through the morning helped to charge the event with meaning. Many were the names of patients, some from the earliest days of the service. They were those who had been most difficult, most loved, or most identified with. A sprinkling of names of teammates was included. Memories flooded the mind and intensified the commitment to the task at hand.

In my opening comments, I reviewed our accomplishments in the three and a half years of operation (555 patient/family PCU admissions; 400 families in Home Care; more than 1,000 consults; bereavement follow-up for a large portion of the families cared for; our research and teaching programs), and I stressed the importance of the retreat for our continuing productivity. Finally, I asked that three premises be accepted by all present: 1) our shared strong motivation to see the service goals achieved; 2) that comments aired during the retreat not be taken as personal criticism; 3) that we each believe that we can be successful in moving forward.

John Little then took over with an interactive session in which he requested and tabulated the perceptions of all in attendance regarding: our present circumstances, how it currently felt to be a team member, and where we were headed. Individual contributions were called out spontaneously, each in turn seeming to enable enhanced candidness from those that followed. The psychiatrist later commented that the unstated question of this opening session was, "Can we dump on the director without him getting angry?" John appeared to be capable, relaxed, and affirming. The director was now on equal footing with all others. I was fair game!

John then challenged us, "If the PCS is to survive, evolve, grow, flourish, and achieve its purpose, what are the things that must be done in the next two years?" The responses were pooled, compared, clustered, and refined into five problem areas: need for improved administration; clarification of roles; improved in-service education; expansion of services; improved management of resources. Each of the five discussion groups was assigned one of these problems to work on during the breakout session that followed. Then it was back to the general assembly to report on the outcomes. And so it went all day. Back and forth.

As the day came to a close, a widespread fear found expression. "Will anything be followed up on? Will this have been a waste of time?"

When asked to give a name to the day there was general agreement: "The Advance Retreat!" As the day ended, there was a general sense of exhaustion and uncertainty, but there was also gratitude and satisfaction and someone in our midst commented, "I am thankful for a team like you."

Supper for the group had been arranged, but fatigue ruled and the hall emptied within minutes. That evening, however, many team members felt an acute need for a "debriefing" and fifteen to twenty gathered at the home of Volunteer Director Kitty Markey. What ensued was a frank, often angry exchange between colleagues too tired and frustrated to be anything but blunt. Yet another reassessment of the service problems took place. At this informal meeting some of the most profound insights regarding our deficiencies surfaced and the seeds for the total restructuring of the PCS were sown.

Twenty-three deficiencies and fifty-one specific recommendations were tabled. Within two months, forty-eight of the stated recommendations were accomplished, embarked on, or decided against. Follow-up reports documenting progress were issued to all team members at the one- and two-month marks following the retreat. There was agreement that the most significant results of the Advance Retreat were: 1) a marked increase in morale and sense of trust between team members; 2) a greater understanding of the perceptions and stressors of colleagues; 3) an important clarification of decision-making process, goals, and priorities; 4) an immediate decrease in staff frustration and distress; 5) more open and consistent communications on the team; 6) a total restructuring of administrative policies; 7) greater confidence in leadership; 8) improved efficiency in all arms of the service; 9) a decision to revise educational programs; 10) an enhanced appreciation of the significance of organizational issues and the potential of organizational-development consultants; 11) a new lease on life and a recommitment to shared goals.[16]

THE LAST DAYS OF LIVING

A late-afternoon phone call from the National Film Board (NFB) of Canada informed me that the board was calling on behalf of colleagues in Sweden who wished to make a film about the Royal Vic PCS. Realizing that we would be unlikely to agree to this "out of the blue" request from strangers, the Swedish filmmakers hoped that the NFB would act as intermediaries by establishing preliminary contact on their behalf. The Swedish enquiry was referred to senior NFB Producer Tom Daly. He was mystified. Care of the dying? Why in the world were the Swedes coming to Montreal to make such a film?

The NFB did its homework and in short order I found myself speaking to Daly. He confided that he felt caught in an ethical dilemma since, while he could recommend his Swedish colleagues as competent professionals, on reviewing the PCS history he felt that the NFB might also be interested in the project the Swedes had outlined.

As a long-standing NFB fan, my response was immediate. If a film was to be made, the NFB would have to be involved. It would be the NFB's decision whether the Swedish and Canadian teams could collaborate.

Following further transatlantic phone calls, there was agreement that a face-to-face meeting involving both companies was required. A film crew of six from Stockholm made the trip to Montreal for a day-long meeting with NFB representatives to determine if a satisfactory plan could be developed. As their closed-door discussion wore on, the emotional investment each had made became increasingly evident. A detached exchange of ideas morphed into earnest negotiations that ended with the conclusion that it would have to be either one or the other team; it couldn't be a forced marriage! Daly summed it up for me. "It would be like trying to ride a two-headed camel. It will have to be them or us." The Swedish team had been aware of the risk. I went with the NFB. We parted as good friends.

Tom Daly was sixty, tall, lean, and soft-spoken, a man who appeared to be comfortable with himself and the world around him. His greying hair framed an open, ever-thoughtful, expression. One sensed that nothing escaped his attentive gaze. Informal and quietly welcoming, he wore slacks and a checkered short-sleeved shirt, its pocket bulging. Ina and I joined him for an introductory chat.

Tom, for that is what everyone called him, had been recruited to the NFB by pioneer filmmakers John Grierson and Stuart Legg in 1940. During the 1950s and 1960s, he was the head of the board's Studio B, and by the time we sat down together to examine our options, he had 285 films to his credit and was widely respected for his legendary skills as a director, producer, and editor. He was a master craftsman! To work with Tom was to recognize a committed student of the inner life and the human quest for enhanced consciousness through heightened awareness and discipline.[17]

Tom's plan for "our" film revealed the careful stewardship for which he was renowned. As we talked, Tom introduced Ina and me to Malca Gillson, who would be responsible for the research, direction, and editing of our film. In preparation, Malca would train as a palliative-care volunteer and then work on the PCU on a daily basis for about six weeks in order to gain familiarity with the ebb and flow of patients, family members, and caregivers.[18] Four weeks of filming would follow, with the camera mounted on a mobile dolly for ease of rapid, unobtrusive positioning in response to a beckoning glance from Malca. All PCU rooms would be pre-lit; each power source could be switched on at a moment's notice. On PCU admission, patients and families would be asked if they agreed to be filmed. There were few if any refusals as a result of their uniform wish to "give back" and be of assistance to others.

Wise, observant, and opinionated, Malca had a warm, dynamic, larger-than-life persona which she usually kept carefully reined in. While she could be outspoken – particularly when jousting with me – she was generous, gentle, and deeply caring with the patients, their families, and her palliative-care colleagues. Malca instantly became my friend and, as she defiantly proclaimed, my "Jewish mother." She was a delight, a creative presence and an insightful catalyst.

Tom's plan proved to be inspired. The film would not highlight a selected group of people chosen for their unusual fortitude, but simply present those who happened to be on the PCU during the weeks of filming. It would soon suggest how consistently people demonstrate courage and grace in facing death. Camera, enhanced lighting, and microphones were quickly forgotten as the film crew became a transparent part of the caring PCU environment. The most nuanced moments in these last days of living would be recorded without resorting to contrived scenarios which could only complicate an already sensitive situation.

"That sounds perfect," I responded, "but there is one thing I must request." I proceeded to tell Tom and Malca about the disturbing CBC television program filmed early in the PCS pilot project, with its dubbed-in, anxiety-producing heartbeat continuo. We couldn't afford to be burned like that again. "The only way I can agree to this is if I have the right to final say regarding inclusion, should I feel that a particular scene is inappropriate." There was silence. Malca didn't move but seemed to have a new-found interest in inspecting her shoes. Tom was silent, his gaze steady. I couldn't read his reaction.

"Well, I'm afraid that is completely against Film Board policy," he commented softly but firmly. "We couldn't make films if we agreed to such a significant loss of control of the creative process." He paused for what seemed an eternity. "*But*, I'll tell you what I *will* agree to in this case. I will accept your condition if *you* agree to be present, at my request, for the critical decisions in the editing process."

"Agreed," I responded confidently, having absolutely no idea what I was committing myself to but thrilled at the idea of seeing these master artists at work. Only later did I wonder if I had detected a slight smile on Tom's face.

The month of filming during the summer of 1978 went smoothly. Throughout, Malca was a warm off-screen presence and compassionate force enabling and supporting many of the most memorable moments. The resulting uncut footage amounted to twenty-five hours of film. "Malca and I will edit it down to a more manageable size, Bal, then you can join us at the Steenbeck," Tom offered casually, referring to film-editing machines at the NFB.

On the appointed day, Ina and I found ourselves on a steep learning curve. Arriving at the NFB filled with a sense of interest and excitement, we were informed that the "more manageable size" consisted of fourteen hours of film!

For those not familiar with the Steenbeck, I ask you to imagine a dark, kitchen-cupboard-sized cubicle in the bowels of the NFB with four wooden chairs more or less fused together in front of a minute table crowded with innumerable spools and reels of film, the whole whirring jumble of equipment surmounted by a compact screen which demanded sustained squinting to maintain a critical eye.

Tom welcomed us with a smile as the lights dimmed and we sardined ourselves into the chairs. He was armed with pen and paper. This was to be a time for note taking, not film editing. As the minutes passed, Tom intermittently offered fleeting comments and at the completion of one particularly touching sequence he mumbled, "Nice, but obviously we can't use it."

"Can't use it?!" I exclaimed in disbelief, already stiff and sore. "Why? It's perfect!!"

In quiet, professorial tones, Tom launched into a detailed analysis of the possible misinterpretations a viewer might have based on that scene. As *he* saw it, the patient and family members would be left vulnerable. *I* thought he was crazy!

That was the first of many such interactions. Humbling stuff! I soon realized that I was in the presence of an unusually perceptive and dis-cerning observer. Time and again his comments revealed a grasp of the intricacies of palliative care and the human psyche that left me in awe. His nuanced observations were astounding. I had gained yet another teacher.

When we were four or five hours into the session, I finally asked Tom to pause, confessed that from here on all judgments were in his hands, thanked him for his patience, and expressed my gratitude for the remark-able masterclass in depth psychology that Ina and I were being treated to. Tom Daly was ... well ... it is hard to put in words but unique, gra-cious, razor sharp, humble, and genius come to mind as apt descriptors.

We then completed our fourteen-hour marathon.

Weeks later, when we sat down for our next Steenbeck session, Tom and Malca had edited the footage down to four and a half hours. Roughly two hours into the screening, I interjected, "Tom, this last sequence is extraordinary! It is infinitely more impressive than when we last saw it. Totally different! Really amazing!"

"Mmmm," muttered Tom. "What do you think we did to it?"

I couldn't be sure but the content and its impact had changed completely. Could they have located footage that we hadn't seen on the first viewing? It was fresher, clearer, had more punch and focus – it was now really quite moving! What had been somewhat lacklustre now sparkled with meaning. "I can't be sure, but you must have done something major. It's *much* stronger!"

He was silent but clearly pleased with himself. "I didn't touch it," he announced with a slight smile. "I edited the segments just before and after it, but I didn't touch the scene itself. It's the *context* that has changed!" I was stunned.

Tom's biographer, D.B. Jones, observed that *The Last Days of Living* "engaged Tom completely," adding, "for a man who saw film as an extension of life rather than an end in itself, offering his total commitment to a project (this late in his career) was getting harder to do, but he had found that level of heightened focus in working on *Last Days*." Jones went on to note that one of the happiest experiences in Daly's career occurred when the NFB held a private (Ina and I were not included) screening of the film for the families of the deceased who appeared in it.

Tom later reflected: "Here they were, all these different families who practically never knew each other but now were meeting together in this common purpose of looking at the film ... The whole evening, for everybody, was a celebration. The families stayed, practically to a person, for three hours, relating to each other and telling their own stories to each other and to us. You could tell that the film was just exactly the honest expression of what they had felt when those events had happened. There wasn't a single example of anybody feeling that it wasn't just the way they had known it. And I was very happy about that. It showed that we weren't over-dramatizing the material."[19]

The final product was breathtaking. Moments of awkward uncertainty were not glossed over; no rose-tinted glasses here. It documented the rich range of potential awaiting us in our last days of living – from anguish to peace, grief to celebration, isolation to reconciliation and depth of community, bumbling clumsiness to awakened grace on the part of all involved – patients, their loved ones, and our team. Dame Cicely called it "the best hospice film I have seen," Colin Murray Parkes, "the best film of its kind to have been produced."[20]

NURTURING INTERNATIONAL INTEREST

According to the biennial timing arranged with Cicely, McGill's Second International Seminar on Care of the Terminally Ill was looming before we knew it. It would be held at Montreal's Queen Elizabeth Hotel on 2–4 November 1978. In my 9 November 1977 letter inviting Cicely to give the opening plenary, I scrawled a hasty P.S.: "I have just made the final decision to discontinue urologic oncology and turn my full attention to the PCS. I am certain it is what I'm meant to do."

Cicely responded: "Many thanks for your letter and the good news that you are now fully involved in the PCS. I am sure this is right. I would be very happy to come to the Second International Seminar and to start proceedings off with *Caring for the Dying*. I would like to stay to the end and have booked off a full week in my diary."

Once again registrants would be seated at tables for ten with a discussion coordinator at each table; each session would include formal presentations, small-group discussions at the tables, and open discussions from the floor. English-French simultaneous translation was planned for all presentations and floor discussions. I was delighted with the program as it took shape.[21]

But I was ill at ease! By the summer of 1978, two other meetings scheduled for that fall would threaten our ability to attract American registrants: a "Forum for Death Education" conference, and, on 5–6 October, the "First Annual Meeting" of the newly formed National Hospice Organization (NHO) and the Fifth National Hospice Symposium, the latter presumptuously titled "The Coming of Age of the Hospice Movement in North America." Both the forum and the NHO meetings were to be held in Washington.

Fired by McGill Seminar paternal anxiety, I thought it grossly inappropriate to term the *birth* of a health-care endeavour as a "coming of age" event, but it was clear that the NHO had attracted a stellar faculty of forty-nine, including such luminaries as Dame Cicely, Senator Robert Dole, Secretary of Health, Education and Welfare Joseph Califano, and, as opening speaker, Senator Edward Kennedy. (Attendance at the NHO meeting was later estimated at "more than 1200.") I was invited to participate on a panel addressing "Starting a Hospice in a State Hospital."

Cicely was seated front-row-centre during the opening session of the NHO meeting, and thus, as a devout Kennedy-phile, I was more than a little concerned as Ted Kennedy strode to the podium with an air of easy confidence to address the topic "Hospice Care." *Given Cicely's presence, what were the program planners thinking? What in God's green earth can he possibly say? This will be embarrassing at best!*

I needn't have worried. At forty-eight, the senator was still youthful in appearance (JFK had died at forty-six, Bobby at forty-three). He was taller than I had expected.

Surveying the audience, Kennedy paused thoughtfully and then, in that unforgettable Boston, New England, brogue, he remarked, with relaxed self-assuredness: "I ... ah ... I am ... ah ... reminded ... of the man who survived the Johnstown Flood!" He was off and running! "In 1889 there was a terrible flood in Johnstown, Pennsylvania. Everyone drowned except for one man and ... ah ... he spent the rest of his life telling everyone who would listen how he had survived the Johnstown flood.

"Then ... ah ... one day, he died ... And he went to heaven where he met Saint Peetah. And Saint Peetah said, 'My good man, what can I do for you?'

"And the man answered, 'I would like you to assemble all the angels and archangels so that I can tell them how I survived the Johnstown flood.'

"Saint Peetah thought for a moment, then answered, 'Very well, it ... ah ... shall be done! But I think I should remind you that in your audience, there will be Noah.'

"Well" continued Kennedy as the uproar settled, "I feel like the man who survived the Johnstown flood!"

The room became blurred. Suddenly, here was all that fondly remembered Kennedy wit and grace; the Kennedy love of oratory and ability to seize the moment; the Kennedy knack in taking a simple idea, polishing it to brilliance, then hitting you between the eyes with it! Totally unexpected. I was deeply moved. Memories of Jack and Bobby flooded the room as it drifted into slow motion. Grief from the depths mixed with a joyful sense of continuity sustained made me swallow hard and look away. Senator Kennedy then proceeded to talk about the need for hospice care in the United States.

The first annual NHO meeting was rich in content, with speakers challenging current norms, planting new concepts, and urging evaluation. Some spoke from experience, some, not so much, but if American Hospice hadn't quite "come of age," it certainly had shown that it had at its disposal a formidable array of talented advocates who would soon foster exciting growth and innovation. All in all, there was a distinct sense that the United States was on the move!

Our Second International Seminar one month later was also a great success. My anxieties notwithstanding, the planned thirty tables for ten were filled to capacity and further registrants were allocated to an adjacent hall equipped with closed-circuit TV. The total registration was Canada 466, United States 256, other 10: Total 732. Table discussions were lively, the formal presentations outstanding, and the discussions from the floor animated.

THE THIRD INTERNATIONAL SEMINAR AND THE RESEARCH METHODOLOGIES IN TERMINAL CARE CONFERENCE, 5–8 OCTOBER 1980

Since my early visits to St Christopher's, Viktor Frankl's insights had frequently come to mind when sitting at the bedside of patients; they were a touchstone reminding me of our potential for transcendence in times of crisis. They had resonated for me as Chip spoke of his journey inward in April 1978, and on countless other occasions.

Frankl's wisdom had been hard-won, germinated as it was in the toughest of schools, Nazi concentration camps.[22] If valid in such a setting, could the human spirit be less relevant for my patients, for me? Frankl had observed, "In spite of all the enforced physical and mental primitiveness of the life in a concentration camp, it was possible for spiritual life to deepen ... to retreat from terrible surroundings to a life of inner riches and spiritual freedom."[23] His epiphany had occurred one frigid morning in early 1945 when he and his fellow concentration-camp inmates were being marched, under threat of whip and rifle butt, to their work site. It was to be a morning that would shape his understanding of quality-of-life determinants, his work as a psychiatrist, and the thinking of his countless students over subsequent decades.[24]

During the pre-dawn hours of that day, Frankl and his fellow prisoners stumbled against icy winds, over boulders, and through puddles, completely silent in the face of weakness and the threatening Nazi guards. Suddenly, the man beside him whispered, "If our wives could see us now! I do hope they are better off in their camps and don't know what is happening to us." No further words were exchanged, but both men knew that each was thinking of his wife. Frankl recalls, "My mind clung to my wife's image, imagining it with an uncanny acuteness. I heard her answering me, saw her smile, her frank and encouraging look. Real or not, her look was then more luminous than the sun which was beginning to rise." The concentration camp was forgotten as his mind filled with thoughts of his wife. It was transformational and he recognized its significance. "Love is the ultimate and the highest goal to which man can aspire. The salvation of man is through love and in love ... For the first time in my life I was able to understand the meaning of the words, 'The angels are lost in perpetual contemplation of an infinite glory.'... A thought crossed my mind: I didn't even know if [my wife] was still alive. I knew only one thing – love goes very far beyond the physical person of the beloved. It finds its deepest meaning in his spiritual being, his inner self. Whether or not he is actually present, whether or not he is still alive at all, ceases somehow to be of importance." Moreover, the compassion and generosity of fellow prisoners had convinced him that we *do* have freedom, even in the direst of circumstances. He had seen too many instances of kindness and grace in the camps to think otherwise, moments of what he interpreted as "spiritual freedom" in facing the horrific conditions engulfing them. All this considered, he resolutely concluded that "everything can be taken from a man but one thing: the last of human freedoms – to choose one's attitude in any given set of circumstances, to choose one's own way."[25]

I picked up the phone. It was 5 June 1979. Professor Frankl was not difficult to locate in Vienna. A woman answered. Yes, Dr Frankl was in and would take my call.

Yes, he would be pleased to participate in McGill's Third International Seminar on Care of the Terminally Ill on 5–8 October 1980. During our rambling chat, he repeated his oft-quoted aphorism, "What is to give light must endure burning." In my follow-up letter I expressed my "profound pleasure and gratitude" that he would be with us and explained that we planned to have him address the seminar on the final day "so as to leave the participants focusing on the meaning of their work both for their patients and themselves." I then closed, wishing him "not only the light but its warmth." Dr Frankl would be a very alert seventy-five years young on arriving in Montreal.

A flurry of pre-conference telephone calls and letters kept the Vienna-Montreal communications open and his concerns pacified over the ensuing months. My last letter, written on 3 September 1980, ended with the P.S.: "Please forgive the haste of this letter [due to] word of my mother's impending death. I must go to Ottawa to be at her bedside."

Meanwhile, the programs for an early October Research Methodologies Seminar and the Third International Seminar were confirmed[26] as, in due course, were the registrants: Canada 456, United States 399, Other (Australia, Austria, Bermuda, England, France, Holland, Hong Kong, New Zealand, Norway, South Africa, Sweden, Switzerland) 43: Total 898. Late arrivals brought the final total to 1,100.

VIKTOR FRANKL AT MCGILL

On Saturday, 4 October, at 3:45 p.m., I scooped up a weary Dr Frankl at the Montreal airport. It was now well past the Vienna witching hour though still mid-afternoon in Montreal. Thrilled to have the great man with us, we had planned a light welcoming meal at our home, inviting psychologist Ron Melzack, his wife, Lucy, and philosopher Christine Allen to join us.

Attention to detail was clearly called for! To establish a calming atmosphere, a tape recording of soft bells was playing on the living-room sound system. It was the relaxation tape that mother had enjoyed during her final days. All seemed perfect, though I must admit Dr Frankl was looking a touch ragged around the edges as Faye greeted us at the door.

A small drink before the meal. Ron, Lucy, and Christine were delighted to meet our highly esteemed visitor. He was, however, fading fast and we had not more than settled into our chairs when he exploded in something just short of a roar.

"Vil yu plees turn off zose infernal bellz?!"

He explained that he had once been the honoured guest at a meeting in Germany – Freiburg, I believe – and was ensconced by his hosts in a lovely inn situated on the ancient town square. All was blissfully quaint until the bells of the historic church chimed the hour at the threshold of pain and persisted in doing so throughout the night!

Following a hasty meal I drove my fragile guest to the hotel. *The problem is the registration desk will be jammed with people arriving for the meeting. This may take hours. I would hate to lose him at this point!*

Leaving the car with the immaculately turned-out attendant at the hotel door, I bundled Dr Frankl – ever-shrinking – toward the front desk where a tall, youthful, blond, unsmiling official awaited. *Lord he looks young! I pray he catches my tone or we may have a medical emergency here!*

"Good evening! This is Dr Frankl from Vienna!! – For *registration!*" I said. "Dr Viktor Frankl! *I believe you are expecting him!!!*"

The young man looked right past me with an air of practised indifference approaching boredom – *It's as if I'm transparent for heaven's sake!*

Bowing ever so slightly to Dr Frankl, he responded, "Guten Abend Herr Dr Frankl. Willkommen in Montreal. Ich hoffe, dass Sie einen guten Flug hatten. Wir haben ein Zimmer bereit für Sie. Wir bringen Ihre Koffer gleich nach oben."

Professor Frankl was suddenly wide awake and looking twenty years younger. He was radiant! I have never felt more proud of the Queen

Elizabeth Hotel – or Montreal, for that matter. I repressed the urge to
hug the young man and beat a hasty retreat to my car. Our guest of honour was in good hands and would sleep well.

In my invitation, I had asked Dr Frankl if he would agree to address
a general McGill audience on the evening prior to his International
Seminar lecture. He would be pleased to comply and chose the topic
"Psychotherapy on Its way to Rehumanization." Enthusiastic campus
sponsorship[27] ensured an overflow attendance at McGill's Leacock
Building amphitheatre.

Refreshed by three nights of sound sleep, ample "downtime" to prepare his comments, and the adulation offered by new friends over good
food, Professor Frankl was in fine form. Freud had pronounced the primary human drive to be the "will to pleasure," while Adler argued for
"the will to power." Frankl, however, concluded that our foundational
search is for meaning, thus initiating "the Third Viennese School of
Psychotherapy." He was on a mission and we were riveted.

His words were charged with a sense of urgency as he examined our
plight during these final decades of the twentieth century. Technology,
he observed, had provided us with endless *means*, but little *meaning*,
leaving us with what he termed an "existential vacuum." We in the West
were educated, wealthy, and awash in all the material goods we could
wish for, yet we found ourselves bereft of solace, engulfed by a sense of
emptiness and on a path toward depression, aggression, and addiction.
Refusing to be told what we *must* do, or even what we *ought* to do, we
no longer know what we *want* to do. Furthermore, he noted that the
sense of meaninglessness didn't just apply to the affluent West but was
found in Communist and Third World countries as well.

Our plight, Frankl suggested, drives us to ask, "What is man? What
distinguishes us from other species?" In response, he stressed that only
man is challenged by a self-awareness that asks the meaning of existence and recognizes our individual capacity to "be." It is this consciousness, Frankl suggested, that uniquely enables a sense of dignity rooted
in discovered meaning, a meaning that must be found through attachment to something greater and more enduring than the self. Meaning,
he observed, enables a sense of wholeness; he identified three paths to
meaning: work (our actions), love (an attachment that celebrates one's
uniqueness), and our potential for transcendence (our capacity to turn
even the most dire predicament into a victory, a tragedy into a triumph).

Dr Frankl was speaking with conviction. He was animated and adamant. He had seen too much to question the ground he was standing on.
Among the horrors of the Nazi concentration camps, he had experienced

love, grace, unspeakable courage, and time-stopping transcendence. He proclaimed with bedrock confidence: "It is possible for all of us to find meaning irrespective of age, sex, race, education, personality type, intelligence, environment or religious beliefs. We have within us the capacity to serve a cause or a love; to rise to a level of personal dignity that celebrates human potential in the face of adversity. We cannot grasp for happiness. The more we grasp for something, the more it eludes us. Happiness cannot be pursued; it must ensue as the product of the work, love or transcendent path we have chosen."

During the International Seminar I had been at the podium just prior to Dr Frankl, and we thus found ourselves sitting together at the completion of his presentation and during the table discussions that followed. I asked him about writing *Man's Search for Meaning* and he spoke in some detail about the manuscript for the book. He had sewn it into his overcoat lining when he was taken to the concentration camps. It was the only possession he took with him. When stripped of his clothes on reaching the camp, the manuscript was forever lost, but, as his internment continued, his experience provided him with further nuances for the now destroyed pages. He came to believe that two factors helped him in his struggle to survive: his need to rewrite that book and his love for both his mother and his wife.

"How long did it take to rewrite it when you finally had the opportunity?" I asked.

"Eight days," he responded. "*Man's Search for Meaning* was written in eight days."

He then turned to me and said with a slight smile, "Here, I have something for you." He handed me two splendid caricatures he had drawn of himself lecturing, one inscribed "For Bal, to remember Viktor in 1980, Viktor Frankl." "Oh, and here's something else," he added. "I did this while you were speaking." It was yet another caricature, this time of me. As we got up to leave, he handed me his lecture notes. "Would you like to have these?" he asked almost apologetically.[28] They were delightfully "Frankl" – penned with vigour, assurance, flourish, and repeated reminders to speak about "the work of Dr Frankl." They are now framed in my study, a treasured memento of this old-style European professor who had become my generous friend.

MAHLER AT THE MOUNTS

Gustav Mahler's Symphony No. 2 in C minor (*Resurrection*) opens with the *allegro maestoso* movement. We find ourselves standing beside the coffin of a man beloved. It is a moment of awe-inspiring solemnity as we consider his life and our own. The struggles of life that are our daily fare give way to intermittent hints of the possibility of wholeness, unity, and healing. But the movement ends with our total, shattering undoing. Our life journey continues through the following movements only to have optimism repeatedly engulfed by the swirling eddies of life's repeated challenges. And yet strains of hope are also recurrent and by the "Wieder sehr breit" of the fifth and final movement those hints have fully blossomed. Our transcendent potential, the possibility of being united with all that is life-giving and life-affirming, can no longer be denied and that glorious reality lifts us beyond the boulder-strewn path that has been our personal journey, toward transformation. By the "Langsam Mysterioso" section of the final movement, all that awaits us blazes into full evidence. We are greeted by the steadfast rock-solid Presence of all that holds us in existence. A Glory that is, at once, both our goal and our reassurance is at hand. In the final phrases of "Mit Aufschwung aber nicht eilen," with the security of the base-continuo on the organ bolstering the brilliance that glints from the shining peaks around us, Mahler leaves us in the all-capable Presence of the Infinite.

I don't recall when I first heard Mahler's Second Symphony, but by the Sunday in early 1979 when Faye and I attended morning service at St Andrew's United Church, it was firmly ensconced in my psyche as a pre-eminent expression of life's most pressing existential questions and the overriding possibility of universal hope. What is life, and what is death? Is there an existence after this one? Is this all an empty dream? Where is meaning to be found? Where love? In response to these questions, Mahler leaves us with glorious reassurance.

The scripture reading at St Andrew's that Sunday was Matthew 25:14–30, the parable of the talents. To our astonishment, during the service the ushers passed down the aisles offering those in attendance baskets of $10 bills – they had been donated by an anonymous church member. We were invited to take as many as we wished. The idea had come from a similar event held at an American church sometime earlier. We were informed that two months later there would be a special follow-up collection when the money plus interest, if any, could be returned. However, no record of the recipients of all this cash was kept. If you needed it, it was yours. No questions asked.

My idea crystallized as the basket of money reached us. I took $40. We would arrange a by-invitation evening concert at our home and present Mahler's Second followed by dessert, coffee, and a voluntary collection.

The formal invitation read, "Talent Night: A Lenten Concert in Aid of St Andrew's Matthew 25:14 Fund."

The date was set for Monday, 9 April. The guest list included twenty-two friends chosen because they were known to be heavily into either Mahler, Resurrections, or both! The particular rendition of the Second that I selected – with the help of urologist colleague and Renaissance man Mike Laplante – was the Decca recording by the London Symphony Chorus and Orchestra, Georg Solti conducting, with soloists Heather Harper and Helen Watts. Our MacIntosh sound system had been tuned to within an inch of its life by cousin Dave. The speakers were recessed into the living-room end wall approximately ten feet above the floor. The sound was breathtaking! The printed program contained a detailed account of Mahler's life, his Second Symphony, and his place in Western music. The seating was theatre-style; our group filled the room to capacity.

At the appointed hour the lights dimmed, leaving us aglow in candle-light. A hush fell on the room. At that precise moment, Michael, a member of the Montreal Symphony Orchestra and the last to arrive, slid into the empty seat beside me. I glanced at him as he took his place. He was turning to page one of the large bound volume on his knee. It was Zubin Mehta's personal copy of the full score.

The electric, tension-filled shimmering of the opening violins sent waves of anticipation through all who knew what lay ahead, then gave way to the rich response of the cellos.

We found ourselves immersed in Mahler's highly charged world as we moved from movement to movement. In the fifth, terrifying questions confronted us. The end of all life, the Day of Judgment, had arrived. The earth quaked as graves burst open and the dead streamed forth in end-less procession, the ego-generated personae of prince and pauper long gone. Wailing filled the air. Fear consumed. Did judgment or forgiveness await? Our senses deserted us with the sounding of the Last Trumpet, but then, out of the silence, a nightingale sang. It was the final echo of earthly life. Trumpets of the Apocalypse rang out and the chorus of saints proclaimed, "Thou shalt arise." The mists of fear cleared as judg-ment gave way to transcendent love ... We know ... We are.

A thunderous quiet filled our living room as the candles flickered. No one breathed. A massive lump filled my throat. I turned to Michael beside me and was about to offer an inane comment, like *Well, what do you think?* but was silenced by his tears. He was staring straight ahead, still in a deeper place; Mehta's score lay closed on his knee as he commented softly, "I have played it many times but that is the first time I have heard it."[29]

EASTER 1980

"Diary Note: Reflections, Sunday, 6 April, 1980, on Mark 4:35–40. Exhausted after teaching the multitude, Jesus slept in the stern of the boat, head on a cushion, as they crossed the Sea of Galilee. It was night. He was spent. The disciples took him with them just as he was. A furious squall comes up; waves break over the boat; they are nearly swamped. The terrified disciples waken him and ask, 'Teacher, don't you care if we drown?' He gets up, rebukes wind and waves – 'Be quiet! Be still!' evoking a total calm, then asks them 'Why are you afraid? Do you still have no faith?'"

Reading that passage of Mark during Easter 1980, I saw it through a perspective modified by two recent experiences: being in the wild storm at sea in early March 1980 when Faye and I went on the medical-lecture cruise/course out of Miami and we felt the fury of the gale and the complementary power and powerlessness of such a situation, and, secondly, being at the bedside of those on the PCU who were facing death. I wrote in my diary:

When Jesus awoke he was confronted by men facing death, by their terror, and by the fury of the storm. They were, some of them, fishermen – men who knew life at sea; he was a landlubber, a carpenter.

To awaken in those circumstances, to face the surrounding night, the surrounding storm, the terror in the eyes of his men – and I believe he would have looked into their eyes – he must have found himself at a crossroads moment.

Then, his words, "Why are you afraid? Have you no faith?" I believe he was not referring to "faith that I will keep you physically safe, that I will calm the storms of life," but instead, "faith that, in the face of death, I am with you always; there is no need to fear, even if death comes. The 'Kingdom' is within. Why are you afraid?" For him, a sobering realization. They hadn't understood, even though he was in their presence.

Broken Open

How strange that the nature of life is change,
yet the nature of human beings is to resist change.
And how ironic that the difficult times we fear might ruin us
are the very ones that can break us open
and help us blossom into who we were meant to be.

Elizabeth Lesser[1]

As springtime 1980 began to flower, there was inescapable evidence of Mother's deteriorating health. The small-bowel sarcoma was gaining an upper hand. Her swelling abdomen and dwindling energy had become increasingly difficult to mask with her customary smile and carry-on-as-usual demeanour. I ached. There were occasional visits back and forth between Ottawa and Montreal; we opened the *Place* in May; and underneath it all we shared an unspoken sense that each day was precious. Her time with us was clearly limited.

Last letters from her sister Marian and niece Joan, dated Long Lake, Sunday, 3 August, 1980, were hand-delivered to "Maudie" at the Island by Jim's daughter Heather and her boyfriend, Frank. Brief and heartfelt, these notes spoke of love, prayers, family, and cherished bonds. Joan quoted Tennyson's *Idylls of the King* and included the opening lines of "The Passing of Arthur," including the frequently quoted "Pray for my soul. More things are wrought by prayer than this world dreams of," and closed with "Oceans of love. xox, Joan."[2]

At the same time, on the home front, each day was tension-filled. The complex nexus of multilayered problems that Faye and I had confronted for a decade were deepening in spite of intense motivation, effort, and anguish. It had been a decade marked by countless discussions and consultations, both personal and professional. Idealistic goals had long since given way to compromise, then alienation and dysfunction. What had

once been nurturing had become toxic. Life-defining choices in the interest of sustained well-being for each member of our family of five must
soon be made. Heavy seas were at hand; the promise of worse lay ahead.
In search of objective counsel, I sought a reference point that I could
count on for direct feedback, a catalyst for insight and growth. I located
just such a person in June 1980.

An analyst or therapist is neither "curer" nor cure; not a guide, nor a
companion. Instead, he/she, at best, is a mirror who reflects reality back
to the seeker, who must remain the active participant in the dynamic at
hand, pointing toward insights that may shed light on all that has been
and what yet might be. A McGill colleague, Irwin Scott Disher, agreed to
take me on. It proved to be an enriching collaboration that would last
twenty-five years.

Dr Disher was a formidable presence – a perennially tousled, probing, interested yet pointedly neutral addition to my journey. During the
Second World War he had served on a corvette in the North Atlantic,
and then, following medical studies, he completed his training in psychiatry in London with Donald Winnicott and his colleagues, including John
Bowlby, Michael Balint, and Marion Milner of the British Psychoanalytic
Society Independent Group. Until his death in 2008 at the age of eighty-
three, Dr Disher was an active member of the Canadian Psychoanalytic
Society. In addition to his private practice, he acted throughout his lengthy
career as a valued teacher and mentor in child psychiatry at the Montreal
Children's Hospital. A man of many interests, he was an equestrian; he
raised sheep on his rustic country estate; he was an ardent African-violet
enthusiast; and, undergirding it all, he read voraciously.

In keeping with psychotherapeutic norms, our relationship was strictly
professional. His personal interests were out of bounds and only gradually seeped into my awareness as the years passed. An exception to this
iron-clad rule occurred the day he introduced me to his cherished fictional comrades-in-arms Captain Jack Aubrey of the Royal Navy and his
accomplice in high adventure, Stephen Maturin, ship's surgeon. In time,
our shared admiration and affection for these two, and for their creator
Patrick O'Brian, would know no bounds. With a nod to propriety, however, it was imperative that *I* be the one to bring up the topic (always
at the end of the session). Then we could enjoy a few moments together
aboard the HMS *Surprise* or one of the other sailing ships we shared
with our two all-too-human heroes, all the while with the clear understanding that any observations I might make concerning their adventures, or indeed any other topic, would be met with pursed lips and a
non-committal nod of his head coupled with a knowing "Hhmmm" that

acknowledged his superiority of insight. "I have, I believe," he casually remarked one afternoon, "read all twenty of the O'Brian novels eighteen times." Stolid and not given to praise, Disher could be challenging. But, then, that was his job! He was an invaluable observer and critic for a quarter-century as together we navigated innumerable lee shores.

On 14 August 1980 the family gathered for Mother's birthday luncheon at 37 Opeongo Road. (By then, she and Dad had relocated to a condominium at 300 The Driveway, and Jim and Ursula had moved into 37 Opeongo.) As she retired to the living room to rest, I gave her the first entry of a journal examining the existential questions she and I had discussed during her illness. We talked as the others finished their meal in the dining room across the hall. These notes were to continue as a source of connection over the days and weeks that lay ahead.

On the 19th of that month, while at the *Place*, I awoke from what some term a "big dream" and recorded it:

I closed my eyes and saw a form
a shapeless angled mass
Brownish
Heavy
Lying still upon the cliff.
self.
And as I watched I opened
and my inner Self escaped.
A butterfly.
Rising happily on lightly beating wings
to freedom
peace.
But alas, 'twas but a dream within a dream.
In the confines of this mass I must remain.
Why, Mother?

On 9 September 1980, at 8:30 p.m., Mother died in the Driveway condo, the family at her side. The undisputed captain gone, the ship felt rudderless; I continued to jot down my experience of those grief-filled hours as Dad and I found ourselves alone, huddled, rumpled, speechless, in the study at 37 Opeongo.[3]

September 10. Conversation:[4]
Head bowed
Gasping sighs through bronchi constricted in protest,

"I feel that I am standing at a precipice," he said.
"The cliffs to south and north,
To east and west, are sheer.
They drop a thousand feet
To blackness."
"Do you feel you will fall, Father?"
"No.
It is the view from Vimy Ridge.
An outlook on
Oblivion."

September 12th, 1400 hours, we gather at Dominion Chalmers
    Church for a service of remembrance.
"I hope to see my pilot face to face
When I have crossed the bar."
We sang at your request
And knew your wish had been fulfilled.
– then we retreated for muted, muffled, tasteless sandwiches and tea.

37 Opeongo Road
I felt this house weep today
In every room.
Thronging with people,
It vainly searched the faces passing through it, for your face.
Panelled walls,
The stairs,
Each corner turned
Provides
Another vista created by your hand.
There the spot where long you sat
Gazing at sailboats on the lake.
How much they meant to you!
"Like birds," you said.
And now, symbolically, that view is overgrown with hedges.
Time obliterates each source of joy – sailboat view, you
your smile
yourself.
One source remains.
Love.
It feels so distant now.

I wander upstairs to escape the crowd.

The Green Bathroom
Unsuspecting
I walked through the door.
I stepped into that room
And outside time.
Your presence overwhelms.
Not just yours – a thousand memories.
In that sink you washed my hair ...
Too sick to go to school today ...
There's the Mitchell's house ...
Where is Pal? ...
Nettie will have the porridge made by now ...
While I sit here I'll review my part, the Lyres Club will sing next
    week ...
High school dance. Decorations were fantastic ...
Judy's chuckling laugh ...
Bob, Dave, Pritch
El and Phyd ...
Time shifts
Same room
Peter slumps, fevered, toward the floor.
I catch him
And from unconsciousness
In whispered tones, he speaks, "Place me horizontal."
– essence of Peter!
In this room
Your loving hands were never far away.
Can't focus.
Who placed this tourniquet around my throat?
Your absence overwhelms.
Reality rudely awakens
And screams the vacuum that is here.
Memories shattered.
The room weeps with me
In emptiness.

It was a month later that Faye and I hosted Viktor Frankl and the
International Seminar. The distraction from the agony ensnaring us

was a relief: it was remarkably easy to slip back into our practised public-teamwork mode. Enjoyable too. But so short-lived. Then, endless walking across acres of broken glass.

Faye concluded, "The only chance we have is a trial separation. You will have to leave; I will not."

We walked arm in arm the few blocks to inspect the rented lodgings where I would stay and immediately felt the pressures lessening. We chuckled and Faye observed, "If the neighbours were to see us now, they would not imagine what this is about."

Crossroad. As late fall gave way to the frosts of winter, Faye and I went our separate ways. It was twenty-three years since our fall 1957 meeting at Queen's.

Anger, disillusionment, breathtaking loss, sorrow. Had we fallen short? Undoubtedly. But not through ill intent. While perhaps inevitable, such an outcome was antithetical to all we believed in and had wished for; it entailed the rupturing of a sacred trust. The roots of our disaster ran deep, their origins shared, as had been our joys, regrets, and cost. Did we pursue all options? To the best of our ability. Were our efforts doomed by virtue of who we were and the shadows of unfinished business? It would seem so. Could we have done more? Probably; probably not.

At that terrible crossroad, the probability of further wounding infinitely exceeded the possibility of healing. Failure admitted; inadequacy recognized; profound grief experienced; growth out of the ashes sought. Faye, Chris, Lauren, Jamie, Bal. Five of us had gained greatly; five of us had paid dearly; five of us lived the phoenix experience and grew, or not, as we were able. Within months, both Faye and I would find lasting relationships elsewhere. Grace received beyond measure or merit. "The goal of the hero ... is to find those levels in the psyche that open, open, open, and finally open to the mystery of your Self, being, Buddha consciousness, or the Christ. That's the journey ... The purpose of the journey is compassion. When you have come past the pairs of opposites, you have reached compassion ... Beyond the world of opposites is an unseen, but experienced, unity and identity in us all."[5] Those few lines by American mythologist Joseph Campbell concisely summarize whatever insights I have been able to glean during the decades that have slipped past since the twinned deaths of Mother and marriage in the fall of 1980.

If our journey through life is irrevocably shaped by even the most insignificant choices at our ten thousand crossroads, those 1980 landmark intersections were clearly epic for each of us who was involved. Would the path we took favour the opening that Campbell spoke of? Though our separation was undertaken in the hope of nurturing healing for all five of us, the months that followed were etched in grey and shattered into countless further broken-glass experiences. Christmas spent with Dad offered a sense of community as he and I faced our respective disorienting maelstrom defined by emptiness. The Christmas Eve service at our church was a boon, *a way through*, but the drive back to my rented rooms was marked by silence.

The emptiness of the rented rooms echoed the bleakness of each day. It was a low point to be sure, but in due course rays of light appeared from unexpected sources. Internist, oncologist, professor, medical philosopher, teacher, and long-time friend Neil MacDonald, who had recently arrived in town, accepted the invitation to share my rented pad while locating more suitable accommodations for his November 1980–July 1981 study leave at the Royal Vic PCS. His months with us were a prelude to developing a palliative-care program at Edmonton's Cross Cancer Institute where he was director. A world leader in whatever he undertook, Neil had founded the Oncology Day Centre at the Vic in the early 1960s and then orchestrated the growth of oncology programs in Alberta. His involvement in our nascent field would provide a shining beacon for our path forward. It seemed too good to be true.[6] A further source of light was soon to appear.

AN OPENING OF DOORS

One solitary, grey March morning, as I groggily thumbed through the *Montreal Gazette* over coffee, a full-page article caught my eye. It outlined the activities of John Main, an Irish lawyer and former member of the British foreign service who had become a Benedictine monk. Father John had arrived in Montreal in September 1977. With the assistance of Laurence Freeman, a youthful Oxford University classics scholar and fellow Benedictine, he planned to establish a centre for teaching "Christian Meditation." *Hmmm, I wonder what makes meditation "Christian?" But, whatever the label, do you suppose it might be helpful for our patients, or staff?* (unconsciously implying *not me, of course!*)

The *Gazette* article noted that Main's fledgling Benedictine Priory of Montreal had recently moved to the "McConnell House," the mansion at 1475 Pine Avenue, a couple of blocks west of the Vic. *McConnell House?* The synchronicity struck me. The McConnell Family Foundation had been the source of the anonymous start-up funding that had enabled development of our Palliative Care Service. Now, here it was once again.[7] I made an appointment to meet with Dom John Main "to explore whether meditation might be useful in Palliative Care."

Though centrally located near the downtown core, the small property that was now home to the priory was surprisingly secluded, tucked away as it was just east of the Montreal General Hospital on a forested wedge of land at the junction of Cedar and Pine avenues. The mansion presented a sense of grand presence, an air of accustomed ease, dignity, and self-assured pre-eminence. (The McConnell home had been among the last in Montreal's fabled Golden Square Mile to be occupied by its founding family.[8]) The winding driveway led to a hidden world of tree-lined elegance as one passed the impressive solarium in approaching the covered stone passageway that sheltered the bronze doors of the main entrance. There was an aura of peacefulness, if not the humility and simplicity one might anticipate in picturing a Benedictine oasis of contemplative prayer.

The grounds were deserted as I parked the car. The classic facade and walls of buff limestone were complemented by verandahs and Mediterranean terraces that offered direct access to the surrounding gardens, trees, and a path that wound its way up to the outbuildings located on the high ground overlooking Mount Royal Park on Cedar Avenue behind the main house. I rang the bell.

I was greeted with quiet warmth by former schoolteacher Doreen Romandini, now oblate and administrative assistant in Father John's meditation community. With my coat disposed of, she led the way down the marble elegance of the cavernous hallway, passing the one-time salon, now a meditation room.

When we reached the far end of the hall, an impressive stone staircase ascended on our left to the floor above, while, to our right, the library revealed yet another example of refined grace. Its coffered ceiling, book-lined walls, and entrance to the verdant solarium were aglow with the warmth created by the hardwood panelling, plush Persian and Turkish carpets, and a welcoming fire in the stately fireplace. Tea and biscuits had been set out.

In hushed tones, Doreen noted that Father John would be joining me promptly, only partially concealing a vigilant mother-hen watchfulness that was the by-product of her fierce loyalty to the prior and a latent capacity to offer a peck here and there when needed to keep the flock in order. Her welcome was genuine, her sense of dedication to every corner of these beloved rooms evident.

Within minutes the door swung open and in strode Father John. Scottish actor Sean Connery came to mind. The room was suddenly infused with a penetrating sense of focus and presence. His erect six-foot-plus frame, confident carriage, and flowing grey and black Benedictine habit were accompanied by an open expression and clarity of eye that suggested a disciplined, alert mind and certainty of mission.

Taking our seats near the fire, we exchanged introductory notions about our respective activities. I outlined the elements of palliative care, the brilliance of Cicely's concept of "Total Pain," and the relevance of the spiritual/existential domain to quality of life in illness and health. He, in turn, spoke concisely about his plan to develop a monastic and lay community based on the practice of meditation with a mantra. He radiated a formality that was courteous yet reserved. *You can take the man from the barrister's bench, but you can't take the bench from the man.* Our visit of forty-five minutes ended with no clear plan to pursue the dialogue. Meditation? *Christian* meditation? A mantra? I was far from clear or convinced as I left the priory.

Both Father John and I, it seemed, had "taken the road less travelled" in our respective professions. How *did* we come to be in that lavish library in pursuit of the same goal – access to the peace, depth, and unity that whispers of its presence within? Who *was* John Main? How did he, an Irish/British lawyer, get mixed up in "monkery," let alone mantra-focused meditation? In like fashion, my journey from urologist to surgical oncologist to caregiver for the dying in the McGill Faculty of Medicine was hardly standard practice. And for that matter, who, theologically speaking, was *I*? In our chats, EKR had described herself as a "vishy-vawshy Protestant." I suspected that might be an apt description of me as well.

Given the social and cultural conditioning provided by a lifetime immersed equally in the mythologies of medical science and the United Church of Canada, what was I certain of? Where did I stand? I had reached a place where even the word "God" was, to my ears, sufficiently encrusted with troubling, archaic baggage that it seemed inadequate, vague, even blasphemous.

On encountering for the first time, some years earlier, the flaming convictions of evangelical creed-bound Protestantism, I had found it all exciting. But before long I felt uncomfortable with the fear-based rigidity and judgment-prone dualistic narrowness and intolerance that too frequently flowers in that garden. I had been burned more than once. To my mind, Christian exclusivity sat awkwardly with the lives of the deeply spiritual saints that I had encountered in a variety of belief traditions – contemplative Judaism, Islam/Sufism, Hinduism, Buddhism, Aboriginal Wisdom, and, truth be told, those adhering to secular humanism or, for that matter, atheism.

Who cares? Why bother with such superstitious nonsense? Surely, at the close of the twentieth century, we are beyond such outworn fairy tales! Yet one *must* "bother," I had concluded, since to ignore the ultimate questions posed by consciousness, love, compassion, transience, and our potential for "peace that passes understanding" in the face of suffering would be to dismiss the authenticity with which Dad and Mother, their mentor Sir Wilfred Grenfell, Marian Anderson, Ken MacKinnon, the Vaniers (Jean, Benedict, and Thérèse), Cicely, Mary Baines, EKR, Viktor Frankl, and countless others attempted to live out such confounding mysteries, not to mention the singular reverence I had always reserved for Jesus of Nazareth.

More than that. To ignore such questions would be to ignore the issues confronting our dying patients and their families. When asked, the majority of those with life-limiting illness list spiritual concerns as an important determinant of their quality of life. How could one accompany our dying patients *without* asking these foundational questions? Not with the goal of finding *answers* per se, but rather in the interest of being a fellow traveller in facing these uncertainties as we all journey toward a deeper lived experience.

Finally, on reflection, I realized that still other issues led me to that meeting with Father John. Why does the church, or much of it, focus with such exclusive urgency on personal, creed-bound, salvation theology rather than on the Nazarene's central teaching about the kingdom within and His foundational challenge to follow Him into reverence, service to the needy, love of others, and selflessness? I had puzzled through the implications of the Apostles' Creed to conclude that I could sign on the dotted line, but *only* after considerable stickhandling around the millennia-old metaphors! How does one move beyond metaphor to discern the truth underlying the remarkable accounts of the Nazarene's lived experience and the claims of His continuing "Presence" in the lives of those who invite it, however that is understood?

And what of John Main?[9] How did London-born Douglas William Victor Main, the third of six children in a traditional Catholic family, find himself living and teaching the contemplative path in Canada? In 1943, at age seventeen, he had joined the war effort as a wireless operator. Following the war, Douglas explored his sense of calling to the priesthood but found the spiritual training he received constricting. His concept of faith was that it should be liberating not limiting and that its ultimate goal should be love. Thus, he left his religious training to pursue a law degree at Trinity College, Dublin, and on graduating in 1954 he joined Her Majesty's Overseas Civil Service and was sent to Kuala Lumpur, Malaysia. There, while delivering a message from the governor general to a local orphanage, he met its founder, forty-five-year-old Swami

Satyananda, a Hindu monk educated in Malaysia and in India where he had been exposed to such towering figures as Ramana Maharshi and Sri Aurobindo. Douglas was deeply impressed by Satyananda's peacefulness and calm demeanour, and, on learning that he attributed this to his meditation practice, he asked the Swami to teach him to meditate. The two men met weekly for eighteen months as Douglas continued a twice-daily meditation practice. He subsequently returned to his sense of a religious calling, became a monk and ordained priest, and, in due course, was sent to be headmaster of St Anselm's Benedictine School in Washington, DC.

At that time, Main explored the history of meditation and discovered its presence in early Christian practice. He was impressed by parallel teachings found in the ancient Hindu Upanishads (800–1000 BCE), the writings of St Paul, the "Institutes" of the early Christian monk and theologian John Cassian (c. 360–435), the traditions of the Desert Fathers in Egypt in the first centuries CE, the fourteenth-century Middle English text *The Cloude of Unknowyng*, and the writings of St Teresa of Avila (1515–82) and St John of the Cross (1542–91). Meditation with a mantra *had*, he discovered, been part of the Christian tradition from apostolic times but later had largely been lost.[10]

The Upanishads proclaimed: "He contains all things, all works and desires and all perfumes and tastes. And he enfolds the whole universe and, in silence, is loving to all. This is the Spirit that is in my heart. This is Brahman." For Father John, "coming to an awareness of the spirit of the universe" meant "an awareness of the risen Christ" in his own heart. When asked about the concept of *Christian* meditation, he would simply reply that for him "there is only one prayer. It is the stream of love between Christ and the Father but this goes on in each human heart irrespective of race or creed. In the depths of the human heart we are one. We are in communion."

Returning to his monastery in London after five years in the United States, he felt compelled to make the teaching of meditation the centre of his life and opened the first Christian meditation centre in London. His teaching was simple. "Sit quietly and lightly close your eyes. During the time of your meditation there must be in your mind, no thoughts, no words, no imaginings. The sole sound will be the sound of your mantra, your word. The word I recommend is 'Maranatha,' the Aramaic word meaning 'Come Lord.'"

In 1977 Father John Main and Brother Laurence Freeman arrived at Mirabel airport and were met by Bishop Leonard Crowley, Quebec bishop for English-language affairs who provided them with a house and initial support to establish a Benedictine priory dedicated to the teaching of meditation. It was a time of political upheaval in Quebec; uncertainty was palpable. Bishop Crowley described his first meeting with Father John: "I shared with him my desire to bring to our city various religious communities, each of which might deepen and enrich the spiritual life of our priests and people with a sense of stability at a time of great political and social unrest in Quebec."

In the months following our first meeting in early 1981, I attended occasional Monday evening introductory meditation sessions. It would, I reasoned, be important to see what it was all about prior to involving the PCS. These weekly introductory gatherings attracted twenty to forty persons from all walks of life. Once we were settled in our chairs against the walls of the spacious basement one-time ballroom, Father John would enter with a low-key businesslike air, offer a word of welcome, and play a brief interlude of quietening recorded music. He sat on a small, slightly raised platform that fostered a sense of personal contact with those present. He then described how to meditate. It was simple – simple, but not easy. "Ma, Ra, Na, Tha ... Ma, Ra ..." My brain chatter was incessant; my mind flooded with thoughts. *Return to the word. Back to the word. Nothing mystical about all this. No dogma; no incense or folderol. Nuts and bolts stuff really ... But I wish I could shut off that bloody brain chatter – even for a second.*

A question period followed the twenty-minute meditation. The questions were the same each week. The prior was patient. His answers were concise, clear, and at times accompanied by a quiet intensity:

"Vision? Madame, if you have a vision, return immediately to your mantra!"

"The *meaning* of the mantra word isn't the issue; the purpose isn't to focus on a Meaning – even a sacred meaning. The purpose is to gently clear the mind; to rest in the deep silence that is within you."

"To find yourself, you must lose yourself. It is the prayer of the heart."

"Meditation is not taught; it is caught. It isn't something one achieves. It is something you receive."

"How long does it take? Well, the first twenty or thirty years are usually the most difficult."

"There is no such a thing as *good* or *bad* meditation. There is just meditation! When the mind intrudes, simply, gently, return to your mantra. Don't judge or fret; just go back to quietly repeating your word."

"Mysticism? Beware of mysticism! It begins with mist and ends in schism!"

"'Holy relic'? Go and give it a good burial."

"The mystery of love is that we become what we delight to gaze upon, and so, when we have opened our hearts to Light, we become light."

He spoke with quiet confidence and matter-of-fact reverence. There was no sentimentality or romanticism. Twice daily, morning and evening, meditation formed an axis around which his – and someday perhaps our – day might quietly rotate. Meditation, he asserted, involved moving beyond distractions of thought, word, or action to access the silence and unity within. It was rather as if he was describing the steps involved in completing a fine woodcarving: precise and gently matter of fact.

One evening, during an introductory session at the priory, a woman to my left asked a question. I don't recall her words, but his response is indelibly etched in my memory. Something about his body language changed, catching my attention. He leaned forward. Her question had taken him to a deeper place. There was silence. He was looking at her, or through her, with a fixed gaze, pausing, as if groping for language to express the inexpressible. "Meditation is like this." He leaned forward a little more, raising his hands, which were about two feet apart in front of his chest, palms facing each other. His gaze was steady, the large grey cuffs of his habit had fallen back. His hands and bare forearms had become indicators of depth in our journey into stillness. Another silence. "Meditation is like this," he repeated, as he slowly lowered his raised hands, bringing the palms progressively toward each other. He was look-ing at her, yet without seeing her. He was intent; hands descending, each one moving toward its opposite mate. "Through the gentle repetition of your word, you clear the mind and descend to the Still Point." His palms were now less than an inch apart. The room was silent. He seemed unaware of our presence – or perhaps profoundly aware, I couldn't be sure which. "You pass through that point: it is a point of pure 'Being.' And as you do," his hand were now palms down and suddenly rapidly moving apart, "you find yourself in a place of unity, a sea of unity, a quantum ocean of Being." I can't be certain of the words he used, but that was their essence. Silence. We sat unmoving.

Linda and Days in Which to Be

Sun's up, uuh huh, looks okay
The world survives into another day
And I'm thinking about eternity
Some kind of ecstasy got a hold on me.

I had another dream about lions at the door
They weren't half as frightening as they were before
But I'm thinking about eternity
Some kind of ecstasy got a hold on me.

Walls, windows, trees, waves coming through
You be in me and I'll be in you
Together in eternity
Some kind of ecstasy got a hold on me.

Bruce Cockburn,
"Wondering Where the Lions Are"

Send the sun in time for dawn Let the birds all hail the morning
Love of life will urge me say you are the new day
Hope is my philosophy Just needs days in which to be
Love of life means hope for me, born on a new day
You are the new day.

The King's Singers,
"You Are the New Day"

Linda whistles. I don't mean that Linda knows *how* to whistle, I mean she whistles most of the time. When I mention it, she tells me that generally she isn't aware of it but claims that it reminds her of her Dad.

"To nurture whistling you must tend it carefully," a wise man once cautioned. Well, almost four decades on, it continues to brighten each of my days. *Dei gratia*.

Faye and I first met Linda Guignion in 1974 when she accompanied her fiancé, Fred, during his visit to our home as a prelude to dog sitting our Samoyed "Nicky" during our family sojourn at St Christopher's that summer. Fred was a candidate for the ministry. He had seen Faye's "Help Wanted" sign on McGill's United Theological College notice board. That August, Fred and Linda were married. Neither Fred's theology plans nor his marriage worked out.

In 1977 our paths crossed again. After her marriage ended, Linda joined our church, Dominion Douglas, to link up with Phyllis Smyth, her minister and friend during Linda's early adult years. At "D.D." Linda became the youngest member of the Wednesday afternoon prayer group for Judy and David Bourke. Faye and I came to know her well. Although it was a horrific, wrenching time, within months of going our separate ways, Faye and I had both entered into lasting partnerships: hers with a man she met while studying theology, mine with Linda.

Linda was the only child of Alice and Robert (Bud) Guignion. Alice Elliott, the youngest of five, in a family with roots in Sussex and Yorkshire, England, became a full-time homemaker after the birth of Linda. Bud was a businessman and, later, a high school teacher whose ancestors had emigrated from Guernsey in the Channel Islands to Gaspé and subsequently to Montreal. The Guignions lived in the east end of Montreal where each of Bud's carefully nurtured hobbies – model trains, the newly minted postwar Montreal Alouettes football team, photography, the United Church, army cadets, art history, computers, and genealogy – enlivened his family presence with understated but infectious enthusiasm.

While Linda and I shared a superficial familiarity resulting from her summer of 1974 dog sitting and, in due course, two years of Wednesday POW meetings, there was a sense of gentle, natural, and quietly reassuring surprise when we finally found an enduring relationship with each other.

We were living in merging worlds. Tall, with light brown hair and hazel eyes, Linda was eleven years younger than me. Given those eleven years, the differences in our reference points in books, music, films, idiomatic expressions, and social norms were a source of recurring amusement. She had been an English major at McGill, a singer in a folk group, and, when we got together, an elementary school teacher for the Lakeshore School Board. Though low key and a self-proclaimed introvert, she had a gift for the unexpected pithy phrase to describe each passing moment, a quick mind, and a quirky sense of humour. The whistling, which at times morphed into humming, was never far away.

During the summer of 1981 we had a round of introductory visits with family and friends. That fall we settled into Linda's upper-floor apartment on Lakeshore Road in Pointe Claire where our changing world seemed to be charged with a surfeit of symbolism bolstered by the fact that our new apartment came with a built-in pathetic fallacy that descended on us several times each day. Our living-room window was squarely on the flight path to Montreal's Dorval International Airport. We could actually wave to the pilots as the giant jets thundered toward us in landing, an experience that can best be described as sobering, hair-raising, and exhilarating.

Chris, Lauren, and Jamie joined us for Christmas dinner 1981. The Reverend Alex Farquhar's words from the Dominion Douglas pulpit that Christmas seemed particularly apt: "The births of life occur in the context of pain. Bedlam / Bethlehem – two potentials within every experience. Was the stable so aseptic? The baby so happy, clean and cooing? The mother so serene? The animals and hay so sweet smelling? The shepherds so clean cut? The wise men so wise? Or was there the pain and sweat of childbirth, the pungent odour of the animals, the fussing of a hungry babe? To omit the pain of the stable is to shortchange the human dimension of the experience. Bethlehem out of Bedlam. Pain as a gift. Pain is never pointless because of Christmas." When each valley is lifted up, every mountain and hill made low, the uneven ground levelled and the rough places made plain, when confrontation becomes collaboration, when anger and depression fade, when the guilt of failure and pain caused to others is gradually reshaped through a reframing of what is possible, when decay surrenders to the healing power of renewed saltiness, when rumination on past and future gives way to a deepening present, there is then a natural slowing, opening, and discovery of joy. There is healing.

Life felt hopeful. As 1982 dawned we found ourselves snowed in at a chalet near Lachute with Jamie and a gifted friend and mentor, the Montreal artist John Francis Williams. With a sense of renewal, I finalized plans for McGill's Fourth International Congress (the name had been changed from "Seminar") on Care of the Terminally Ill. The faculty was to be memorable: Cicely, Mary Baines, Thérèse Vanier, Derek Doyle, EKR, Kathy Foley, Ed Shneidman, and Dom John Main as well as additional speakers from the international community including Sir Ferguson Anderson, Glasgow; Lea Baider, Jerusalem; Luis Jose De Souza, Bombay; Paul Pruyser, Topeka; and, from Temple University, psychiatrist and poet Michael Simpson, who would act as congress Poet Laureate reading a just-written new work at the close of each session in response to the content of the plenary. It proved to be a novel way of monitoring the evolving internal milieu as the meeting progressed. Our focus was on the whole person, whether patient, family member, or caregiver, as it had been since 1976.[1]

It was a busy year as Linda and I acclimatized to life together. Lauren moved in with us following our move to a downtown apartment convenient to the hospital and to Lauren's high school.

A trip to attend palliative-care meetings in England and Sweden was looming.

In London with Linda, its sights, sounds, smells were familiar yet so new: the National Gallery, Trafalgar Square, and Kew Gardens; London cabs snaking through the maze; news hawkers bawling out details of the unfolding Falklands War; a hearty lunch with John Fryer, a colleague in the International Work Group on Death, Dying and Bereavement, at The George – the storied inn noted for its galleried architecture, fine food, and earlier clientele, including Shakespeare and Dickens; participating in the St Christopher's International Conference '82; evenings of London theatre that left us filled with wonderment.

It was Peter Shaffer's *Amadeus* that was my undoing! It is, of course, a magnificent work, a masterful weaving of Mozart's music and biography, or rather, his biography as it *might* have been. My undoing was not so much the music or the story per se, it was instead the searing soul-searching prompted by Salieri or, to be more precise, the incomparable English actor Paul Scofield *as* the court composer Salieri. Toward the end of the play, an embittered Salieri, whose self-esteem had been shredded by his sense of inadequacy when compared to Mozart's greater gift, walks to the stage apron and stops. He stands there, facing us. The house lights come on! *What is happening? The play isn't over, is it?* ...We theatre goers are now alarmingly exposed before him, specimens to be examined, pinned to our seats in full view! He studies us. *This is most uncomfortable!* ... Salieri speaks. Actually, he addresses *me*! I felt totally exposed. Dripping with sarcasm prompted by the "unachievable, uncaring God" who had ignored him in favour of Mozart, Salieri confesses that life no longer holds any meaning for him, and then he adds, in case I had missed the point: "Now I go to become a ghost myself. I will stand in the shadows when you come here to this earth in *your* turn. And when *you* feel the dreadful bite of your failures ... I will whisper my name to you: 'Salieri. Patron Saint of Mediocrities!' and in the depth of your downcastness you can pray to me. And I will forgive you. Vi Saluto."

Next stop Sweden for the meeting of the IWG hosted by the Karolinska Institute's Loma Feigenberg. It offered memorable encounters with old friends as we struggled to establish international standards of care and untangle the web of issues surrounding "death education."[2]

Our return to Montreal led to a summer of further Linda introductions at various family gatherings and then a week with Lauren at music camp. Years hence I would recall those busy months with their frenetic mix of remorse and gratitude, hurt and healing, on reading the words of a new and gifted fellow traveller, Lou Gehrig's disease victim Philip Simmons:

> Life is both more and less than we hoped for. We've known earth's pleasures: sunlight on a freshly mowed lawn, leaves trembling with rain, a child's laugh, the sight of a lover stepping from the bath. We've also seen marriages sour and careers crash, we've seen children lost to illness and accident. Beyond the dualities of feast and famine we've glimpsed something else: the blessings shaken out of an imperfect life like fruit from a blighted tree. We've known the dark woods, but also the moon. This book [his masterwork *Learning to Fall: The Blessings of an Imperfect Life*] is for those ready to embrace this third way through loss to a wholeness, richness, and depth we never before envisioned.[3]

JOURNEYING INWARD

On returning to the PCU I noted that an aura of concern had replaced the usual warm welcome that awaits our visitors. While I was away the team had admitted our teammate, bedrock night orderly Don MacGowan, the same "Magoo" who had reassured his patient that "a void is better than nothing at all." He had been referred to us from the Neurological Institute where they had diagnosed an inoperable brain tumour. Engulfed by the sinking sense of disbelief that accompanies the news that a loved one is in extremis, I went to see him.

Typically, irrepressible Magoo had notified his disparate friends of his new status by posting over his bed a sign that read "Waiting for Godot" and then sending a message to Father John at the priory that visits would be welcome. Somewhere along the way, it seems, Don had added Benedictine oblate to his lengthy list of vocations: student, vagabond, hippy, philosopher, bon vivant, world-renowned unpublished poet, palliative caregiver, and now Benedictine oblate.

Father John had been a regular visitor to Don's bedside in the days prior to my return from the United Kingdom. While his PCU visits were always discreet, they nonetheless managed to be stately bordering on epic, given the sweeping flourish of his flowing habit, his towering physical stature, and his delightfully Irish ability to celebrate the moment. Don, with his unfailing eye for a "happening" was, one imagines, as delighted by the theatre of these encounters as refreshed by their spiritual content.

This was the first time we had admitted a team member to the PCU, one of our own, so to speak. I had been at St Christopher's during similar circumstances but this was different. This was family – *our* family!

With Don's death, Father John agreed to conduct the memorial service. It was to be held in a chapel at the historic St Patrick's Basilica and would bring together a striking cross-section of humanity representing the various lives Don had celebrated: jaded young intellectuals; members of the street-partying and drug sets; philosophers; students; businessmen; healthcare professionals; Benedictine oblates. We were there to honour a man who had added an edge to life for each of us. Magoo would be missed.

As we gathered, I was surprised to see that Father John was absent. How odd. He had been replaced by a young monk who introduced himself as Father Laurence Freeman. Meeting Laurence left an immediate impression: his bright, youthful, open face, already receding hairline, articulate expression, and incandescent warmth suggested liveliness, joy, and attentive presence, even in these muted circumstances. I could not, of course, fully appreciate the future significance of this meeting, but I did sense our immediate ease in relating. For my part, I was struck at first contact by his boundless energy, his quick eye and dizzying creativity, his capacity for simultaneously initiating countless schemes, his encyclopedic knowledge of English literature, and his towering, questioning intellect.

Leaving the basilica following our farewell to Don, I realized that Father John's absence remained unexplained: fearing something was amiss I made my way to the priory. Doreen greeted me at the door with an expression of relief. "Oh, I'm so glad you are here. Father John is upstairs. He is in a great deal of pain."

I was ushered to his room on the second floor. A delightful touch of irony was evident, one that, I was certain, he must have enjoyed on happier days. The prior occupied what once had been Mrs McConnell's boudoir. The alterations he had introduced spoke of the broad interests and insights of this intelligent, witty, cultured man. The spacious bed-sitting room of old had been transformed into an orderly private office complete with a number of carefully placed reference books, while the frolicking nude nymphs splashing joyously across the frescoed ceiling of the ensuite bathroom had been allowed to frolic on.

My patient and his bedroom were, however, nowhere to be seen. His private quarters, it turned out, were behind the oak door near the northwest corner of the office. What had previously been the compact dressing room of the lady of the house was now the monk's bedroom. This approximately twelve-by-eight-foot space was bare save for a cot against the near wall, a simple wooden chair, and a plain bedside stand. That is all. A second doorway on the end wall of this cubicle led to the shelves and clothes hooks required to meet the modest needs of a monk's personal attire. Art history and architecture had been respected, the monk's humility and simplicity of needs honoured.

The warmth of his greeting as I reached his private nook spoke for itself. He was, however, experiencing severe low back pain which he attributed to an old disc problem. Following my physical examination, I telephoned a senior colleague at the Montreal Neurological Institute. He would see him promptly.

Late on the day of that appointment, my phone rang and a rather puzzled, if not disconcerted, colleague put it to me as politely as possible that I might have mentioned to him that Father John had a known malignancy which had spread to his spine. I was astonished yet had to smile in realizing that, although Father John had spoken with apparent candour about his history of disc disease and the severity of his distress, this reserved, very private man had neglected to mention that in recent months he had been under treatment for cancer. In speaking about it later, he pointed out with sincerity and humility that he had preferred that others did not know about his critical state: he feared it would complicate relationships by drawing attention to himself and away from his work. From that point on, our PCS Home Care team was involved, always at the discrete distance dictated by the patient.

On 6 October 1982 Father John was to deliver the closing plenary address at our Fourth International Congress. Though I offered to arrange for an alternate speaker, he insisted on honouring his commitment, asking only for an elevated bar stool at the podium to enable conservation of energy. It would be his last public address. Only later did we learn that throughout his talk he was in pain. He preferred physical discomfort to risking compromised clarity of expression due to analgesic medications. His remarks, later published as *Death – The Inner Journey*, began: "*The person who would find his life must lose it*. A paradox is a frightening reality to confront because we are faced with two equally true forces each contradicting the other and yet holding each other in place." As his presentation closed, the audience could not know the personal depths he had mined on their behalf:

What are the practical conclusions that we can draw from all of this? Conclusions that are relevant to all of us present here – those who care for the dying and for all of us who are on the road that requires that we each face death. I think they are quite simply these: First, we must all prepare for death. Just as we prepare for life by our education, so must we prepare for death. Secondly, to live fully we must live in relationship with others. We must live our lives with love. To learn to love we must learn to die to self. Thirdly, meditation is the perennial wisdom that appears in all ages and all traditions leading us away from egoism and its limitations, into love. And finally, meditation is, therefore, well-called in the tradition – *the first death*. It is essential preparation for the second death which is our definitive entry into eternal life.

In caring for Father John during his final weeks, Sue Britton, our highly experienced nurse, remarked on two features that distinguished him from other patients. "While he was experiencing some physical pain, nevertheless he seemed to have sublimated the pain to a higher level. I attributed this to his disciplined life of meditation. [Furthermore,] he was not hanging on but was letting go. This memory has helped me immeasurably in preparing others for death."

Father John died on 30 December 1982 with the members of his community at his bedside. He was fifty-six years old. Laurence Freeman, on whose shoulders had fallen the colossal task of building and shaping Father John's pioneering centre for Christian meditation, was thirty-one. He had just lost his father figure, teacher, mentor, colleague, project founder, and friend.

In the months following Father John's death, Laurence and I established a routine of taking an hour-long early-morning walk on Mount Royal each Wednesday. While we covered a wide range of topics as the months passed, we found particular food for thought in sharing the parallel challenges of our respective vocations. These rambling explorations proved to be richly rewarding for both of us. A rare privilege for me, they continued for a year or so, revealing my companion to be a man of absolute integrity, singularity of purpose, and unflinching courage in the face of daunting challenges. Laurence's new mantle was weighty, the community needy. Certainly, the disciple was apt and able, but he was the first to recognize the impact of so great a loss.

COMING HOME: BRICKS, MORTAR, AND COMMUNITY

Life was filled with dizzying newness. On 26 March 1983, with the support and presence of choir, family, and friends, Linda and I were married at our church, Dominion Douglas United, by the Reverend Farquhar. In August we left for a combined honeymoon and lecture tour of Tahiti, Australia, and Japan.

That fall, our home acquired a new "commander-in-chief" and long-term boarder, West Highland White Terrier "Vickie."[4] We moved to a larger flat on Victoria Avenue so that Chris could join us. Then, in February 1984, Jamie moved in as Chris moved on. Finally, in February 1985, we settled into our permanent home at 4018 Marlowe Avenue. In every sense it was a profoundly joyous "coming home." With the tireless help of Linda's parents, Bud and Alice, we began restorations to life and lodgings by scrubbing and painting throughout, stripping away layer upon layer of paint to expose glorious oak panelling that had been long buried according to the taste of former times. Our beloved paintings were carefully hung and the ground, both in back and front, was prepared for Linda's gardens. We were home.

That same month, Ina presided over our RVH PCS 10th Anniversary Seminar.[5] As we gathered for that special celebration, I scanned an incomplete list of colleagues who had worked with us over the previous decade.[6] They were the reason for the success of our pioneering experiment. Reflecting our primary goal, we had initiated, under Robin Cohen's leadership as director of research, the development of the McGill Quality of Life Instrument, identifying progression toward improved quality of life, or QOL, as "healing" and regression toward a decline in QOL as "wounding."

Throughout these years we visited the priory for Laurence's Monday evening "introduction to meditation" sessions, although I still felt a faltering need to guard my Hans Kungian evaluative stance concerning the Catholic tendency to hang on to "medieval theology, liturgy, church law and the power structures emanating from Rome." My resistance was, however, proving to be increasingly vacuous given my deepening bond with the three Vaniers: Trappist Monk Father Benedict at Oka, Thérèse at St Christopher's, and Jean at L'Arche Troisly Breuil, France.

One sunny late July afternoon, our doorbell rang in the midst of Jamie's birthday party on the back deck. With eight rowdy teenagers at the picnic table devouring hot dogs amidst gales of laughter, I hurried to the door. There stood Jean, hair ruffled, a questioning smile present on that magnificent craggy face.

"Bal, I am here without a place to sleep. Will you take me in?"

"Jean, welcome! What a pleasure! I'm afraid you'll have to put up with a bit of bedlam. We're in the middle of a birthday party – Jamie's 17th."

"That's perfect. Parties are what we do best at l'Arche."

We went through to the back and squeezed onto the crowded bench. Jamie and his friends, as well as Chris and Lauren, had no idea who had just joined us. He was simply one of the gang. And I found myself wondering how often I, too, am blind to the presence of grace, greatness, and the transcendent.

By the late 1980s, Linda and I left our church to become unofficial adherents at the priory and, later, aspiring "Protestant-Benedictine Oblates." The priory seemed to enable softening of perspective, ease of community, and an opening to mystery. *But the question remains. How does one silence the brain chatter, even for a second or two?*

Over these years we grew ever-closer to Laurence. Music and lingering meals over a bottle of wine at our home or at the *Place* were accompanied by endless discussions that found joy in dissecting the gifts and challenges facing each of us, as well as the priory and its lay community[7]; delight in parallel passages in the wisdom literature of the various traditions; niggling debate regarding the potential of psychotherapy as a helpful accompaniment to meditation (Bal, yea; Laurence nay); celebratory moments cheating at Scrabble; swimming around the Island; and sharing twilight Mass on the screened-in porch as the gold of dusk faded into the deepening blues and blacks of pine and sky to the accompaniment of the inevitable loon somewhere down the lake.

But a bumpy road lay ahead as Laurence attempted to implement Father John's dream of a Christian meditating community. Linda and I were drawn into negotiations through our bonds to Laurence, our deepening, if neophyte, practice of meditation, our closeness to members of the priory community, and our clear memory of Father John and his expressed goals. The path was tortuous, often painful, but always instructive. Laurence was to teach us a great deal about stewardship, grace, forgiveness, and unswerving commitment, and in so doing he would have a deep impact on our lives and those of countless others.

During the September 1990 John Main Seminar given by Jean Vanier in London, I joined Laurence and an informal working group of supporters in seeking advice from Jean regarding the way forward for the international community of meditators. My mind was filled with images of the Jean Vanier I knew – the quietly thoughtful listener, the man of infinite patience and grace, the consummate pourer of oil on troubled waters. In a way, all of that was still there in spades, but, in addition, I was awestruck to encounter a Jean Vanier I had *not* seen before, a man of extraordinary executive ability, an astute philosopher able to dissect complex subjects and cut through affective encrustations to the crux of each issue. Shrewd, probing questions were asked; insightful advice given. Here was intellect, grace, wisdom, compassion, clarity of thought, depth, and discernment. The potential for a global monastery without walls was becoming clear.

During the final session of that London seminar, there would be the sole opportunity for registrants to discuss with Jean the rich material he had presented over the preceding days. The questions were astute, his answers clarifying and insightful, gracious, and mind-expanding. In Jean we encountered a scholar who had the ability to speak with both simplicity and depth about the spiritual life.

The session was nearing a satisfying conclusion when a burly, tousle-haired Irish priest in a bulky Aran-knit sweater made his way to the microphone. His expression suggested great anguish; he was flushed, his face contorted with emotion – Anger? Sadness? Dejection? Disillusionment?

"Jean Vanier, I don't understand you at all! I just don't understand you! You have been in the church all these years. You *know* its hypocrisy! And yet you say nothing!" He wasn't shouting, but his rich Irish brogue was loud and choking.

I was moved by the man's distress. Here was someone who had suffered some unidentified injustice. My head swivelled to see Jean's expression, anticipating the deep compassion, the soul-probing depth I had seen characterizing his listening in the past. But he was smiling. *Smiling?* Actually, gently laughing! *My God Jean, don't laugh. Can't you see he is suffering?* Before I could turn back to observe the man's reaction to this unexpected response, Jean spoke through his smile. His voice was gentle.

"But my friend, don't you understand? The church is just you and me and a couple of other guys." What more was there to say?

Medical Students and the Denial of Death

Depend upon it, sir, when a man knows he is to be hanged in a fortnight, it
concentrates his mind wonderfully.

Samuel Johnson[1]

But first, that's alright, go ahead and cry.
Cry, cry, cry your heart out.
It's love. It's your only path.
O people, I am so sorry.
Nothing can be hid.
It's a circle in the round.
It's group theatre,
No wings, no backstage, no leading act.

Ted Rosenthal,
How Could I Not Be Among You?

My urology teaching responsibilities sometimes seemed to be simply another task in a busy day. Let's face it, whatever my personal interest in the topics at hand, most students found that my enthusiasm for issues genito-urinary had little relevance to their personal professional plans. Not so with palliative care. From the first, I found palliative-care discussions with the medical students a highlight in my week.

The reason became clear early on as I listened to these would-be doctors in small group sessions. They reminded me of the overwhelming neurosis-inducing challenges and pressures that colour their daily experience. These bright, achievement-oriented young men and women, who generally come to medical education with at least one science degree tucked under their belts, not to mention awe-inspiring past accomplishments as community-service volunteers, competitive athletes, award-winning musicians, or Himalayan mountain climbers, find themselves immersed

in a maze of interactive issues spiralling from macroscopic, to micro-
scopic, to quantum. They inhabit a world overwhelmed by data that have
been refined in a multitude of fast-forward laboratories, data that are
animal-tested and whose efficacy is verified in randomized clinical trials
and then processed through the Cochrane Review strainer to be spewed
out as evidence-based "best practice" standards of care. *A never-ending
tsunami of factoids that someone's life could depend on me knowing!*

When we chat in small group sessions, I learn that most of these discerning, driven, compassionate young people chose to study medicine
because they wanted to help others. Simple as that. But somewhere along
the way the people part is eclipsed. Once trust is established and defences
are down, the flow of their angst may run something like the following:

> Such a jungle of details to consider if I am ever to treat a patient
> – even *one*! The consultant this morning asked me, "What about
> her kidney function, *Doctor*? Do you think her renal perfusion is
> irrelevant?" And all I could think of was that I didn't have a chance
> to read that chapter last night. It was, after all, 2:30 A.M. and I had
> to be back on the ward before 8:00! What about the effects of her
> ageing? Her co-morbid conditions? Her alcoholism? The fact that
> she is a smoker? There are whole *chapters* of life-or-death determin-
> ing factors hanging over her head, or rather, over *my* head! And by
> the way, did you notice how disdainful Dr T. was when I hadn't a
> clue about that recent *Lancet* article?

The woman that student had hoped to "help" no longer existed. She
had dissolved into the pathophysiology of her disease. Furthermore, this
aspiring young colleague was discovering that his/her own personhood
had also been sacrificed on the altar of medical science. In addition, there
was yet another issue working against these students, the unconscious
death anxiety that plays a roll in everything we say and do.[2]

What is the impact of this depersonalizing cascade on that student
and her/his colleagues? On their patients? How equipped are they to
deal with the inevitable subliminal ache of personal transience? What
defences can they call on? Knowing the "science" may help, but it isn't
the whole answer. Something deeper is being threatened day by day.

Palliative care, indeed all patient care, must embrace a broad spectrum
of goals: to recognize the person in the patients, their families, and ourselves as caregivers; to grasp the differences between experienced illness
and disease; to understand the complex array of contributors to suffering and how to identify those relevant in this individual; to ask what

"healing" means; to question whether we can die "healed"; to consider the determinants of healing for each member of the therapeutic triad (patient, family member, *and* caregiver); to examine critically the caregiver-patient relationship, its significance and its potential; to reflect on why Carl Jung and the wisdom traditions of the great religions differentiate between ego-related *self* and our deeper potential *Self*; to monitor our personal battle fatigue as caregivers and the daily cost of that fatigue to our inner journey toward wholeness. In short, to acknowledge the art as well as the science of medicine and the fine balance between the two.

How can one "teach" all that? There were two sessions I felt privileged to give in the first-year medicine curriculum at McGill on an annual basis that consistently provoked open dialogue concerning these issues.

Psychologist Herman Feifel published his landmark book *The Meaning of Death* in 1959. Featuring contributions by a galaxy of eminent thinkers, it shed light on death and suggested that our culture is ill-equipped to deal with transience, ageing, and dying. That conclusion seemed consistent with the findings of our 1973 Royal Vic study, and thus, in the early years, I presented a half-hour examination of these issues during my student lectures.

That was to be only the beginning. Once aware of our endemic death-denying stance, I began to recognize evidence of its presence everywhere. Driving home one day I heard the same theme voiced in a popular song on the car radio. Before long I noticed another. Songwriters, it seemed, had particular awareness of this domain. I made lists of the best examples of death denial and, as time passed, I came to realize that this thread of discomfort runs through the very fabric of our daily lives.

The original half-hour student session expanded to one and a half-hours followed by a discussion that occupied at least another half-hour. "Death, Our Silent Dancing Partner: North American Attitudes to Death and How They Got to Be That Way" was shoehorned into the McGill medical-student curriculum and was offered in other settings as well. It combined an avalanche of cultural/historic observations, images, pop-music segments,[3] and recordings of the spoken word, among them: Hitler ranting before hundreds of thousands of rabid Nazi supporters; Martin Luther King's prophetic words spoken hours before his assassination; the observations of a grieving widow during a radio phone-in show – a conspiracy of silence regarding her husband's cancer prognosis had destroyed their customary open communications during his final months. In the last case, the exquisite clarity of the widow's anger and pain, caused by the doctor, was devastating to hear.

We began to appreciate the unexpected relevance in our daily lives of the probing confrontation between Zorba the Greek (Anthony Quinn) and the young scholar (Alan Bates) in the 1964 film:

"Why do the young die? Why does anybody die, tell me."

"I don't know."

"What's the use of all your damn books? If they don't tell you that, what the hell do they tell you?"

"They tell me about the agony of men who can't answer questions like yours."

Ted Rosenthal was thirty when he was told that he had acute leukemia. I first encountered him through the prize-winning Public Broadcasting System (PBS) documentary film *How Could I Not Be Among You?* during its late-night television screening and then later through his poetry and prose in his 1973 Avon book of the same name. His story became the subject of my second lecture addressing end-of-life issues.

Rosenthal was an arresting figure. His broad forehead was framed by long, dark, now thinning, post-chemotherapy hair and his still abundant beard and moustache. He was wrapped against wind and world by his duffle coat, its shielding collar turned up. He was a man on fire with earnestness, urgency, and a message that he needed to share. He wanted us to benefit from the cliff-edge drama engulfing him, his wife, and their two small children as he found himself in a world of thermometers, boredom, and racing "mud thoughts" as well as the daily trivia that repeatedly interrupted his numbing reality with an urge to "vomit the mind." He had much to teach us. In his last words he urged us to "keep moving, people," but then he asked in awe and wonderment, as we all must, "How could I not be among you?"

Each year the first-year class and I hunkered down in Rosenthal's world and as the film ended we were surrounded by intense silence. The discussion that followed was always thoughtful, self-disclosing, rich, and at times raw. Handwritten student letters in follow-up were not uncommon.

Jan. 12

After sitting through your lecture today, I am totally unable to concentrate on details (the small ones – like head & neck anatomy) ... You know the syndrome. I find one part of myself screaming both emotionally and mentally for life and answers, while another feels the need to respond to a comment made in class. Before I lose this energy, I think I'll do the latter. I really want you to hear this.

Following the film today, many interesting things were said. It is one of these that I wish to address. A well-spoken classmate of mine raised the issue that we, as directed, ambitious, forward-looking youths, had little in common with this starry-eyed hippie dreamer (excuse the paraphrase) – that we, as future-oriented people could not feel empty or dissociated from expectation simply because of our station in life.

Somehow, although I had not the energy to challenge this statement in class, I would like you to know that not all of us are so incredibly directed or practical. Some of us felt that Ted Rosenthal was not simply an example of an undirected person who is facing death, but rather that he was one of the most sane and perceptive people we'd heard speak lately. For myself, I can say (quite honestly) that the emptiness he spoke of is mirrored in my life (when I decide to allow myself to see it), as is the effusive joy at the wonders of *life*, of nature, of simply *being*. I am intensely bothered by the belief that by selecting medicine as my course of study and career, I have begun to squelch my humanity – that by directing my life in this way I have chosen to suffocate the present in view of some wondrous and glowing imagined future. I know that I am not alone in this train of thought and that many of my classmates consider themselves a bit star-struck as well.

In any case, I'd like to thank you for raising these issues and forcing me to think (again). Also, (as the practical medical student), I'd like to ask you where I can find Ted Rosenthal's poetry. If you have any leads on this please let me know. Thank you for your time, energy and perspective. M.B.

Sharing our visceral response to death and dying with the students consistently gave way to an intimate exchange of thoughts about life, death, meaning, our values, and our chosen profession.

It was, I believe, largely based on these memorable shared moments that the McGill medicine class of 1983 requested that I give the convocation address at their graduation. This landmark family occasion was to be celebrated in the grand splendour of Salle Wilfrid-Pelletier at Montreal's Place des Arts. It felt like a unique opportunity. I held the students in such high esteem! What focus would do justice to this most special occasion? It mustn't simply be the usual trite platitudes. What important reality should we consider together in this, our last, meeting?

The personal demands exacted during the physician's professional lifetime came to mind. I had frequently discussed the challenges that

face every busy doctor and his or her family with my longtime friend
and colleague Merv Vincent. Now a few decades into his career, Merv,
a respected psychiatrist, had cared for three hundred medical colleagues
who were alcoholics. He knew the cost of a life lived in the shadow of
Hippocrates. His data on the high incidence of alcoholism, divorce, and
suicide among physicians were troubling and had been confirmed by
others. In congratulating our graduates, perhaps I could add a timely
cautionary word about the risks as well as the rewards that lay ahead
and the need to look after both themselves and their families.

The splendidly turned-out parents and distinguished guests had settled
with a respectful, if quietly excited, hum just in back of the empty seats
reserved for the row upon row of new medical graduates who then filed
into the hall dressed in their plain black gowns. The expectant, beaming
parents seemed to swell visibly as they craned to pick out of the throng
"their son (or daughter) the Doctor"!

On entering the vast magnificence of Salle Wilfrid-Pelletier as a member of the officiating party, I was impressed by two things: the size of
the venue when viewed for the first time from the vantage point of the
platform party, and the fact that the approximately three-thousand-seat
auditorium appeared to be full to overflowing.

We, the members of the academic procession, were undoubtedly suitably impressive in our academic dress. Solemn. Even stately. We entered
to the strains of a subdued but heraldic overture. With our full-length
gowns, colourful, university-specific hoods, and appropriate academic
caps, tams, or bonnets in place, we presented a dazzling spectacle, each
telltale set of markings boasting (to those knowing the secret code)
the particular identity of one or another of the finest centres of higher
learning in the world. Preceding me in this august procession was the
honorary-degree recipient, an internationally respected, white-haired
octogenarian. We were elegance writ large as we found our place in our
individually labelled seats on stage as the ceremony began.

Now to be fair to myself, I *had* realized that my sobering warnings to
our graduates must be accompanied by a more traditional note of celebration, so I added a clarion call to "ascend to the mountain tops," or
some such thing, in my closing phrases.

All I remember of my convocation address was the progressive blanching that transformed the sea of beaming faces peering up at me as we
considered the likelihood of alcoholism, depression, and suicide. *This is
not going well!* I attempted a mid-course correction by adding particular emphasis to each mountain-top-related word, but I am afraid that,

this late in the game, my call to the heights provoked first a sprinkling of guffaws and then frank laughter in disbelief.

All stood as the platform party finally filed off the stage and I pondered how magicians manage, with apparent ease, to disappear at will. We were nearing the exit stairs and a deeply longed for escape when the newly honoured octogenarian LLD at my side leaned over and pronounced with feeling in my ear, "*That* was the *most* remarkable convocation address I have ever heard!" I felt a very faint flush of uncertain relief. Then he added, with particular emphasis, "and *certainly* the most inappropriate!" I walked-ran the five miles home, successfully avoiding contact with all life forms. *Perhaps there might be an opening at another university, or perhaps a small village somewhere.*

A postscript. In 1979–80 one of the students attending the "How Could I Not Be Among You" session was Dave Williams, who was a member of that 1983 graduating class. Fifteen years later, on 17 April 1998, Linda, our daughter Bethany (whom we had adopted three years earlier), and I were Dave's guests at the Cape Kennedy Space Center for the thunderous, fiery, earth-shaking, heart-stopping lift-off of the space shuttle *Columbia* carrying Mission Specialist 3 Dr Dave Williams. With his STS-90 Neurolab colleagues, Dave was to carry out twenty-six life-science experiments on the effects of microgravity on the brain and nervous system while orbiting the Earth 256 times, covering 6.3 million miles and logging 381 hours in space. It was an unforgettable experience. An invitation from a member of *that* class seemed akin to an unexpected commuting of a death sentence.

But there was to be more. Nine years later, on 8 August 2007, Dave was a member of the STS-118 crew aboard the space shuttle *Endeavour* as it lifted off, bound for the International Space Station where, standing on the end of Canadarm2, he would complete three space walks entailing seventeen hours and forty-seven minutes of extravehicular time.

The *Canadian Medical Association Journal* issue of 23 June 2009 contains an essay by Dave describing his second space walk four days into the mission. He explained that he was to remove, then replace, a malfunctioning gyroscope, one of four that were critical in maintaining the orientation of the space station. He was accompanied by his fellow crew member Rick Mastracchio.

Dave's *CMAJ* account conveyed the moment-to-moment attention to detail involved in coordinating the precision choreography between the space walkers and the crew operating the complex robotic arm from inside the space station, noting that "a single mistake can start a chain of catastrophic consequences." Two years of training had gone into each manoeuvre by the crew of seven.

The pilot driving the arm that would carry Dave more than thirty metres to the shuttle's payload bay asked if he was "ready for motion." Dave's *CMAJ* account continued:

"Ready for motion," I reply. I've said the words hundreds of times in training, but today is the first time I'll actually ride the famous arm.

Controlled by our seasoned pilot, the arm starts to move. Our 350 kilometre altitude provides an astonishing view of Earth moving beneath us 25 times the speed of sound. We're traveling 8 km per second, faster than a bullet. Far below, whole continents drift by in minutes.

Years ago, in another millennium, during my medical studies at McGill University in Montreal, Quebec, I read poet Ted Rosenthal's book, *How Could I Not Be Among You?* chronicling his emotional response to the terminal phases of leukaemia. For Rosenthal, the final phases of death provided profound insights. His value of living "in the moment," capturing forever the joy, wonder and beauty of each moment in our lives has guided me for 3 decades. Standing alone on the slowly moving arm, suspended in space, I finally understood the significance of his words.

Turning slowly to my right, I look over the gleaming white shuttle into the infinite void of space. There is blackness no earthly experience has prepared me for. There is nothing to be seen, no stars, no planets, just the vast unforgiving, cold, emptiness of space. To my left I see a fine latticework of clouds scattered over the Pacific. The sun is beginning to set, highlighting the thin turquoise layer of the Earth's atmosphere. Beneath me is home. Home to all of us struggling to live together in countries separated by borders that I cannot see. The entire history of all species including ours, has taken place on the blue sphere turning far below. I look back to my right at the infinity extending beyond our solar system, beyond known and unknown galaxies. I wonder if life existed somewhere in that vastness. In seconds that will stay with me a lifetime, I truly sense what it means to live "in the moment."

"Call the stop and let me know when you're ready to go to the worksite." ... [The call of pilot Charlie "Scorch" Hobaugh] brings me back to the task at hand. As I ease toward the shuttle, the sound of my breathing blends with the quiet hum of the suit's fan. The significance of our mission is dwarfed by the magnitude of infinite space and cosmic time. It is an extremely humbling experience, yet I feel satisfied with the realization of the truth in Rosenthal's words that "whatever it is you have, you've already got. Right there. And it makes that moment an eternity." In one brief eternity, I felt embraced in the 4.5 billion-year history of our planet.[4]

The Eighties: Wounded Healers a Decade On

*The conclusion is that the care of the dying and their families can be
greatly improved. The cost involved is minimal – insignificant in the light of
the suffering alleviated. There is, in fact, a saving in costs per patient treated.
A palliative care service can make it possible for more patients to die at home.
It can free active treatment beds in an acute care hospital and increase the
number of teaching beds in institutions where that is a priority concern.
The success of this project is a magnificent testimony to the dedication
and enthusiasm of a remarkable team.*

Excerpt from the Preface to the
Royal Victoria Hospital Palliative Care
Service Pilot-Project Report

1984

The year 1984 brought both personal and global reminders of transience: the Ethiopian famine claiming 400,000 lives; a massive acciden-
tal explosion of missiles in the USSR, heightening global awareness of
the risk of war, intentional or otherwise; the defoliant Agent Orange
causing hundreds of thousands of birth defects and the deaths of countless servicemen; Indira Gandhi's assassination in New Delhi; an estimated 16,000 dead resulting from a methyl-isocyanate gas leak from the
Union Carbide plant in Bhopal, India.

On the home front, the term "Palliative Care Service" and the McGill
program bearing that name celebrated its tenth anniversary. The year
1984 was to be a time of change and renewal. Yvonne Corbeil replaced
senior administrator Dottie Wilson, Mary Coughlan replaced Kitty
Markey as volunteer director, and, in response to my suggestion that we
recruit a new PCS director, McGill Dean of Medicine Richard Cruess

offered me a one-year sabbatical. For me, it was to be a time of renewal through study, reading, drawing, and painting.

Pope Jean Paul II visited Montreal that September. I was closing the newspaper on the morning he was to be in town when I noted that he would be at St Joseph's Oratory in an hour or so. "Joe's Place," as it is affectionately known, was nearby. Linda was teaching. It seemed silly not to bicycle over and have a look.

Queen Mary Road was blocked off for the occasion. The streets, in fact, were empty. Leaving my bike against a nearby fence, I stepped onto the street to lean against the barrier at the point where the motorcade would turn into the oratory grounds. I was alone: no police, no press, no spectators.

Just then, the papal procession came around the corner. John Paul II was standing in his "popemobile," and, as it reached the sharp turn directly in front of me, it slowed to a crawl so as not to spill its cargo. As a result, the pope and I found ourselves standing perhaps ten feet apart, alone and facing each other. There was a sense of personal contact, but neither of us spoke. I suspect I smiled; he acknowledged our meeting with a penetrating gaze and apparent interest. I felt that he was the "good man" I had anticipated. The next day I used a newspaper photo taken at the oratory as a model for a quick sketch. It was a crossing of paths that some years hence I would have cause to reflect on.

Letters from Cicely during those months continued the frequent contact that I valued so highly. She wrote to say that her husband (since 1980), Polish artist Marian Bohusz-Szyszko, though unsteady, would be able to attend a private audience with the pope in Rome. In a later note she observed: "We are well and cheerful – at least Marian's fine – I'm recovering from another of my falls – battered and bruised but not broken. I literally fell into the Motor Neurone Disease Association where I was speaking."

About the same time, Ken MacKinnon, who had left Montreal in 1982 to take up a new post at the Halifax Infirmary, wrote: "Bal, you are so right in your stance on transience – my intensity of awareness is rapidly accelerating. My present admin. job here will continue – perhaps 2 years. Do you think I might then find a role in Palliative Care (part-time)? How long a training experience would I require?" His query proved to be the initial overture that would lead to his involvement in the development of palliative care in Nova Scotia.

McGill's 1–3 October 1984 Fifth Biennial International Congress on Care of the Terminally Ill zeroed in on the topics of current concern in our field. As in the past, registrants sat at round tables for ten, and plenary presentations were discussed at each table followed by open discussion from the floor.[1] In addition, nineteen submitted films were offered for registrant viewing and a special plenary session was convened to explore issues related to the threat of nuclear war: "Concerns for a Terminally Ill Planet."

Initially, I had hoped that Mother Teresa[2] might participate in the 1984 Congress. Perhaps, I mused, McGill might give her an honorary degree. Clearly, that would be more than fitting given her unique contributions to the global community. Such ceremonies, however, are held during faculty convocations which would not coincide with our October Congress dates. Nevertheless, after further discussion with the principal and vice-chancellor, he suggested that I "proceed with the invitation and we'll work out the details if she agrees."

How to reach Mother Teresa? I found her Circle Road, Calcutta, address in Malcolm Muggeridge's 1971 book *Something Beautiful for God* and picked up the phone, asking for the overseas operator. To my utter astonishment, the voice of my assistant was that of comedian Lily Tomlin's infamous creation, telephone operator "Ernestine." *Exactly* Ernestine!

"Hello, how may I help you?" she snorted. Though perhaps less condescending and a fraction more sympathetic than the Ernestine I knew on the radio, the effect was distracting. *Phoning Mother Teresa? With the assistance of Ernestine? This can't be happening! I'll have to make this very official, or it ain't gonna fly!*

"Yes, well, I'd like to speak to Mother Teresa on Circle Road in Calcutta, India. Unfortunately, I do not have the telephone number. I'm calling on behalf of McGill University," I proclaimed in the most official tone I could muster.

"I'll have to go through Bombay to get that number. Do you want me to call Bombay?" Ernestine responded in her usual semi-dismissive Ernestine tone, which managed to convey that she handles several calls for Mother Teresa daily.

Do I want you to call Bombay? Why else would I ...? "Yes, please." There followed a dial ... dial... dial.

The voice answering in Bombay was incomprehensible.

Ernestine interrupted her Indian colleague in English, completely unfazed. "This is Canada calling for the number for Mother Teresa, Circle Road, Calcutta."

Following a long pause our Bombay friend responded in English. "The number is ..." I wrote it down. Ernestine interjected, "The number is ... Do you want me to put the call through to Calcutta?"

Do I want you to put the call through? "Yes ... please!"... dial ... dial ... dial.

A young woman answered on the second ring: "Sisters of Charity," she said. Her voice was gentle, remarkably expressive, even lyrical. For some reason, those three words, coming from her, spoke volumes. I found her words grace-filled and unexpectedly moving.

"Canada calling Mother Teresa," trumpeted Ernestine.

"Mother is not here. She is in Rome. She is at the Vatican. Do you want her number there?" asked the quiet angelic voice.

"Mother Teresa isn't there. She is in Rome at the Vatican," repeated Ernestine. "Do you want her number?" *Good grief ... At the Vatican? ... With the pope? ...*

Do I want her number? It would seem callous to interrupt ... But I have come this far ...

"Yes ... please."

"Yes, we would like her number in Rome," repeated Ernestine.

"Mother's number at the Vatican is ..." said the angelic voice. I wrote it down.

"Mother Teresa's number at the Vatican is ..." repeated Ernestine. "Do you want me to call the Vatican?" *I know. I heard her! Good grief!* "Yes ... *please!*"... dial ... dial ... dial.

The answering voice was male, authoritative, and loud. He was speaking Italian.

"Canada calling Mother Teresa," sailed in Ernestine, in English.

"Mutha Teresa isa nota heah," the Vatican official intoned. "She's ona retreata in aSpain. Do you wannah her numbah in Spain?"

"Mother Teresa isn't ..." parroted Ernestine.

"I know!" I shouted. "I heard him." By this point, I was perspiring profusely.

This is ghastly ... I can't bother her... I mustn't! On retreat, for God's sake – literally! ... That would be unthinkable ... But, I have come this far ... "Yes, please," I whispered.

"Yes, we would like the number," said Ernestine in her unflappable monotone.

"Mutha Teresa's numbah ina Spain isa ..." I wrote it down.

"Mother Teresa's number ..." started Ernestine. "I KNOW!" I protested.

"Do you want me to call ..." *Oh Lord!*

"YES!" I roared. ... dial ... dial ... dial.

"Mother Teresa speaking."

My throat went dry. Totally dry. I literally couldn't speak. I cleared my throat and swallowed hard.

"Mother Teresa, I am so sorry to bother you while you are on retreat. My name is

Mount, Dr Mount, I am calling on behalf of McGill University in Canada and the

Palliative Care Service for the dying at the Royal Victoria Hospital. We would like to invite you to be the keynote speaker at our International Congress, 1–3 October this year. McGill would be honoured by your presence and the university would like to offer you an honorary degree at that time."

"Oh, Dr Mount," her voice was calm, her response instantaneous. "How kind. But you know, Dr Mount, you don't need me. The only person you need is Jesus."

"Well, we were sort of hoping to have both of you," I responded hesitantly.

She chuckled. "He'll do just fine."

DAD

Dad's eighty-eighth birthday was on 13 February 1984; four months later, his loving sister, Veda, turned 90. He would not accept the invitation to move in with either Jim or me. Instead, as his frailty increased, Vera Kestner, a patient during the early days of his practice, was recruited by ever-vigilant Veda to be Dad's housekeeper. With Veda and Vera's support he could remain safely ensconced in his eighth-floor condominium at 300 The Driveway, enjoying the daily memory-rich liturgy of winding the grandfather clock and the graceful tree-lined panorama of waterway and passersby far below. How each piece of furniture, each painting, each richly textured area rug, each carefully planned living space reminded him of Mother! Her clothes still hung in the closet.

Although blind in the left eye, Dad could still manage serviceable penmanship and his mind was generally alert. We wrote each other at least twice a week. Both long and short-term memory were intact: he could describe a handful of pivotal moments in our early family life with great clarity. At the same time, he had pointedly questioned me about my impending sabbatical leave. "Have you made definite plans as to who will take over your leadership in your absence?"

His long-standing restlessness and enquiring mind remained, causing him to observe, "I always need a bone to chew on!" He was puzzled by his increasing weakness.

"Frankly, I cannot evaluate my problem and do not recall having ever had such a group of symptoms outlined by any patient I have ever seen professionally – my general weakness is associated with a decrease in desire for food and almost constant sensation of 'pins & needles' penetrating my feet & legs with no cessation." In each letter he reflected on his loneliness, Mother's perfection as wife and mother, and the affection we shared for her.

He remained engaged in life during the early months of 1984. "I plan to go to the YMCA today. Each Friday the luncheon speaker is on for noon. It is a very excellent weekly experience." As the year drew to a close, however, his strength decreased as his restlessness and episodes of clouded thinking increased. With Christmas approaching we moved him to Jim and Ursula's home at 37 Opeongo. He was increasingly forgetful and had progressive weakness and periods of drowsiness and edginess, yet he remained characteristically concerned that he was not "suitably attired" if he was without a tie when family pictures were taken.

"But, Dad, I don't have one either," I reassured him.

"Yes," he responded coolly. "I noticed."

New Year's Eve, 1984, brought a peaceful sense of community that I could not have imagined hours earlier. Dad had rallied. Linda and I were with him. We shared a pot of chocolate fondue with fresh fruit and a bottle of chilled champagne as the three of us celebrated the occasion with delight and quiet joy. We chatted. "The Island," he mused quietly. "How Maude loved the loons!" He wanted to hear our up-to-date news. We complied: Wren's seventeenth birthday and graduation from Westmount High School had been followed by a trip to England to volunteer at Sheila Cassidy's St Luke's Hospice in Plymouth, then backpacking in Wales; Chris had turned twenty, moved into his own apartment, and taken a job at the Ritz Carlton while puzzling over his future – maybe some English courses to sharpen his songwriting skills; Jamie, fourteen, was coming into his own – taking apart the Johnson 4 outboard motor at the Island, diagnosing the problem and improvising repairs; he was a tireless worker, born mechanic, skilled impersonator, and avid fisherman. He loved sailing and waterskiing. Jamie was the glue in the family.

"Why I've never heard tell of material like this!" Dad enthused, as he layered waves of rich dark chocolate sauce on a section of tangerine. "It is most unusual. I've never had anything like this before. I can't recall a more fitting and appropriate evening." Linda and I caught each other's glance. Neither could we.

Dad peered over his champagne glass with a smile. "Let's have a little more of that material." He nodded toward the fondue pot. "It has been a wonderful evening – and a memorable year, for that matter."

A FURTHER OPENING OF DOORS

With a decade behind us, my PCS priorities turned to our sister hospitals in the McGill system. The presence of Ina and later Anna Towers, who had been director of the Family Medicine program at McGill, ensured that the Royal Vic PCU had a clinical director who was consistently available on a day-to-day basis.

Following discussions with Executive Director John Charters at the Montreal Children's Hospital, I was invited to explore the possible development of a pediatric palliative-care service there. At the same time, as interest in palliative care increased locally, nationally, and internationally, my list of speaking engagements suggested the need to be more selective in responding to the growing tidal wave of requests.[3] The year 1985 provides an example: *May*, lecturing in Norway at the Second National Norwegian Conference; *June*, speaking at the Third St Christopher's International Conference in London; *July*, initiating, with PhD nursing colleague Linda McHarg, the Montreal Children's Hospital Palliative Care Needs Assessment Study; *August*, lecturing in Adelaide, Australia; *October*, lectures in Winnipeg, Richmond, Virginia, and Los Angeles; *November*, resigning as RVH PCS director as Ina assumed that responsibility[4] and speaking at the Cleveland Clinic and Nijmegen, Holland; *December*, Ken MacKinnon arrives to train with us for a month. A number of indelible experiences from those months live on with graphic clarity these decades later.

A TASTE OF NORWAY

In May 1985, following flights from Montreal to Amsterdam, then on to Stavanger, Norway, Chris, who had just turned twenty-one, and I boarded a shuttle flight heading north to Bergen. The ragged shoreline and surrounding awe-inspiring peaks formed an arresting mosaic of islands, bays, channels, fjords, and lakes. Bergen, the capital of Norway until the early fourteenth century CE, was a trading centre from as early as 1020. Dr Stein Husebo at the Haukeland Hospital and the University of Bergen suggested that I give a lecture at the hospital and then join him and his colleagues on a six-hour bus trip north through Norway's west-coast fjords region to the village of Loen some 125 miles inland at the easternmost tip of the majestic Nordfjord. There we would join colleagues from across the country for the 13–15 May "2nd National Conference on Palliative Care" hosted by the Norwegian Cancer Foundation at the elegant (1884) Hotel Alexandra.

Stein was a slim, wiry, 5'11" bundle of energy and charisma. His lean frame, sharp eye, and restless, inventive mind betrayed his addictions to hiking, long-distance running, skiing, fishing, and dog walking, not to mention his "Renaissance man" passions as philosopher, poet, art lover, classical-music connoisseur, and ardent reader of fine literature in several languages. He had a whimsical, overflowing capacity for life. Was he Peer Gynt, the romanticized Norwegian man of the mountains? Who knew? But one could be certain of his predilections. He was richly influenced by his three Norwegian mentors – romantic composer Edvard Greig, intense artist Edvard Munch, and edgy realism playwright Henrik Ibsen, who observed, "A forest bird never wants a cage." Stein sailed an exciting course coloured by these three as he moved through life's harrowing adventures with a buoyant "Life's not so bad, eh?" and "Life's not the worst we have!" personal creed. When asked how he was doing he would simply respond, "I'm wonderful."

The village of Loen, nestling fjord-side in long-established order, is surrounded by some of the oldest farms in Norway. With the May air crisp and bracing, the sky presented a brilliant blue high above the lofty snow-capped peaks, while the compact community breathed Norwegian stewardship and hard-earned stability, situated as it was in the shadow of mountain-face scars that spoke of landslide tragedies past.

Inspired by the surroundings, Chris and I stowed our luggage in our hotel room and set our sights on scaling the impressive, if unstable, steep-shale incline just behind our lodgings. It was a venture that earned us medals for stupidity *and* honorary Norwegian citizenships from a delighted Stein, as well as his promise to introduce us next morning to our imposing neighbour, the 5,640-foot Mount Skala. We could, Stein enthused, climb it during the pre-conference early-morning hours.

It was to be a climb that involved snow to the groin (for those weighing more than Stein), loose rocks, cut arms and legs, sunburns, and serious misgivings about our sanity. Up the face toward the deceptively near-looking summit we climbed, with lingering thoughts about heart attacks as we became soaked with sweat amid repeated stops for rest, changes of socks, and countless gulps of water. We climbed for six hours, then slid back down to the tree line in thirty minutes!

During that exhilarating descent, there was a stop-time moment when I looked back at Chris who was still far above me. His arms were outstretched as he slid down the steep grade, half standing – sudden memories of a slide in New York's Central Park how many lifetimes ago? I felt a deep ache from somewhere on the underside of consciousness as the passing years were mirrored in his outstretched hands.

On reaching the tree line, co-host Ulla was waiting for the slow-moving Mounts to inform us that Stein had run on ahead to make the meeting on time. *Run! Run? ... Unbelievable!* We were hardly able to walk down the knee-breaking last half mile ... or was it 100 miles? ... Would we ever walk again? At the meeting, Stein introduced us to the audience with typically exuberant élan and a triple salute, "Henceforth it will be called Mount Balfour. I award you both honorary Norwegian passports, *and* with my admission that I am tired, and *that* doesn't happen very often!" The conference was a celebration of Norwegian competence in palliative care and hospitality.

Two days later, I made a post-conference mountainside house call accompanying home-care nurse Bente Rambolt as she visited a family she had been following for some time. The near-vertical winding trail up to the farm of Akslund Asebo, his wife, and their little post-neuroblastoma daughter afforded a spectacular view of the mountainous panorama surrounding their home. Akslund and I stood together gazing down the precipitous slope that constituted his farm. He was soft-spoken and quietly at ease.

"Is it an old farm?"

"Yes, quite old."

"How old?"

"We're not sure."

"Approximately?"

"Well it started in the eleven or twelve hundreds." Then he added almost apologetically, "But there have been some changes since then. They changed that paddock boundary down there about 150 years ago."

"I see."

Later, Akslund and I met in town in response to his invitation to attend a confirmation and baptism service at the 1837 Lutheran Loen Kyrkje. All present were in traditional Norwegian attire. In the graveyard of the church stood a thousand-year-old cross marking the spot where Christians are thought to have first assembled in inner Nordfjord.

As I review this account, I recognize that I have self-consciously omitted part of my conversation with Akslund. As we stood surveying his farm, he turned to me and asked, "What do you think of magnetic resonance imaging [MRI]?" I was stunned. It was 1985. The first MRI reports were published in 1980. We were on mountain top in rural Norway. I was speaking to a local farmer – a remarkable man to be sure, but ...

"Akslund, I don't believe that I can give you an informed assessment. But, how in the world do you know about magnetic resonance imaging?"

He shrugged, "Oh, there was a very good article in a recent issue of *Scientific American*."

Before leaving the region, Chris and I joined our Norwegian colleagues in a trek along country paths to view the great Birksdal Glacier as I sketched and Stein took yet another swim, this time in the foreboding, motionless, turquoise meltwater lake with its floating blocks of ice at the foot of the glacier.

I believe it was as we chatted in Stein's hotel room among the piles of notes, bottle of scotch, pens, markers, scribbled drawings, letters, poems, and books that I met the deeper Stein. Like his hero, German novelist, poet, and artist Hermann Hesse, author of *Siddhartha*, *Steppenwolf*, and *The Glass Bead Game*, and winner of the 1946 Nobel Prize in Literature, Stein was engaged in a wonderfully open search for authenticity, self-knowledge, and spirituality. I would have expected nothing less – his cathedral was a remote mountaintop ski cabin and the natural world around him, his liturgy, salt air inhaled in gulps. It was in that hotel room that Stein introduced me to the work of German printmaker and sculptor Kathe Kollwitz. A copy of her *Woman with Dead Child* was lying on the desktop heap of mementos that follow Stein everywhere. I couldn't take my eyes off it: the distraught mother, hunched over and nude, is wreathed in shadows as she cradles in desperate grief the dead child in her arms, its sunbathed face fallen back toward me, eyes closed, as time stopped.[5]

I was moved by the artist's craftsmanship, but there was much more than that – *so* much more. Her drawings, etchings, and lithographs informed me about suffering that I had not known. She opened my eyes. I examined one of her self-portraits. Her unwavering gaze was staring straight at me, with left hand raised to her forehead, deep in thought. She was asking, asking, asking. And I was left searching for answers.

As Stein and I were saying goodbye, he presented me with yet another gift, a lavishly illustrated volume of the life work of Edvard Munch. As we parted, I realized that I would henceforth travel enlightened by Kollwitz and Munch, and that, when confronted by stop-time moments, I would think of Stein.

FRANCIS BACON AT THE TATE, LONDON, JUNE 1985

During a free afternoon in the schedule of St Christopher's International Conference, I joined Colin Murray Parkes and American sociologist Robert Fulton in a visit to the Tate Gallery to see a one-man show of the works of Francis Bacon. *Francis Bacon? The sixteenth-century philosopher? At the Tate?* I had no idea what lay ahead.

We emerged from the taxi and passed beneath the Tate's imposing columned facade to be greeted by a large black-and-white photograph of the artist. He was staring at us wide-eyed, his gaze challenging, penetrating, and evaluative – and *yes,* it *does* require all three adjectives. The introduction was arresting, if not somewhat numbing. *Who in the world is Francis Bacon?*

We were told that this was the second major retrospective exhibition at the Tate for this Irish-born British artist. *Second!* Remarkable; a rare occurrence, I was told. The cover of the pamphlet for the exhibit featured the dismembered head and torso of a middle-aged man against a black background. His red-rimmed eyes were closed; a swath of white paint swept down from the bloody outer corner of the right eye and forward under his nose to end on the bulbous upper lip. Beneath it, the cheek, mouth, and swollen lips remained intact but sagging for lack of underlying boney structures of cheek and jaw. Skin flaps dangled where chin had once been. His neck had been torn open to expose the larynx just above a formless smudge of blacks and blues.

I noted with incredulity the gushing evaluation in the Tate handout: "The timeless quality of his paintings allows them to hang naturally in our museums beside Rembrandt and Van Gogh, while his main themes are conveyed with a poetic appreciation which can be compared with Shakespeare or the Greek tragedies." Bacon's themes include nihilism, suffering, homosexuality, mortality, violence, existential isolation, meaninglessness, dismemberment, bowstring emotional tension, despair, the unsettling potential for emergence of the beast/human hybrid within us, and crucifixion – crucifixion not in pious Christian terms, but instead, that suggested by the splayed meat and unconscionable suffering of the abattoir. Each room in this apparently endless exhibit of graphic horrors was illuminated to operating-room intensity. Ted Rosenthal's quaint phrase "vomit the mind" swam into my consciousness.

There was something about Bacon that struck a personal chord. Why? How? Bacon, I concluded, faces us with a world of familiar, if largely unconscious, existential angst. It is a world we know all too well, yet it generally passes unrecognized given the immense effort we expend minute by minute, hour by hour, and day by day in shoring up our vulnerable egos.

Bacon is an observer who is sufficiently open and honest to express the largely unnoticed violence generated by our daily lives: our quest for success, our nihilism and worship of the fiscal bottom line; our blind eye turned to crooked politicians and swindling investors (the sharks of Wall Street), child-molesting priests, organized crime, and "kick-backs";

our global addiction to conflict and gridlock politics; the swelling ranks of the homeless and unemployed; the outrageous salaries and bonuses of CEOs, film stars, entertainers, and athletes; our mute acceptance of tax-avoiding offshore bank accounts and Third World low-cost manufacturing; burgeoning terrorism fuelled by religious extremists; the growing enclaves of the dispossessed, the chronically hungry, poverty-induced malnutrition, obesity, and diabetes; tidal waves of refugees; our racism, sexism, homophobia (and antibodies to all that is LGBTQ); our readiness to ignore the psychologically wounded and desperate; our breathtaking capacity to ignore climate change and global warming – even deny its existence; our tendency to see the planet as ours for the raping, as we clear-cut, frack, and denude once-pristine wilderness to feed the unquenchable greed of unfettered capitalism and its need for continual growth in the face of decreasing non-renewable resources, increasing cost of living, and the accelerating global population explosion. Always in need of *more*, our racing minds generate endless restlessness as we calculate yet another path to this or that Holy Grail and a way out of the meaningless maze. And it all passes as the norm. Violence? We humans have killed in excess of one hundred million fellow humans in the twentieth century alone.[6]

In 1985 the United States officially became the world's largest debtor nation, with a deficit of $130 billion.[7] Francis Bacon forced me to recall the anguish of my Université de Montréal colleague Michael Strobel as he bemoaned the fact that no one had listened to the 1970 MIT "Limits to Growth" warning. It would be another seven years before I heard Bacon's message voiced with razor-edged clarity by Leonard Cohen in his prophetic song "The Future"[8] and, a quarter-century after that, when the United States elected a president who appeared to support many of these dark ends.

LIVE AID AND THE MONTREAL CHILDREN'S
HOSPITAL PCS NEEDS ASSESSMENT

In July 1985 two issues became my preoccupation: "Live Aid" and a study documenting the need for a Montreal Children's Hospital PCS.

On 13 July the world witnessed the sixteen-hour global telecast of the transatlantic Live Aid benefit concerts for Ethiopian famine relief from Wembley Stadium, London, and John F. Kennedy Stadium, Philadelphia. This event was viewed by an estimated audience of 1.9 billion people across 150 nations and raised approximately $283.6 million. Mother Teresa commented to Live Aid's organizer, Bob Geldof, during their brief meeting in the airport at Addis Ababa: "I can't do what you can do and you can't do what I can do. But we both have to do it." I saw Live Aid as an important response to Francis Bacon's critique of our dysfunctional social consciousness and felt it should be celebrated. That led to a Mother Teresa/"Saint Bob"/Ethiopian youth collage that became the poster for our 1986 McGill International Congress.

Meanwhile, as the summer of 1985 progressed, it became clear to me that the nurses in the MCH's Neonatal Intensive Care Unit combined ICU skills, gentleness, compassion, and concern for family needs to a degree that I had not previously observed in our adult-serving McGill hospitals. They welcomed me with interest when told that their hospital would be examining (1985–87) the need for a palliative-care program, but their expressions were somewhat quizzical. Was there a need? The MCH had already carefully developed facilities and support programs for most of the children and families facing death. They had already been assigned a high priority.

As we chatted, a problem relating to one of the newborn infants under their care reached crisis proportions. The senior pediatric fellow interrupted my conversation with the ICU nurses to request their assistance in his third attempt to establish intravenous access via a scalp vein in the tiny newborn boy. A chromosomal abnormality had caused the little fellow to have multiple heart and intestinal malformations resulting in life-limiting problems. His life expectancy was a few days, a week or two at most, since any oral intake or secretions from his mouth passed directly into his lungs. Repeated attempts by the doctor to set up an intravenous line for hydration were causing the newborn (and the nursing staff) considerable distress. The nurses opposed another attempt; the fellow was adamant. "Nothing is more troubling than dehydration and thirst. We have to help this little chap!" Escalating tension and frustration were palpable among these competent and empathetic teammates. For their part, the young parents of this doomed infant were completely unable to visit their son and watch as their dreams were dashed.

Knowing that a moist, clean mouth prevents thirst in spite of dehydration in dying adults, I suggested using small water-soaked sponge applicators to create the same conditions here. It wouldn't hurt to give it a try. The doctor was skeptical but agreed to a trial prior to his next attempt to gain intravenous access.

After his mouth was cleaned and moistened and he was placed in a bassinet alongside a cassette-tape recorder playing soothing music, the baby settled immediately. In those days the tape recorder surpassed the baby in size, resulting in the tiny babe and music source completely filling the bassinet; the intravenous line was not needed. Benefiting from the nursing staff's considerable experience in supporting parents, the agitated, grieving young couple who, until then, "simply wanted to get this over with" gradually started to visit their baby and found their way toward something approaching a sense of calm as they came to terms with this disastrous end to a long-awaited pregnancy. For my part, I was intrigued that the lessons we had learned in adult palliative care were so dramatically relevant in the pediatric setting. I was hooked. The Children's Hospital study should be done. We all had a lot to learn.

The Montreal Children's Hospital Palliative Care Needs Assessment Committee was convened in July 1985 to assess end-of-life care in four target areas: symptom control; whole-person care; loss and grief for patient, family, and staff; and staff stress.[9] From the summer of 1985 through March 1987, when the final committee report was tabled, I devoted four half-days per week to the MCH study while nursing colleague Dr Linda McHarg was a gifted full-time participant. Multiple factors proved relevant to the anguish-filled ambience of this tragic setting: the tragic nature of childhood death; the complex nexus of problems encountered in meeting the highly charged issues involved; the youth and high turnover rate of the pediatric nursing staff; the brief preparation time for most parents experiencing the loss of their child; the rich mix of cultures and languages in the urban population being served; and the uncertain pattern of bereavement support available. Many grieving parents were left with the feeling that "we were surrounded by caring people who didn't know what to do or say."

One morning, I received a phone call from Dr Dixie Esseltine, a senior pediatrician and member of the Palliative Care Needs Assessment Committee.

"Bal, I have three young patients I think you should meet. As it happens, they are all in the clinic today. I have spoken to each of them about our committee and they have agreed to chat with you. Actually, now would be a good time. I've finished seeing them and it's their 'social time.' They get together whenever they can – a sort of Three Musketeers kind of thing."

Gregory, Pierre, and Jill had settled into three over-sized chairs. They were relaxed, even welcoming, once introductions were behind us.

"Hi folks," I offered, seeing in them the kids in the Teens Club that Faye, Phyllis Smyth, and I had run. Each of them was seventeen; each had a brain tumour; each was beyond any hope of cure. "Mind if I join you?"

They were in jeans. The two boys – make that *young men* – were perhaps 5'8" or so; Pierre was a little taller and the heaviest of the three.

Greg looked tired; he wore a baseball cap, backwards. Jill was pale but the most animated.

We opened with the small stuff. "How's it going? ... I really appreciate meeting you ... Tell me about yourselves ... In return, if there's anything about me that you think wouldn't bore you to death, feel free to ask!" *Groan! ... bore you to death? Well, that was brilliant, Bal, you twit!*

They had become "the gang of three" over their months of treatment. Now, they graciously included me in their group. An "outsider" who was not a member of the MCH staff yet was a doctor (who had also had been a cancer patient) seemed like a good person to dump on. I felt privileged and told them so. Although, as events unfolded, we would meet only three times (the last without Greg), they taught me a lot.

Yes, they admitted, the cancer was always there in the back of their minds, but that didn't mean that they didn't have a life – a *good* life. While their days had many tough moments – lonely, boring, sick ones – there were also good times. What did they enjoy most? "Easy!" They all answered at once. "It's when our friends, you know, from school or the neighbourhood, include us and treat us as if we're normal. When they pick us up in a car and take us with them on a Friday evening – just to sit around and sip milkshakes and hang out down at the corner joint where we like to go. To be *normal* for a while!"

"And the worst?" The *worst* part was when people treated them as if they were fragile and about to break, or as though they were weird and abnormal, or when others whispered knowingly to each other about them at the fringes of their presence. But the *very* worst part was that they were causing their parents so much pain! "Their tears and turmoil are never far away. We would do anything to help. Anything! But there's nothing we *can* do."

What did they want most? "Just to be treated like we are normal and to be included by our friends. To do normal stuff with them."

I was moved by their grace and grit. They taught me something about the well of courage within that enables us to face almost anything and the importance of community in helping us grasp that inner resource. I loved and admired those kids. I associate them with the words of Bob Geldof: "Mankind at its most desperate is often at its best. When the physical is reduced to an ugly irrelevance the possibilities of blinding human beauty emerge."[10]

Further teachers followed the Three Musketeers. Mike, age nineteen, was angry and everyone on the ward knew it. Cystic fibrosis (CF) had controlled his life and relationships. It had mangled his options at each turn for as long as he could remember. He was in a private room on the adolescent ward, the door always closed. Mike knew that the median life expectancy for CF at that time was about twenty-five years. That was the *median!* He knew the clock was ticking.

"It's a bitch!" was the epithet he used to describe pretty well all aspects of life. While the other young people with CF generally selected a caregiver advocate on their treatment team to be their special confidant and friend, Mike isolated himself from family, staff, and fellow patients.

I was particularly moved by the plight of the CF kids. Their courage and tireless commitment to "keeping up the fight" was a daily reminder of how to face adversity. I mentioned to more than one of them my admiration, repeating the old sport slogan, "When the going gets tough, the tough get going." Sometimes it seemed to help. They tended to grin and nod. Mike, however, hated upbeat visitors who came by to parrot yet another cliché to cheer him up.

During rounds, one of the nurses suggested that I might have a go at getting to know Mike – see if we could "hit it off." She thought that a quiet approach by someone who was ready to listen might do the trick. I had dropped in to see him once or twice and was met with icy indifference, but perhaps she was right. Perhaps if I went in simply to listen, I might get through that wall. *Low key … that's the ticket. Listen! Be a presence! Watch a movie together? Just sit?*

I entered his room, circled the bed, and leaned against the window sill. "Hi, Mike," I mumbled quietly, in an offhand kind of way.

"*What?*" he challenged indignantly. *Keep it low key. Keep it quiet; hang in.* I was about to respond with my best "quiet-presence" demeanour when the door burst open and slammed against the wall.

In strode four or five guys. They looked like they were in their twenties. They were dressed in slacks, loafers, and gaudy open-neck sport shirts – swaggering, loud, laughing, boisterous – but beneath all that I thought they looked a little nervous.

This is the damnedest thing I have ever seen! I could kill them! Completely inappropriate! What do they think they're doing?! Blast! Who the hell are these guys? Whoever they are they're a way out of line! Someone needs to get them out of here!

At that very second, the guy who seemed to be the ringleader strode around the foot of Mike's bed and barged in front of me, pressing me back against the window. He hadn't even noticed me. *Doesn't this jerk know I'm a doctor? Here to see my patient? Who the hell does he think he is?*

As he stopped, the intruder swung something across Mike's bed. It hit both raised metal bedside rails at the same time with a resounding crash that reverberated down the hall. I was dumfounded. It took me a moment or two to see that the missile was a hockey stick. *This is nuts!* Then, the shameless young upstart roared at Mike, "Here Mike, this is for you! It's signed by the whole team." And it was. I could see that now.

Mike broke into a wide grin. He seemed to grow in size. He was taller. He was beaming now. Head held high.

These guys are from the Montreal Canadiens! Of course!

I silently slid out of the room as each of the Habs greeted him and shook his hand.

It was humbling to see someone get it right, for once. The nurses said it was the first time anyone had seen Mike smile.

Our committee report recommended that the MCH develop a palliative-care service to complement existing services. A March 1987– November 1988 implementation program was suggested. I returned to the Royal Vic on a full-time basis.

It had been a challenging experience. To enter the world of dying children, their parents, loved ones, and their Montreal Children's Hospital caregivers was to be confronted with many of the problems we encountered in the adult setting but somehow, in addition, they seemed magnified by the haunting presence of suffering in the very young, the agony of parental loss, and the oppressive burden of lives never lived. I came away with a sense of awe for the immensity of the challenges when a child dies, and with unqualified respect for my MCH colleagues who address these needs on a daily basis.

LEO EITINGER

McGill's Sixth International Congress on Care of the Terminally Ill was held 27 September–1 October 1986. It attracted an international audience of thirteen hundred delegates. The opening plenary speaker was Professor Leo Eitinger of the University of Oslo. I had heard him speak in Loen, Norway, fifteen months earlier and, having already decided that our 1986 opening plenary address would be titled "Things I Have Learned from My Personal Experiences with Death," I concluded that Dr Eitinger was a providential answer to my quest for just the right speaker. I invited him at the conclusion of his Loen presentation. Happily, he agreed, "health permitting."[11]

Dr Eitinger sat alone at the somewhat austere linen-covered, microphone- bedecked, speaker's platform during the music and slide-show images of autumn transience that opened the plenary session. Marcel Boisvert, PCS physician and session chairman, was standing silently beside him. As the house lights swelled, he slowly and deliberately poured the professor a glass of water as the packed amphi-theatre watched in sustained silence. Eitinger sat transfixed, his gaze on the glass. The moment was unhurried, the warm legacy of the music and images still fading in our minds.

There was something about that moment: the intentional pause in the proceedings, Marcel's solemn formality and obvious respect both for Professor Eitinger and for this moment when one thousand people were coming together for their first taste of the 1986 International Congress community. Though brief in duration, the moment was timeless. There was a hint of the sacred in the shared focus, the slight smiles, and total silence of these two men. Eitinger was about to captivate us though his rare combination of wisdom, rhetorical eloquence, and equal portions of humility and grace. A man of medium height and calm demeanour, he smiled easily as he surveyed us, his lively eyes peering attentively through wire-rimmed glasses. As with many of our faculty that year, one felt priv-ileged to be in his presence.

Leo Eitinger's awareness of transience was hard won. The youngest of six children of a religious Jewish family, he had studied philosophy and medicine, graduating from Masaryk University in his Moravian home-town of Brno when he was twenty-five years old. He was soon con-scripted into the Czechoslovakian army but chose instead to participate in humanitarian efforts assisting groups of Jewish children attempting to reach Norway in the face of the gathering Nazi storm.

He immigrated to Norway in 1939 in the wake of his eviction from Slovakia as a Jew. On receiving a work permit (he was fluent in Norwegian, English, French, and German), the young doctor was appointed to Norway's northernmost psychiatric hospital at Bodo, nar-rowly escaping the Nazis who had just invaded Oslo. In early 1942, however, Eitinger was arrested and, as a Jewish doctor caring for Jews, was singled out for harsh treatment.

In February 1943 he was transported to Auschwitz where, because of his training and linguistic skills, he was charged with maintaining pris-oner health and death records. When they fell ill, patients in the camp had to achieve a "fit and cured" status within fourteen days or they were sent to the gas chamber or given lethal intracardiac injections. Eitinger's practice of falsifying medical records saved many lives. He was later transferred to a small Auschwitz "hospital" where he worked alongside a Czech surgeon, doing what they could with their meagre available equipment. In the winter of 1944, with the Russian army approaching, the camp was evacuated and the ten thousand prisoners were forced to cross the snow-covered countryside on foot.

In January 1945 Eitinger was in the last group to leave Auschwitz. He was sent to Buchenwald where all Jews were ordered killed. Forging his own death certificate, he took the name and number of a Czech prisoner who had died the night before. (Prisoner "Leo Eitinger" died on 6 April 1945.) Within days, the Americans liberated the camp. Of the 762 Norwegian Jews deported to German concentration camps, only 23 survived, Leo Eitinger being one of them.

Following the war, Dr Eitinger took a position at the University Psychiatric Clinic in Oslo, becoming professor and department head in 1966. Throughout his career his focus was the study of human suffering, "victimology," and disaster psychiatry. He published a landmark paper on "Concentration Camp Syndrome" in 1964.[12]

In his 1986 Congress plenary address, we joined Dr Eitinger as he relived his horrific daily confrontations with death and the recurrent dilemmas faced by a Jewish concentration-camp doctor in having to choose between evils as he attempted to live each crossroad moment both thoughtfully and compassionately, according to his values.

As the prolonged applause following his remarks came to a close, Marcel grasped his hand with warmth. Again there was silence in the room, then Marcel said softly, "Professor Eitinger, we envy your grace. We don't envy how you got it." A muted morning coffee break followed.

Our Congress organizer, Eddy Polak, later told me about the private conversation he shared with Dr Eitinger during that mid-morning pause in proceedings. By chance, six months earlier, Eddy had organized a meeting on "Peace and Security" convened by one of my friends and mentors, McGill Faculty of Education Professor Bill Lawlor. One of the speakers on that occasion was Elie Wiesel, who had just been awarded the Nobel Peace Prize. Following Wiesel's presentation, Eddy had the opportunity for a private chat with him, similar to the one he would have six months later with Dr Eitinger during that Congress coffee break.

In his discussion with Elie Wiesel, Eddy disclosed that his father had also been a Holocaust survivor, leading Wiesel to ask if his father had ever told Eddy what got him through the ordeal. Eddy recalled that his father had concluded that random *chance* seemed to play a role in his survival on more than one occasion. Wiesel had nodded in agreement, then added, "There were times when it was very difficult for me to keep going. Indeed, on one occasion when I felt I could go no further, by chance, a fellow inmate, a doctor, happened by. He saved my life. Without him I wouldn't have survived."

Now, six months later, Eddy found himself alone with Dr Eitinger. In their ensuing exchange they talked about the extreme difficulties of camp life and the role that chance played in determining survival in the experience of Eddy's father. Eddy told Elie Wiesel's story that, when things were at their darkest, he met, by chance, a doctor who saved him. Eitinger turned to Eddy and paused before commenting quietly, "I was that doctor."[13]

EASTER AT CHRISTMAS 1986

Our Children's Hospital study had carried on through 1986 and it was now 16 December. I was heading along the dimly lit hospital corridor at MCH. *Oddly quiet for a Tuesday morning.* I was on my way to the largely deserted interns' residence where I had a temporary office. It was an overcast day; a snowstorm was predicted and I was lost in thought, my mind focused on the week past and the Christmas festivities that were imminent.

Glancing to my right as I passed a patient's room, I caught my breath and slowed in wonderment at the tableau beside me, then quickened my pace so as not to disturb the three figures wrapped in their private world. The patient was a lovely young woman. She was sitting in near-coma drowsiness, cradled by her mother's supportive presence at her back while, facing and leaning over them with outstretched, embracing arms, was the girl's father, thus completing a circle of unconditional love.

The patient, Geneviève, was sixteen. Time had stopped at that most magic of moments when the loveliness of a little girl blooms before your eyes into the unspeakable grace and beauty of a young woman. A transcendent moment and a rare gift to witness to be sure, but in this case that breathtaking, grace-filled transition was star-crossed by impending death. I kept walking.

On reaching the office I did a simple stylized sketch of that family trinity and pencilled above it:

Trinity in Suffering (16 Dec. '86, 11 a.m.)
Easter at Christmas.
The gift of unconditional love
Bridging the abyss
Between
This world
And the infinite.

Returning to their room, I handed them the drawing as a token of my gratitude and respect.

The end was near. Yves, her father, had just asked Geneviève what her Christmas wish might be. She had answered, "To see our tree one more time." As I arrived with the sketch and handed it to her mother, Yves picked Geneviève up, as if she were weightless, and carried her to the elevator. She was radiant, flushed with illness, her own blooming, and the timelessness of the greater transition at hand.

I had one last glimpse of her gossamer nightgown, closed eyes, and flushed face. Radiant. Cradled in her father's arms with her mother, Louise, at their side. The elevator doors closed.

Yves walked, he later told me, out through the hospital main entrance with the snow now falling heavily in billowing gusts as he lifted Geneviève into a taxi that was at hand. On reaching their home, he carried her through the blizzard, up the outdoor staircase, and into the living-room warmth where he laid her on the couch. As, in silence, they turned on the Christmas tree lights, Geneviève opened her eyes, smiled warmly with deep contentment, and died.

Linda and I visited their home a day or two later in response to their phone call to inform us that my hasty sketch had become their announcement to friends of Geneviève's passing.

So many circles completed. It was, indeed, Easter at Christmas. A week before, on Tuesday, 9 December, Dad had telephoned to ask if I would come to see him at the veterans' hospital in Ottawa. I responded that I would be there Saturday morning.

"That won't be soon enough," he answered.

"Dad, I'll be there on Saturday. That's just four days. I'm so looking forward to seeing you." He sounded strong.

The Friday morning telephone call from Jim on 12 December left a deep sadness and sense of shame. Dad had died quietly that morning. Neither Jim nor I was present. Why had I not listened? My team had "ears to hear"; *they* would have heard! Linda and I got in the car and drove to Ottawa. I had a deep need to see him.

At the National Defence Medical Centre, we went to his ward and asked for him. The startled nurse explained haltingly that he had died. His body had been wrapped and would soon be moved to the morgue. I told her that I was a palliative-care physician and that we wished to spend some moments alone with him. She called the nursing supervisor who led us to a small closet. It contained the stretcher on which Dad's wrapped body lay.

There was a sense of presence as I folded back the plastic shroud. His eyes were closed. His dear face carried an expression of great calm: all the lines of worry, all those countless "bones to chew on" that he had both enjoyed and perpetually fussed about, all the problems of countless patients that he had been delighted to ponder – all were gone. He looked twenty years younger. I found it healing. I kissed and thanked him. And thanked him again, as Linda and I stood with him in that tiny closet shrine. His ninetieth birthday ten months past had seen his work complete.

The drive back to Montreal that night was filled with silence, regret, memories, and gratitude. It was four days later that I would encounter Geneviève, Louise, and Yves. Louise Primeau, Geneviève's mother, would later become a volunteer on our team, then our director of volunteers. Alice arrived from Cambridge for Dad's funeral service on 20 December.

1987: THE UPS AND DOWNS OF IT

With the dawning of 1987, the global community faced instability on many fronts. As we neared the two decades' mark since the *Limits to Growth* warning by Meadows et al., their predictions continued to hold true. The world population had reached one billion circa 1800, the second billion was added in only 130 years (1930), the third in less than 30 years (1959), the fourth in 15 years (1974), and the fifth in 13 years (1987).[14] As the subsequent years passed, six billion was reached in 1999[15] and 7 billion in 2011.[16]

In addition, it had become clear that global warming far exceeded that associated with the glacial advance and retreat cycles of the past 650,000 years. Shrinking polar-ice masses, rising sea levels and global surface temperatures, with an increase in ocean warming and acidification, and extreme weather events were among the outcomes.[17] Climate scientists agreed that these trends were very likely due to human activities[18] and Canada ranked in the top ten nations contributing to this unfolding disaster, the United States being the worst offender.[19] Only Saudi Arabia, Kazakhstan, and Iran joined the United States as greater offenders than Canada.[20]

The 1987 stock markets provided another reminder of precarious instability. On Monday, 19 October, unpredicted rash selling in the Asian markets led to panic among New York stockholders who sold off millions of shares, causing world markets to lose more than $500 billion US in a matter of hours. The impact was worldwide. The Toronto Composite Index dropped a record 407.2 points, a loss of 11 per cent, and a total of $37 billion. It would be nearly two years before the index would rebound to pre-crash levels.[21]

There were, however, glimmers of hope on the political front. The Cold War, which had strained international relations since 1945, was showing hopeful signs of transition to a new season of rapprochement. Mikhail Gorbachev, general secretary of the Central Committee of the Communist Party of the Soviet Union, campaigned for *glasnost* (openness) and *perestroika* (reconstruction); American President Reagan visited Berlin to mark its 750th anniversary and called on Gorbachev to tear down the Berlin Wall; and Reagan and Gorbachev met in Washington to sign a treaty banning all short- and medium-range nuclear weapons in Europe.[22]

Meanwhile, health care in Quebec was facing turbulent times. While early in the decade the new Royal Vic executive director, Steve Herbert, had reduced operating expenses at the hospital by $5,000,000, thus avoiding threatened receivership,[23] this encouraging fiscal picture was soon to be eclipsed by continuing reductions in provincial health-care funding. The hospital's annual reports documented the impact of these draconian cuts: "preoccupation of the board, senior management and medical staff was required to monitor the risk to quality of care" (1982); "ongoing underfunding" (1984); "a new fiscal deficit of $2.4 million and the painful need to close almost 100 beds" (1986). Heightened strain continued in the face of static income from government (1987), while hospital operating expenses almost doubled during the 1980s largely because of inflation. Indeed, there was substantially less real expansion in hospital activities during this period than in any previous decade in the Royal Vic's history.[24] These were grim times. Colleagues who saw palliative care as lying outside the teaching hospital mandate favoured the closure of our programs.

It was during this 1987 crisis that the *Montreal Gazette* published a series of personal attacks on Steve Herbert. I responded with a letter in his defence that found its way to the newspaper's front page. The day after my letter was published, an attending staff colleague remarked as we passed each other, "By the way Mount, if you crawl out on a limb too far, someone will cut the branch off!"

"Was that a threat?" I queried. But he was gone. Tensions were running high.

That same year, Dr Dale Dauphinee was named chief of the Department of Medicine at the Vic. The fiscal tensions of this period were suggested by a telephone conversation early in his tenure.

"Bal, Dale here. I'd like your input. I have to close one of three wards – the Medical Intensive Care Unit, the Cardiac Intensive Care Unit, or the Palliative Care Unit. Which one do you think I should close?"

"Dale," I replied, "I think you're asking the wrong question." That proved to be the case. The three units survived. But I had few illusions about the depth of support for palliative care in our cash-strapped hospital.

As the months passed, there was good news from our international hospice/palliative-care colleagues. The field was coming into its own. In 1987 the Royal College of Physicians of London and Edinburgh recognized palliative medicine as a new medical specialty. Correspondence with friends around the world was equally encouraging.[25] As 1987 drew to a close, new Christmas traditions found their way into our PCS routine. According to mythology, it all started with "the stocking affair." Shirley Baxter, the PCU nurse in charge that Christmas morning, was distributing the early-morning medications. Mr Ambrose, a crusty amputee in his late sixties, wakened quickly as Shirley touched his shoulder. Taking his bearings, he looked up at her and winked knowingly. "Quick, take me to the solarium," he beamed. "You never know what Santa has left under the tree." Shirley was dumfounded. Ambrose's only relative was his sister, whom he always addressed in a brusque, demanding tone. Both were single. She was exhausted. Their relationship was strained at the best of times, and she had not been in to see him for several days. There was certainly nothing for Ambrose or, for that matter, any of our other patients, under the Christmas tree in the PCU family lounge.

As Ambrose reached for his housecoat, Shirley stalled, suggesting that he should take his medications first, muttering that she would have to return to the desk for a moment. Following a sleight-of hand-concealment of one of Mr Ambrose's socks, she hurriedly consulted the other nurses. Candies, a pack of cigarettes, and some other odds and ends were hurriedly stuffed inside the old sock and a colleague swept it off to the solarium as Shirley returned to Ambrose with the meds. Moments later Shirley assisted him down the hall. He was aglow with anticipation. At the tree he stopped. He visibly shrank and started to tremble as he sat down, tears glistening. "What is this?" he blurted with anger and bewilderment. "That's not from Santa! It's a fake." The tears were running freely now. Awkwardness and stunned silence reigned. This was beyond the pale, but who could have predicted it? Ambrose returned to bed without another word and cried the rest of the morning.

Shirley was both crestfallen and determined. Ambrose had reminded us of the importance of traditions established early in life and of the child that remains within each of us. Shirley took two actions. She swore she would never work on Christmas day again and she telephoned Dolores Nickerson at home.

Dolores was both nurse and volunteer. A Royal Vic nursing grad of 1961, she had heard Ina speak on palliative care during a North Sydney, Nova Scotia, nursing refresher course in 1981. That did it. She and her husband, Harold, had their child-rearing years behind them: she would become a palliative-care nurse. She applied to join our team in 1986. At that time, however, the nursing staff was more or less complete, so Dolores signed on as nurse two days per week and PCU volunteer one day per week.

How to describe Dolores? She was competent, giving, and energetic, with a flair for attention to detail. She was also flexible. When nursing she was a nurse; when a volunteer, she never stepped over that line. Dolores was a practising Catholic – an increasing rarity in secular Quebec. Someone quipped that, with her iron-clad faith, cheerfulness, and peaceful yet dynamic demeanour, she risked giving the church a good name! She seemed always to have on hand an endless supply of small red hearts (candies, cards, paper weights, bon-mot books ... all manner of things, so long as they were heart-shaped) or, if not hearts, angels (poems, stories, lapel pins, small statues, cards, medallions). Dolores personified compassion and a listening ear. Who better for Shirley to call? Besides which, Dolores knew Mr A.

As it happened, Ambrose wasn't the only somewhat cantankerous man on the ward that Christmas. Mr C., down the hall, had a distressed, depleted family – a threadbare wife and two boys eight and ten years old. Neither man, A. or C., seemed to be aware of their own belligerence or the stress their family members were enduring.

One mid-December evening as she worked an evening nursing shift, Dolores suggested to each man that he might want to give his family members Christmas presents, adding that she had a gift cupboard at home and would be happy to bring in some things for them to choose from. "Why would I do that?" asked Mr A.

In the end, both men gave in. There was bubble bath for Mrs C and games for the boys. Mr A.'s sister couldn't believe it when her brother gave her his present. Later, during bereavement follow-up, she said, "The gift I received from my brother has touched me more than you will ever know. It was such a surprise. I get the warmest feeling when I think about it. That is how he told me that he cared for me."

On listening to Shirley's tale of PCU Christmas-morning woes, Dolores had an idea. Next Christmas there would be a stocking on hand for every patient and they would be distributed at 6:00 A.M. Christmas morning so that, as Dolores put it, "when the meds are given out they'll wake up with that touch of Christmas magic already there." And there was more. The profound sense of meaning experienced by the A. and C. families as a result of "receiving a gift from him on his last Christmas" had been deeply moving for our team. The following year, each patient would be offered the chance for "bedside PCU Christmas shopping." There would be a gift cart piled high with donated gifts and wrapping paper. Gifts could be chosen without charge for as many loved ones as each patient desired. Patients would select their gifts, watch as the volunteers wrapped each one, and then be helped, as needed, in writing the accompanying cards. If the patient was too ill to participate, loved ones would be invited to select their own gift from the cart. Annual PCU Christmas shopping was instituted for Christmas 1988.[26] When there were enquiries about the cost of the gifts, the answer was, "Hugs, please."

Each year during October (early in order to avoid the business of the holiday season), volunteers Bea Crawford, Sally Kauser, and Linda Merrill would meet at the Nickerson home to prepare the sixteen stockings donated by the firm that made them for the Montreal Children's Hospital. The collection of gifts for the following year commenced shortly after each Christmas.

Over the years, a host of memorable bedside-shopping moments brought smiles to the team. In one case, no sooner had the gift been wrapped than the patient said, "Could you please unwrap it so I can see it again? I will want to look at it often between now and Christmas."

On pondering the many treasures available on the gift cart, a frail patient commented, "I don't want anything that my husband will have to dust. I'd like to give him this box of linen handkerchiefs." Some months following her death, a volunteer spoke to her grieving widower at the memorial service on the PCU. Weeping, he said, "My wife gave me this handkerchief, you know. I feel that she is with me when I cry, and it helps." The volunteer was pleased to tell him the story behind his wife's choice and her thoughtful insight in wishing to minimize his dusting duties.

The following year, there was a destitute fellow from a homeless shelter who, when reassured that there was no cost, asked if he might choose more than one gift and then proceeded to select twenty-three, one for each PCU caregiver who had made a difference. And there was also the young mother who, during her bedside-shopping spree, chose a locket for her five-year-old daughter, among other things. While dictating the gift card to accompany the locket, she was interrupted as her husband unexpectedly arrived on the scene for a visit; she dissolved in laughter, hurriedly stuffing her selected presents under the quilt. Such experiences taught us that the satisfaction and joy to be found in celebrating personally meaningful events may eclipse dwindling physical and mental capacities. Indeed, special events may even acquire new meaning through the opportunity to provide one more testimony of shared caring.

In palliative care, the multilayered complexity of need and context may blur the lines that customarily define professionalism in other clinical settings and, as a result, call for flexibility in response. The Simons family comes to mind.

Tom Simons, a young husband and father, was dying. His wife, Carolyn, felt completely isolated as she battled to support him, care for their two children ages five and seven, manage the needs of their home, and monitor her own personal resources. She was an extremely capable woman who radiated strength, spoke five languages, and projected an aura of competence. She had to hold it all together! "I'm fine," she would reply, even when things were at their worst.

One morning, when Dolores was working the day shift as a PCU nurse, a deeply concerned volunteer reported to her that Carolyn was crying: it was hardly her norm. Dolores thanked him and, on her way to lunch a few minutes later, went to the room.

Mr Simons was asleep in a reclining chair and Carolyn was stretched out on his bed, weeping quietly. To Dolores, it seemed a golden opportunity. As she entered the room, she said, "Carolyn, I have a fifteen-minute lunch break now and I'm going to stay here with you." With that, she lay down beside her on the bed. Although she had never done such a thing before, it seemed to be what was needed. It released a pent-up flood. Carolyn sobbed, "I'm the one always giving! I'm so alone! I'm so alone!"

They were still talking some time later when Tom Simons woke up and saw them lying together on the bed. He started to laugh. The ice had been broken and the opportunity created for sharing at a deeper level.

Always the professional with a sharp eye for standards and propriety, Dolores later questioned her own intervention and reviewed what she had done with Dr Margaret Scott, the physician involved in Tom Simons's care. Margaret, an excellent clinician with a penchant for personal privacy, was typically concise in her assessment. "It was what was needed." A door had been opened, needs had been expressed, and as a result there had been movement toward healing. When pressed, Dolores added a postscript. "You know, Carolyn and I stayed in touch after that and when, some years later, she remarried, Harold and I invited them to use our condo up north."

BEYOND SYMPTOM CONTROL

A pioneering hospice physician once claimed that palliative-care doctors should limit their concerns to symptom control. Symptomatologists? Is that sufficient? *Au contraire!* There were daily indications that psychosocial and existential/spiritual issues were critical quality-of-life determinants for those receiving our care.

The felicitous move of the PCU to the Ross Pavilion with its spacious solarium and family room led to new initiatives toward improved
whole-person care. We added afternoon teas on Tuesdays and Thursdays,
complete with home baking and music, often live. Personal tea-time invitations to both patient and family were extended and reinforced by the
welcoming warmth of our volunteers, the sense of relaxed community
that these gatherings generated, and the natural patient-to-patient and
family-to-family discussions and friendship that flowed from them. The
success of the teas quickly led to similar events to celebrate birthdays, anniversaries, Valentine's Day, Easter, Chanukah, and other special occasions.

Regular Wednesday "Happy Hour" celebrations soon followed.
They added an upbeat change in routine, with their choice of wine or
cranberry-juice cocktails served in attractive glasses accompanied by
tasty hors d'oeuvres. The same was on offer as "room service" for family members who wished to remain at the bedside rather than join the
shared festivities in the lounge.

In due course, the families themselves began to plan and host similar
events. A patient commented, "I feel so healthy when I come to these
parties. They remind me of being well."

As I passed the volunteer director's office one afternoon, Mary
Coughlan beckoned, "Bal, got a moment?" With her usual matter-of-
fact directness, Mary continued, "Do you know Dolores Nickerson?"

"Sure," I responded.

"Well," she went on, "I think you might be interested in having a word
with her. She has had experiences with patients that no one else reports –
some sort of near-death experiences, it seems." I thought of Miss Vallor
at St Christopher's and her radiance as she spoke of being with Jesus and
his disciples by the Sea of Galilee. I also thought of our patient who, a
few days before she died, "dreamed" that she was floating near the ceiling of her room, above her body, looking down on herself.

A series of chats with Dolores ensued. Yes, she responded with her
customary openness and penchant for clinical detail, she had often had
chats with patients who described being visited by deceased loved ones.
"How often has this happened?" I asked.

She paused and thought back, finally commenting with a shrug, "I
would say about forty times."

"Forty?"

"About that. It's quite frequent."

"How come nobody else has these experiences with patients?"

"Oh, I think they do, but they don't say anything, either out of fear
of this leading to a psychiatric consult and medication changes such

as increased sedation, or, perhaps because they feel it is a very special, private, even sacred experience for the patient and the visitor and that they should keep it private." Dolores paused, "You know, a while ago one such episode was reported and the patient's medications were changed. It was very distressing for him."

"Do both men and women have these experiences?"

"Yes. And they may happen on repeated occasions with a given patient; they tend to find them very comforting."

"Dolores, would you describe your most recent such experience?"

"Well, earlier this week, as I was driving to the hospital, I went through my usual routine of quietening myself in preparation for being on the unit as a volunteer – praying really, but not in words – just sort of being focused, being conscious of wanting to be of service to the patients that I would see that day."

I was interested in her choice of words. Identical words had been used to describe his mental preparation by another palliative-care volunteer, Keevin Robins, a businessman whose friend Barry I had operated on several years earlier. Keevin had spent six years at an ashram in India as a youth.

As a surgeon, I had similarly prepared for cases during my pre-operative scrub procedures. It involved developing intentional presence and focused awareness, but there was more than that, something of a "handing over." It was, at the same time, a condition of being alert, calm, and energized, with a sense of focus and openness that is not easy to put into words.

"Dolores, on that occasion were you going to the hospital as a volunteer or to do a nursing shift?"

"Oh, a volunteer. It *only* happens when I am there as a volunteer. When I am there as a nurse, there is, perhaps, a different sort of purposeful, goal-oriented quality to my presence.

"Tell me about what happened."

She described which PCU room the patient was in, and then continued:

His light had been on earlier so I went to see if he still needed anything. As I approached his room I was doing my usual silent inner preparation. At the doorway, I knew someone was there in addition to the patient and me. It is hard to describe. There is just such serenity and love and joy, a sense of bliss. This is not something that I had created; it was already there in the room. On sensing it, I paused. The room was permeated with love – a swelling to overflowing. I said to him, "I can see you are busy, shall I come back later?" And he said, "No, she doesn't leave when it is you ... but if others come she goes away." He was looking at the empty chair in the room with such love. And I said to him, "She's here now isn't she?" and he said, "Yes." ... I just stood against the wall silently. They were in rapid-fire communication with one another. When she left, his face was aglow and I just said to him quietly, "I'm so happy for you." He asked me, "Did you see her?" and I said "No." And he replied, "Well, she saw you."

"Dolores, you said their communication was 'rapid-fire,' yet no words were spoken. What made you think it was 'rapid-fire'?"

"Because so much was exchanged between them. The whole time was not more than two or three minutes but for him it could have been two hours. It was an experience of out-of-time perception, not time as we know it. It's a rapid, almost simultaneous, exchange of thoughts. For him it had seemed like a long time. He told me how lovely she looked, said her hair was up in a braid wrapped round her head."

"How come I've never had such an experience?" I asked with a grin.

The diplomat that she is, Dolores didn't suggest that this might have something to do with me. She simply commented, "Well it is far more frequent for me when I am calm myself." She added that she had respect for such "sacred" moments, which left her feeling "richly blessed."

Our discussion was coming to an end; there was a pause as Dolores searched for anything she may have omitted. Then she added, "It seems to have something to do with breathing. I become aware that I am breathing with them. I recall one woman I went to see who was dying with lung cancer and having immense trouble breathing. She asked me if I would breathe with her to help her breathe and I told her I already was. She started to relax and finally fell asleep but I felt I had to keep breathing with her. It was exhausting, but eventually she stopped breathing. It was a peaceful death. Sympathetic touch and massage can have a similar effect."

THE DECADES GO AND COME

The final two years of the 1980s featured many landmark events. Some were encouraging: Reagan and Gorbachev dialogue continued; the USSR began to destroy medium-range nuclear missiles and announced a unilateral cut of 500,000 troops over two years; thousands of East German refugees escaped to West Germany via Hungary, leading to the demise of the Communist government of East Germany, the collapse of the Berlin Wall, and, in due course, the unification of the two Germanies; eighty nations agreed to stop production of chlorofluorocarbons (CFCs) by 2000 to combat ozone layer depletion and global warming.

Other events were horrific: a Libyan Islamic terrorist bomb brought down Pan Am Flight 103 over Lockerbie, Scotland, killing 270; the Exxon Valdez oil tanker struck a reef in Prince William Sound, Alaska, with a record oil spill of eleven million gallons creating an ecologic catastrophe; pro-democracy students occupied Tiananmen Square, Beijing, in a protest that was crushed by tanks and assault rifles, leaving thousands dead; meteorologists proclaimed 1989 the warmest year on record and attributed it to the greenhouse effect; the United Nations predicted that the world population would reach 14.2 billion by 2100.

In Montreal, it was Wednesday, 6 December, 1989, a drizzly, cold afternoon. Linda and I were delivering boxes of citrus fruit marking the end of that year's very successful annual palliative-care fundraising campaign. We would drop off a box at the home of Faye and her husband, Pierre, and then head to the east end, the back of our compact Toyota Tercel wagon still filled to overflowing. Sales had gone well. A satisfying day! We were in high spirits. Our volunteers were tireless!

Turning onto avenue Édouard-Montpetit, we were confronted by a tangle of flashing lights. Ambulances and police cars were strewn across the street and onto the Université de Montréal campus. The École Polytechnique lawns were swarming with the shadowy figures of first responders scurrying ant-like in apparent random confusion. Night had suddenly descended, sucking both oxygen and joy out of the afternoon air. We switched on the car radio.

A twenty-five-year-old, rejected student applicant had entered a class of sixty engineering students armed with a .22-calibre rifle, separated the men from the women, ordered the men to leave the room, and then opened fire, shouting "I hate feminists" while jumping from desk to desk to aim at his cowering victims. His rampage eventually covered three floors as he killed fourteen young women in forty-five minutes. Then he turned the gun on himself. A pall of meaninglessness and overwhelming loss smothered the city.

QUALITY-OF-LIFE DETERMINANTS AT THE END OF LIFE

From the beginning, our goal was to "palliate," that is, "to improve the quality of." But how were we to measure success? How does one measure a change in quality of life? Apparent QOL determinants include such unmeasurable variables as love, compassion, and meaning. While from our earliest days we collected quantitative data where possible, there were some things we just couldn't measure and, in the judgment of skeptics, qualitative research seemed prohibitively soft around the edges.

The phone call from McGill psychologist Ron Melzack was a god-send. "Bal, I have someone you should meet. Her name is Robin Cohen. She has been one of my graduate students; her PhD is in psychology. She has a great mind and is a hard worker."

Ron understood our problem. His work in developing the gate-control theory of pain with Pat Wall had approached the challenge through a holistic lens. It was how he saw the world, how he functioned. He viewed the components of lived experiences through perceptive eyes. I met with Robin. She agreed to join us as a post-doc fellow, and ultimately, having established herself as an investigator, she would be hired by McGill in 1996 as our director of research. Having her on board changed every-thing. She took a student internship on the PCU, working shoulder to shoulder with the team, our patients, and their families, and in the pro-cess she befriended the colleagues she would later call on as research collaborators. She came to understand their goals and perspectives.

Robin and I began a series of discussions about the nature of illness and suffering as she immersed herself in the relevant literature. She lis-tened to the patients and their families with low-key, shrewdly insightful discernment and openness. We discussed the need to engage the team in research, reviewed strategies for capturing the nuances of their observa-tions, and clarified the necessity of eventually aiming toward multi-centre trials given the limited number of patients in any one program. A series of publications followed.[27] We were off to a good start.

As these activities evolved, Robin and I reviewed the quality-of-life instruments in current use. None included the existential or spiritual domain. I found that problematic. Indeed, in the development of one of the most widely used QOL instruments, the patients who were surveyed had stressed the importance of spiritual issues but this had been ignored in the process of designing the instrument because, as the responsible investigator commented, "nobody funds research on spiritual issues."

"The McGill Quality of Life Questionnaire" (MQOL) was developed by Robin, validated in a series of trials, and then used to evaluate QOL in patients with cancer and Human Immunodeficiency Virus (HIV). It was the first QOL instrument to demonstrate that the existential/ spiritual domain is an important determinant of QOL for persons with advanced illness. While such issues were not of particular significance in the early stages of HIV, later in the illness, when the patient had full-blown AIDS, the spiritual domain was the *most important* determi-nant of their QOL.[28] Robin had earned credibility within our team and within the broader international palliative-care research community. How could we further deepen our understanding of the QOL of our patients, their families and ourselves as caregivers? Our next catalyst would be Dr Pat Boston.

HEALING CONNECTIONS

Psychiatric nursing consultant Pat Boston gave the weekly two-hour "Family Nursing" program that was attended by our PCS nurses during the late 1980s. Her focus was on family-systems theory and the family as the unit of care. Following nursing training at the Radcliffe Infirmary, Oxford, Pat had worked at the Middlesex Hospital in the United Kingdom and then in New York and Montreal prior to earning a humanities and sociology degree at Concordia and a PhD in education at McGill. A low-key, unassuming presence and calming demeanour complemented Pat's keen eye and uncanny ability to understand people and situations with penetrating insight. In a word, Pat was wise. Her assessment was invariably on the mark. She offered her observations and opinions quietly, thoughtfully, and only if asked. She brought grace and charity to each deliberation. In earning her PhD, Pat had focused on qualitative research under the tutelage of postmodern feminist and sociologist Professor Nancy Jackson, who, with Pat, had helped to uncover some of the modifiers of quality of life at the culturally diverse Royal Vic with its fifty-seven spoken languages and dialects.

At Pat's urging, I joined the twenty to thirty students enrolled in the qualitative-research course given by Dr Jackson at McGill's Faculty of Education. Jackson was articulate, grounded in her subject, and possessed oodles of no-nonsense confidence in the research ground on which she stood. Yet, listening from *my* quantitative medical-sciences background, I experienced the ideas she championed as falling somewhere between fairyland make-believe and "wishful thinking." *Smoke and mirrors! A sort of, Let's make up the truth; if you can't evaluate it with REAL science, make it up; pretend, but sound convincing and be sure to develop a complex in-house lingo to mystify the great unwashed!*

The pretense to significance that qualitative evaluation offered, I was convinced, was seriously misleading, somewhat embarrassing, a waste of time! Then, slowly, during one of Professor Jackson's lectures, the light began to dawn, ever so slightly. *Well that would be useful – if it were only true – and reliable.* From there it became mildly interesting, then almost convincing, then fascinating, and eventually exciting, if not addictive. *By Jove, this is great. A new world!* I was hooked.

Jackson's class assignment was to submit a hypothetical research proposal. Mine was not hypothetical. It was the first draft of a study to examine whether there are demonstrable predisposing factors underlying QOL in dying. Perhaps there are common themes shared by those of us who die in a state of extreme anguish and suffering at the lower end of the QOL continuum, and likewise, themes common to those at the other extreme of the QOL spectrum, those who, in dying, experience unusual peace and a sense of wholeness and equanimity.

Response shift theory was becoming well established[29] and recent QOL research had come up with some counterintuitive findings. Those near death might describe themselves as "heathy," even "very healthy." What was driving those unexpected evaluations? Moreover, a study by Bower and colleagues examining the long-term experience of HIV-seropositive bereaved men following their partner's death from AIDS had resulted in intriguing observations. Bereaved men who engaged in "active cognitive processing" (implying personal, intentional, in-depth, analytic examination of their own loss and grief) were *more likely* to find meaning in their life. Furthermore, those who *did* find increased meaning showed more sustained immune protection and lower rates of AIDS-related mortality.[30] This study was the first to show an association between mortality and the experience of increased meaning and the first to report an association between meaning and a physical-health outcome that does not appear to be mediated by health behaviours or other explanations assessed in the study. *Exciting stuff! Can finding new meaning really enhance immune response and lengthen life? And if so, what issues are involved?!*

Pat and I discussed collaborating on my proposed study, but my timing was bad (or, as it turned out, fortuitous). She had just been offered a teaching position in Vermont. I found a salary for her. She stayed at McGill. We fine-tuned the study, pursued research funding, and informed our Royal Vic nursing and physician colleagues of our need for end-of-life subjects.

To be selected for inclusion in the study, patients were required to have life-threatening illness and to stand out from their peers by virtue of either their dramatic sense of equanimity and well-being or, conversely, their marked existential anguish. The purposive sampling technique afforded a unique perspective on the dynamics of adaptation. Conjoint interviewing that involved both Pat and me appeared to contribute significantly to the enrichment of the interviews, field notes, and analysis. I found qualitative research eye-opening; it offered a fresh, focused, intimate picture of the life-shaping experiences that had overtaken the generous people who agreed to meet with us. Accepted qualitative-research strategies would be employed in the study.[31]

Interviewing study participants gave way to transcript analysis, then detailed iterative dialogue toward synthesis. Gradually emerging themes across cases began to edge into focus. The importance of meaning-based adaptation to advanced illness was substantiated. But meaning, it became evident, was not an end in itself. Instead, it was the means to an end. The real brass ring, it seemed, was not the specific *source* of meaning so much as the sense of connection that was enabled. Man's search, we concluded, is for connectedness, not meaning per se, though one may well correlate with, or lead to, the other. Four sources of connectedness were noted: an increased sense of connection to Self, to others, to the phenomenal world (experienced through the senses), and to "ultimate meaning" (God, the Other, Reality, however perceived.) A new-found sense of connection through one of these domains frequently appeared to enable increased openness to the other three.

As analysis of the themes across cases continued, we identified five shared themes at each QOL extreme. Those experiencing *suffering and anguish* (the low end of the quality-of-life continuum) generally had: a) a sense of disconnection from self, others, the phenomenal world, and ultimate meaning; b) a crisis of meaning, an existential vacuum and inability to find solace or peace; c) a preoccupation with future or past; d) a sense of victimization; and e) a need to be in control. Conversely, those experiencing *integrity and wholeness* (the high end of the QOL continuum) were likely to have: a) a sense of connectedness at one or more of the four levels; b) a capacity to find meaning in the context of suffering; c) an ability to find peace in the moment; d) an experience of a sympathetic, non-adversarial connection to their disease; and e) an ability to choose their attitude to adversity, a capacity to find potential in the moment that was greater than the need for control.

Cast in this light, the caregiver's opportunity to act as a catalyst toward healing connections became evident. To limit one's goal simply to being a "symptomatologist" would be to ignore totally the importance of aiming toward this potential for meaning, considered by many to constitute the *art* of medicine, and to fail to capitalize on the precious transformative possibility that may be there. We had come to see *man's search for meaning* as a quest to enable attachment to something greater and more enduring than the self. And we were coming to understand how this might relate to palliative care.

Four years after the publication of our paper on "healing connections," an insightful, ever-giving colleague, Harvard psychiatrist and neuroscientist Greg Fricchione, director of the Massachusetts General Hospital's Division of Psychiatry and Medicine and of the Benson-Henry Institute for Mind Body Medicine, shone a dazzling light on these issues in his book *Compassion and Healing in Medicine and Society: On the*

Nature and Use of Attachment Solutions to Separation Challenges. In a groundbreaking inquiry based on an evolutionary understanding of the brain, its purpose, and its effect on the body under conditions of stress (separation) and solace (attachment), Greg concluded that attachment responses to life's recurrent separation challenges constitute the driving force behind evolution and also present a golden opportunity for us to be midwives for healing through relating. He suggests that the essence of medicine lies at the confluence of three rivers: knowledge, meaning, and healing, and that this fact offers an incalculable gift if we accept the risks and challenges inherent in entering that potential-ladened transitional zone with the patient.[32]

THE CHALLENGE OF CARING

Having examined the inner-life experiences of our patients, we explored the same issues as they pertained to us as caregivers. Selected colleagues with ten to twenty-five years of palliative-care experience agreed to participate in three weekly meetings of two and a half hours' duration. Discussions were audiotaped, field notes documenting non-verbal aspects of the meetings recorded, and the data analyzed.[33] Emerging themes included: the factors involved in creating openings for depth discussions, our cumulative grief, healing connections, issues of transference and counter-transference (the unconscious attribution of one's own feelings, attitudes, or desires, positive or negative, to the other person in the caregiver-patient relationship), the importance of "spirituality" (with admitted difficulty in defining the term), personal vulnerability and frailty as "wounded healers," the need to sustain a healing environment for ourselves as caregivers, and, finally, the costs and benefits of these intimate moments in our daily work experience. The candour of our long-standing colleagues suggested both the need to unburden and the high degree of trust existing among us.

Challenging circumstances were discussed. A colleague recalled: "I remember a patient who was very angry and he said to the volunteers, 'You're all self-serving bitches. You're all self-serving. Don't come and bother me with your kindness. When you have something positive to say – like *a cure! ... then* come and smile!'" Another member of the focus group responded. "It's interesting ... you know, we can say 'Good for him for expressing himself' – it's fine in theory. I agree, 'Good for him!' – *but* to be face to face with someone and you're trying to be nice, and that person speaks like that ... It's not easy to deal with." A third member of the group added: "Our patients have many reasons to be angry, but

if they know we are there for them ... and when they see that we come
back the next time they call, whatever their needs ... they begin to trust
... that yes, it is just disgusting to be dying when you are fifty with bags
draining your stool on one side and urine on the other: it's very humiliat-
ing. But when they can voice all that, it seems to bring down their anger
and it may make it easier for them to express [it all] as sadness. A link
[can be] established through our caring, a door opened."

Our insightful music therapist, Deborah Salmon, spoke of intimacy and
her feelings of closeness to the patients when sharing music with them.

When I'm there, within the patient's spiritual space – in that intimacy –
it feels great. Because it's close, it's connected, it's authentic, it's intense,
it's deep – it's all the things we thrive on – it's sharing! But I think that
what is *hard* is to keep going there ... to keep getting there and then to
go from one patient to another. What do you do with it all? If you're
running from one to another, and you don't have time to process, and
then you go home and there's kids and homework ... and you fall into
bed and then you start all over the next day. And that's where burn-
out starts to happen ... So, being there is great, but I think we have to
process it. We have to do something with it and we have to find places
where it's not always about death ... To keep going without allowing
for the processing and self-nourishment is dangerous.

The challenge of caring runs deep for each of us in the patient/family/
caregiver therapeutic triad. Risking intimacy may confront us with unexpected vistas of need and support. A PCU nurse who was very wise,
respected, and fondly regarded by all her colleagues recounted her experience in caring for her dying patient following the suicide of her own adult
son.

I think what our patients feel toward the end is a lack of purpose, a
lack of meaning. You want to give them back that feeling of purpose
... My patient was deteriorating day by day and she was more angry
with each loss. Her sister was trying to help her without much success. Many of the nurses felt very impatient with her but she was my
primary patient so I was the one regularly caring for her.

      As day after day passed I felt we were making a little progress,
but it was really slow. Then my son died and I left the hospital for a
few weeks. But I felt bad leaving her, so after a few days I went into
the hospital to see her, even though I wasn't returning to work ... I
felt I owed her something ... I told her what had happened – with no

secrets – I told her my son had committed suicide and I cried with her. Now, at that time she was not getting out of bed ... and I told her she would be in heaven soon and I wanted her to look after my son. And she responded, "When I die, give me the picture of your son in my coffin." And she cried and told me she never had a son and that I could trust her that she would look after him. And she took over right away I guess, because from that moment on she was calm ... I think once you have discovered that you are vulnerable, that you are fragile, it makes you very humble. And I think from then on, you don't look at your patients in the same way. You see them – their vulnerabilities and suffering – in a different way, and I think you are more compassionate.

The Nineties: Closing the Millennium

It was the best of times, it was the worst of times,
it was the age of wisdom, it was the age of foolishness,
it was the epoch of belief, it was the epoch of incredulity,
it was the season of Light, it was the season of Darkness,
it was the spring of hope, it was the winter of despair,
we had everything before us, we had nothing before us ...

Charles Dickens, *A Tale of Two Cities*

THE WORLD SCIENTISTS' WARNING TO HUMANITY (1992)

Two decades had passed since the prophetic *Limits to Growth* warning out of MIT first sent a chill down my spine. The concerns, first voiced to me in 1973 by Université de Montréal colleague Michael Strobel, had been well founded. The 1992 warning from the world's leading scientists was stark. It left no room for hedging one's bets. Their assessment included a detailed analysis of the Earth's atmosphere, water resources, oceans, soil, forests, and living species, including the escalating global human population. Their statement regarding the corrective measures to be taken was concise, their tone urgent. The implications of the facts at hand were beyond comprehension. Like lemmings, we are mindlessly racing toward mass destruction. As a novice sailor, I sensed the relevance of a further metaphor: the winds defining our future are hurricane-strength, the lee shore is at hand, and we *all* are in the boat. No sane person could persist in upholding the outrageous fantasy that all is well.

Did we listen? Did *Canada* listen? No.[1] It could have been different.[2] As would eventually be reported by the Washington-based Center for Global Development, which tracks the record of twenty-seven wealthy nations regarding their commitment to seven areas that have a positive impact on the world's poor, Canada came thirteenth in the 2013 survey.[3]

Denmark led the list, followed by Sweden and Norway, with Japan and South Korea at the bottom. Canada had dropped from twelfth place a year earlier and, in the environmental-protection category, ranked twenty-seventh. Every other country made progress in this area except Canada. When a global perspective is adopted, it is the worst of times. As a physician caring for the dying, how much more relevant, from my perspective, could our global crisis be?! Those at risk are ALL of us!

PALLIATIVE MEDICINE: A RECOGNIZED DISCIPLINE

For myself, the 1990s did indeed prove to be "the best of times and the worst of times." An emotional roller coaster seemed never far away. While the high stakes warned of in *The World Scientists' Warning to Humanity* documented our rush toward ecological catastrophe on a global scale, the closing decade of the millennium also involved extremes in multiple domains that I had not anticipated.

Palliative medicine was recognized as a specialty in the United Kingdom in 1987, leading Edinburgh's pioneer in the field, Dr Derek Doyle, to observe:

> This enabled us to attract colleagues of the highest academic caliber. Moreover, it gave us a shoulder to shoulder seat at the table with the leaders of all other medical and surgical specialties. Henceforth, we will be there for the critical discussions shaping British Health Care. Our patients and their families will now have a voice. That was fundamental. While our nursing colleagues generally knew that end of life care was inadequate, our medical colleagues were absolutely certain that the care *they* were providing was perfect. We faced a wall of ignorance and unrecognized need. Making Palliative Medicine a specialty of the Royal College and getting it into universities was a huge move forward.[4]

What about Canada? In October 1992 Ken MacKinnon agreed to chair a task force to study issues relating to the formation of a Canadian Society of Palliative-Care Physicians and the recognition of palliative medicine as a Canadian specialty. Working with the Royal College of Physicians and Surgeons of Canada and the College of Family Medicine, this task force suggested a cooperative model according to which *either* college would be a recognized route of entry into a two-year post-certification palliative-medicine training program. This would be precedent setting for Canada.

The task force's report, *Palliative Medicine: Toward Recognition as a Discipline in Canada*, was finalized in September 1994 following critical review and input by the appropriate directors of both colleges. Perusal of the final document led a senior Royal College spokesman to call it "the strongest application for discipline recognition that the Royal College has received in a decade."[5]

All good news indeed, but I foresaw roadblocks looming in our path. Massive federal and provincial deficits suggested the probability of further health-care cuts. Palliative care was generally viewed as being of low priority when compared to "established" disciplines. We were left in a position of vulnerability.

To complicate matters, there were very few funded full-time academic palliative-medicine jobs in Canada and even fewer qualified candidates for those positions. This was not surprising. Because it was not a recognized discipline, there was no secure funding mechanism for physicians wishing to practise in the field. As a result, many opted for minimal palliative-care involvement while earning an income through other activities. We were losing good physicians, promoting an ad hoc image of palliative medicine, and stifling the development of the discipline in Canada. In contrast, the British experience demonstrated that recognition of palliative medicine as a specialty led to increased physician recruitment, enhanced credibility of the field, and the protection of palliative medicine during rationalization of scarce health-care resources.

We needed to break the vicious cycle. In particular, it was imperative, in my opinion, that the Canadian Royal College follow the example of its United Kingdom counterpart. While the College of Family Medicine should be invited to participate, I felt that Royal College recognition should not be delayed if negotiations with Family Medicine became problematic.

Incredibly, given its "best in a decade" assessment of our application, the Royal College acquiesced to the Family Medicine proposal for a one-year training program which offered successful candidates a certificate but no specialty status. Professor Neil MacDonald voiced the task force's assessment of this conclusion: "In [my] view, the wrong-headed decision of the Royal College – a decision seemingly made for administrative/ political reasons rather than a clear analysis of existing and future palliative care needs – has grievously hurt Canadian Palliative Care. Our burgeoning role within medical schools was set back, our ability to sit as equals at the table with academic peers was hampered, our profile as specialists with defined skills and responsibilities was diminished and the creation of well-defined Palliative Care posts has been limited."[6]

The Royal College, and in particular its Committee of Associate Deans, had betrayed the sickest patients in our health-care system and had done so for petty political reasons related to its nascent dialogue with the College of Family Medecine, as well as personal financial concerns. It represented a shameful lack of stewardship that cost Canadian palliative medicine twenty critical years. The Royal College of Physicians and Surgeons of Canada finally recognized palliative medicine as a new subspecialty of medicine in October 2013.[7]

L'ABRI

An unexpected embarrassment of riches blossomed into being when it became evident that the growing number of Mounts anxious to be at our family island, the *Place*, could no longer be accommodated during the few annual weeks of summer sun. Selling my half of our beloved island to my brother, Jim, Linda and I purchased a tiny scrap of Quebec minutes from Mont Tremblant in the Laurentians north of Montreal. It was discovered on our behalf by real estate agent and PCU volunteer Bob Picard. "Sure, Bal, I'll be happy to see what I can find." Easy-going, 5'10", 250-lb.-plus Bob lived in a lakeside chalet in Tremblant Village. For two years he had made a weekly Wednesday pilgrimage to Montreal to volunteer at the PCU. These sojourns would eventually become a seventeen-year gift of benevolence. Bob had a way with people that had been burnished into perfection through years of dealing with the public as a heavy-equipment representative in the construction sector. His relaxed, jovial, low-key manner with prince and pauper alike instantly put PCU patients, family members, and staff at their ease. He was to become a lifelong friend.

Henceforth known as "L'Abri" (the shelter), our new lakeside one-acre plot with its single-room cottage quickly became as cherished as it was diminutive. Situated at the northern end of Lac Mercier, L'Abri had a balcony that overhung the shoreline, providing a picture-postcard vista that featured the forests cloaking the low hills on each side of the lake and the picturesque church nestled among the trees in Tremblant Village on the far shore, one and a half miles south of us.

We were surrounded by a seasonal kaleidoscope of changing colours: from the early-spring patchwork of delicate translucent greens that deepened as the months passed to the riotous chaos of deciduous fall yellows, reds, and oranges interspersed with the deep blue, almost black, hues of the stately conifers, finally to become the haunting, misty, gossamer mauve of etched-bare branches through the winter months – all of it framing the moment-to-moment changing moods of lake and sky.

There was a feeling of lightness and a softening of neck and shoulder muscles each time we pulled into the driveway at L'Abri. *I had no idea I was tense. Smell the pines; feel that breeze off the lake.* With each arrival we found ourselves pausing involuntarily in reverential awe as we shut down the car, wordless on finally stepping outside, hushed into stillness as we experienced the gently shadowed quiet and sense of perennial calm and changelessness among the towering pines

B.C.

Linda and I, accompanied by our two West Highland White Terriers, Vicky and Pebbles, headed north to L'Abri on a Thursday evening with an eye toward hours of decompression involving music in front of a crackling fire. Bliss. It was mid-November, chill and grey. Too late for sailing my Laser or taking out *Ruah*, my beautiful cedar-strip canoe; too early for skiing.

That Saturday morning we headed into Saint-Jovite to pick up groceries and a couple of early Christmas presents. As I waited in the car while Linda retrieved some cash at the nearby banking machine, I watched with detached interest as a large dog left the side of his apparent owner and crossed the road in front of me. A passing car slowed as the driver yelled, "Hey, mister, you should keep a closer eye on that dog of yours." The man walking past my car shouted, "It's not mine: never seen him before."

As I watched, the dog's revised goal became obvious, a family-ladened station wagon parked across from me on the other side of the road. He stood on his hind legs, pawing the window. When they shooed him away, he crossed back across the road and carried on.

Later, as our vet dispensed some medication for one of the Westies, I described the independent stranger to her. "He was impressive, quite magnificent, black with a white blaze on his chest, long haired, wide head – could be a Lab/Golden cross." No, she didn't know of such a dog, but she wasn't surprised. "Lots of people abandon their dogs before heading back to the city at the end of the summer. He could have been on the run for some time, foraging through garbage and what not." We agreed it was a shame.

An hour later, Linda and I emerged from a shop on Saint-Jovite's busy main street, purchases tucked under our arms. The traffic was bumper to bumper – heavy trucks, transports, buses, cars, and the intermittent, self-promoting, thunderously revving, end-of-season motorcycles – all jacked up a notch or two by the chill of the impending first frost.

Dumbfounded, I stopped in my tracks as I saw that same dog weave without concern through the growling lines of traffic in both eastbound and westbound lanes. He was heading toward us. "Hey, mister," a fellow snarled at me disdainfully, "if you don't take better care of your dog than that, you won't have him very long."

The dog plastered himself against my leg and stopped, expectantly. I patted him. He kept pressing, hard. He was perhaps sixty pounds. *Given his imposing frame, he should be over seventy.* I decided to risk it and picked him up. Picked him up? *This is nuts! He's a big, intact, male, a total stranger; he doesn't know me from Adam!* I did it anyway.

Amazingly, he didn't resist as I carried him up the nearby outside staircase to the second-floor office of our vet. "*This* is the dog," I announced, with more than a hint of pride and self-satisfaction. She ran her hands over him.

"He's lovely." But, no, she couldn't keep him and there was nowhere else in town where he could stay. She phoned the Society for the Prevention of Cruelty to Animals (SPCA) in Sainte-Agathe. They had a place. It would take us a couple of hours to drive there, drop him off, and return. She gave us a cord and pulled a ragged collar out of a box under her desk. "Take these ... if you have the time to go all that way."

"Why not?" On opening the back door of the car, he jumped in and lay down on the seat. Not a sound. We headed for the Autoroute. A few minutes later, with the silence from the back seat deafening, I turned my head to see if he was still there. He was standing. His head was inches from mine. His great brown eyes peered deeply into mine without wavering. I had seen those eyes before. As crazy as it sounds, they were Mother's. I turned to Linda, "We'll take him to the SPCA, but if no one claims him in four days, I'm keeping him." There was something about my tone that stifled her looming misgivings. Lauren accompanied me at week's end to pick him up.

Linda had never owned a big dog. She admitted that she was afraid that this formidable newcomer would eat the Westies! An elaborate plan was established. The three dogs would meet at "Triangle Park," the small grass intersection with a park bench at the junction of three roads a couple of blocks from our home. Pebbles growled. Vickie was incensed. She was, after all, a *Westie!* and thus the Alpha Being in the universe. Our new family member totally ignored them both. The growling and posturing of the diminutive duo stopped over the first week or so.

Why do I go into all this detail, you ask? In a word, I can't believe I have progressed this far in my tale without disclosing the important place dogs have always had in my life: their great souls, their unconditional love and loyalty, their deep wisdom, their sense of humour, their capacity for unfailing larger-than-life bonding, their patience, their desire to please, their willingness to learn from us and to teach us if we have ears to hear and eyes to see.

Having him adopt us was a major crossroad. What would we call him? He clearly had been "shipwrecked at the stable door." We named him B.C. for *Big Circumstance*, as in the Bruce Cockburn song. After all, we had gone to a Bruce Cockburn concert with four friends during the first evening Linda and I had shared. B.C., or "the Boy," or simply "B," as I usually called him, was to be one of the great loves of my life. Our adventures were to be unending.

If you buried your face in the Boy's coat, you could just faintly detect a slight odour – not of dog but of a gentleman's smoking jacket. His dignity was omnipresent. While deferential to others as circumstances indicated, from the outset, B.C. was the self-contained, self-confident master of the house. I liked to think that we met as equals, at least during those moments when he was moved to give me the benefit of the doubt.

During the almost fifteen years that we were a team (B died in March 2006), the Boy and I developed a solemn routine that we both took very seriously. Out-of-town lecturing commitments took me away from home on eighty occasions over our partnership years. While I looked on those trips as a privilege, an opportunity to spread *the gospel according to St Cicely* both nationally and internationally, it was also an onerous task, both in preparation time and in the frequent absences from home and hospital. My journeys took me across Canada and the United States, to the United Kingdom, Europe, Japan, China, Australia, and New Zealand. It was something I could do to further the field, I reasoned, something I *had* to do. But, as already noted, those holding the fort at hospital and university (never Linda, who was always supportive) saw my life as glamorous and they let me know it – often! *They* carried the load; *I* was on a grand tour! However, from my end, it rarely felt that way.

B.C.'s arrival lightened the burden in a way I hadn't expected. The evening before each planned departure, he and I would walk to Triangle Park and sit together on the bench – a position he assumed with great seriousness. I would tell him where I was going and how long I would be away and remind him that I counted on him to keep the home fires burning and Linda safe. During these special chats he always listened intently with a serious expression. Anthropomorphizing? Perhaps. But these Triangle Park business meetings deepened the sense of partnership for both of us, I am certain of that. On my return home from these frequent trips, he would, without fail, greet me at the door and sit with me as he "delivered his report" in a quietly dignified manner.

Over the years, I watched B.C. break up several fights, usually by simply coming between the two adversaries, a compulsion I haven't seen in other dogs. Where did this pacifist habit come from? My only hint at the genesis of this gallantry was his cowering reaction when finding himself close to an innocently swinging broom. Had he been beaten as a pup?

In 1994 both Westies died. Within a week, we returned to the Sainte-Agathe SPCA and brought home a lively black pup of perhaps three months. Out of our profound grief – a grief that only a dog lover would understand – and with thanks for Katherine Paterson's brilliant children's story about bereavement, *The Bridge to Terabithia*, we named her Tera. While B.C. had completely ignored the Westies, he was smitten by this new playful pup whom he quickly adopted and trained with fastidious attentiveness.

During his years with us, B.C. was never aggressive. He did, however, scold others on two occasions. Both were at L'Abri. I was the first object of his displeasure. Having just discovered that Tera had helped herself to a healthy portion of my treasured copy of the Karsh classic, *Portraits of Greatness*, I chastised her, with eyes undoubtedly bulging, by waving a rolled-up newspaper in her face while informing her that this was "never to happen again, or I'll skin you alive!" Suddenly, in mid-rant, my left arm was frozen in space. I couldn't move hand, arm, or body. I was startled. What was going on? I looked down at the newspaper and found those big brown eyes looking up at me. B's jaw was gently but firmly locked around my wrist, a mere caress in force and yet I couldn't move my hand an inch. His tail was wagging. He was grinning, but he was clearly telling me, "Leave her to me. She's *my* puppy." I nodded, trying to conceal my smile.

His second disciplinary action came some months later when Tera succeeded in provoking his displeasure. As she grew to equal B in size, Tera continuously terrorized him in a relentless effort to engage him in play during their off-leash walks along the lakeside park. B put up with her nips at his heels as long as he could and then would simply outrun her toward home. But, in due course, her pace equalled his. We became chagrinned: her nips were starting to hurt him.

We were about a mile from L'Abri the day he took control. Now, as it happened, while Tera loved nothing better than swimming and would delight in a galloping run to jump off the end of the dock, the Boy didn't like to swim. He did, however, enjoy trolling in the shallow waters near the shore where he could attentively watch the minnows and other tiny creatures dart back and forth around his paws. He never chased or snapped at them. He simply trolled with undiluted fascination.

One memorable day, B was trolling when Tera attacked him. He left the lake and started his homeward run. She nipped persistently at his hind legs, delighted by his repeated yelps. Suddenly, he turned, stopped, and drove her into the lake. She was surprised, startled, alarmed. He wouldn't let her return to land. He then walked off, as if to head for home, and Tera slunk onto the path behind him. He instantly whirled and drove her back into the lake. Again and again this repeated itself. Having been forced to wade the mile home through water and rocks, Tera never bothered him again

TREVOR

Another L'Abri-associated blessing for Linda and me was Trevor. A telephone call from the University of Ottawa offered me an honorary degree during the 1993 spring convocation. "We would like you to give the convocation address," the regent added.

As I fumbled for the appropriate words, he continued in an apologetic tone, "The only thing is, it will need to be less than five minutes." I laughed; he explained.

"You see we have a second recipient. Trevor Pinnock will receive a degree immediately following yours and he has agreed to play for us as *his* "convocation address.""

"*The* Trevor Pinnock?!" I blurted. "In that case I'll speak for less than one minute." We both laughed.

Maestro Pinnock had been the principal conductor and artistic director of Ottawa's National Arts Centre Orchestra (NACO) since 1991. As founder and conductor – from the harpsichord – of Britain's fabled Baroque orchestra the English Concert, and as pioneer in the original-instruments renaissance in Baroque and early classical music, he was recognized as an icon of period-music excellence. His 6 June 1993 "Convocation Address," a Mozart quartet, was to be delivered with three NAC colleagues.

We found a mutual bond at the pre-convocation gathering and in the subsequent hours of celebration later that day. All I recall of my own convocation address was my opening comment on how meaningful the event was for me. "After all," I observed, "who would ever have thought that I would be asked to open for Trevor Pinnock at the National Arts Centre?"

As he and his colleagues presented *his* "address," he was seated at the keyboard of the magnificent grand piano not three feet from me. It was awe-inspiring. I had not previously experienced similar musical transcendence that close at hand. My mind went back to Marian Anderson.

As we parted, Trevor suggested we keep in touch; we exchanged phone numbers. Weeks later, I answered the phone and the voice announced, "Hello, Trevor Pinnock here."

Over the ensuing months we found ourselves partners in many walks on the park at L'Abri, exchanging memories of our disparate early years in Canterbury and Ottawa. Trevor had been a boy chorister at Canterbury Cathedral, later serving as a church organist. He had taken up the harpsichord when he was fifteen. At nineteen he was awarded a scholarship to the Royal College of Music.

In time, we found ourselves discovering unexpected similarities in challenges and rewards as we discussed our experiences working with teams of talented musicians and caregivers, respectively. To Linda's and my delight, Trevor turned out to be a superb chef with an astonishing ability to concoct a gourmet feast out of trifling refrigerator leftovers. From the outset, Trevor, Linda, and I became a family threesome.

"When did your parents first know there was something different about you?" I asked during one L'Abri lakeside stroll – phrasing my query rather awkwardly.

"I can't recall how old I was," he replied, "but I was able to walk. I was with my parents in a park and a brass band was playing with gusto at a nearby bandstand. I had not heard live music before. The effect on me was electric. Music was not a feature of our home. I was mesmerized. They couldn't pull me away." He paused in thought, then continued. "A later experience stands out as another very early memory. I was perhaps four or five. I recall running into the kitchen where Mother was preparing a meal and with great excitement I asked her if she could hear the carrot tops singing. When she answered that she couldn't, I was totally devastated. For the first time I understood that the most important person in my world did not experience life as I did. It was a crushing blow."

As the months passed, Linda and I were to be Trevor's guests at NAC concerts and post-concert dinners, and he ours, at L'Abri and in Montreal. We quickly learned to turn off the music on CD player and radio on these occasions. He had given at the office.

We were now a family of three – well, *six*, when Chris, Wren, and Jamie were around. No, *eight* actually, when we included the Boy and Tera – and *they* were always included!

YO-YO MA

I was scheduled to be in Ottawa for a Thursday, 5 October, 1995 Health Canada research meeting and was delighted when Trevor called a couple of days earlier to say that he had managed to get me a ticket to attend his National Arts Centre concert with Yo-Yo Ma on Wednesday evening. The concert, followed by a late dinner and time with Trevor, an all-too infrequent event, *and* the privilege of hearing Yo-Yo Ma play was an offer of sublime potential.

Arriving at the NAC at 7:30, I joined the gathering throng awaiting the opening of the hall when a chance glimpse of the interior beyond the closed doors revealed Yo-Yo Ma alone on the stage playing to an empty house. It didn't strike me as odd, nor did it dawn on me that anything was amiss.

The doors opened and we, the expectant audience, trooped in to confront an empty stage. It was 8:05 P.M. but the orchestra was absent – no warming up and tuning of instruments, no chatter of anticipation. The packed house included the prime minister but the stage was empty.

A microphone was hastily set up and the NAC's executive director, Joan Pennefather, announced with regret that Maestro Pinnock was ill and unable to conduct but that, happily, Victor Feldbrill had been contacted in Toronto and was willing to help out. In fact, she noted with a nervous laugh, at that very moment his plane was landing at the airport. She then added, "In the meantime, our very special guest Yo-Yo Ma has kindly agreed to play for us while we await Maestro Feldbrill." With that Yo-Yo Ma walked on stage to say that he would play the Bach Cello Suite No. 1 in G Major. The audience uttered what was by then its third collective gasp.

The thrill of hearing those familiar notes played by Yo-Yo Ma live would have been more than breathtaking had it not been for my anxiety about Trevor. My imagination ran wild. Nightmare! But I was unable to leave my tenth-row centre seat to check backstage.

With the completion of the awe-inspiring Bach, our supremely gifted soloist announced that Maestro Feldbrill had arrived. "So," as he put it, "let the concert begin." He left the stage to thunderous applause. The orchestra filed on, tuned up, and on walked Feldbrill.

The collective drama inherent in the moment was multilayered. Worry and uncertainty about Trevor was mixed with a sense of anguish due to the fact that Victor Feldbrill's wife, Zelda, who had been dearly loved by the NACO musicians, had died just three weeks earlier. A week following her death, Trevor had opened the NAC season with the Mozart *Requiem* and telephoned Feldbrill before the performance to tell him that he, Trevor, and the orchestra were dedicating this performance to his wife. Feldbrill, who had guest-conducted the NACO since its earliest days, was deeply touched. The performance of the *Requiem*, which Linda and I had attended, was memorable. A further aspect of that evening rendered it particularly moving. Although the *Requiem* had been scheduled by Trevor many months in advance, it wasn't until August, only days before its performance, that it dawned on him that it was rather odd to have booked a requiem to *open* the NAC season. He then realized that at an unconscious level he had booked it to honour the fifth anniversary of the tragic death by drowning of his beloved younger brother, Melvin.

As the *Requiem* ended on that season-opening evening, Linda and. I had watched from the audience as Trevor stood with head deeply bowed, hands tightly grasping the podium, his back to the audience. In response, there was a stunned silence for what seemed an eternity before Trevor slowly raised his head, glanced at the back of the score, and motioned for the choir to stand. He later confessed to us that when the audience remained silent he became confused and wondered if he had completed the work – thus he had stolen a peek at the last page of the score. He had been completely unaware of his deeply contemplative stance.

Because the two Yo-Yo Ma concerts were sold out months in advance, the celebrated cellist had suggested to Trevor that they make the Wednesday morning practice session an "open rehearsal," with proceeds from the reasonably priced tickets going to support the orchestra fund. The plan was hurriedly announced on Ottawa radio stations and one thousand people attended. Trevor was delighted with both the attendance and the rehearsal when we talked by phone Wednesday noon. Shortly after we spoke, he felt unwell and was taken to the Civic Hospital.

It was, to say the least, an unpredictable turn of events: a recently bereaved conductor poised to conduct music he had not reviewed let alone rehearsed; an orchestra concerned about their conductor's health; a guest appearance by one of the world's premiere soloists. The tension that Wednesday evening was not lessened by the drama of the opening offering, Beethoven's *Coriolan Overture*, but it was later soothed by Haydn's Symphony 102.

At intermission I went backstage to be handed a message from Trevor to meet him in his room at the Château Laurier after the concert. His worrisome health crisis had been dealt with. Relieved, I returned to my seat for the remainder of the performance.

The unspeakable beauty and intensity of Dvorak's Cello Concerto in B Minor took on additional depth and meaning given the circumstances. I had not attended a Yo-Yo Ma concert before and was mesmerized. While he is unquestionably a virtuoso musician of rare genius, there was something more – his joy, his other-centred grace, his absence of ego and focused listening to his fellow musicians. He drew the listener into an experience of unity with the music. When not playing, he turned his back to the audience to listen to each section – strings, woodwinds, brass – listening to each individual musician, it seemed, with profound attention and respect. They, in turn, responded with playing that was breathtaking. Walter Suskind, the music critic, was to comment following the Thursday evening concert that he had never heard the orchestra sound better. It was a tribute to Trevor and his colleagues, but also to the grace of Yo-Yo Ma: a humbling glimpse of an open soul.

Following the concert, I made my way to the Château, where Trevor and I shared a late meal in his room. As we chatted, he told me of his first meeting with the revered cellist on Tuesday afternoon.

As they met, amidst the bustle of the hallway near Trevor's dressing room, a member of the NACO staff burst from a nearby room shouting in dismay in response to the radio announcement that former National Football League player O.J. Simpson had just been acquitted of the murder of his ex-wife. There was a sense of disbelief among the milling musicians.

Trevor and Yo-Yo found themselves unexpectedly shaken by this apparent travesty of justice. They had not met before and now they found their first moments together coloured by awkwardness and disbelief. Yo-Yo suggested they go for a glass of wine. There ensued a personal exchange about their respective life journeys and about death. It was an interchange that otherwise would not have happened. All of this, as it turned out, occurred only a brief time before they would both be wondering if Trevor's life was in jeopardy.

It had been a great disappointment for Trevor to miss the Wednesday concert. Would he be well enough to conduct Thursday evening? A medical test was booked for that morning at the hospital. His physicians would advise after seeing the results. Victor Feldbrill was there if needed.

We met early Thursday morning in the private dining room on the Château's fourth floor and were well into breakfast when, glancing past me, Trevor observed, "Here's Yo-Yo now. Yo-Yo!"

We were introduced and, as I thanked him with considerable feeling for the concert, he turned the topic to me and Trevor and our friendship. No, he couldn't stay for breakfast with us, he had some calls to complete in his room. He then knelt beside Trevor, engendering a sense of privacy, and asked him how he was feeling. In response to Trevor's account of the pending test, he urged him not to push it. "We'll have further opportunities to play together."

Later, as we chatted, Trevor commented that it was so typical of Yo-Yo to have acknowledged my feelings of appreciation for the concert, then to have turned the conversation away from himself. He had gracefully changed the equation from an inherent admiration-based monologue to a discussion among equals.

At the hospital, the doctors gave Trevor a passing grade: there was no contraindication to his conducting if he felt up to it. We drove up into the Gatineau Hills to an inn where, two days earlier, Yo-Yo and Trevor had shared a memorable roadside lunch on the outdoor patio. Totally delighted by the medical report and the brilliant foliage surrounding us, Trevor made his decision. He would conduct that evening. I took him back to the Château for an afternoon sleep.

My ticket was again tenth-row centre. It offered me a direct view of Trevor and Yo-Yo Ma, and also of my brother, Jim, who was in the third row with his wife, Ursula, and their son, Matthew. Trevor's appearance, after the well-publicized scare of the previous night, was greeted with exuberant applause. The orchestra was in fine form. That evening they played as if unseen hands had added an invisible overarching dimension of magic. The "superb" of the night before became "dazzling."

The Dvorak Cello Concerto was once again beyond description, my enjoyment enhanced by watching Jim's face as he, in turn, responded to the grace of the soloist who, when not playing, again turned in his chair to savour the playing of others, beaming with rapt attention at each in turn as he cradled his silent cello. The bond between him and Trevor felt palpable. Great music. But greater than that was the example of a transcendent human spirit, grace personified. We were at the Deep Centre, a place of Union. "Wasn't that extraordinary?" I stammered to Jim afterward as the crowd dispersed, the applause still echoing in our ears. Flushed, he shook his head, barely able to speak, "That doesn't begin to describe it."

Trevor and I drove, largely in silence, through the enveloping darkness of a chill fall rain to the post-concert reception at the home of our NACO hosts, a cellist and his violinist wife, as we discussed the remarkable talent we had witnessed. Trevor noted the presence and attentiveness Yo-Yo had for each person he spoke to. He had, Trevor observed, an intuitive ability to "read" situations and those present.

On arrival at our destination, I commented to our hostess, whom I had come to know over the several years Trevor and I had been friends, "Isn't he special? I was watching your reaction when he turned to listen as you were playing."

"Good grief," she replied, her face flushing, the eyes of this seasoned professional brimming. "I thought, if he looks at me one more time like that, I'll burst into tears!"

Yo-Yo arrived at the party about half an hour after the rest of us. There were perhaps thirty present. I was the only non-musician. Few present knew why I was there.

When Yo-Yo arrived he carried a box of glasses through to the kitchen, to the accompaniment of spontaneous applause from his NACO colleagues. He once again smiled in that open, guileless way that somehow managed to deflect the attention from himself. He turned toward me in the adjacent sitting room and commented lightly but warmly, "Well, you're quite a person aren't you? I hear you stayed up until 2:00 A.M. to call Kim [Trevor's partner in London] to let her know that Trevor was all right." Until that moment there had been a reverential distance between all present and Yo-Yo. These professional musicians had placed him on a pedestal. With his easy-going comment to me, the least identifiable person in the room, the pedestal had evaporated and we were suddenly all just folks standing around chatting and enjoying a glass of wine. The normality of relating thus established, he had become a welcome guest among friends.

Late in the proceedings, I walked over to the buffet table as one of the musicians helped herself to a last serving of food. She didn't see me approach; she didn't know me. I had noticed her over the years of attending concerts. She frequently seemed unhappy and brusque with her NACO colleagues. Without a word of introduction I leaned quietly into her ear. "He's an amazing guy, eh?" She turned. Her face was a dusky burgundy and contorted with emotion; our heads were inches apart.

"He's not like anyone I have ever seen. He's from another planet," she responded with a whispered earnestness and openness I could not have imagined. It was a profoundly moving moment. "It's true," I thought. "Healing begets healing, begets healing."

When Trevor invited me to join their conversation toward the end of the evening, I asked Yo Yo, "Would you like some feedback?"

"Always," he replied with that engaging smile.

"I have been watching you give to others. You are a remarkable healer. Your openness and presence to others brings real healing."

"I think that is what the music is all about," he smiled. "Don't you?"

"May I ask you a personal question?" I added. He nodded. "Of course."

"Do you meditate?"

"I do a kind of breathing exercise," he responded. "You know, it is important that we empty ourselves."

Two days later, on Saturday, it would be his birthday. "I'll be forty," he observed in response to my question.

In parting I told him that within two weeks Linda and I would be in China to claim our deeply anticipated daughter, five-month-old Bethany Yao.

Trevor and I drove in silence back to the Château. The rain was still falling. Trevor quietly exclaimed, "We are so lucky!" I could think of a thousand reasons why this was true but simply responded, "Lucky?"

"The music! We have all this music! And it is such a mystery. Even those of us who make the music for a living cannot explain it."

YAO YAO

Our Marlowe Avenue neighbour had stopped Linda for an impromptu January 1995 curbside chat, asking, "Is your son Chinese?" It took Linda a moment to make the connection.

"Oh no, Jamie is a member of the Dene Nation in the Northwest Territories. Why do you ask?"

"Laurel and I are adopting a little girl from China and we wondered about his nationality." In fact, Rob and Laurel would eventually become a family of four, their daughters Zoe and, in due course, Kiri both having been born in China.

Our efforts to have a baby had failed. Over supper that evening, Linda told me about her conversation with Rob. She was always ready to shift her personal needs and desires to the backburner, but this time she persisted. "I think I'd like to adopt a baby." I had realized from the first that she would be a loving, attentive mother; it didn't need deliberation. "Let's go for it!"

The telephone call came on 14 September. "Your baby girl Yuan Yao was born on May 19th in the city of Yichun in Jiangxi province." The news was as heart-stopping and moving at fifty-six as it had been at twenty-five, and twice thereafter.

I phoned Linda at Allancroft School where she was teaching grade one. The secretary, guessing the message, asked me to hold the line, arranged for coverage of Linda's class, and told the expectant mother she had a phone call. When I heard Linda's voice on the line, neither of us could speak.

An hour or two into the Chicago-Tokyo segment of our 19 October 1995 Japan Airlines (JAL) flight, I began to develop right-leg pain, then swelling, patchy ecchymosis, and erythema in the calf. Deep-vein thrombosis (DVT). That led to nine hours lying on the floor of the 747 upper cabin, my leg propped up with back packs.

The JAL flight crew refused to comply with my repeated requests that they notify Dr Shigeaki Hinohara of my developing predicament. They found it impossible to imagine that I could know this revered national figure. The renowned doctor and his team had visited the PCU and we had stayed in contact as he championed palliative care in Japan. Physician to the emperor in earlier years and now director of St Luke's International Hospital in Tokyo, Dr Hinohara was a celebrated icon and an internationally respected leader in the development of whole-person care.[8] When we arrived in Tokyo, I finally managed to reach him and I was admitted to St Luke's for anticoagulation while Linda, a timid flyer at best, flew on to China to meet our precious daughter Yuan Yao.

I was concerned about Linda. Prior to a fateful flight several years earlier, she had been an enthusiastic flier. Then, a mid-Atlantic announcement by an Air Canada pilot that they would be returning to London because of "unexpected difficulties" changed all that. How would her current fear of flying adapt to winging her way unaccompanied across China? But, fearful or not, she wasn't about to miss the rendezvous with her baby.

The St Luke's staff was gracious, competent, hospitable to a fault, and unilingual. My Japanese was less than non-existent. A sense of isolation was descending when I recalled that Faye's nephew David and his wife, Hiroko, lived in Tokyo. They were a most welcome godsend. Their daily kindness and generosity knew no bounds. There was nothing they wouldn't do to transform my Tokyo hospital room into a home away from home.

When, in error, the delightful, obsequious, anxious-to-serve resident physician gave me ten times the recommended anticoagulant dose (it had been carried to the bedside with liturgical formality on a red-satin pillow by a shy young nurse, the doctor proceeding to the bedside two steps behind her), David and Hiroko helped me calm the young doctor's deep remorse and feeling of loss of face. What would I have done without them?

A second even more unlikely link to my personal world then came to mind. Trevor and the English Concert would, at some point, be touring Japan. *Was that this fall?* I called his partner, Kim, in London. "Kim, where is Trevor?"

"What time is it?"

"About 2:00 P.M. in Japan – if that is relevant."

"Well, let me see. He should be landing at Narita Airport about now."

"Will he phone you when he arrives?"

"I believe so."

"Could you let him know I am a patient in Tokyo's St Luke's Hospital and would love it if he had the time to drop by?"

Within hours, Trevor walked into my hospital room. The next evening he dedicated the English Concert's first Tokyo performance to *Bethany Yao Mount* – our "Yao Yao.'"

Sitting at my Tokyo hospital bedside a day or two later, Trevor became reflective. "Interesting isn't it? Five weeks ago I called Victor Feldbrill about his wife, and in that conversation I represented life and he represented death. Then, two weeks ago, at the concerts with Yo-Yo, we found ourselves in contact again, but this time Viktor represented life and I death. And it is the case with you and me, as well. Now here we are, halfway around the world and the tables are turned again. How transient it all is. What a gift life is."

Trevor visited me daily and phoned Linda in China regularly during what turned out to be rather harrowing, if memorable, days.

Linda, Bethany, and I were finally united at Narita Airport. Linda looked wan and exhausted as she sleepwalked her way toward me in the line of arriving passengers. Unable to manage Chinese delicacies, she had survived the ten days on a diet of Chinese beer. The small bundle strapped into the pouch on her chest was quiet and sported a black Mohawk haircut, the legacy of months spent in her earlier centre of care. We three were united for the first time. Weary, grateful, and overwhelmed by a dizzying surfeit of unreality, we were deeply thankful for David and Hiroko's guiding presence.

On 30 October 1995 Linda, Yao Yao, and I were somewhere over the Pacific between Tokyo and Vancouver when we heard the results of the Quebec sovereignty referendum launched by the provincial Parti Québécois government of Premier Jacques Parizeau. Quebecers had narrowly voted against the sovereignty option that would have resulted in their separation from the rest of Canada. Of the 4,671,008 votes cast, 49.4 per cent had voted *for* separation, 50.6 against. A small group of family and friends were waiting at the gate in Montreal. How good, on all accounts, to be home.

Yuan Yao quickly became Bethany Yao and in due course Bethany. But, since the Chinese form of endearment is to repeat the given name, to her Daddy she became, and always shall remain, Yao Yao. It is our exclusive bond, even as, to me, her sister is "Wrennie," her brother "Jamie," and Chris simply "Chris." Father Laurence baptized Bethany in our living room in the presence of a small legion of colleagues: Trevor, Laurence, Phyllis Smyth, my PCS colleague Bernard Lapointe, and Linda's friends Pat and Kathy Philips, all of whom agreed to be godparents.

MICHAEL

There was to be yet another link cemented at L'Abri that would influence my perspective on life. A mentor and friend, palliative-care physician Michael Kearney, and I were invited to co-author a chapter on "Spiritual Care of the Dying" for the planned Oxford University Press *Handbook of Psychiatry in Palliative Medicine*.[9] To get the ball rolling, in October 1994, following McGill's 10th International Congress on Care of the Terminally Ill, Michael, B.C., and I headed north for L'Abri.

These decades later, when asked by me, Michael estimated that our L'Abri sojourn had lasted "a week to ten days, or so." I agreed. A recently recovered record from the period noted, however, that it had been a "two day working retreat." *Two days?* Our mutual error in recalling the duration of those intense hours speaks volumes. That L'Abri retreat kick-started a dialogue that continues today.

During those intervening years, Michael moved from Dublin to Montreal (in 2001–03 he was a visiting professor for the McGill Programs in Whole Person Care) and then on to Santa Barbara, California, while our conversations evolved from chats over home-brewed Chai, to handwritten letters, faxes, and telephone calls, to e-mails, and finally to Skype calls.

Two years prior to our seminal hours at L'Abri, the journal *Palliative Medicine* published "Palliative Medicine – Just Another Specialty?" It was Michael's challenge to those in our field who suggest that palliative medicine could meet its mandate if it simply produced "symptomatologists" and nothing more. Such an approach, Michael argued, would ignore something indispensable, the "something more" that is front and centre when we attempt to understand existential suffering – both our patients' and our own. Our L'Abri tête-à-tête with B.C. was to lead to multiple McGill International Congress presentations and workshops over the subsequent years.[10]

Spiritual Care of the Dying. What meaning, if any, do those words have in this secular age? The *Oxford English Dictionary* defines *spiritual* as "relating to or affecting the human spirit as opposed to material or physical things," or again, "having a relationship based on a profound level of mental or emotional communion." Thus, I tend to link *spiritual*, not to religion per se (although for many that may be the primary association that comes to mind), but to an experience of the *existential* in the sense of having the capacity to affect one's experience of existence. The potential of the inner journey to foster both healing and wounding continues to amaze me. The following examples come to mind.

L.T., a bumptious seventy-four-year-old widow, was admitted to the PCU with weakness, irritability, and pain related to bone metastases. While her pain rapidly responded to medication adjustment, she continued to be restless and to register a variety of daily complaints. She was cantankerous. The nurses commented, "We just can't seem to get anything right." Nevertheless, as days passed and her general condition deteriorated, the team began to notice a gradual softening in her mood and easing of her anguish. Some months after she died, a letter addressed to our nursing staff arrived from L.T.'s daughter, her only family member. It read: "Thank you for giving me the mother I never had. Our last days together were precious to me beyond words. In them, we were finally really there for each other. Somehow, that made it all worthwhile. It was a gift I cannot adequately describe."

A lonely, chronically dishevelled, spinster in her sixties was dying in the PCU. She spoke only Polish and had no relatives or friends. The distinguished, quietly dignified man down the hall spoke only English and was blind. He was also dying. In each other, these two starkly contrasting individuals found a healing presence that was profoundly moving to observe. The PCU's environment of tranquil safety made possible a paradoxical relationship, a bond of deep mutual caring that was enabled, rather than hindered, by the barriers of language and sight that were theirs.

Joyce provided yet a further example. There was something about Joyce, a forty-two-year-old woman with advanced abdominal cancer, that didn't add up. Her nurse noticed it the day she was admitted to the PCU. "Her consistent equanimity seems too good to be true." Days later, in the wake of massive fecal incontinence, Joyce's ability to hold her world together dissolved. "This is the last straw," she cried. "Do you call this 'dying with dignity'? If this is a sign of what is to come, I want it over now."

Over the next twenty-four hours, her distress remained extreme and her demands for euthanasia became increasingly strident. Her only relief came from intermittent sedative medication, but each time she awoke she appeared even more agitated.

During the team meeting, there was agreement that her emotional distress suggested existential/spiritual pain. She seemed stuck. How might the team reach the root of her suffering? Michael was part of our team while Joyce was with us. He had been trained in image work and explained to Joyce what was involved in that approach to care, suggesting that it might be helpful, if she was agreeable.

"I am willing to try anything that might help," she replied.

In the quiet and privacy of her room, Michael then asked her to close her eyes as he led her through a gently unfolding journey into the present moment through active imagination.

> Joyce, imagine yourself standing on a grassy hill. It's a summer evening and the sun is beginning to set in a clear sky. It's still warm. There is a faint breeze, which you feel on your face and in your hair. As you look around, you can see, in the middle distance, a river. It's a large river, wide, and obviously deep as its surface is still and smooth and its black waters hardly appear to be moving. You are enjoying the warmth and the swaying grass and flowers as you walk down the slope toward the river's edge where, standing by the water, you encounter someone who knows you and cares deeply about you. The person may be someone you know well or someone who is unfamiliar, but you know the person to be wise, someone who knows the river well, someone who is able to guide you safely in this next stage of your journey.

Michael went on to suggest that there was a little wooden rowboat tied at the river bank nearby and that the guide was offering Joyce safe passage across the river. Michael asked if Joyce would like to accept the offer. It was her choice.

At this point, Joyce nodded and began to weep quietly. Michael asked if she was all right. Joyce nodded again, murmuring, "Yes." He sensed that her tears were those of relief rather than desperation and continued to describe Joyce and her guide getting into the small boat, then gently proceeding out onto the enormous river.

> You know that you are with someone who knows about the boat and who understands the river. You do not know where it will bring you, but you do know that you are with someone who knows the way there. You have done all you can. At this stage you can choose to trust yourself to this guide and to trust yourself to the river. Let your guide lead the way. Let the river carry you. Allow yourself to be carried, to be held by this deep and silent river that is flowing into the next stage of your journey. Be aware, notice, experience how this feels. Allow this experience. Allow yourself to be carried.

Joyce was now lying utterly still, breathing slowly and evenly as if deeply asleep.

She opened her eyes briefly and recalled having met her husband by a river. Her tears now seemed those of sadness. "I asked my husband to help me to die," she continued. "He said he was with me, and that we would be together." She then smiled and, looking deeply relaxed, asked Michael if she could sleep now.

As he left the room he reassured her that she would be watched over while she slept: her needs would be met. From then on, she needed no further medication. At one point she opened her eyes briefly and smiled at a nurse. Her family was at her side. She died in the early hours of the following morning.[11]

Paradox. At the end of life, in a setting of crippling decline, it is possible to encounter healing and a new experience of wholeness. It is possible to die healed. The potential for healing through competent care coupled with the healing potential of an I-Thou relationship, the bonding that occurs when we are present to Self and each other at the deepest level, continues to astonish me. The impact is observed daily where there is care that is both competent and compassionate. Indeed, palliative care is the practice of presence. American educator Parker Palmer favours the wording of Annie Dillard, who writes: "In the deeps are the violence and terror of which psychology warned us. But if you ride these monsters down, if you drop with them farther over the world's rim, you find what our sciences cannot locate or name, the substrate, the ocean or matrix or ether which buoys the rest, which gives goodness its power for good and evil its power for evil, the unified field: our complex and inexplicable caring for each other, and for our life together."[12]

Michael was an important guide as I came to understand more fully Annie Dillard's words. L'Abri, B.C., Trevor, Yo-Yo, Yao Yao, and Michael. It was the best of times.

EUTHANASIA AND PHYSICIAN-ASSISTED SUICIDE

Gersh, one of our PCU patients, was cruelly trapped. Over the previous year, cancer had shredded each aspect of his life. Now, he was unable to talk as a result of brain metastases that had rendered all speech agonizingly garbled at best.

During my ward rounds one afternoon, Gersh and I unexpectedly connected across our mutual sense of impotence.

Would I please get him a pen and paper, he asked. I did.

At the bedside, I watched as he wrote in large, childlike letters.

Ge ... er ... rsh.

"Gersh! ... Your name is *Gersh*," I observed. He nodded.

I h o/ ... oor // ho o ... r // ho // I hor ... nn ... I hro.

"Horse. Horse? ... Gersh, are you saying '*I horse*'?" He nodded again.

"Gersh, are you saying, if I was a horse you would shoot me! Why do you let this go on?"

In an explosion of relief, his right hand struck the bed as our eyes locked and he bellowed a deep, anguish-filled affirmative, *Uuuuhhhh!!!*

His plight was achingly clear. He was asking for euthanasia.

Over the half-hour or so that followed, we cemented a new level of understanding. I acknowledged the terrible plight facing him and listened as he expressed his anguish both non-verbally and in staccato grunts. Then, I explained that, instead of ending his life, our team would do our best to end his suffering.

With the hard reality facing us expressed, an unexpected nuance seemed slowly to appear in our relationship. There was a new and unforeseen sense that we were becoming "brothers in arms" and it began to edge out our former doctor-patient relationship. Was that imagined on my part? Was it wishful thinking? As the minutes passed, it became clear that we both felt this encouraging change. We were now in this together. A new sense of mutual caring was evident to each of us.

I do not imply that there was some sort of rose-tinted journey into bliss. Rather, we both experienced a transformation that was the product of a new meaning that the journey facing Gersh now held for both of us. We had discovered a fresh sense that we would be taking this challenge-filled trip together. Man's search for meaning had uncovered new resources, a new depth, as it were, through our discovery of community. In that process, the possibility of sharing the load had suggested a glimmer of hope for new light and lightness. The mountain ahead would be steep, but it might all become possible. The notion of euthanasia had been sidestepped by both of us, but not the granite walls of anticipated suffering that lay ahead.

As I left his room, the question remained in my mind. Euthanasia? Physician-assisted suicide? To be or not to be. Society was faced by a crossroad decision about the nature of medical care. Does killing the patient belong in the medical-practice toolkit?

Those opposing euthanasia have been viewed by an increasing cohort of Canadians as callous, if not completely unfeeling, religious fanatics who are anti-democratic and incapable of respecting individual autonomy. *After all, whose life is it anyway? It's my right to die that we are talking about.* Indeed, opponents of euthanasia seem inconsistent. *They would euthanize their suffering pet, but not people who are suffering.* Furthermore, notwithstanding the widely held religious stand against euthanasia, some religious heavyweights, including Hans Kung and Bishop Desmond Tutu, have held a pro-euthanasia position. Indeed, some palliative-care providers are in favour. Long-standing Harvard palliative-care pioneers Drs Andrew Billings and Susan Block remain advocates, as does my widely respected Royal Vic PCS colleague Dr Marcel Boisvert. In fact, as already noted, Marcel observed with particular irritation that Dame Cicely and I loved to proclaim, *One should meet patients where they are, not where we think they should be.* Nevertheless, when the patient asked for euthanasia, our high-sounding rhetoric was soon forgotten. We were fair-weather theorists – inconsistent at best, dishonest at worst.

Why do I oppose euthanasia? I find it difficult to believe that society has not transcended the pro-euthanasia stance given all that is now possible. We note that euthanasia supporters in the general public are frequently unaware that they have the right to refuse unwanted treatment. Furthermore, they are not aware of the current effectiveness of palliative care and the availability of palliative sedation for unrelieved suffering. Moreover, referring to euthanasia with the euphemism "physician-assisted dying" or the Canadian version, "Medical Aid in Dying" (MAiD) is misleading. Medical aid in dying? That is the definition of palliative care. Medical aid in dying suggests that the alternative must be *no* medical aid in dying. What we need is education about what is now possible and we need universal access to skilled, competent palliative care.

The obfuscation continues. If it isn't "physician-assisted dying" the public is being sold by the euthanasia enthusiasts, it is "death with dignity." *Goodness, I'm for that! Who wouldn't vote for making that legal?* Or they are being sold "the right to die." *They even want to prevent my right to die after all I've been through! When they fool with my rights and liberties that really gets my dander up.*

There is no question raised about the potential impact permissive legislation might have on the doctor-patient relationship. *Might he kill me?* There is no discussion of the slippery-slope potential. *Oh, so you have legalized E/PAS for this particular age group and that specific clinical situation. But what about those who are suffering intolerably but don't quite fit in those categories? They have rights too, you know!*

There will be, however, according to euthanasia advocates, strict guidelines and built-in safeguards against abuse, in spite of the mounting experience that these have turned out to be meaningless ruses. The risk of slippery-slope extension of euthanasia criteria has become evident in Holland and Belgium. Furthermore, the risk that such legislation poses to the most vulnerable in society is also clear – those who fear they are a burden to loved ones; those unable to speak for themselves; the seriously disabled – mentally or physically; the depressed; those deemed unworthy based on their inability to live productive lives; those without access to state-of-the-art palliative care.

On 5 June 2014 the Quebec National Assembly became the first Canadian province to legalize "doctor-assisted death," meaning euthanasia. In February 2015 the Supreme Court of Canada ruled that parts of the Criminal Code would need to change to satisfy the Canadian Charter of Rights and Freedoms. The parts that prohibited medical assistance in dying would no longer be valid. On 17 June 2016 medical aid in dying by physicians and nurses and their assistance in that act by others was legalized in Canada.

When, in the 1970s, Cicely and I chatted about the legalization of euthanasia, her position was concisely expressed: "I am against it because it places at risk the most vulnerable among us." Her point was made not on religious grounds but on a broader, time-honoured cultural prohibition against killing in general, and in particular against physician-involvement in killing their patients. For Cicely, that would constitute a fundamental distortion of the doctor-patient relationship.

Two patients frame my position on E/PAS. I admitted to the PCU a refined, articulate accountant with advanced cancer. He was in his late fifties and was accompanied by his caring wife, who, on introduction, informed me as she held her husband's hand that they would like to "end this suffering." She added, "He has been through enough; the time has come. I am speaking for both of us because he is tired."

I assured her that we would get to know him over the coming days and establish the sources of his suffering. Our conversation would then be better informed, based on my clearer understanding of the problems involved. Having taken his history, carried out a physical examination, and written his orders, I attended to my other patients.

Later that same afternoon I returned to my new patient's bedside to see how he was settling in. His wife had left. We chatted. He was quiet, alert, responsive, and engaged. After perhaps a quarter of an hour I remarked, "You know, Tom, I am puzzled; some things just don't seem to add up. As I see it, you are not a man who wants to die, but instead, one who would like to live if you could be comfortable. It seems to me that you have spent a lifetime supporting your wife and two sons. You have participated in meeting the needs of society, and now, in your time of illness, you need society to care for you, to ensure your comfort and ensure *your* security. I don't think you want to die. I think you want to live."

His eyes filled with tears. "You are right. But I don't want to be a burden for my family." Our chat reassured him that he need not be a burden.

His remaining weeks were comfortable, and, one might say, rich: rich in the sense of being accompanied into the unknown with a feeling of security through skilled, caring, and consistent support. He did not become "a burden" to his wife, sons, or himself. He lived his last days thoughtfully and peacefully.

N.J. was in his mid-sixties when admitted to the PCU on transfer from the Montreal Neurological Institute with an advanced brain tumour. He was unable to speak. He had been hemiplegic for weeks, leaving him completely unable to move his right side. His left arm was widely bruised, caused by days, if not weeks, of violent flailing about in his attempts to express himself. He had been drifting in and out of coma for several days. The wedding picture on his bedside table suggested his grace and dignity in earlier years and the awesome magnitude of his recent losses.

Among the medications I ordered to control symptoms was a large dose of intravenous steroids. To our profound delight, over the ensuing day he regained his ability to speak. My feeling of elation was, however, short-lived as the continuing depth of his anguish and frustration found voice. I sat with N.J. and his wife and discussed the options that would face us during the coming days of declining consciousness. "Should you wish, I could give you medication that will put you to sleep. You would be comfortable and would not awaken during your remaining days, if that is what you prefer. We would accompany you and tend to all your needs, but you would be asleep."

"That would be more humane," he smiled. Pneumonia followed within three or four days. The palliative-care treatment goal – optimal quality of life – had been upheld without the need for euthanasia. The rights of the most vulnerable in society had been protected and N.J. spent his final hours in comfort thanks to skilled care and palliative sedation.

For Cicely and me, the question facing us was not a religious issue, but, as already noted, a much broader moral issue with far-reaching implications. One must ask, "Why now? In all the centuries since Hippocrates, why now?" Why did Hippocrates, 2,400 years ago, in spite of his extremely limited means of symptom control, find it important to include a specific prohibition on euthanasia? Why does our anxiety about "personal rights" come to particular prominence at this juncture in human history? Our capacity to relieve suffering is greater than ever before, but so is our need for control. How does that relate to our death anxiety and what we now understand about terror-management theory?[13] Do we really believe these issues are unrelated? Our desperate need for an illusion of control appears to be infinite. Again, why now?

Within weeks of what I considered to be a disastrous decision on the part of the Supreme Court of Canada, I wrote a letter to each of the nine justices.

A Letter to Each of the Nine Supreme Court of Canada Justices:
The Honourable ____   March 4, 2015
Supreme Court of Canada.

Dear Justice ____
A skilled Palliative Care physician asked me, "In light of the recent Supreme Court of Canada ruling, how do we respond to the patient who has been under the care of our team and yet asks for Euthanasia or Physician Assisted Suicide (E/PAS)? How do we reply with caring and compassion? Just saying that "we don't do that here" may be one answer, but that has its own issues. It will be hard to transfer away from our Palliative Care Unit someone who is well known to the team. I really don't have a good answer!"

You don't have a good answer? The answer is clear: palliative care.

Four decades ago, England (St Christopher's Hospice, London, 1967) and Canada (Royal Victoria Hospital Palliative Care Service, Montreal, 1975) pioneered the first comprehensive programs featuring Inpatient Wards, Home Care, Outpatient Clinics, Bereavement Support programs, research and teaching, as well as a consultation service to the active-treatment wards of the Royal Vic, a McGill Teaching Hospital.

How would we respond if confronted by the hypothetical situation my colleague describes? I would sit down at my patient's bedside and say, "Tell me, Joe (Helen), what is the worst part for you today?" I would sit ... and sit. I would listen carefully with the bedside curtains drawn to assure privacy. I would need to be *radically* present because this is the soul-to-soul stuff of the Hebrew prophets; this is First Nations Great-Spirit-at-one-with-the-Universe stuff; this is at-the-foot-of-the-cross stuff; Atman-to-Atman stuff; Buddha's emptiness-that-is-a-plentitude stuff; together-in-the-Sufi-dance stuff; standing-naked-in-our-helplessness and vulnerability stuff. It presents simultaneously imminence and transcendence as we confront our separation challenges in search of attachment solutions. Socrates said it well, "Wisdom begins in wonder," and again, "A system which is based on relative emotional values is a mere illusion, a thoroughly vulgar conception which has nothing sound in it and nothing true."

Facing persistent suffering we would question – *for the hundredth time* – the patient's sources of meaning. We would start over! We would review every aspect of his/her anguish and Total Pain: the complexity of the needs; the care we are providing. We would *yet again* search for enhanced effectiveness in the face of physical, psychosocial, existential/spiritual distress.

What then? *Then*, should all our efforts fail, I would ask a special colleague to step in for me, take my place. Forty years ago at the Royal Vic I asked Dr Ina Cummings or Dr John Scott. At St Christopher's, I asked Dame Cicely Saunders, Dr Thérèse Vanier, Dr Mary Baines, or Dr Tom West. In other words, I sought out a colleague who would relentlessly examine, with what Dame Cicely called "a beady eye," the Gordian knot facing us.

What then? If my colleague's insights had not shed important new light on the suffering, *then*, we would ask ourselves, "Is it time for a trial of palliative sedation?" I would say to my patient, "Would it be easier for you to be asleep?" and would explain our individually optimized titration of hypnotics in the face of uncontrolled suffering. We use individually optimized doses so that our suffering patient is *just* asleep and comfortable, this being an intervention that could give way to a trial reversal of sedation at any time, should intuition suggest that exhaustion was a significant aspect of the problem. If ongoing sedation is required, death would occur in a short period of time, with family and friends at hand.

Our aim would be as it has always been, optimal quality of life. There would be no need for E/PAS. Our therapeutic goal would not have changed; as always, it is *quality* of life. The intent is to kill the suffering, not the sufferer. Palliative sedation, as described, is legal and does not require new legislation or a change in goals. It does not expose society to the slippery slope currently facing Holland and an increasing number of other jurisdictions. If someone asks why we do not kill (E/PAS) people here, we tell them as many stories as they wish to hear concerning the risk that such an action would pose for the most vulnerable among us. Not only those who may experience enhanced quality of life as a result of our indefatigable efforts, but also, the disabled, the demented, those unable to speak for themselves and, in particular, those who "don't want to be a burden" to loved ones.

"You don't want to be a burden, you say? But, my friend," I would respond, "You live in Canada. We do not kill people here. You are precious to us. You are not a burden. You are why our

Palliative Care Service is here. A burden? You have no need to worry about that. We will care for you. Your family and loved ones can visit as they are able, without being 'burdened' by your life."

"But what about my individual rights? Surely this is a matter of autonomy."

"Well, my brother, you are perhaps forgetting something. You already have the right to refuse any treatment, as well as the right to competent Palliative Care. Moreover, from the earliest times, society has recognized that individual rights have limits, even in the most caring society. Community rights must take precedence over the rights of the individual. That is why over the centuries we quarantined those with leprosy, the plague, smallpox, ebola, and so on. We think of it, *not* as curtailing the rights of a few, but as honouring the rights of all, and in particular the most vulnerable among us. That is why we provide the care I have just described to you. You need not be abandoned with unrelieved suffering. It is called Palliative Care! It should be offered to all Canadians because each of us matters, and we matter until the very end of our lives. You will not be left alone. We are with you always, and if it remains as hopeless as it feels today, we will help you sleep."

Today in Canada, universities have been revising their Medical Faculty curricula to include the Whole Person Care I have described above. After four decades of Palliative Care in Canada the Royal College of Physicians and Surgeons of Canada and the College of Family Physicians have established (October 2014) a two year Palliative Care Certification program for candidates licensed in either of these Colleges.

The end-of-life healthcare crisis in Canada does not arise from a need for E/PAS legislation. It is the result of the shameful forty years-long failure of provincial and federal politicians to support the provision of universal access to Palliative Care for Canadians.

The notion that E/PAS is the appropriate corrective for political failure and an unquenchable need for personal control is madness; a needless, unqualified catastrophe! When we struggle to this particular summit of apparent reason and peer with misgivings down the other side, we will find a slippery slope of cascading consequences that we had not anticipated awaiting us.

Sincerely,

Balfour M. Mount OC, OQ, MD, FRCS(D), LLD,

Emeritus Eric M. Flanders Chair of Palliative Medicine,

McGill University

I sent my letter to each of the nine Supreme Court of Canada judges. I did not receive a single response.

The suffering of people at the end of life has been enough to legalize E/PAS but, interestingly, not enough to mandate excellence in palliative care for all Canadians. This is an ongoing need and, in my view, a tragedy. An international wave of permissive E/PAS legislation was and is washing up on shore after shore in the international community, as is the predictable detritus that follows in its wake. It was and is the worst of times, and that has been, and currently is, unnecessary.

RITES OF PASSAGE

It was in 1994, but I don't recall the exact date when I first became aware of the dynamic duo. D.G. had replaced Dale Dauphinee as the RVH physician-in-chief and M.K. was named director of nursing for the RVH Department of Medicine, including the PCS. What I *do* recall with clarity was the day I was stopped in the hall by a colleague in the wake of a meeting of the chiefs of the Department of Medicine Service.

"Bal, I would keep an eye on M.K. if I were you. At the meeting just now she announced that her number one goal as director of nursing would be to close the Palliative Care Service. I thought you should know."

It was a memorable opening salvo from this newly minted dyad who would have a defining impact on PCS functioning over the months and years that lay ahead. Although the cavalry charge was led by M.K., D.G. was complicit in that he did not contradict her stated objective, then or later. While the PCS was not represented at senior administrative meetings, concerned colleagues kept me informed.

In fairness, one must consider the context: a weak Quebec economy had necessitated hospital budget cuts and home care of the dying had been transferred to the newly minted Centre Local de Service Communitaire (CLSC) community-based clinics in Quebec, a resource that was, to be charitable, ill-prepared for the task.

There was a further strike against us. In spite of the documented inadequacy of end-of-life care, the demonstrated PCS track record of excellence, and our recognized strength in research and teaching, many colleagues in the Department of Medicine regarded the concept of palliative care as an anathema and foreign to the hospital mandate. *In these days of fiscal restraint why in God's name can't they be cared for in nursing homes? They certainly don't need to be in a tertiary care teaching hospital!* A Vic physician was expected to be a world-class, finely honed, subspecialist in his or her particular Royal College-accredited field. Uncertainty regarding our PCS lineage was understandable. When the PCS opened, Ina and Marcel were the only two family physicians on the Royal Vic staff.

Maurice McGregor, a South African, was the only "outsider" (that is, non-McGill graduate) in RVH's eighty-year history to be named director of the Department of Medicine (1974–79). He had served as dean of medicine (1967–72) and was the RVH's chief of medicine as we admitted our first PCU patient. Over the ensuing decades, on at least a twice-yearly basis, Maurice would pause on seeing me approaching, then comment in his characteristically thoughtful manner, head tilted, hand stroking his chin, "Bal ... sometime you must tell me what you are up to, what 'palliative care' is about." That was Maurice – direct, honest, enquiring, probing – always challenging, always asking for the data that supported your hypothesis, but always open to innovation. That was what made him an honoured medical scientist, a thoughtful administrator, and a respected dean. Dr Sylvia Cruess, the RVH's director of professional services, pointed out years later, "If Maurice hadn't supported the PCS pilot project, it would never have been given the green light."

In our rare fleeting encounters, Nursing Director M.K. was a taciturn force of nature with a granite mien. Chief of Medicine D.G., on the other hand, presented himself as a quietly affable colleague. It was difficult to picture him as an adversary.

Close the PCS? In the wake of a twenty-year track record of documented need and excellence in the PCS response to that need? During one of our rare chats, D.G. commented, "Bal, we're on your side, you know." But those words rang hollow given M.K.'s oft-repeated position concerning the PCU. Neither of these two colleagues ever demonstrated interest in the PCS, discussed our function, or included me in discussions regarding options when funding became tight. M.K. was a woman on a mission. The fox was in charge of the henhouse.

During the week of 20 June 1994, I received a request from D.G. for an analysis of the impact that closure of four of our sixteen PCU beds would have on our ability to function. On 27 June he received my detailed response emphasizing that the tighter the hospital budget, the more urgent was the need for a fully functioning PCU to ensure optimal RVH bed utilization and patient care in *all* pavilions (Medical, Surgical, and OB/GYN). A four-bed PCU closure, I pointed out, would *increase* the number of active-treatment beds "blocked" by dying patients based on the proven effectiveness of the PCU and PCS home-care programs which served to lengthen the duration of home-based care and diminish hospital length of stay. I argued that, since closing PCU beds would undermine patient care across *all* RVH pavilions, any such closure should be decided by a hospital-wide consensus. In addition, I noted that the PCS "pays its own way" to a greater extent than any other clinical service since I was raising more than $185,000 annually through community donations to cover salaries for team members involved in our clinical-care programs.

My detailed analysis resulted in a follow-up letter but no face-to-face examination of alternatives. D.G. noted, "Overall I agree that the preferred course of action would be to maintain the status quo but clearly a four bed closure on the PCU would be a possible, although unpleasant, course we may have to follow." On 5 July I was informed that he had already recommended the four-bed closure.

On 11 July, I wrote the RVH president, P. Aspinall, concluding:

> It may well be that there are no alternatives left but to undermine a flagship program for which the Royal Vic is known worldwide. It may well be that the long-range plans of "Palliative Care McGill"[14] need to be rethought and that the fiscal pressures facing us make the time required for inter-hospital dialogue concerning the rationalization of Palliative Care services a luxury we can't afford. All that may be true. It is a concern, however, that the process to date does not allow us to draw those conclusions. In fact, I believe that the process reveals a lack of the kind of long-range planning and vision that are urgently needed. As we all know, we face further budget cuts in the coming years. If the current ad hoc piecemeal whittling away of programs is allowed to continue current areas of excellence will be destroyed ... In closing, I would like to recommend that the PCU at the RVH be considered for an expansion in the number of beds to a thirty bed ward to accommodate the rationalized patients from the Montreal General Hospital and the Montreal Neurological Institute. I would also like to pose a question to you and those who receive a copy of this letter.[15] At what point do we exercise leadership and take to the public the reality that further budget reductions are incompatible with sustaining the standards of excellence for which the RVH has been known over the past century?'

The four PCU beds were closed on 20 October and the numbers of patients awaiting PCU admission throughout the hospital increased as I had predicted.[16]

On 2 November, the RVH president received a letter from an anonymous donor in the community. It stated:

I hereby commit $98,000.00 to fund the immediate re-opening of the four PCU beds for the coming year. I furthermore make a commitment to keeping these beds open over the next three years. In making these donations it is my expectation, however, that appropriate internal adjustments will be made to enable the ongoing presence of sixteen PCU beds at the RVH, funded from customary budgetary sources following this three year period. In this way these donations will not represent an uncomfortable precedent through which the public assumes responsibility for the cost of inpatient care. I want this donation to be referred to as a token of public support for Palliative Care by the Montreal community. The vision and concern for the most vulnerable members of society demonstrated by the RVH in opening the PCS twenty years ago has been greatly appreciated. It causes us great concern to realize that hospital support for this program may be waning, particularly in view of the evidence that the presence of a strong PCS enhances patient care and helps the hospital to use most effectively its decreasing number of active treatment beds.

The beds were reopened on 21 November 1994. There was no acknowledgment by either D.G. or M.K. of this remarkable community support and of the PCS excellence that it suggested.

KAPPY

Meanwhile, our future was being shaped in ways we could not have imagined, thanks to a process that had its inception three years earlier 5,500 miles away in Jerusalem. On a clear, sun-drenched day in December 1991, Marcia Flanders and Dr Ted Fink were in the gardens of the Hadassah Medical Center Hospice, Mount Scopus, in Jerusalem. The sweeping vista before them as they chatted took in Ramat Rachel Kibbutz directly ahead and Bethlehem farther to the south. Beyond all that, the sweeping expanse of sand, dunes, and the Dead Sea loomed large. The view was majestic but their thoughts were elsewhere. Dr Fink, a retired British physician, was the volunteer medical director of the Hadassah hospice program; Kappy (Marcia's nickname since early childhood) had returned to Jerusalem for a respite visit in the wake of the death of her husband, Eric, the previous June. They had been married thirty-four years.

Eric, a prominent Montreal businessman, had died with lung cancer following surgery and chemotherapy at the Montreal General Hospital. Kappy had been supported through their whirlwind ordeal by Eric's surgeon, David Mulder, and oncologist Michael Thirlwell. Their attentiveness included home visits during Eric's final illness and they had become Kappy's lasting friends.

"Did he receive palliative care?" a friend asked Kappy early in her Jerusalem visit. "What's that?" Kappy responded. After offering a brief explanation, her friend added, "You really should see Dr Fink at the Hadassah hospice. He can tell you all about it."

Not one to ignore a lead with creative potential,[17] Kappy sought out Dr Fink: thus their hospice-garden chat. On hearing his description of their palliative-care program, she was determined. "If I can find donors to cover your expenses, would you come to Montreal to speak to our doctors about palliative care?"

Dr Fink replied with surprise. "But Montreal is where I learned about palliative care. They invented it."

On her return to Canada, Kappy's telephone enquiries were fielded by ever-astute Yvonne Corbeil, who had replaced Dottie Wilson as PCS chief administrator. A lunch with Kappy, Yvonne, Volunteer Director Mary Coughlan, and me followed. Shortly thereafter, Dean of Medicine Richard Cruess organized an informal chat with Kappy and me in his office. As Kappy left, Dick acknowledged that she was indeed a remarkable woman, a person of vision, one who could be a great help in our efforts to improve patient care.

In October 1994 Kappy brought into being the Eric M. Flanders Chair in Palliative Medicine at McGill. On 15 December Principal and Vice-Chancellor Bernard Shapiro presided at the inauguration of McGill's newest Faculty of Medicine chair. The venue was McGill's Osler Library, described by Dean Cruess as "the soul of the medical school." Kappy had composed "A Letter to Eric" for the occasion which she read during the proceedings. In it she commented, "The reasons that brought us to this evening were not happy ones but we hope that the benefits that others will derive from this Chair will have made our sacrifice worthwhile." In a similar vein, Eric's daughter Susan stated, "The Chair does not make [Dad's] death easier to bear. It does, however, give it some meaning. While Dad will always live in our hearts, the Chair will allow him to touch and affect the lives of many others as well." In response, I observed, "Some acts have ripple effects far beyond the dreams of the person who first threw the pebble into the pond. I predict the ripple effects of this pebble will exceed our greatest expectations."

On 11 December 2004, at the ceremony to mark the tenth anniversary of the Eric M. Flanders Chair, I recalled the many ripples resulting from Kappy's vision, noting, "To paraphrase Churchill – Some pebble! Some toss!"[18] The M.K.-D.G. threat had been dealt an important blow. Circumstances may dictate the closure of clinical programs, but the probability is likely to be reduced if there is a university chair attached.

In addition to the Eric M. Flanders Chair, the year 1994 had featured other promising highlights. Canadian oncologist Neil MacDonald returned to Montreal, following a twenty-three-year absence, to assume dual activities at the Université de Montréal's Centre for Bioethics (focus on ethical issues) and McGill (focus on palliative-care research and teaching). Neil was a larger-than-life Renaissance man, his academic activities balanced by his knowledge of history and current affairs, music, and film as well as his enthusiasm for sports. He didn't bother to keep an agenda: he unfailingly retained phone numbers and future commitments in an ever-updated mental file.[19]

Also in 1994, Anna Towers, director of family medicine at McGill, was recruited, thus significantly bolstering our clinical, teaching, administrative, and research resources, the latter dealing with the management of lymphedema in patients with malignant disease. Discussions with long-time medical scholar John Seely, then dean of medicine in Ottawa, regarding his return to McGill to join our palliative-care team were, it seemed, reaching finalization, an initiative enthusiastically supported by Dean Cruess. Robin Cohen was named director of research, Palliative Care McGill, as she continued to refine the McGill Quality of Life instrument and generate an array of other studies. Finally, McGill's 1994 Tenth International Congress on Care of the Terminally Ill attracted 1,400 delegates from 28 countries. It was the best of times.

CHALLENGES TO A NEW DISCIPLINE

As 1994 morphed into 1995, recent encouraging palliative-care developments were submerged by the cumulative effect of a series of menacing edicts initiated by the Quebec government, the Royal Vic's Department of Medicine, and the McGill Faculty of Medicine. Taken together, they threatened the PCS's ability to function, forming a perfect storm of issues that would leave palliative care at McGill and across Quebec in ruin if left unchecked. Finding myself completely unable to fulfill my mandate under these circumstances, I was confronted with three options: simply ignore the realities now at hand, attempt to stamp out each successive brushfire until the smoking ruins became evident to all involved, or resign, thus serving notice to those in a position to salvage palliative care in Quebec, at the Vic, and in the McGill Faculty of Medicine.

While the visionary action almost twenty years earlier, by the Quebec Ministry of Social Affairs, in pioneering a salary mechanism for palliative-care physician reimbursement deserved commendation, by June 1995 the ministry had presented us with four prohibitive roadblocks:

- Further palliative-care program development in Quebec had been frozen since 1991.
- In October 1994 the ministry banned palliative-medicine physicians from providing home care unless requested by the patient's primary-care physician, and then only for matters pertaining to pain control. This was unacceptable. Many Quebec patients did not have a primary-care physician. Furthermore, family-physician-staffed community clinics were generally closed weekends and from 5:00 P.M. until 9:00 A.M. on weekdays and, in addition, their existing workload frequently precluded early attention to new patients. In contrast, our Home Care physicians and nurses were available seven days a week, twenty-four hours a day. Moreover, dying patients are among those with the most complex and challenging needs, and thus the ministry's suggestion that consultation could relate only to pain was remarkably naive: What about malignant bowel obstruction, profound multifactorial dyspnea, unresolved existential anguish, and a seemingly endless list of other issues?
- Quebec medical specialists interested in practising palliative medicine were obliged to seek permission from their provincial subspecialty committee to obtain a clinical salary. This direct conflict of interest scenario was untenable. For example, when in April 1995 University of Ottawa Dean of Medicine John Seely agreed to return to McGill to assume a palliative-care leadership role, McGill's Dean Cruess offered to support the position with an academic salary. Nephrology, the relevant subspecialty, refused. Dr Seely was thus unable to join us.
- On 31 May 1995 I received a letter from the provincial government informing me that PCS family-physician coverage must be cut, effective 1 May 1995, from its existing level of 244 hours per week to 126 hours per week, and furthermore, that night and weekend coverage would no longer be reimbursed. This edict meant that our three family physicians must each diminish their work week to thirty-five hours, while a fourth colleague who was currently returning to the PCS, having completed a master's degree in epidemiology at McGill, would be restricted to twenty hours per week. It seemed painfully ironic that the ministry had declared that palliative care was one of their "ten priority issues for 1995."

In the early 1990s, provincial fiscal pressures required bed closures in Quebec hospitals. Data accrued over the two-decade PCS experience had clearly demonstrated that optimal "through-put" of patients was fostered if "active-treatment" beds, *rather than* palliative-care beds, were closed. Nevertheless, as we have just seen, on 29 September 1994 one-quarter of the RVH's PCU beds were closed in spite of the predictions that such a move would decrease effectiveness of bed utilization throughout the institution and undermine patient and family care. The four-bed closure resulted in the predicted negative consequences and led to a striking increase in the daily number of patients waiting for hospital admission, from a norm of two to four patients to as many as eighteen. When four PCS beds were reopened 21 November 1994, due, as we saw earlier, to an anonymous $98,000 donation from the community, the backlog of RVH patients awaiting PCU admission immediately dropped to initial pre-closure levels.

At the time of the PCS bed closure, I was assured that the PCS had sustained more than its share of cuts and would be spared during future bed closures. However, six months later, without consultation, our consult-nurse position was cut. This position had, in the twenty years since its creation by Director of Nursing Lorine Besel, been central to the smooth interactive functioning of the four clinical arms of the PCS. Trish Hunter, our last consult nurse, was, like her predecessors, Pierrette Lambert and Glynis Williams, an astute clinician and teacher, a thoughtful adviser to the staff on the acute-care wards, and an effective liaison person between the PCU, the acute-care wards, and the Home Care service, thus maximizing efficient patient flow. In response to the remarkable suggestion by the chief of medicine that accepting cuts to the PCS was important if we were to be "perceived as belonging to the culture of the hospital," I suggested that that was a shallow rationale for poor administrative decisions which undermined patient care and the efficiency of bed utilization.

On top of everything else, in 1995 the McGill Faculty of Medicine entered the first year of a mandate that required a 20 per cent budget reduction within five years. Toward that end, the University Academic Strategic Planning Group was to undertake a comprehensive budgetary review. Fortunately, its stated "Faculty Principles for Planning" guidelines included seven foundational criteria in which palliative care excelled.

We were at a crossroad. I argued that McGill must decide whether or not palliative medicine was a priority program to be protected, nourished, and supported and that, given the small size of the program, *any* decrease in palliative-care support would be fatal; indeed, without *additional* support for palliative-care teaching, research, and academic growth, our survival would be endangered, if not rendered impossible. Faculty decision makers were supportive, as they had been for two decades, but the stakes were high and the odds were not encouraging.

Others, both within our McGill community and in the national and international community who were monitoring our track record as we pioneered the integration of a palliative care/hospice in an academic centre, appeared to be unaware of the overwhelming implications of all the above threats to palliative care. I was left with no option but to resign. On 5 June my letter of resignation from the Eric M. Flanders Chair and all palliative-care programs was sent to the McGill principal, the chancellor, and the new dean of medicine, Dr Abraham Fuks (Dean Richard Creuss had retired in May after fifteen years in office), as well as to Kappy and the appropriate administrators and department heads at the RVH. I also notified Cicely and selected colleagues in the international palliative-care fraternity whom I felt should receive the news first-hand.

In response, McGill Principal and Vice-Chancellor Bernard Shapiro scheduled a 16 June meeting to include the appropriate university, faculty, and RVH representatives.[20] It was agreed that I would present my concerns, answer any questions that might arise, and then leave the meeting in the interest of facilitating frank discussion. Three colleagues offered to attend the meeting at their own expense in order to express their opinions and respond to questions regarding the significance of this crossroad for the international community: Dr Eduardo Bruera, professor of oncology, Alberta Cancer Foundation; Dr Robert Dunlop, medical director, St Christopher's Hospice, London; and Dr Kathleen Foley, chief, Pain Service, Memorial Sloan Kettering Cancer Center, New York City. A closed session involving university and hospital representatives was to follow.

At the 16 June meeting I offered an outline of the problems facing those who might wish to continue palliative care at McGill following my resignation and my observations concerning the necessary steps to be taken if the PCS, as we knew it, was to be salvaged. A document spelling out the details of the crisis at hand was distributed.

I deleted a final paragraph of my planned statement since the central issue it addressed was already deeply familiar to all in the room. The days were ticking down toward an approaching Parti Québécois referendum that would ask Quebec voters whether the province would proclaim national sovereignty and become a state independent from Canada. The polls suggested that the results would be too close to call. The omitted paragraph read: "As a Palliative Care physician for twenty years, my estate is somewhat more limited than might otherwise be the case and, in fact, in large part consists of my NDG [Notre-Dame-de-Grâce] home. In this referendum year I find the value of my property dropping with each passing day and varying inversely with the number of 'For Sale' signs which seem to grow like weeds on the lawns of our community as the weeks pass. For this reason and also because of the difficulties imposed through the uncertainty of the current process, I will have to arrive at a final decision prior to 30 June."

The results of this meeting were:

· ongoing assessment and negotiations in the targeted areas;
· a flood of concern and support generated by the *Montreal Gazette*, the *Canadian Medical Association Journal*, and the leaders of the international palliative care/hospice network;
· a sufficient increase in the number of physician hours awarded to the RVH PCS to allow a PCS physician, Dr Pauline Lavoie, to return to active duty on our team;
· clarification by the Ministry of Health that "the prohibition of Palliative Care physicians from participating in home care except when invited by the 'treating physician' and then only for purposes of pain management" did *not* apply to the RVH PCS;
· affirmation of the intent "to support factors that permit academic excellence in Palliative Care at McGill";
· a continuing review of McGill commitments to palliative care to be undertaken by Dean Fuks and Dr Leyland-Jones, director of the McGill Department of Oncology;
· creation of a task force chaired by neurosurgeon Joseph Stratford to examine the future of palliative care in the wake of the planned amalgamation of the RVH and the Montreal General, with Dr Stratford promising that he would recommend a structure that would ensure that the resulting palliative-care service or department would not be unduly vulnerable compared to other clinical programs.

Clinical funding for Quebec specialists doing palliative care remained unresolved pending the outcome of negotiations to establish palliative medicine as a recognized discipline in Canada and Quebec.

The dangerous erosion of the RVH PCS had been brought to the attention of the stakeholders, including the public at large. While most issues remained a "work in progress," we appeared to be standing on much firmer ground, and so, on 7 September, I withdrew my resignation, noting in my letter to the principal: "While the progress is encouraging, it should be noted that to date we have failed to reach a satisfactory conclusion in any of the problem areas. I look forward to [further] creative solutions arising from the above." I would continue to work with Dean Fuks, as I had with Dean Cruess since the early 1980s, to recruit an academic leader to guide our PCS programs into the future.

JOHN

John Seely (1937– 2009) was the most "compleat" (in the classic, quintessential sense) physician that I have known. McGill's loss, through the failure of Quebec's nephrology leaders of the day to fund him via existing mechanisms, was a deplorable example of self-interest trumping insight. It was an unforgettable, unforgivable, totally avoidable lost opportunity, the worst of times writ large! Having trained at McGill, the University College Hospital, London, and Yale, John was named director of the Division of Nephrology and professor of medicine at McGill prior to accepting the position of professor and chairman of the Department of Medicine (1984–89) and later dean of medicine (1990–95) at the University of Ottawa's Faculty of Health Sciences. In 1996 John resigned the last position and became director of the University of Ottawa Institute of Palliative Care. Sadly, McGill and Quebec had dropped the ball.

A consummate clinician, teacher, researcher, administrator, and catalyst for healing in all he laid his hand to, John was a William Osler of his day. He uniquely combined head and heart to the betterment of his patients, their families, his students, colleagues, academic institutions, friends, and family. Indeed, throughout his career, John was a thoughtful leader in administration and education for the faculties of medicine he served, and for the Royal College of Physicians and Surgeons of Canada on whose behalf he carried out countless discerning academic assessments at centres of excellence across the country and in the international community. As a clinician, John regularly gave his pager number to nurses and junior staff so that they could reach him on a 24/7 basis, whether or not he was on call. He treated each person he met, whether patient, family member, or caregiving colleague, with profound respect that was the product of the uniqueness he recognized as theirs.

Beyond all that, John was a man of catholic interests: from the works of Richard Wagner and the Bayreuth Festivals, to the insights of Virginia Satir and American critical thinker Werner Erhard; from lakeside cottage maintenance to making jam and world-class knitting. He was gentle, introspective, discerning, and humble. His thoughtful quest for the life fully lived led him to in-depth explorations of Quaker practices, Buddhism, and meditation, the latter including ten-day silent retreats. To all of that John brought enthusiasm, a buoyant sense of humour, and consistent presence to the moment.

For four years prior to his move to Ottawa, John had been my weekly Sunday morning tennis partner, and then, during his Ottawa years, he became an honorary member of the Mount family, with weekend visits to Montreal several times each year during the remainder of his life. Our deepening bond on the winding road that lay ahead of us was a consistent support. The deepening of our shared paths, in health and illness, was to be among the unexpected benefits experienced in times of celebration and challenge.

The privilege of accompanying John during his final months, both at Ottawa's Lord Lansdowne Residence and later at the Maycourt Hospice, led to countless memorable moments. Most unforgettable, perhaps, was the joy shared one afternoon as he and I sat, transfixed, watching Christopher Nupen's staggering film *The Trout*, which features a remarkable pick-up group of friends in their early twenties – Daniel Barenboim, Itzhak Perlman, Jacqueline du Pré, Pinchas Zukerman, and Zubin Mehta – performing Franz Schubert chamber music. In those magic moments we experienced the gift possible when the youthful exuberance and dazzling genius of those five was allowed to wash over and place in perspective the challenges and uncertainty of illness. Transcendence experienced.

The Existential/Spiritual Domain Revisited

In the way of God thoughts count for little, love is everything.
Brother Lawrence

Your own Self-Realization is the greatest service you can render the world.
Ramana Maharshi

One touch of nature makes the whole world kin.
William Shakespeare

Cicely's concept of "Total Pain" posits that human experience is *always* modified by every aspect of our being – physical, psychological, social, and existential/spiritual.

While assessing physical and psychosocial factors may be challenging, we at least are able to discuss such issues with a shared understanding of the relevant vocabulary. That is not the case, however, when existential, meaning-related spiritual matters come under scrutiny. In our increasingly secular age, the mere suggestion of a "spiritual domain" is likely to carry us onto thin ice; dialogue frequently becomes guarded. The unexpressed brittleness tends toward, *Where is he coming from? What does she think she is talking about? What is the underlying bias here, the fantasy?*

What defines *my* sense of existential meaning, my spiritual home, so to speak? While over the decades, in my teaching, I have payed lip service to the significance of the helpfully vague category of spiritual/existential factors, unless I am specifically asked, my personal beliefs have been high on the list of topics I avoid in lectures or when speaking to colleagues, patients, and their families. Meanwhile, these life-defining issues are inevitably shaping my experience and that of each of us.

What is my position? I consider myself a Christian and endorse the "New Creed of the United Church of Canada." Nevertheless, I have long felt uncomfortable with the word "God" given the millennia-old baggage the word carries. I resonate to the words of John Spong, retired Episcopal bishop of New Jersey, who was once asked, "If you had to name one belief of yours that has evolved or grown the most over the last ten years, what would it be?" He answered, as I would, although, I must confess, without his clarity and precision:

> I believe it would be the way I think about God. God is no longer a person, a being or an entity to me. God is rather a presence in whom, to use words attributed to St. Paul, "I live and move and have my being." The "old man in the sky" was the first image to go, then the heavenly judge who kept record books and finally the father figure who desired praise and whose mercy I implored. The invasive, external heavenly deity faded and new images began to intrude themselves into my consciousness. The interesting thing to me was that, while these old images were fading, the God intensity within me remained steady and steadfast. Today I am a God-intoxicated person, but my definition of God is anything but crisp and well defined. I struggle to find words big enough to use when I try to talk about God. God to me is now more of an experience of transcendence, or perhaps the source of life, the source of love and the ground of all being. An experience to me is vastly different from a being who might be described externally. People hear these concepts sometimes as simply words. I hear them, however, as a call to transcend all human limits and all human boundaries. God to me is a call to live fully, to love wastefully and to be all that I can be.
>
> A redefined Jesus still stands at the centre of my God experience. He is not the one sent to be my saviour, redeemer or rescuer. Jesus is not to God what Clark Kent is to Superman, a deity masquerading as a human being. He is rather a God presence through whom I am empowered to be open to the life, love and being that flows through me.
>
> I now call myself a mystic because in my understanding of God I have gone beyond words into a kind of wordless wonder, awe and mystery. This is not where I was a decade ago. I doubt if it will be where I am a decade from now, but it is where I am today and it represents the evolving, growing frontier of where I was ten years ago.[1]

In a conversation with Cicely early in her final illness, she observed, "Bal, I find that as time passes I have fewer beliefs, but I am believing them more deeply." She continued with typical deliberate thoughtfulness as she told me about the great comfort she was finding in the W.H. Vanstone book *The Stature of Waiting* and asked me what I thought of it.

In a detailed textual analysis, Vanstone describes how aging and then dying take us from active to passive (action to passion), from working to waiting, from subject to object, in a journey, he notes, that follows that of Jesus as recorded in the Gospels. Cicely had found both challenge and comfort in recognizing that the author had illuminated the path she found herself on. She could identify with the waiting and the need for openness, patience, acceptance – and dare one say, celebration – in moving from *self* toward *Self*, from the pressures evoked by ever-dominant ego demands to the succour available at the Deep Centre.[2] In referring to the biographical narrative of the final weeks and days of the life of Jesus as interpreted by Vanstone,[3] she remarked, "I think that is probably an accurate interpretation of what happened, as well as how and why."

I thought of Florence, our feisty, creative, and respected PCU patient who had fought through a similar transition in coming to terms with amyotrophic lateral sclerosis (ALS). One day during ward rounds, in response to my enquiry, Florence spelled out on her alphabet board, using a straw held firmly between her lips, "I used to scream for attention, but now I long for solitude."[4] In her words I heard her observing that, if we can begin to let go of our ego-generated clinging and reactiveness, we may begin to find our "way through" in opening to the depths, and once again Viktor Frankl's hard-won wisdom came to mind: "Everything can be taken from a man but one thing: the last of the human freedoms – to choose one's attitude in any given set of circumstances, to choose one's own way."

DIGGING DEEPER

During the 1990s, a series of events beyond those already described served to inform my sense of the existential/spiritual inner journey. They brought to mind the depth of meaning underlying Cicely's concept of "Total Pain" and in particular the integral part played by the existential, spiritual, relational, meaning-rich, and attachment/healing aspects of our moment-to-moment experience of Being. Existential issues were being nudged to my personal centre stage by a number of interactions during this millennium-completing decade. The cumulative impact of these experiences was to shape my response to the unexpected events that awaited me. I must begin with Bede Griffiths.

The 1991 John Main Seminar in New Harmony, Indiana, brought together approximately eighty meditators from the international community. The speaker was the eighty-five-year-old British Benedictine monk, author, philosopher, and mystic Bede Griffiths. During his undergraduate years at Magdalen College, Oxford, young Alan Griffiths formed a lasting friendship with C.S. Lewis, who observed that Griffiths was "one of the toughest dialecticians of my acquaintance." In his long, reflective, and enthusiastic life, Griffiths's brilliant, enquiring mind and radiant spirituality drew on varied sources: an analytical reading of the biblical narrative, the "perennial philosophy" of the East, the Buddhist teaching of Dzogchen, Transpersonal Psychology, the Creation Spirituality of Matthew Fox, and, through David Bohm and Fritjof Capra, modern science. His fecund legacy includes the books he authored[5] as well as his impact on the thousands of pilgrims who came to his ashram in Tamil Nadu, India, and those privileged to hear him at meetings such as the John Main Seminar.[6]

In 1955 Bede immigrated to India to adopt the monastic tradition of *sannyasa*, a life of utter poverty and abandonment to the spirit, of which Francis of Assisi is the most famous Western exemplar. In India he learned Sanskrit and adopted the customs of the Indian monastic tradition, walking barefoot, wearing the saffron *kavi* robe of the sannyasi, sitting on the floor, and eating with his hands. It was a quest, Bede observed, "in search of the other half of my soul." The product of his journey was the Shantivanam ashram where he developed a model of worship that celebrated a more interior, less institutionally centralized Christian tradition, a form that he believed could be relevant for the future.

Bede Griffiths was regarded by many as a prophet, a sage, even a saint. He both loved the church and was deeply critical of it, yet he never strayed from his unshakeable belief in Christ and Christianity. Lord Yehudi Menuhin referred to Bede as "a highly charismatic monk, [who] became the great reconciler of the world's religions and a man whose wisdom radiates around the world." In like manner, the Dalai Lama observed, "His vision has guided him to open the hearts and minds of mankind to gain understanding and acceptance of all the major religions with respect and dignity, to gain a sense of peace and unity to further the cause and goodwill of all people."[7]

Father Bede brought to New Harmony a rich historical, philosophical, and spiritual feast that took us from the Rig Vedas and Upanishads of millennia BCE to the depersonalized, science-based rationalism of today, all of this as background for his examination of the contemplative path in Christianity and the other major religions. The lectures he gifted us with had been carefully handwritten on lined legal-length paper, their delivery punctuated by spontaneous digressions, explanations, anecdotes, and giggles of delight. Three themes struck me as being of particular personal interest: his notion of the "marriage" of East and West, his elaboration of the contemplative path toward spiritual depth as a universal practice, and his concept of "the Cosmic Christ."

Bede considered our Western preoccupation with aggression, rationality, and power to be "masculine" traits and sought their marriage with the "feminine," intuitive aspects of the mind. The future of the world, he suggested, would depend on the "marriage" of these two minds, the conscious and unconscious, the rational and the intuitive, the active and the passive. But, he challenged, this "marriage" must first take place within the individual. Such personal transformations were a prerequisite to any lasting external union. While he tended to be gently self-referential rather than dogmatic, I sensed an urgency as he spoke of the Western mind's tendency toward rational dominance and our need for a balancing openness and intuitive presence if we are to nurture our access to deeper levels of Being.

He viewed the contemplative path as central to realization of our potential and noted that, while it can be traced back to apostolic times in Christianity, it had more consistently been followed over the subsequent millennia by the Eastern religions. Indeed, Bede's understanding of Christianity resembled a rich tapestry in which the contributing threads of each wisdom tradition – including science – bring their own unique light to our understanding of the transcendent mystery at the heart of Reality.

He spoke to us with dynamic earnestness:

The great spiritual teachers of all religions have practiced and taught mindful-ness. To be mindful is to live in the present moment, not to be imprisoned in the past, or in anticipating a future that may never happen. We have to learn to step back from these tendencies into the freedom and possibility of the present. Meditation takes us within ourselves. It is a process of inner withdrawal, a centring in the place of inner detachment, a staying of the mind on the transcendent. It is found in Aboriginal traditions, Buddhism, Taoism, Hinduism and is followed by the Sufis of Islam and the Jewish Kabbalah ... Recall that what the Christian tradition has referred to as "Original Sin" is the "fall" into the duality of the ego. Christ came to set us free from that dualism through the unifying Spirit. He broke through the dividing wall, thus opening the Divine Mystery to everyone. He restored humanity – not just for Jews, or Christians, but for all humanity – those of *all* faiths. We are part of one single organic living whole. Gaia: the Unity spoken of in John – *that they may all be one; even as thou, Father, art in me, and I in thee, that they may also be in us.* That is, a Unity of Love, in the Hindu sense of "Advaita" or non-dualism, an understanding that nothing exists apart from the spirit ... God is not a simple monad, you know, but a "Being-in-relationship" – Jesus saw himself *in relationship* with the father; the Spirit is the love that flows between them.

In reference to "the Cosmic Christ," Bede observed: "In the historic figure of Jesus we see mirrored, and perfectly revealed, the Cosmic Being, the principle of the Godhead active in all history. The Cosmic Christ may be seen moving in and through all the great religions in every age."

Years later, Bede's words came home in a new way when I reconnected with a former colleague who was now living with advanced cancer. During the 1970s, Maurice Dongier was a respected scientist and director of the McGill Department of Psychiatry. His support of the Royal Vic PCS as it struggled into existence was critical. Now, still active at age ninety, he had, until recently, been pursuing his academic interests, albeit at a more leisurely pace. A friend informed me of his illness, adding that Dr Dongier was now a meditator. Perhaps, our friend suggested, we would enjoy meeting after all these years.

Maurice welcomed me warmly as we met in the stately front hall of his home. He was shorter now and was pushing a walker, but what astonished me – stopped me in my tracks, actually – was his radiance. He actually radiated light, peace, quietness, joy, and openness, a sort of inner stillness. We meditated following a brief chat, and then he asked if I would join him for lunch at the kitchen table, offering an elegant wedge of Stilton blue cheese and a small glass of fine red wine. We sat in silence.

"How long have you been meditating?" I asked, anticipating decades.

"Perhaps four years," he estimated thoughtfully.

"How about you?" he enquired. I gulped. Now, I must confess, no one has ever accused me of radiating peace and calmness. I felt embarrassed. I thought back to my introduction to meditation and visits with Dom John Main during his final illness. Off and on, I had been an inconsistent meditator for more than three decades.

"Oh, about MMSHDUH years," I mumbled inaudibly behind my open hand and a concealing cough.

"How *often* do you meditate?" I queried after an incredulous pause.

"Constantly," he responded with a quiet smile. "When I cross the room pushing my walker, I meditate; when I brush my teeth, I meditate. When I visit the lab, it is a sort of meditation." I thought of St Paul's counsel to "pray without ceasing" and offered a simple nod … What could one say?

"Would you have some more cheese?" he asked lightly, then, after a thoughtful pause, adding quietly, "Bal, I should tell you, I am an atheist.

No, not an atheist, perhaps an agnostic ... I don't believe in God. I simply believe in love."

Over the weeks that followed, we continued to meditate as Maurice grew weaker.

His evident calm and openness continued. Our final visit was on a Thursday, two days before he died. He was asleep when I arrived. A little later he opened his eyes and on noticing me his face broke into that radiant smile. We chatted. He did not fear death. He was at peace. He slept briefly, then he opened his eyes again, beamed, and said, "Let's meditate." It was our last conversation but the meditation continues.

As the 1991 New Harmony seminar with Bede drew to a close, a group of us met with Father Laurence Freeman and Bede to discuss the future of the scattered global meditation community that was the legacy of John Main's teaching. The tortuous discussion seemed endless, the points raised disjointed. Then, rather unexpectedly, order emerged out of chaos. We would found a community to carry forward the practice of meditation as taught by John Main. Laurence would be the teacher of the new community, an ambitious concept since that would call for him to circle the globe continuously, rather like a latter-day St Paul. What would we call our community? "What about the World Community for Christian Meditation" (WCCM)?[8]

Less than two years later, Father Bede died in a simple hut at Shantivana, his Benedictine ashram beside the sacred River Cauvery in South India, Laurence having ministered to his final needs.

DEATH, THE WORM AT THE CORE: THE TERROR MANAGEMENT THEORY OF BECKER, YALOM, PYSZCZYNSKI, SOLOMON, AND GREENBERG

Palliative care presented me with death on a daily basis. In his 1973 Pulitzer Prize winning book *The Denial of Death*,[9] American cultural anthropologist Ernest Becker examined death anxiety as a foundational product of the "catch-22" dilemma posed by our two irresolvable realities, our innate inclination for self-preservation and the inevitability of our death. It is a conundrum that may generate paralyzing terror. Death anxiety, Becker observed, leads us to search for adaptive strategies of coping. Death is, indeed, "the worm at our core." We seek symbolic personal immortality through cultural world views that offer meaning through solutions that are more enduring than the self.

In the same vein, Stanford University psychiatrist Irvin Yalom identified four key challenges that haunt our daily lives: *death* (existential obliteration), *isolation* (the unbridgeable gap between self and others), *freedom* (the experience of an absence of external structure), and *meaning* (in a world of uncertain meaning). He agreed with Becker that, in coping with death anxiety, we adopt a cultural world view that aims at achieving symbolic immortality.[10] How do such insights affect us?

In one of those happenstance moments that shape life, Linda came across a brief newspaper article reviewing the work of three American social psychologists – Tom Pyszczynski, Sheldon Solomon, and Jeff Greenberg. Their research concerning death anxiety and "Terror Management Theory" builds on Becker's observations. I invited them to present their work at McGill's Ninth International Congress on Care of the Terminally Ill. As a result, Jeff Greenberg delivered the 3 November 1992 plenary lecture "At Different Times in Different Ways, We All Board the Same Train," presenting their groundbreaking studies that have helped to clarify the central role of death awareness in shaping human behaviour and our psychodynamic response to heightened death anxiety.[11]

Terror Management Theory has demonstrated that: 1) death anxiety is ever with us; 2) we are generally "unaware" of its presence because it remains in the unconscious, repressed by a *protective buffer system* comprised of two components – a) belief in a world view (or *culture*, as Becker termed it) consisting of a set of beliefs, shared in community with others, that gives life *meaning* and access to symbolic, if not actual, *immortality*, and b) belief that we are doing a good job in upholding our cultural value system, thus providing *self-esteem*; 3) when either personal culture or self-esteem are threatened, or our mortality salience (awareness of personal mortality) is increased, even if we remain unaware at a conscious level, it causes us to reinforce the buffer system through enhanced bonding to our culture and/or aggression against other cultures, as well as actions that bolster our self-esteem.

Thus, in one study, municipal court judges with enhanced death anxiety (even though unaware of it) set a bond for prostitutes that was ten times higher than the bond set by a control group of judges without death-anxiety enhancement. Likewise, Christians with increased death anxiety were more condemning of Jews, and death-anxiety-enhanced students became more protective of symbols of their culture (such as a Christian cross, or an American flag) and more aggressive toward those of other cultures. Similarly, post-9/11, Americans attended church in greater numbers and were more punitive toward foreigners.

While providing palliative care may increase caregivers' mortality salience, at the same time, the succour, benevolence, dignity, hope, and decreased suffering it affords may augment the caregiver's cultural sense of meaning and self-worth. Furthermore, when palliative care brings one's fear of death into consciousness, it may at the same time enable reflection and foster a life lived more intensely in the moment. Also, as the caregiver supports a lessening of death anxiety in the patient and family, he/she may experience enhanced quality of life through the realization of personal cultural norms. Moreover, given the omnipresent reality of impending death, palliative care may call forth humility and gratitude in each participant, whether patient, family member, or caregiver, and, through that awareness of community in shared vulnerability, may allow them to experience a sense of healing. Again, we may recognize that, even as wounding begets wounding begets wounding, healing begets healing begets healing.

TREVOR AND MUSIC AS A SPIRITUAL EXPERIENCE

The power of music! It can transport us to a place of awe, an awareness of those aspects of life that defy description, an experience through which we pass out of time into timeless Presence.

Sitting in silence, my mind had been elsewhere. I hadn't noticed the organist take her place at the console. Suddenly there was a soaring, indeed, a *roaring* from the majestic Beckerath Tracker Organ. *Building!* Then, building still further! *Exquisite*. Hair raising in fact! Breath stopping yet also triumphant! Suddenly, I was radically present. As the thunderous waves rolled over me. I then, had a sense of panic as the fleeting thought crossed my mind. *What if there had never been a pipe organ?! What if it had never been invented?! Buxtehude could not have expressed this* in *any other way; there would be a black hole in Creation, in all that might have been.*

The power of music! For Trevor Pinnock, Bede Griffith's experience of the "Cosmic Christ" is encountered through Papa Haydn, Mozart, Bach, Handel, and the other mentors who accompany him to the keyboard or podium. During the 1990s and beyond, he has taken Linda and me into that Presence on many occasions – at performances of Handel's *Messiah*, Mozart's *Requiem*, Dvorak's Cello Concerto with Yo-Yo Ma, and J.S. Bach's *St Matthew Passion*, among many masterpieces. Trevor still hears the carrot tops sing and, with endless grace, transmits that gift to those with ears to hear.

He put it in words when he phoned me from the all-engulfing backwash of his three Gewandhausorchester Leipzig performances of J.S. Bach's sublime Mass in B minor.

"How did it go?" I asked, delighted and surprised to hear his voice on the other end of the telephone line. There was a pause. When he answered, his voice was measured; he sounded – exhausted? Elated? Centred?

"I'll say more later ..." he paused. I waited. "It went well ... Sold out ... 2,000 at each performance." Then he added quietly, "Bal, we have just served Mass to 6,000 people ... You know," he continued in a respectful, measured tone, "it is very special with that orchestra ... With many orchestras, in preparing a major work, if you speak of the sacred, spiritual or transcendent you quickly lose their attention: they *are* 'professional musicians' you know! They just want to get on with it. But it is not so with the Gewandhausorchester. They are right with you. They understand ... When I spoke of these aspects of the Mass in B at our rehearsal, they were right there. They are like that. They have played at that level for centuries. They hold that sacred ground. They are *there* in a very special way."[12]

ROBIN COHEN AND ANN LYNCH AT THE RVH, 1993–97

Head and *Heart* are needed. David Tasma was right when he told Cicely that what he needed was what was in her head and heart. Nevertheless, during the early 1990s, instruments designed to measure quality of life excluded the existential/spiritual domain with few exceptions. Why? How could that be? The significant role played by the "heart"/spiritual domain/Self/Deep Centre, however understood, seemed clearly evident. Indeed, a decade earlier, in 1982, American medical scholar Eric Cassell had observed, "Transcendence is probably the most powerful way in which one is restored to wholeness after an injury to personhood."[13] Nevertheless, in 1990 a leading researcher still cautioned that QOL assessment should stick to the patient's "physical, psychological and social response to disease and its treatment." He went on to label the term QOL "a misnomer" and "imprecise," claiming that "it conjures up images of religiosity, life satisfaction and ambition and makes pretence of representing deeper philosophical notions underlying living."[14] My response was, "You bet it does!"

In 1993 our director of research, Robin Cohen, and I re-examined the determinants of QOL. The result was the "McGill Quality of Life Questionnaire," which documented the important role played by the existential or spiritual domain in influencing QOL during illness.[15] It was to be the first of many contributions Robin would make to palliative care.

With MQOL, my commitment to further exploring the determinants of the inner-life journey, the journey that Chip had spoken of with such clarity two decades earlier, became a central personal quest at the bedside, in discussions with grieving families, in research, in teaching medical students, and in all lecture presentations, whatever the setting. It wasn't about pushing "religion" or "spirituality," but it certainly *was* about the deeper philosophical notions underlying living. Evidence of the foundational importance of the existential/spiritual domain accumulated on a daily basis. Cicely was right again; all one needed to do was listen to our patients and their family members.

"Listening" for existential/spiritual issues became a higher priority across the Royal Victoria Hospital in January 1996 when Ann Lynch became the director of nursing for the Medical Pavilion. Deeper philosophical notions underlying living and excellence in whole-person care now found important support where previously they had, for a period of time, been lacking. Ann would continue to nurture that awareness through her lengthy career of nursing leadership at the Vic and later at the combined McGill University Health Centre.

FATHER LAURENCE AND DEAN ABE FUKS

Laurence and I arranged to meet in Houston in mid-November 1996 for two days of reflection, teaching, and planning. It was good to reconnect. It always is. His quick mind, perennial bubbling creativity – so evident in his sensitive, story-within-a-story photography – his instinctive grasp of the slightest potential at hand, and his ever-ready sense of humour can be counted on to recharge tired batteries. I always leave our encounters energized and with ten fresh, untouched issues on our "next time" list.

In addition to our seminar at Houston's St Luke's Episcopal Hospital on "Transformations: Meditation as a Way of Living and Dying," there was a workshop the following day on "Care of the Dying Patient" at the Texas Medical Center Hospice and an invitation to return four months later for lectures at the MD Anderson Cancer Center.

It was as Laurence and I were discussing how we might work together more closely in the future that he informed me that a meditator in Napanee, Ontario, planned to donate his home to the World Community for Christian Meditation. Since Napanee is situated just minutes by car from the Kingston hospitals and the Queen's University campus, would I consider starting a meditation centre there in conjunction with clinical work, teaching, and research within the Queen's Faculty of Medicine and its palliative-care program under Dr Deborah Dudgeon? The dean of medicine at Queen's was supportive, as was Deb Dudgeon. A move to Kingston or Napanee seemed rich in potential.

An appointment with our newly minted (1995) McGill Faculty of Medicine dean, Abraham Fuks, followed. I viewed it as an opportunity to express my heartfelt gratitude for the decades of support at McGill and to inform him about my plans.

"Have a seat, Bal. Tell me more about what you plan to pursue at Queen's." Abe, who was practical and open, brought a critical, assessing lens to the table. I spoke of my proposed search for a deeper under-standing of the less evident QOL determinants that seem relevant to whole-person care.

"What can you do there that you couldn't do here?" he asked and pushed my thinking further by suggesting that a similar program might be developed at McGill. "Have you signed anything, Bal?" I had not. "Don't sign anything before Friday. Let's meet again then."

When we met, Abe laid out a proposal. "I would like to suggest that we create a McGill program similar to the one we discussed. There is space for your offices in the Oncology Department. The financial arrangements will need adjustment and that can be achieved through the Flanders Chair."

Sometime during those days of decision, the Napanee homeowner backed away from his offer. That advantage of the move had been lost. My interest in pursuing the inner-life implications of our MQOL findings at McGill would be happily congruent with Dick and Sylvia Cruess's work on "professionalism" and with Abe's own medical- education interests. I opted to remain at McGill and the McGill Programs in Whole Person Care was born.

HIS HOLINESS THE DALAI LAMA, FLORENCE, ITALY, MAY 1999

In 1980 Tenzin Gyatso, His Holiness the Fourteenth Dalai Lama, met John Main at the Montreal Benedictine Priory. It was to be their only meeting but it engendered a sense of mutual understanding that was perhaps predictable. Both men were perceptive, analytical, and incisive; both knew the deep silence of those committed to the contemplative path yet were men of action. Both enjoyed a wide range of interests; both radiated authenticity. Both valued personal privacy yet could show appealing openness that others found highly engaging. In addition, both had an eruptive sense of humour that enlivened countless occasions. This was evident in Father John's deft impersonating skills and mastery of storytelling in the Irish tradition. It was seen in equal measure in the Dalai Lama's sparkling joy that is never far from the surface. For example, in response to a question from Laurence regarding how he chose his daily scripture reading, His Holiness quipped, "The Buddhist scriptures include 4000 Sutras. I hope someday I can read them all!" then burst into a fit of giggles before pausing to add a comment by the ancient Buddhist monk Shantideva: "As long as space endures and as long as sentient beings remain, may I too remain and dispel the miseries of the world." Wit, humility, and teaching had been neatly combined.

Building on their earlier priory bond, Laurence invited the Dalai Lama to comment, for the first time publicly, on selected passages from the Christian Gospels. His response was the 1994 John Main Seminar in London.[16] Subsequently, in 1998, Laurence and the Dalai Lama met at Bodh Gaya, India, at the traditional site of the Bodhi Tree where, some 2,600 years earlier, Prince Siddhartha is said to have sat for six years, becoming enlightened and henceforth to be known as the Buddha.

During their discussions, Laurence and His Holiness agreed to further meetings in the interest of promoting a deeper understanding between their spiritual traditions. They would call these encounters "The Way of Peace." The next such gathering was held in May 1999 at the Villa San Leonardo al Palco Prato in the Tuscany hills a few miles northwest of Florence, Italy. There were eighty of us, an equal mix of Buddhist and Christian-aspiring contemplatives, several wearing the yellow and red-ochre robes of Buddhist monks.

The hilltop Villa San Leonardo was surrounded by sheltering trees – olive, cypress, and palm. Its terracotta-tiled roof bore a modest tower with two bells. The cream-coloured stucco walls were punctuated by regimental lines of small dark windows marking the upper two floors. The overall impression of grand, if somewhat sombre, solidity was softened by the gentle breeze, the moderate mid-May climate, and the cloudless blue skies that brightened the surrounding rolling landscape of vineyards and spring fields. The ancient path ascending to this oasis of silence somehow invited respectful hushed tones as we greeted friends, old and new.

We were settled in our compact, spartan lodgings when His Holiness arrived, walking up the path accompanied by a cluster of devotees. I was struck by his evident humility, simplicity, and warmth as he stopped to greet the shy, apron-clad kitchen staff who were peering expectantly through their cracked-open doorway. This particular Nobel Laureate clearly lived out his oft-claimed identity as "a simple Buddhist monk."[17]

Cameras were not allowed. I was to be the lone photographer. This edict had been announced by Laurence in an effort to meet two objectives: lessened distractions during our time together, and cost-cutting in the

wake of an earlier WCCM event that had opted for the financially crippling services of a professional photographer. I had spoken up blithely,
"Laurence, I'll be the photographer if you like, and there won't be *any*
fee," thus unwittingly substantiating Alexander Pope's adage, "Fools
rush in where angels fear to tread."

I wanted to express my gratitude to this iconic model of charity and
service to humanity and knew of his childhood delight in repairing old
watches. As a result, when Laurence introduced us, I pressed a small
gift into his hand. It was the long-silent watch Dad had worn at Vimy
Ridge and Passchendaele eight decades earlier. With my explanation of
its history, His Holiness urged me to rethink my gesture. "This should
remain in your keeping." I said that I wanted want him to have it, and
Dad undoubtedly would have as well. He responded with a long, assessing gaze, then answered quietly, "Well, I thank you."

We found ourselves shoehorned into a small, modestly lit, steeply
sloped amphitheatre that was filled to capacity. The Dalai Lama and
Laurence sat facing us on simple straight-backed armchairs with wicker
seats, their feet alternately on the ground or disappearing under their
robes as they drew them up into a lotus position. They were accompanied by a scattering of flowers, recording equipment, microphones, His
Holiness's translator, Thupten Jinpa, and several Buddhist monks who
sat quietly against the wall behind them. Our proximity to Laurence
and His Holiness produced a sense of community and goodwill as they
discussed differences in Buddhist and Christian scriptures, the use of religious images in their respective paths, and the core tenets of the two traditions. Periods of meditation in the villa's cloisters, gardens, sheltered
walkways, and chapel complemented the daily meetings. Meals were
enjoyed at tables accommodating ten to twenty in the spacious, brightly
lit dining hall. The general sense of calm was tinged with an ever-present
hint of delight and anticipation.

Laurence spoke. "It takes peace within to make peace. We are here,
not for dialogue regarding beliefs, but to enter into joint meditation,
contemplative prayer; to be seriously committed to the way of peace."

His Holiness followed, speaking in resonant, short, sharply cut phrases
varying from brief bursts to paragraphs that ranged in pitch from a low
rumble to unexpected highs delivered with animation and intensity, as
well as ripples of laughter and chuckles. He was at ease and relaxed
but, at the same time, intent and overflowing with energy. He observed,
"We retreat to provide a space where one can distance oneself from our
usual thoughts and conceptual activity by setting a boundary so that we
can return to the world in a different way – strengthened. One is free to

take a religion or not, but once taken [it must be] taken seriously and sincerely, otherwise you cannot get a deeper experience."

His Holiness explained the core teachings of Buddhism.[18] The dialogue between Laurence and His Holiness was informative as they examined similarities and differences in their traditions: creation, causality, natural law, dharma, the concept of God, the role of faith, the impact of prayer, and the place of images.

As the session ended, Laurence asked, "Were you to look at a crucifix, what would that [image] mean to you?"

"For me it would speak of the Buddhist ideal of self-sacrifice for the sake of others." He continued, "Similarly, the image of the Virgin Mary carrying the baby Jesus is a powerful representation of compassion."

"And were there to be an image of the risen, resurrected Jesus, what would that say to you?" Laurence asked.

"That isn't really foreign to us. There are parallels in the Tibetan tradition. For example, the famous Tibetan meditator Milarepa appeared to his disciples after his death."

"How would you understand visions?"

"We would think of them having three origins – three kinds. They may arise at a sensory level, at a mental level, and at a deeper spiritual level. But even at the sensory level, if there are a number of people present, some may not have the vision."

"Your Holiness, at the end of St Augustine's book *The City of God*, written in the fifth century, he has a description of the vision of God I think you might enjoy. He says, the people in heaven will enjoy the vision of God, but not sitting in the audience looking on a throne, but [instead] they will have the vision of God when they turn and look at each other – at each other's faces and into each other's eyes."

"Wonderful."

It was the afternoon of our second day and His Holiness was to make his way to Florence where he would be made an honorary citizen of that cradle of the Renaissance. The city had originated as a Roman military garrison under Julius Caesar in 59 BCE. In due course it was destined to become Firenze, the home of Leonardo da Vinci, Michelangelo, and the Medici and Machiavelli families, a veritable cauldron of history, architecture, art, and culture. Laurence would be accompanying his honoured friend to this auspicious ceremony. "Bal, why don't you join us as the photographer?"

Five black sedans were waiting in a tight line at the door. His Holiness and Laurence were offered the back seat of car number two. I was to join a Buddhist monk in car number four. Our chauffeurs drove as though this wasn't the first time they had been behind the wheel; all save the four of us in the rear seats of cars two and four were police or blank-faced, suit-attired men of very husky build. They had us covered, so to speak.

We headed down the hill toward the main divided highway. By this time the sirens that our vehicles were equipped with were wailing and a sixth car had joined our procession to travel "shotgun" beside the Dalai Lama's car. Each time our single-lane road narrowed to the point of certain death, the shotgun car slid in behind the Dalai Lama's without anyone bothering to slow down. Our speed was blinding. It was then that I noticed two new factors. The traffic on the packed multi-lane highway that we were fast approaching was at a standstill in both directions as far as the eye could see. The police had blocked all access and egress points. In addition, a final piece in the equation had been added. A helicopter was now directly above us, flying very low directly above car number two. With skillful manoeuvring we crossed the blocked highway and headed into Florence, where we were engulfed in a chaotic, adrenalin-pumping mix of speed, whirling helicopter blades outside our window, car six weaving in and out of our line as circumstances demanded, and blaring sirens. It seemed possible, if not probable, that life might be very brief.

On entering the city, we plunged into a complex spaghetti nexus of narrow, winding, intersecting streets that snaked between the overhanging ancient buildings. With parked cars on each side, collision seemed not farther away than the thickness of an additional paint job on any of the vehicles, but our speed didn't lessen – at all!

Car six was now required to take it up a notch, from remarkable to miraculous. The thundering siren blasts were ricocheting off the buildings just feet from our ears, then eerily falling off as the echo was lost at each intersection. The helicopter was still with us, but in attempting to hang on I lost sight of its position.

We turned a corner and suddenly emerged into the sun-bathed Piazza della Signoria, the L-shaped square in front of the Palazzo Vecchio. We had stopped at the city hall.

A vast sea of wildly cheering, joyfully waving spectators roared their greetings from behind sturdy barricades. On reaching the impressive mass of stone beside us on our right, we glided to a stop. The sirens and helicopter had disappeared; they were replaced by the stirring heraldic blasts of long, silver, banner-bedecked, valve-less trumpets sounded by five men in scarlet and white medieval dress boasting the city's fleur-de-lis coat of arms.

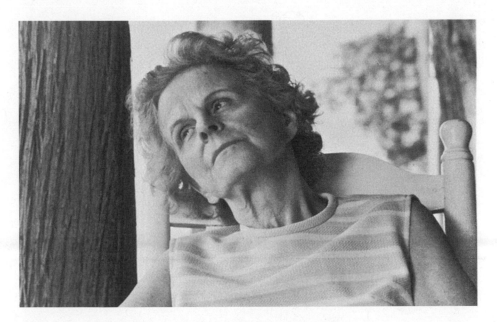

Last moments: mother at the *Place* during the summer of 1980.

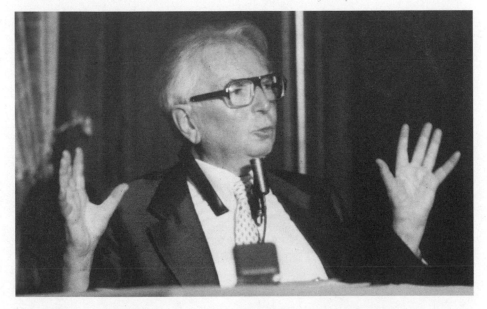

Viktor Frankl: neurologist, psychiatrist, author of *Man's Search for Meaning*.

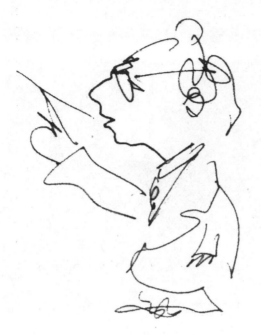

An impromptu gift:
Frankl's self-caricature inscribed
"For Bal, to remember Viktor
in 1980. Viktor Frankl."

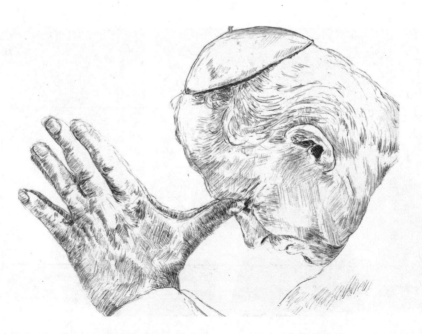

Pope John Paul II, Montreal, 1984.

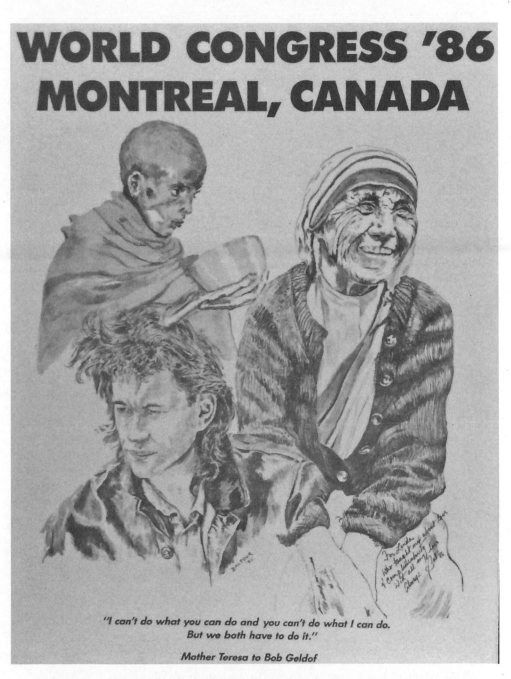

World Congress 1986 reminder of Mother Teresa, Bob Geldof, and Ethiopian hunger.

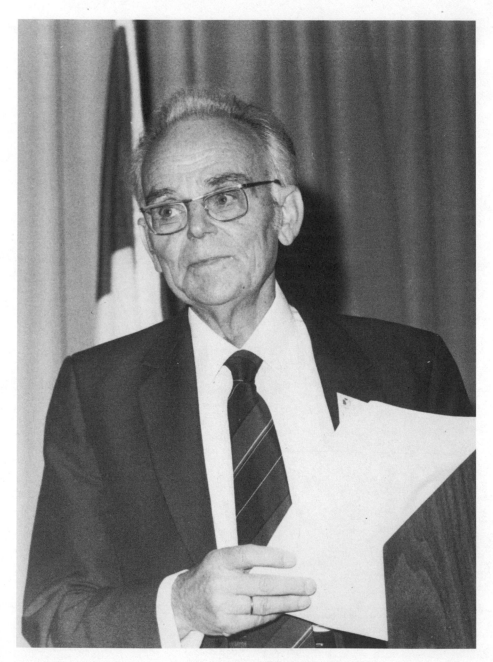

Leo Eitinger: Holocaust survivor, psychiatrist, educator, man of grace.

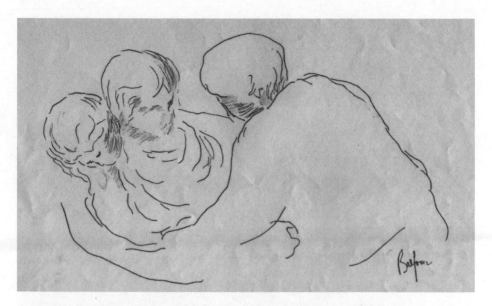

Easter at Christmas with Geneviève, Louise, and Yves.

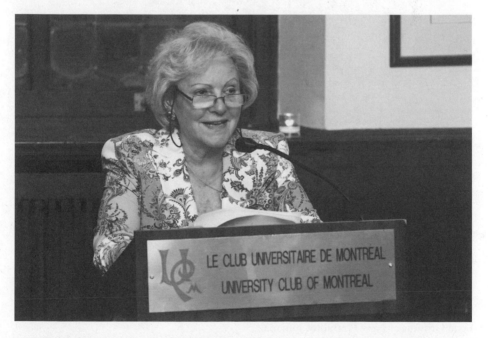

Kappy Flanders: founder of McGill University's Eric M. FLanders Chair in Palliative Medicine and ever-attentive benefactor of those in need.

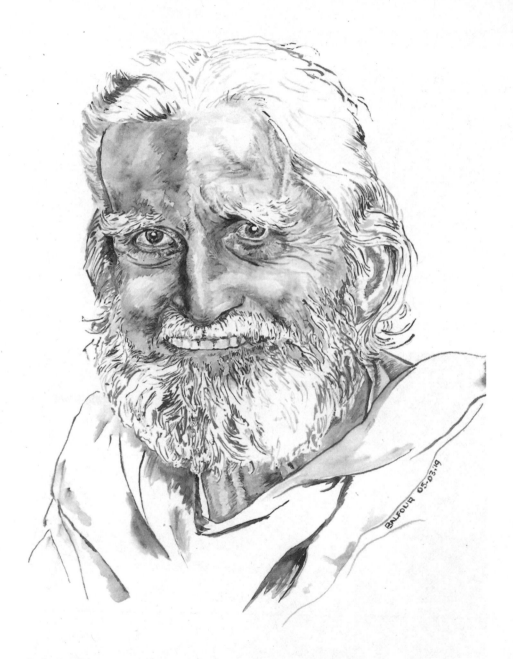

Bede Griffiths at New Harmony, Indiana.

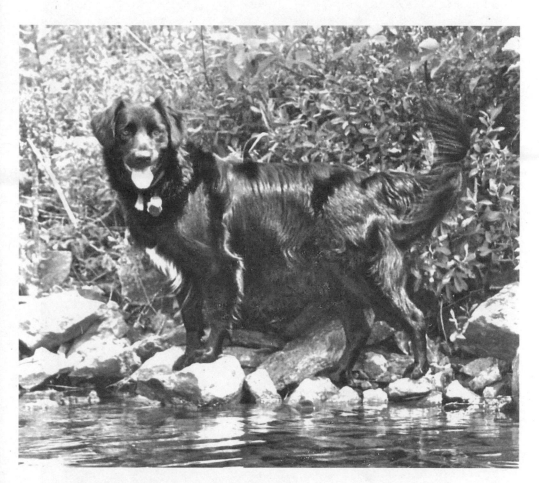

"B.C." ("The Boy") on assuming leadership of the Mount family, November 1992.

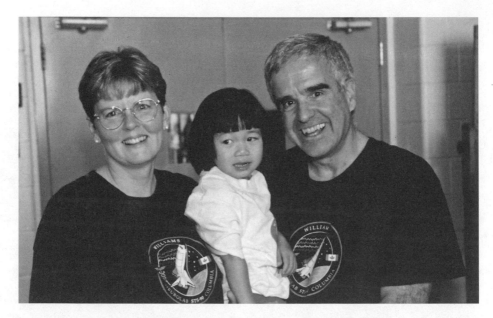

Linda, Bethany, and the author attend the 1998 launch of spaceflight STS-90 as guests of astronaut and mission specialist Dave Williams, a McGill medical graduate.

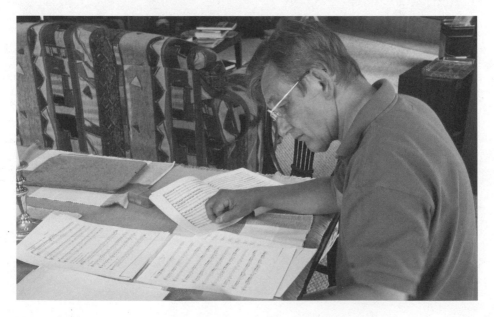

Trevor finishing up a little homework at our holiday cottage.

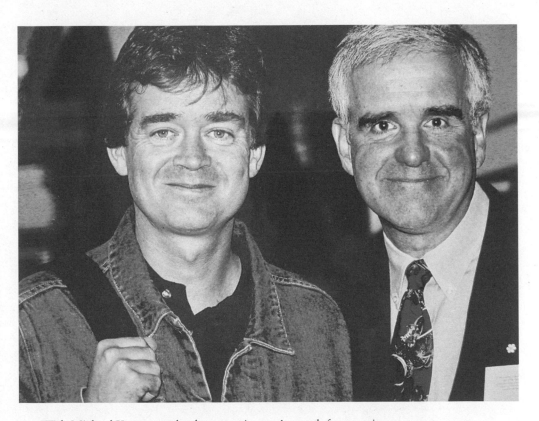

With Micheal Kearney, valued partner in man's search for meaning.

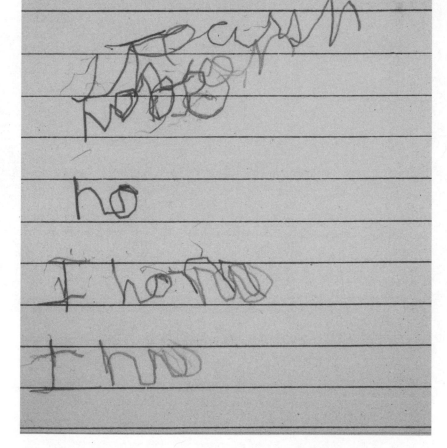

ROYAL VICTORIA HOSPITAL
MONTREAL, QUEBEC H3A 1A1

— PROGRESS SHEET —

Gersh's plea, *I horse*.

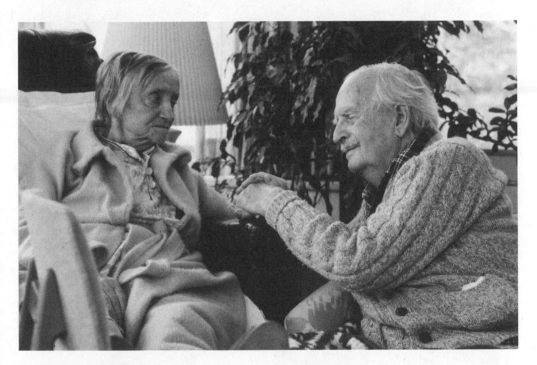

Contact at the end of life across barriers of language and sight.

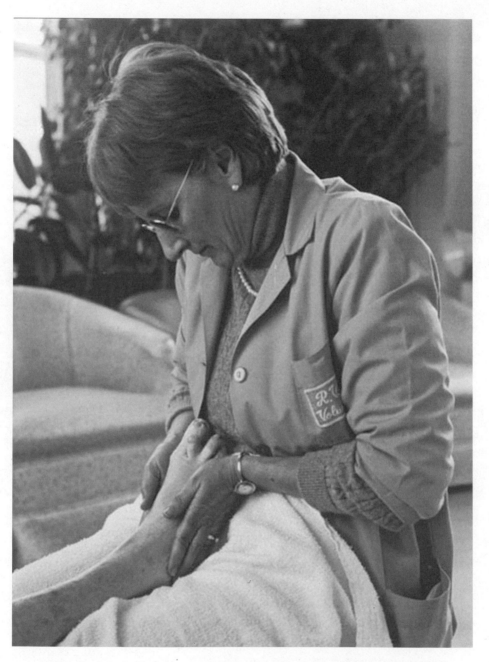

Dolores Nickerson: PCU nurse, volunteer, and discerner of the existential/spiritual dimension.

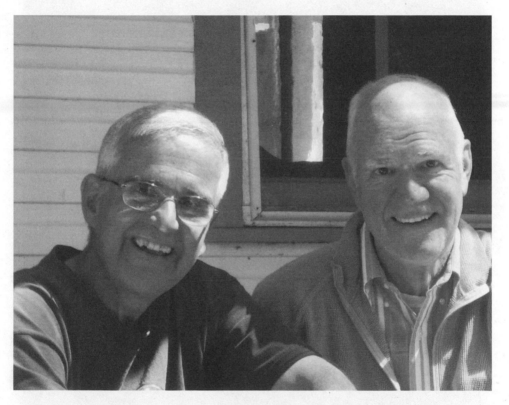

With John Seely: internist, Ottawa's dean of medicine, man of grace, and insight.

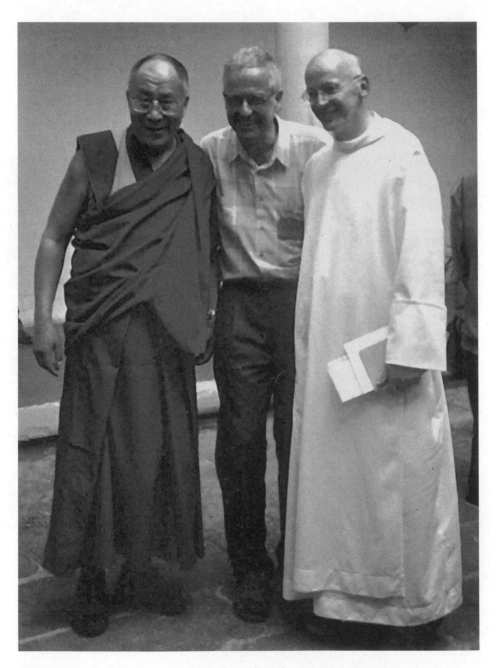

His Holiness the Dalai Lama: in Florence with Father Laurence Freeman.

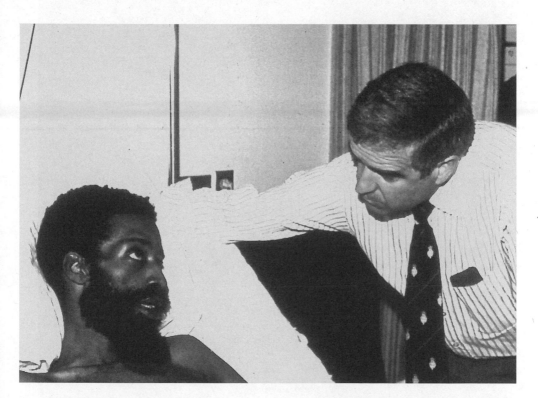

Ken Jackson: the discovery of unexpected and deeply cherished bonds.

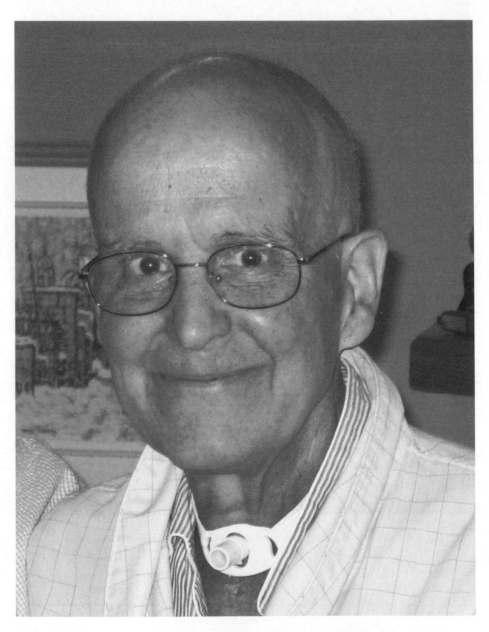

The author post-tracheostomy, esophagectomy, radiation therapy, and chemotherapy.

An oddly serene host opened the door of car number number two and the Dalai Lama stepped out, followed by Laurence. The sun was blazing. The crowds cheered enthusiastically, His Holiness warmly acknowledging them with a beaming smile.

Laurence in his flowing white habit, the Dalai Lama, my car number four companion in his robes, and I started up the historic stairs of the Palazzo Vecchio. At the second stair a heavy hand barred my way and two policemen started to drag me toward the throng of bystanders.

"*Laurrrenceeeeee!*" I cried, but my voice seemed minuscule and a thousand miles away. Laurence turned. "He's with us. He's the photographer." They glanced skeptically at my modest camera and reluctantly let me go.

Attempting to regain some semblance of dignity, I staggered through the towering doors into the relative gloom of the cavernous interior. Construction of this epic symbol of civic power had begun in 1299, *exactly* 700 years ago! If "surreal" implies strange, unusual, and having the quality of a dream, this was the most surreal moment I could recall. Any pretense of belonging to this cast of characters, or of being a *real* photographer, had long evaporated. Mother's immortal phrase, *What in God's green earth am I doing here?* rushed to mind! As my eyes accommodated to the subdued lighting, I was determined not to lose track of Laurence.

In due course, official greetings had been pronounced, the assembled dignitaries had applauded, books had been signed, His Holiness had delivered his remarks, and we headed for the door. Well, to be more accurate, His Holiness headed for the door. Remarkably, the others were momentarily distracted by the grandeur of place and event.

It suddenly occurred to me that the Dalai Lama was leaving, not in order to escape, but to greet the massive, cheering throng waiting in the Piazza della Signoria. I fell into step, just behind his left shoulder. The two of us were now on our own and I suddenly realized that this was about to be a photographer's dream. I steeled myself. *Mount,* BE *a photographer!*

The ancient door was opened for us and we were momentarily blinded by the dazzling light. The roar of the crowd peaked. His Holiness and I started down the five or six steps. Even from my position just behind him, I could see that he was beaming.

We were crossing the empty square and approaching the delirious throng when it happened. Above the din a single male voice rang out, *Vive le Québec Libre!* I was stunned. Was I hallucinating? It couldn't have been! Had the Quebec independence movement gained new life? Was it a cry for support from His Holiness? My distinguished partner didn't seem to have heard it. I was a step or two behind. *I must catch up.* We were almost at the barricades. *Still just the two of us ... this is bizarre!* and I was gripping the camera, planning my shot. Then, it happened again! It came from somewhere off to my left in that massive crowd. *Vive le Québec Libre!* I tried to refocus my attention as we approached the ecstatic faces; I was right at his shoulder; my shutter was clicking away. In an instant, the moment had passed. Laurence and the others had arrived at the cars; the entourage was leaving.

It wasn't until I was back in Montreal telling Linda this tale that clarity dawned, prompted by Linda's eyebrow raised in disbelief. "But *didn't* you hear what he was saying? It was "Vive le *Tibet* Libre!" *Of course, Mount, you idiot!*

Back at the villa, when we finally had a moment alone, I asked Laurence, "How did you enjoy our ride to the Palazzo Vecchio, and how in the world did His Holiness react to it?"

Laurence paused. "You know, I thought we were all going to be killed. It was amazing. But perhaps my strongest memory of this whole retreat will be how he responded during that drive into Florence. The moment the car door closed, he closed his eyes and started to meditate. He was in a place of peace. He didn't move until the car door opened at the Palazzo Vecchio. At that moment he resumed his presence with us as if nothing had happened. I shall never forget it."

In the end, the photographs had been dutifully taken. Holding a rosary that Laurence had given him, the Dalai Lama settled into his place of peace. I clicked the shutter.

Although I had maintained a focused presence to issues photographic, I later realized that I had missed many of the insights that had been conveyed to others by His Holiness. I wondered how often at the bedside I mistake physical presence for depth listening. What His Holiness *did* convey to me with great clarity, however, was his capacity to explore reality at a depth that embraced both the transcendent *and* science, both recognition of our brokenness *and* potential for a union that is beyond the dualism we cling to.

ZHANG HONG, TIANJIN, BEIJING, AND GUO WEI

The red and white banner over the entrance to the Conference Centre in the sprawling port of Tianjin in northeast China proclaimed in both Mandarin and English: "A Warm Welcome to the Opening of International Palliative Care Conference." It was 2 June 1999, my first visit to mainland China.

Looking out over an endless sea of faces as I commenced my keynote address, I experienced with a jolt the stark contrast between that moment and the far more intimate and bilingual Hospice Congress hosted by my friends Enoch and Daphne Lai in Taiwan, where I had been a speaker in July 1995. Translation facilities had been present then; here, they were apparently absent. It was one of those "abandoned in the wilderness" moments of near panic. I was in a foreign universe, the odd man out, to the disadvantage of all present.

The facts of the case seemed oddly relevant. China's population was 1.2 billion, Canada's 30 million. The friendly but somewhat blank faces stretched to the horizon. I knew I would be completely unable to share adequately the lessons learned over the preceding quarter-century. While these worst fears were undoubtedly realized, my audience did their best to convey interest. It was painful.

Zhang Hong was a thoracic surgeon in the Oncology Unit at the First Teaching Hospital, Norman Bethune University of Medical Science, in Changchun, China, approximately 430 miles north of Tianjin. He had flown to the Tianjin meeting with a special mission in mind. Would I, he asked, drive with him to Beijing where a lung-cancer patient on whom he had done a pneumonectomy was now dying and in a great deal of pain? It would be a drive of seventy miles. Hong could arrange for a car.

I liked Hong. He was thoughtful and insightful, his handsome countenance open, earnest, and perennially engaged. His eyebrows were finely tapered at their proximal ends, approaching each other just over his nose. A baseball cap fully concealed his head of dark hair. He was perhaps ten years younger than me. I believe that part of his training may have been in the United States.

We chatted easily that first day; I suspected that Hong was probably both a competent surgeon and a compassionate physician. As time passed, it became clear that the sole reason for his rather arduous trip to Tianjin, then to Beijing and back, was to request that I see his patient. Here was a man who dared to *go the extra mile*. Remarkable.

The drive northwest to Beijing found us on a crowded, narrow, auto-littered secondary road that, I quickly realized, required driving skills that I was completely unaware existed. Hong was unperturbed but totally focused on the task at hand. Tangles of dented cars and irate drivers were commonplace. First-responder vehicles with their sirens coarsely blaring were to be seen here and there, mired like everyone else in the morass of traffic. There was no idle chit-chat as Hong volunteered some now forgotten data on the frequency of automobile accidents. I don't recall if our car had seatbelts.

On finally arriving in Beijing, we were to proceed directly to one of China's most renowned hospitals. It had been in the international news recently owing to the admission of an important official. Night was falling. Hong for some reason was having trouble locating this respected centre of medical excellence in the maze of winding streets, bicycles, and milling pedestrians. We made our way at a snail's pace. Then, unexpectedly, he pulled over and parked. Turning off the car lights, we found ourselves in semi-darkness. We had arrived.

The streets were now empty. The pedestrians had vaporized. But the stone stairs leading up to what was obviously the front door of this famous hospital were occupied by men alone or in small groups of two or three. They were clad in the faded garb of patients. Some were smoking. All were coughing and spitting onto the stairs beside them. Silence prevailed as we passed. No one moved. No one spoke.

After some difficulty locating our patient, we were directed, with some uncertainty, to the second floor. There, we encountered a cavernous grey hallway extending to a shadowy infinity in both directions. This long passageway was lit by a single 60-watt light bulb dangling by a cord from the high ceiling some hundred yards to our left. Twenty or thirty yards to our right was what must have been a nursing station. It was deserted and completely empty. Indeed, during more than an hour on the premises, we encountered only one member of staff, the quietly confused figure Hong had asked for directions at the front door.

After a long door-to-door search, Hong found his patient. His wife was at the bedside. They were worn and pale. *Maybe in their thirties*, I judged, then, recalling the youthful appearance of many Asians, *or maybe forties*. Their pleasure at seeing Hong was deeply touching.

Hong introduced the patient as Guo Wei, saying that it means "can be strong" or a variant thereof. He added, "I call him that sometimes; you can too. It is not his real name but you would find that difficult to pronounce." The profound deference of the man and his wife deepened my concern about whether or not I could meet their expectations. Hong had informed me that the stoic couple had a clear understanding that his days were numbered and that my visit, if it could be arranged, would be in the interest of improved pain control. What was already clear, however, was their joy in reconnecting with Hong. His entry seemed to brighten both their faces and the simple bareness of the room.

With Hong translating, I took a history and examined Guo Wei. We reviewed his current medications. Regular, individually optimized four-hourly doses of his painkiller would almost certainly bring relief without side effects. Hong would discuss my suggestions with the doctor in the morning.

My parting moments with Guo Wei and his wife were brief yet filled with a tangible warmth that bridged the gaping chasm that ran between our worlds. He looked exhausted, but the evident mutuality of our bond did not need words. Indeed, it struck me that the closeness experienced between the four of us transcended the barriers imposed by race, language, and the grave prognosis at hand. Hong had "gone the extra mile"; we all had reaped the benefit. My Tianjin friends had taught me a great deal about grace.

That message was underscored the next day when Hong took me to a stall selling local handicrafts. There he bought a kite that featured a magnificent eagle. He inspected each minute aspect with great care. It was for Yao Yao, our Bethany. His exact words are now long forgotten but their meaning remains clear. "For us, the symbol of the eagle is very important. It means 'Hero,' as do the hawk and the bear. Bethany will have this eagle to remind her of her homeland and the special life that lies ahead of her."

ISRAEL

If I experienced multiple events in the early to mid-1990s as replete with windows on the inner journey – from ego to Deep Centre, from self to Self, from separation challenge to attachment solution, from the abiding intrusion of past and future on the mystery of the radical present, from left-brain dominance to the augmented enhancement of a right-brain assist – such windows were once again memorably evident as the decade ended.

The 2nd Annual Bella Sebba Lectures in Palliative Care at the Shaare Zedek Medical Center, Jerusalem, were to be held on 13–14 October 1999. The theme was pointedly phrased: "Spirituality and Meaning versus the Kevorkian Options of Assisted Suicide and Euthanasia."[19] My Memorial Sloan Kettering colleague Nathan Cherny, director of the Shaare Zedek Pain and Palliative Medicine Service, invited MSKCC nursing consultant Nessa Coyle and me to participate. My three presentations were to be on "Existential and Spiritual Suffering," "Attitudes toward Death in the 20th Century," and "Clinical Issues in Palliative Care: Case Presentations," a challenging trio of topics anywhere, but for me, this was particularly the case in Israel given the value-added meaning of the historical context of the locale.

Shortly after accepting the invitation the phone rang. It was Kappy.

"Bal, I hear you will be speaking at the Shaare Zedek Conference."

"Yes, it should be interesting."

"I'll be there."

"Kappy, you're kidding! That's great. What a happy coincidence. I hope we can get together at some point during the conference."

"You don't understand. I wasn't *intending* to be there, but I want to see your face when you see Israel for the first time!"

It took me a while to grasp the meaning behind her words. Kappy had invited Nessa and me to join her on an exhaustive tour of Israel. We would have as our personal "tour guide" Mike Hollander and his comfortable white touring van "Doris." Mike, a former Canadian, was considered the best in his trade as he "opened" the many timeless, yet ever-evolving, meanings of Israel. He proved to be a font of knowledge, a source of endless point-specific maps, diagrams, historic anecdotes, and factoids relevant to each bend in the road, and, in addition to all that, he was just plain fun to be with.

Thanks to Kappy's deft negotiations with the no-nonsense armed authorities in the milling arrivals area, we moved through the crowd in Tel Aviv's Ben Gurion Airport without undue delay and made our way by car through the rural countryside to Jerusalem.

Somewhere on those busy city streets during that first day, I spotted two young men deep in conversation. They were dressed exactly as in my 37 Opeongo Road sidewalk dream of Jesus and his companion decades earlier. Was it unconscious programming in my interpretation? Probably. But my thoughts were elsewhere. Israel, that crammed, teaming, tiny, archaeologic museum-cum-country, has perpetually lived its colourful, dynamic, conflicted life in a state of chronic agitation. Israeli occupation of the West Bank and Gaza had led to the 1987–93 intifada and subsequently the 4 November 1995 assassination of twice-Prime Minister and peace activist Yitzhak Rabin by a Jewish ultranationalist enraged by Rabin's support of the Oslo Peace Accords. Threats of annihilation come from without and within Israel's borders. Constantly. The Nazarene was not among my conscious concerns as we had entered that milling throng.

Despite the turmoil, Israel remains precious beyond measure, a fact underscored by the growing list of World Heritage Site designations within this tiny fleck on the planet's surface. The country offers examples of intimate multi-millennial and cultural co-existence that are mind-blowing. As we approached the holiest of all Jewish sites, the Western Wall, built by Herod the Great in 20 BCE (now all that remains of the great Temple that was to hold the Ark of the Covenant), Mike stopped to draw our attention to the three buildings lining the nearby street. A solid, recently built, four-storey Armenian apartment building replete with a shower of satellite dishes sprinkled across the roof stood to our left. Attached to its wall was a mosque boasting a hefty towering minaret, and next to that, a modern, stylish, upscale block of condominiums: Armenian Christian, Muslim, and Jew living and worshiping as cheek-by-jowl neighbours.

We turned to face the tumble of massive squared-foundation stones strewn among the debris from the 70 CE destruction of the Temple. Nearby was the "Western," or "Wailing," Wall, with its clusters of men in black, broad-brimmed hats, beards, and long coats, their bowed heads rhythmically bobbing as they recited the daily services, while others tucked personal prayers into the recesses marking the revered ancient stone surface.

A tapestry of graphic memories floods my mind as I recall our week together: the sense of timelessness that colours the clearing mists over the Sea of Galilee; the receding, blanched stillness of the Dead Sea; spotting at Qumran, far up the roadside cliff face, the entrances to the caves that had sheltered the Dead Sea Scrolls over the millennia, while awaiting the scrolls' discovery by a Bedouin shepherd boy in 1947; the Golan Heights and their strategic, all-encompassing view of the Upper Galilee and our encounter with the unmistakable, ordered discipline of an Israeli Army convoy rolling through that highland vantage point; my late-evening solitary walk by the unexpectedly modest Jordan River a stone's throw from the Syrian border and the kibbutz where we spent the night; the Negev desert and the warm hospitality offered by palliative-care physician Yoram Singer, his wife, Tammy, and their children in Beersheva; Yoram's clinical practice, half Jewish, half Bedouin, suggesting his efforts to form bridges of compassion and healing; our visit to the Bedouin Co-op where women from five tribes chatted and sold their handicrafts under the leadership of a gracious young Muslim social worker whose otherwise inconceivable McGill master's degree had been made possible through Kappy's support; Caesarea, the largest port in the eastern Mediterranean (the site where Pontius Pilate governed, Simon Peter converted the Roman, Cornelius, and St Paul was tried and imprisoned for two years), with its meticulous archaeological restorations and Roman amphitheatre built by Herod the Great; the nearby Herod's Kosher Restaurant, complete with adjacent minaret to cover all the bases; Tabgha, on the northwest shore of the Sea of Galilee not far from Capernaum, previously known also as Heptapegon or "place of Seven Springs," a locale of lush vegetation, algae-rich water, and plentiful fish; the surrounding hills, the traditional site of the Nazarene's local teaching and miracles; the narrow Kidron valley southeast of Jerusalem and the

Monastery Mar-Saba, founded in 483 CE by the Cappadocian monk St Saba. A timeless tapestry, but three experiences focused my attention as had no others.

First, Yad Vashem. The sacred and profane were irretrievably entwined in the grotesquely calm, heart-stopping, icy silence of the Yad Vashem Holocaust Memorial to the victims of the Holocaust. In anticipation, one steels oneself against the horror of it all – *I have seen those horrific photographs, don't you know* – but, such pretenses to personal equilibrium notwithstanding, it completely overwhelms as one is surrounded by man's unspeakable inhumanity to man.

At Yad Vashem the evil wrought by Nazi Germany, hinting at the same potential lurking within each of us, erupts afresh at every turn. It hits you in the gut. There is a hollowness, a sick emptiness, drawn from the inescapable presence around us of the more than 6 million victims, an estimated 1.5 million of them children. They are present in the stark, dimly lit, tomb-like Hall of Remembrance where one is surrounded by the names of twenty-one concentration camps displayed on individual black-basalt slabs. They are present in the central placement, in that vast emptiness, of a casket filled with ashes from the cremation ovens. And they are in the eternal flame that burns above it. Their presence underscores the searing tragedy of a letter displayed nearby on the wall, written by the Canadian delegate to the March 1938 Évian Conference held in response to the plight of the increasing number of Jewish refugees fleeing Nazi persecution in Europe. It reads: *The trouble is that the more that is done for them the more of them there will be ... So nothing will be done by Canada.*

And the murdered children are present in the Janusz Korczak Memorial recessed into one of the walls. All I could make out on first glancing at the sculpture was the light reflected off the lifeless, ragged, vertical lines that etched the black bronze. Then I saw it: a large, drained, grieving face and the surrounding hand that embraced the vertical lines. It was coming into focus now. As I moved closer, everything leapt into terrible clarity. I was peering at Janusz Korczak – Polish Jew, pediatrician, educator, and children's author – as he cradled a cluster of his broken, diminutive, starving charges: children once alive with potential, now shrivelled into lifeless bronze.

Since 1911 Korczak had developed and nurtured the Warsaw orphanage for Jewish children. In 1940 he and the children were moved to the Warsaw Ghetto. In August 1942 German soldiers transported the 196 children and their doctor to the Treblinka extermination camp. He was offered an escape but refused and went to his death with those to whom he had given his life. Their wasted faces and thin bodies were clear to me now, as was his haunting, questioning, undaunted gaze, thrown into high relief by the love conveyed in his embracing hand and the awful vacancy in the faces of his once youthful loved ones.

The second experience that gripped me was our visit to Gethsemane. Have you ever experienced a transformation in understanding when issues long-contemplated are passed through the corrective lens of direct experience? I have. As our second or third day was drawing to a close, Mike asked if we had any further local goals on our sightseeing wish list. "Bethany," I responded, uncertain of the distance involved and more consumed with thoughts of my four-year-old daughter, Bethany Yao, than Lazarus. It was to be a crash course in the indecipherable mix of fact, fiction, faith, fantasy, and historic sleight of hand that enshrouds each of the venerated sites in the "Holy Land." Bethany was the storied town where Lazarus and his sisters Mary and Martha lived, providing Jesus with a "home away from home" when he visited Jerusalem. But in my request to visit there I had not fully appreciated the Jericho/Bethany/ Mount of Olives/ Gethsemane/Temple Mount geographic links until I personally experienced them.

Bethany is the site, believers claim, where Jesus raised Lazarus from the dead four days after his burial. Others postulate that the story is an account either of an actual miracle or of an historic event that was later elaborated into the reason for the decision of the religious leaders to kill Jesus. Alternatively, the story has been assessed by some to be an entirely fictitious tale used by John the Evangelist as a vehicle for introducing some particular points of Christian teaching.[20] Such claims prompt a sense of reverence in some and skepticism in others, but in all they provoke a sense of awe and fascination at the vast sweep of history each of these narrative conclusions involves. A Franciscan church stands at the traditional location of the biblical miracle. Built in 1954, it is the fourth church to mark the site. The first is said to have been constructed in the mid-first century, the second in the post-330 CE Byzantine period, and the third by Crusaders between 1138 and 1144 CE. The traditional tomb of Lazarus is marked by a Greek Orthodox Church which replaced a sixteenth-century mosque at the same location.[21]

Three landmark features run in a northwest-to-southeast direction parallel and adjacent to each other. From west to east they are: Jerusalem's Temple Mount; beside it, the narrow (perhaps 600 feet or so wide) Kidron valley; and, just east of that, the Mount of Olives, on the lower slope of which (facing Jerusalem across the Kidron valley) is Gethsemane.

Heading for Bethany, we left the Old City, crossed the Kidron valley, and proceeded south on the "Old Road to Jericho" that rounds the south end of the Mount of Olives, the total distance being less than six miles. Given the lateness of the hour, our only stop in Bethany was at a small roadside shop where I purchased, for a very modest sum, an exquisite hand-carved olive-wood bust of Jesus.

Driving back toward Jerusalem, Mike stopped by a gate adjacent to the sloping incline of the Mount of Olives. A stately camel attended by his camera-bearing Arab companion watched us intently, hoping in vain for one last late-afternoon tourist in search of a "that's-me-on-a-real-camel" souvenir.

"Through that gate is the Garden of Gethsemane," Mike commented. "They close at 5:00 o'clock so you only have a few minutes if you want to have a look." Ignoring the forest of monuments to faith that dot the hillside,[22] I stepped off the main path into a stand of young olive trees, each cluster surrounded by wooden beams to ensure their protection.

Gethsemane. Shutting out the intermittent announcements of the number of minutes to closing time, I selected the closest wooden beam as my meditation cushion. I was determined not to miss the opportunity, if only for a few minutes, to journey deeper at this historic crossroad that had heretofore been an image constructed in my imagination.

At this closing-time hour, I was alone. As I settled, I found myself looking across the Kidron valley at the Temple Mount in Jerusalem directly in front of me, and surprisingly close at hand. Thanks to the intervening barren expanse of the Kidron valley, my Gethsemane vantage point among the trees offered, as it would have done two thousand years ago, an intimate, unobstructed view of the only Jerusalem landmark Jesus had any interest in – the Temple. It was one of those moments when the reality of the geography instantly casts a new light on old imaginings. With the surrounding trees, this contemplative spot would render one completely hidden. Here was a secluded place of quiet that afforded a private sense of presence to his "Father's House" without being noticed by others.

And there was more. There was, and still is, a path that led directly from this sheltered Gethsemane hillside grove back over the Mount of Olives summit to Jesus's "home" with Lazarus, Mary, and Martha in Bethany. His adopted Bethany home thus provided access, not only to Gethsemane and this quiet place of contemplative reflection, but also to the Temple and the city. Moreover, on journeying here from his northern haunts in the Galilee, he could bypass any brewing hostility in Samaria by opting for the trans-Jordan route south, crossing back across the Jordan in the region of Jericho and from there going directly to his friends in Bethany.

One could visualize Jesus working through the daunting implications of his mission as he understood it. Gethsemane offered silence, privacy, and immediate proximity to the Holy of Holies. The geography of the events that were to unfold at this site – give or take 150 feet or so to my right or left – was now crystal clear. Long-held, somewhat vague understandings suddenly morphed into concrete historic and geographic realities. *Goodness, it actually all happened! And it happened here!*

Finally, there was Capernaum. The Scriptures recount:

And passing along by the Sea of Galilee, he saw Simon and Andrew the brother of Simon casting a net in the sea; for they were fishermen. And Jesus said to them, "Follow me and I will make you become fishers of men." And immediately they left their nets and followed him. And going on a little farther, he saw James the son of Zebedee and John his brother, who were in their boat mending the nets. And immediately he called them; and they left their father Zebedee in the boat with the hired servants and followed him. And they went into Capernaum; and immediately on the sabbath he entered the synagogue and taught. And they were astonished at his teaching, for he taught them as one who had authority, and not as the scribes" (Mark 1:16–22).

The Evangelist Mark wrote this chronicle in Rome during the late 60s CE. It is the earliest surviving narrative of the life of the Nazarene.[23] Mark continued his account by describing the miraculous healing by Jesus of a man "with an unclean spirit." News of the presence, teaching, and actions of Jesus, including his healing of the sick, "spread throughout all the surrounding region of Galilee," that is to say, the region on the west and north coast of the Sea of Galilee. "And in the morning, a great while before day, he rose and went out to a lonely place and there he prayed ... And when he returned to Capernaum after some days, it was reported that he was at home" (Mark 1:35, 2:1)

Kappy, Nessa, Mike, and I descended in "Doris" from the Golan Heights on the northeast shores of the Sea of Galilee to head west across the shaggy grasslands where a small herd of cows was grazing contentedly. Mike casually commented, "Capernaum, or, Capharnaum if you prefer, is just over there, if you'd like to have a look."

The site of the ancient village of Capernaum had been abandoned a millennium earlier to be buried under the detritus of the passing centuries. Archeological discovery, when it came, was remarkably recent as measured against the sweep of history involved. Preliminary excavation of the ancient village of Capernaum occurred during 1906–15, detailed research not until 1968–86. The lakeside community had acted as an important crossroad for travellers leaving and entering the Tetrarchy of Herod Antipas; a detachment of Roman soldiers was stationed there as well as a tax collector. The large amount of coinage excavated at the site revealed primary commerce with the northern regions of upper Galilee, Golan, Syria, Phoenicia, Asia Minor, and Cyprus.

The remains of a white-limestone synagogue dating from the late fourth century (thus more than three hundred years after the period when Jesus lived there) were uncovered at the site, and beneath its foundations the remains of a more modest black- basalt synagogue from the first century. The latter was, the archeologists concluded, the synagogue that had been built for Capernaum by the centurion of the local Roman detachment, and that Mark identified as the location where Jesus worshipped, taught, and performed healing miracles. Unlike "traditional sites" scattered throughout Israel where biblical events are *thought* to have happened, here was the *exact* location where history gave rise to legend, whatever one makes of the related events and their spiritual and secular significance two millennia later.

In addition to the first- and fourth-century synagogues, the researchers identified the site of the home of Simon Peter and discerned the details of daily life in that ancient village, all the while meticulously documenting their conclusions through text, photographs, and isometric drawings related to each building and artifact.[24] The homes in Capernaum were modest, consisting of a walled open courtyard entered from the public street through a single doorway. The courtyard served as the main living, cooking, and sleeping area. Adjacent to each courtyard was a cluster of roofed rooms. Stone stairs against one wall offered access to the roof. Walls and pavement were constructed using local black-volcanic basalt stones without true foundations or the benefit of strong mortar. Given the proximity to the lake, there were no washrooms, drainage systems, or water cisterns as seen in larger cities at that time.

The remains of an octagonal church were identified at Capernaum in the early years of the twentieth century. The church, it was concluded, had been erected on the site of St Peter's home. Stanislao Loffreda summarizes the archaeologists' findings:

The house of St Peter, often mentioned by the Synoptic Gospels in relation to the activity of Jesus in Capharnaum, and recorded later on by pilgrims, was rediscovered in 1968 under the foundations of the octagonal church some 30 meters south of the synagogue.

The history of that house where Jesus lived can be summarized as follows: (1) the house was built in the Late Hellenistic period (323-31 BCE); (2) in the late first century CE it was changed into a "domus-ecclesia", i.e. became a house for religious gatherings; (3) in the fourth century CE the same "domus-ecclesia" was enlarged and was set apart from the rest of the town through an imposing enclosure wall; (4) in the second half of the fifth century CE an octagonal church was built upon the house of St Peter and remained in use until the seventh century CE; (5) the identification of the house of St Peter is based on the combination of archeological data and literary sources which run side by side in a wonderful way.[25]

The decor and artifacts of the original central room in St Peter's home occupied an area of 130 square feet of pavement covered by at least six layers of white plaster as well as some painted fragments originally decorating the inner walls of the room. Fragments of Herodian lamps dating from the second half of the 1st century CE to not later than the beginning of the 2nd century CE were found imbedded in the white plaster pavement. This was the only example of plastered pavement and walls in Capernaum. A modern church was erected over the site for the purpose of protecting the ancient artifacts while at the same time leaving them untouched and enabling improved viewing from above. It was dedicated in June 1990.

As we drove away from the site, I found myself subdued by what we had seen. There had been a lot to absorb. And everything was somehow rendered more impressive by the complete absence of theatre and commerce that would have accompanied a site of similar pedigree in North America. An unpretentious booth offered Loffreda's book for sale to those fortunate enough to locate the vendor. That was all. The first-century discoveries, both at the synagogue and in the home 100 feet closer to the lake, left me with a longing for certitude and at the same time a sense of quiet, stillness, and wonderment. Of course, certainty of the kind I sought does not rest on first-century basalt stones but arises out of less easily defined determinants.

Israel! Someone recalled the observation of David Ben Gurion. "In Israel, in order to be a realist, you must believe in miracles."

MICHAEL AND SAINT COLMAN MACDUAGH

On my way home from Israel, I was a guest speaker in Dublin at a seminar on "Meditation and Personal Wholeness." A bonus arising from this commitment, and for me the main attraction of the visit, was the fact that Michael Kearney would be in Ireland and we could spend two or three post-seminar days together on the west coast of that magic isle.

Michael's compact, stone-walled, thatch-roofed cottage was nestled in a quiet corner of the seaport village of Kinvara, County Galway. The welcoming informality of its Dutch door complemented the smell of wood smoke drifting from the fireplace and the warmth of the comfortable furnishings.

Perhaps it was that first evening over a second mug of Irish coffee that I asked Michael to tell me about the symbolism of the "Celtic knot." As we studied the flames and settled ever deeper into the evening, he spoke with a soft, understated eloquence about that treasured ancient symbol that brings to mind, with its absence of beginning and ending, the timeless nature of our spirit and the infinite cycle of birth and rebirth in realms physical and ethereal. We were off to a good, truly Celtic, start.

In addition to exploring the charms of Kinvara and a trip to a seaside pub for lunch and "black stuff" (Guinness) in the harbour village of Ballyvaughan, Michael had planned a memorable afternoon trek into the distant past. "Let me show you the Burren," he said.

We parked the car and set off cross-country on foot, leaving the rural roads, picturesque thatched-roof cottages, and weather-worn farms with their grazing cows and emerald-green, stone-walled pastures to confront a veritable moonscape of desolate rocky wilderness – "the Burren."

A craggy, scarred cliff face reached from horizon to horizon before us in the middle distance. Between us and this formidable wall there spread a tumultuous half-mile expanse of higgledy-piggledy limestone slabs punctuated by occasional hints of plant life – a scraggly tree here, a tuft of grass or thorns there.

But something was tugging at my unconscious. We were being watched! I was sure of it. Weird. There was no one else evident on this barren planet. Then, after minutes of standing still and scanning the higher reaches of the stolid rock face, we saw him. An imperious, large, white feral goat, standing on top of the cliff face, had us fixed in his regal gaze and above him a Burren eagle circled in and out of sight. We stood in respectful silence.

"St Colman Mac Duagh was born in County Galway, in 560 CE, the son of the Irish chieftain Duac – and thus the *Mac* Duach in his title," Michael explained quietly. "He was a man whose life journey was marked by mystical events. We are on the way to the site of his monastery. I thought you'd be interested."

We picked our way through the rock slabs as he continued. "He went on to become a bishop in the early Irish church, a man of solitude and great compassion ... There are many legends about him: the rooster, mouse and fly he had as pets; the fountain that bubbled up from the earth so that there would be water for his baptism – later to become his well – which we shall see shortly."

Michael went on to speak of Kerry-born poet, philosopher, and mystic John Moriarty, who had observed, "Myth not math is mother tongue," and he reflected on the shared respect he and Moriarty had for the *Red Road* of Native American Indian wisdom and spirituality, while considering the possibility of it leading us once again to walk beautifully on the earth with a renewed sense of the unity of all things.

As we drew closer to the desolate cliff face, we found ourselves passing through an open forest of hazel and birch trees. There was no path, no sign that anyone had ever passed this way before. Then, without warning, we came upon a well and, a few yards farther up the sloping rock, a cleft in the limestone.

I stooped to enter St Colman's Grotto, or *Leaba Mhic Duagh*. The "cave" is about fifteen feet long and four or five feet at its greatest width. I could almost stand erect at its point of greatest height, but it accommodated only one of us at a time. It has remained perfectly preserved over the more than fourteen hundred years since Colman sat in this same spot contemplating creation. Some called him a hermit, a recluse, but in that timeless moment a vastly different perception brought to mind the observation in the Tao Te Ching: "Ordinary men hate solitude. But the Master makes use of it, embracing his aloneness, realizing he is one with the whole universe."[26]

19

One More Case

You matter because you are you
and you matter to the last moment of your life.
We will do all we can,
not only to help you die peacefully,
but also to live until you die.

Cicely Saunders

The cry of loss may not expect or want an answer
but only a silent listening.

Cicely Saunders[1]

It was a balmy mid-May afternoon. The Mount Royal maples and summit oaks were in full leaf under the warming sun. A variety of locals – a blue jay, some flitting chickadees, a robin – were busily going about their business nearby, quite oblivious to the quiet tableau on our side of the PCU family-lounge windows.

We were huddled at the far end of the room's welcoming grace, a panorama view of Montreal's downtown elegance before us, the sloping Mount Royal forest ascending to our right. My exhausted, greying companion and I were at her husband's bedside as he drifted in and out of consciousness, nearing the end of his long journey. Encased in these syrup-slow moments, the silent room seemed cavernous but safe.

A volunteer came to enquire whether I could take a telephone call at the nursing station. It was from Saskatchewan.

The caller was a palliative-care colleague who asked if we would accept a patient in transfer. The young man, he explained, had been referred by Prince Albert Maximum Security Penitentiary. He was from Montreal, in his early thirties, now dying with kidney cancer. He had asked if he might be transferred home so that he could be closer to his family during his final days. The prison authorities agreed; my colleague thought it a reasonable request. Would we accept him? I concurred and, pending confirmation of practicalities at both ends, we tentatively arranged for his transfer to the PCU on the following Friday afternoon.

"What's he in for?" I asked in closing.

"Bank robbery," my colleague replied, then added that our patient was losing ground rather rapidly and was receiving continuous subcutaneous medication for pain.

"Perhaps," he added almost apologetically, "if it's not too much trouble, would you mind mailing our syringe driver back to us when it is no longer needed?"

"Shall do," I replied.

German author Werner Herzog once observed, "Civilization is like a thin layer of ice upon a deep ocean of chaos and darkness." Prophetic words. On informing our seemingly unflappable PCU nursing team about the planned admission, all hell broke loose. Three of our most competent nurses immediately announced that they would refuse to care for him. In each case their stand was based on a painful personal experience caused by "that kind of person." The three were not palliative-care newcomers. Each, in fact, was an expert of long standing; each I considered to be a candidate for veritable sainthood. I was dumbfounded by their stand! But worse was to come.

If I was dumbfounded, Jacques Voyer, our universally loved and respected quadriplegic psychiatrist, was outraged.

"Refuse to care for a dying patient?" he roared. "Under ANY circumstance?"

Given his personal vulnerability, his anguish seemed achingly justified. On the other hand, the stand of each of these palliative-care pillars of nursing excellence was also understandable when their personal experiences were considered.

The solution arrived at by Rhoda Hoffman, the nursing captain of our PCU ship, was to name our potentially crusty Australian nursing teammate Anne Patterson as the patient's primary-care nurse, accept the complete distancing from his care demanded by our expert trio, and shift nursing schedules to enable alternate coverage in Anne's absence.

But there was still more! The Royal Vic administrative nursing hierarchy proclaimed, sight unseen, without the benefit of any risk assessment or information concerning the patient's current status, that a hospital attendant must at all times be posted at the door of the patient's room, an edict that resulted in increasingly bizarre, if not laughable, circumstances, as the clearly ill-trained, often elderly "guards" kept watch over an obviously dying young man.

Given the mounting furor, I decided that I would be his physician. While miffed by this "tempest in a teapot," I don't recall being outraged. Perhaps, however, there was just a smidgen of unconscious determination to show *how Cicely would handle it* – a sort of *What would William Osler, or, for that matter, Jesus, have done?* stance – but, of course, I steadfastly refuse to acknowledge that I would ever embrace such an Olympian fantasy.

Anne admitted the patient on cue and informed me that he was now awaiting my medical assessment, his father at his bedside. I proceeded to the room with empathic determination, treading the moral high ground from desk to door, the bit firmly clenched in my teeth behind a fixed welcoming smile.

The bed was empty. The only person in the room was a man in his sixties who was leaning somewhat unsteadily against the wall near the foot of the bed, bathed in the unmistakable aroma of what must have been several stiff, morale-boosting, drinks.

Smiling beneficently, I entered the room, enquiring, "Mr. Jackson?" He nodded toward the washroom beside me. At that moment, the bathroom door swung open and the occupant strode past me, at the same time directing a remarkably powerful broadside with his elbow that sent me reeling into the wall. Without further acknowledgment, or so much as a glance in my direction, my assailant proceeded past his father to the window on the far side of the room and stood peering pensively at the forest below. I was stunned.

"JACKSON, YOU TWIT!" (In fact, the invective I used was stronger by several leagues!) I bellowed in a voice that would shatter glass, to the total astonishment of all three of us. "I don't know where that chip on your shoulder comes from, but you damn well better get rid of it fast, or I'll send you back to where you came from!"

With that I wheeled and returned to the nursing station without looking back. Simultaneously, my mind was spinning, *Where did that come from? I'm a dead man! Did I really say that?* Only then did I recognize the anxiety I had so totally concealed under a charade of objectivity and cool moral superiority.

Within minutes his father appeared at the nursing station.

"Doctor, I want to apologize for my son's behaviour. He is anxious – sort of unsettled, you know."

I looked at him as he nervously thumbed the counter searching for words.

"My dear man," I replied with an embarrassed self-conscious smile, "you have no need to apologize. It is *I* who should apologize. Your son isn't here to meet our needs; we're here to meet his."

I returned to my patient's room and pulled up a bedside chair to have a better look at the cause of this "deep ocean of chaos."

It was clear at first glance that, in his day, Ken Jackson had projected a handsome, commanding presence. He was 6' 2" or so, and his striking Afro-Canadian complexion, knowing brown eyes, and regal bearing had undoubtedly assured respect and deference from his peers. His curly black hair and matching eyebrows, lashes, beard, and moustache added a striking aristocratic air. Former stature had, however, given way to profound weight loss, fatigue, and weakness, and the "in-your-face" mask of aggression present at our opening joust, a prerequisite for prison survival, he later explained, had now faded. We were now simply two men meeting across a chasm of need.

It soon became clear that the Montreal "family" that Jackson wished to return to for his final days was the gang of bank robbers that had comprised his community. During his stay, the members of this all-Caucasian gang intermittently showed up, five or six at a time, forming a self-conscious line marshalled along the wall.

Only much later did I meet their soft-spoken leader, an impeccably attired, quietly evaluative young gentleman who resembled nothing quite so much as a successful business executive. The "family" parked their high-end cars at the front door to the Ross Pavilion. They were never ticketed or towed away but instead were apparently considered untouchable on this traditionally sacrosanct real estate. Our patient, we later learned, had been the "enforcer" of the gang. I did not ask what that title had entailed.

His medical history and physical examination completed, notes from the penitentiary reviewed, short-term goals drawn up with Anne, orders written, a frail, greying "security guard" propped up in a hallway chair by his door, and it was "game on!"

The idea hit me as I drove home. Since it was Friday, "Tippy" would be one of the volunteers on the ward that evening. Perfect!

Retrieving her various phone numbers, I reached her at her office. Like "Ross III-Stella," Tippy Firlotte was a force of nature. A successful business woman and owner of a prestigious interior-decorating firm with offices in Place Bonaventure, she was of a certain age and perhaps five feet in height, certainly not much more. Natty in dress and pleasantly welcoming in demeanour, Tippy was shrewd in her assessments, generous by nature, and whirlwind-quick on the uptake. Although PCU volunteers were never assigned to specific patients (and certainly *not* by anyone other than the PCS director of volunteers!), I felt that this situation somehow merited special consideration.

"Tippy, it's Bal, you'll be on the Unit tonight, eh? ...Well, we have a new patient who is rather special ... hard to describe in a few words but he has special needs and I think you're the person for the job. Would you please be sure to pop in to see him?"

It would be a day or two before I got the unvarnished details of the ensuing interaction. On arriving that evening, Tippy had listened to Rhoda's taped early-morning volunteer report with its brief comment about the new patient to be admitted later that day, then headed for his room. On entering, she was confronted by an odd formation of enigmatic expressionless figures leaning shoulder to shoulder against the wall in a line reaching almost to the window. Facing them, and Tippy, from his throne of pillows, the bed-bound Grand Inquisitor was wearing a singularly sinister expression.

Tippy paused, and then, without missing a beat, commented with easy grace, "Well, Mr Jackson, I can see you are busy right now. I'll try to get back to see you later this evening."

Without pausing for a response, she turned to leave, but at the door she stopped, bent forward at the waist as if to enable a better look, and pivoted to face the scowling patient, exclaiming, "My God! Are you gorgeous, or are you gorgeous!" With that she turned on her heels and was gone, leaving the room awash in stunned silence, mouths agape.

During the following days, I made rounds frequently. We were now conversing with ease and had become "Ken" and "Mountain man" (a moniker of his devising). While the content of these chats is no longer clear in my memory, they did not deal with his criminal record or his "family." Whatever his past, the present provided a space for deeper bonds that soon evolved into "Ken" and "Bal" and I was increasingly impressed by the man behind the mask.

A similar bond was forming between Ken and Tippy. It was later that week that he asked her, "Teepee, would you come back to tuck me in tonight?" (He always called her "Teepee.") *Tuck me in?* Tippy wondered. *What might that entail?*

Later that evening, she straightened his bed covers and was chatting rather absently when Ken said, "Teepee, can I kiss you goodnight?" While she wasn't quite sure what he had in mind, she agreed. "Of course, Ken," and, leaning down, she turned her cheek toward him. She then felt the lightest, most tender, almost imperceptible peck – nothing more than the faintest brush of lips on skin. She was deeply moved. Her instant image was that a small child had just said goodnight to his mother.

While Tippy and I were experiencing these deepening ties, with Anne it was a different story entirely. She became the focus of his residual pent-up rage. Nevertheless, Anne, who had a well-known short fuse when it came to negative feedback from her patients or colleagues, responded to his aggression with consistent, uncomplaining grace. Indeed, as the days passed, Anne was transformed as, with each of his assaults, a greater and more impressive level of patience and kindness surfaced. While I didn't discuss this with her, I was in awe.

Gradually, it became important to me for Linda to meet Ken, though I had never introduced her to other patients – a precedent that evoked yet another storm of angry protests from one or two of our nurses. It was on a Tuesday that Linda and I made our early-evening visit. When we entered his room, something I had heard on the six o'clock news came to mind and I casually mentioned, "Oh, by the way, Ken, do you know what happened today?"

"No, what?"

"Rajiv Gandhi was assassinated."

If the remark had any forethought at all, it was simply to use an off-hand news update as a prelude to introducing Linda. I thought it was highly unlikely that Ken had heard of the former prime minister of India and felt a fleeting twinge of guilt at having unwittingly "tested" him in that way. I like to think that it had been unintended.

"Really!" he shot back, his eyes narrowing in concentration, his mind racing. "Really! Well! Let me see ... that would be the Tamils that did it."

I was astounded.

That Ken would know of the militant Sri Lankan Liberation Tigers of Tamil Eelam seemed inconceivable. The breadth of his knowledge and familiarity with the nuances shaping word affairs astounded and humbled me.

A nun who came to visit Ken while he was on the PCU gave us the back story we did not know. When his mother was pregnant she was in prison. Following Ken's birth, she was returned to prison and the baby was cared for by a local religious community. They grew to love him and were deeply impressed by his great promise.

One afternoon on Rounds, not long after that, I noticed that Ken appeared disturbed. He looked deeply concerned.

"What's up, Ken?" I asked as I pulled up my chair. "What's on your mind?"

"Bal ... are we friends?" His serious expression caught my attention. I had no idea what lay behind the query. His eyes were locked on mine.

"Well, Ken, I don't know what else we would call it. Of course we are. Why do you ask? What's up?"

"Well, I was awake most of the night wondering about what we could do together if I wasn't sick ... and if I had my old life back ... and you, yours ... How could we have been friends?! What would we have in common? What could we have done together?"

We pondered the question for a few minutes without much headway. Then I asked, "Ken, do you play tennis?"

"Well, a little. I'm not very good."

"Me either. I used to play each week with a friend, John Seely, who moved to Ottawa, but neither of us was very good. Maybe you and I could play tennis."

Ken relaxed. "Yes, we could play tennis."

Our conversation continued. It was at a deeper level now. His caring was evident.

"Bal," he whispered, his tone earnest. "If you are ever in a bank when a robbery happens, do exactly what they say. Lie down on the floor; don't move. They're on a high. Do what they say. Otherwise you'll risk being killed."

My pain is that I can't recall the details of Ken's last moments. I like to think it was peaceful, a gentle easing out of a life that had been short-changed and too deeply troubled. What was, and still is, clear to me, however, is that I lost a valued friend.

Many moments bring Ken to mind. I think of him when I confidently pass judgment on others, and when I take for granted the countless opportunities that have come my way in life. And again, he turns up when I complain about the multiple daily challenges of life with aging. What benefits, I wonder, could have come to society had Ken Jackson's talents been nurtured toward creative ends? In a host of settings I am left feeling a mix of gratitude and determination and I realize once more how easy it is to "throw away my shot." I feel more keenly the admonition that of him to whom much is given, much shall be required. I also realize that I deeply loved that guy, and still do. He had become a brother.

As I was leaving the PCU the day Ken died, the leader of his "family" stopped me in the hall as he offered a slow, very firm handshake while pressing a piece of paper into my palm, saying with particular emphasis, "I want to thank you for everything you did for Kenny. If there is ever anything I can do ... I mean ... *anything* ... let me know." His phone number was on the paper. (How often, over the subsequent years, when experiencing moments of intolerance, utter frustration, or anger, have I wished that I had kept that phone number!)

The funeral service had been arranged by Ken's "family." I took down the address of the Catholic church, all the while imagining, given my understanding of Ken's stature in his profession, an epic Mafia-style funeral complete with flower-bedecked black limousines, scores of men in black suits and dark glasses, crowds of curious onlookers, and camera-toting Mounties high up telephone poles recording the identity of attendees.

When I phoned Anne and Tippy to suggest we go together to pay our last respects to our friend, both declined, stating that they had decided not to attend. With a little pressure, however, both agreed that it was important for us to be there, and to go together.   At the appointed hour, the street in the industrial district that matched the address I had been given was empty. Furthermore, there was no church. We circled the block. *Well perhaps that humble structure squeezed between its neighbours might be a church, but where are the lines of limousines, parked cars, traffic cops and police officers?*

We parked in front of the compact chapel and made our way in, feeling subdued and somewhat depressed. Mine was the only car on the street. A closed casket stood alone in front of the altar. The sanctuary was empty save for one person, a stranger. His clothes, age, heavy coat with turned-up collar, not to mention his shifty uneasiness as he inspected us on arrival, identified him as a "family" informant, present to report back to the boss. We four were the sole celebrants in the empty pews as the tall, distinguished, greying priest arrived to welcome us. He brought abundant grace and evident pastoral presence, but, when he spoke, it was with a distracting speech impediment. I reacted with spontaneous defensive anger – my friend was being short-changed by life one last time! Then it came to me. How appropriate! It was, in fact, the completion of a circle: the wounded offering healing attention to the wounded, on behalf of the wounded.

20

The View from Here

*It takes a shock
to make us see our lives afresh.
Life, after all, is a terminal condition.*

Philip Simmons[1]

*I have found that if you love life,
life will love you back.*

Arthur Rubinstein

A century completed, or rather, left incomplete, yet offering promise in ever-hopeful hearts for better things to come in this conflicted world. To mark the moment, Michael sent me a photo of his daughter Mary-Anna as she welcomed the rising sun on 1 January 2000 at Dublin Bay.

1 January 2000. A new day. A new year. A new century. A new millennium. A reminder of the unknown potential that lies ahead of us and our freedom to choose our response in all circumstances. The latter was about to be tested.

CROSSROAD ENCOUNTERS

January 2000: *What is that unpleasant taste?*

It was intermittent at first. Then it became a nuisance. "Linda, you know what?" I mumbled as we were going about our business, "I think I have gastric cancer." An odd thing to say. We discussed it in an offhand manner and returned to our daily preoccupations.

25 February 2000: "Bal, you have a small ulcer in your esophagus." Then, after a pregnant pause, my doctor corrected himself. "No, you have a *large* ulcer in your esophagus."

Peter, a colleague of several decades, had anticipated a short, rather trivial endoscopy: obtaining a culture from a documented duodenal diverticulum, perhaps a biopsy for Celiac's disease, "a quick in and out" as the saying goes. But this was both quicker and more epic than we had planned. An esophageal ulcer!?

"Peter, you mean I have carcinoma of the esophagus."

"Well, not necessarily, Bal," he fumbled. "It could be a viral infection," then adding, "but I do think that you should see a surgeon while we wait for the biopsy results."

I was thankful for Peter's mix of professionalism and caring. He cleared away the instruments, filled out the pathology requisition, and spoke briefly to the nurse as he wheeled my stretcher out of the small outpatient operating theatre and into the screened-off recovery area, pulling the curtains around us to provide a modicum of privacy.

"Bal, rest here until the premeds wear off."

Alone with my new reality and knowing all too well the implications of the diagnosis, I was surprised to find that I was smiling. *Why is this man smiling?* I thought, and I found myself saying aloud to the empty cubicle, "However this ends, it won't get the best of me!"

Where in the world did that *come from?* The answer was immediate, *Mother*. It had her tongue-in-cheek ring to it. Nevertheless, my upbeat response surprised me, particularly because it felt more than skin deep. I had accompanied far too many patients in their dying to ask, "Why me?" My question instead had always been, "Why *not* me?" But now there was a sense of deep calm that went beyond that – a sense of numbness as well.

Esophageal cancer? A *large* ulcer? Cataclysm. Yes, I felt calm, but everything had changed: suddenly life was "slip slidin' away," as Paul Simon might say, dissolving before my eyes. Laurence once observed about such a crossroad that it "was terrible at the time, but looking back, I'm glad it happened. It taught me something. It made me grow in a way I would never have grown otherwise. It awakened something in me that changed the direction and meaning of my life." Perhaps that was something to hold on to.

10 March 2000: A passing succession of ceiling lights silently saluted me as the attendant wheeled my gurney down the endless corridors to the OR. The sense of calm persisted – *the premeds perhaps*. I transferred onto the OR table and watched the intravenous lines being established as Dave Mulder and his team scrubbed up.

Linda, Kappy, and her daughter Susan were in the adjacent family room, waiting for the long day to inch past.

The thoraco-abdominal, "three hole approach," total esophagectomy – *a rather indelicate term*, I thought – was topped off with a vagotomy, pyloroplasty, and an unscheduled splenectomy necessitated by transgressed adhesions, the souvenirs of Whit's 1964 retroperitoneal lymph-node dissection. Then, the modified stomach remnant was attached through a neck incision to the lower end of the oropharynx, adjacent to the vocal cords – or rather, vocal cord, for only one remained functioning as a result of the invasion of the esophageal cancer which had been full-thickness.

Opaque blackness. The recovery room? My eyes were fixed shut under protective gauze; tubes and masks prevented speech. As I began to swim upward through the vortex of deep anesthesia, I felt Linda squeezing my hand – once ... a second time ... a third. It was her signal – "I love you." I signalled back in kind. The next thing I heard was the voice of Dick Cruess. "*BAl! ...* You're doing just fine!" Linda had reassured him that I was aware and encouraged him to announce his presence.

The dean had spoken! Now I *was* certain, this ordeal wouldn't get the best of me! Still today, years later, I recall my sense of gratitude for Dick's supportive presence with a clarity that suggests its impact at the time.

Two ICU days later, I was visited by the surgical residents as they made morning rounds. One of them approached as the others huddled indifferently at the foot of my bed.

He looked particularly young – perhaps an intern. He came closer. I couldn't speak easily, given the uncomfortable tubes in every orifice and my just hanging-on state, but I longed for him to speak to me, to acknowledge my complete awareness. I hungered for contact with the world. But he offered not a glance in my direction; not a word was spoken. He had stopped by my side to examine the urine output. Then, having checked the numbers on the vital-signs sheet, he returned to the safety of the pack and muttered his observations. I felt a sinking sense of abandonment, of being invisible.

The residents were, it seemed, behind a virtual glass wall. They were standing less than eight feet from my searching gaze as they turned to move on to the next object of their data-collection travels when one of them commented to his neighbour, "It's such a shame, but I guess he may have two or three good months left." For them, the invisible glass wall was sufficiently thick to lead them to presume that their words were inaudible. My sense of isolation was total. They moved on, unaware of what they had just done, and what they had completely failed to do.

The team returned on a subsequent morning, still apparently oblivious to my conscious state. The senior resident, a flint-eyed young woman, commanded her underlings in an imperious tone, "Discharge him to the ward."

There had been not a single word to me, no enquiry about how I felt, no comment about how I was doing, not the slightest encouragement or acknowledgment that I was a sentient being, let alone a colleague who had been one of their teachers, one who was achingly aware of each proceeding microsecond.

"He's bleeding quite heavily through the nasogastric tube," the junior intern interjected, almost apologetically.

"Discharge him anyway. It will stop," Flint-eyes retorted, as she spun on her heals.

Screw this! I decided. Having neither a gun to shoot her with, nor a voice with which to engage her, I rang for the nurse.

When Dave Mulder arrived, he cancelled the resident's order, tended to the gastrointestinal bleeding, and chatted away amicably in his customary reassuring manner. I had once again gained a foothold in the land of the living.

On transfer to the thoracic ward, I was struck by its efficient attentiveness. I had lost forty pounds since striding confidently into the hospital while waving goodbye to Linda that fistful of days earlier.

I was now profoundly weak. Coughing to clear the constant airway secretions and avoid pneumonia led to prohibitive incisional pain. My innate will to charge forward into healing had melted in the face of my overwhelming inability to fend for myself. "Just ring the bell if you need anything," the head nurse reassured. And they did indeed respond promptly. That is, unless it happened to be the change of shift.

That evening I received a graphic demonstration of the impact of government budget cuts and understaffing. The bell rang: there was no one to respond. *I'll have to hire an attendant for tomorrow night. I can't go through this again.*

On her arrival the attendant introduced herself from the doorway, put on a protective pair of heavy, kitchen-style, rubber gloves, pulled up a chair in a distant corner, and promptly drifted into a sound sleep. She simply couldn't be roused. The next three nights, Anita Mountjoy, friend, neighbour of four decades, and retired Surgical head nurse, shepherded me through the tedious hours with quiet, rock-solid presence. Oh blessed, blessed presence! Oh Anita, dearest friend!

During this post-operative period, Dave Mulder suggested we consider chemotherapy, noting that the current protocol was quite effective with my particular tumour.

"Does it impact on the five-year survival rate of responders?" I asked.

"No," he replied.

"Then I think I'll save it until the need is evident." We both knew the minuscule survival rate that accompanied the pathology at hand. The die had been cast.

Home again. Back to normal. But it was a new, withering normal. Trouble swallowing, repeated aspiration of oral intake into the lungs, the need to sleep in a sitting position to prevent bowel contents running into my mouth, the weakness that is inevitable following a rapid forty-pound weight loss, the need for repeated dilatations to correct the recurrent strictures in my throat. Inability to vomit. *Of course! We need esophageal reverse peristalsis to vomit.*

It was a slow uphill battle with help found in unexpected places, such as the time I accompanied Lauren to see the newly released film *Gladiator*, which prompted reflections on the movie's various portrayals of facing death with courage and meaning, and then appreciation of the final notion at its conclusion. "But not yet ... not yet."

Enter Home Care nurse Joan Foster with her personal whirlwind of efficiency, reassurance, good humour, and upbeat presence. "Don't expect any great improvement until forty days have passed," she warned. "It's that biblical thing! They knew. It takes forty days ... Now, let's try walking again and I want to see you getting in more of that dietary supplement." Confident, informed, and clearly in charge, Joan brought with her a daily tsunami of nursing competence, insight, and support.

Letters, cards, and warm greetings from family and friends provided encouragement. Among them there were two postcards. One, sent by Trevor, on concert tour in Italy, featured the photograph of *Cristo della Trincea*, a marble bust of Christ crucified, from the basilica at Aquileia. The second bore a head-and-shoulders photograph of the Hindu Saint Bhagavan Sri Ramana Maharshi.

The latter came from Laurence, who had been visiting Bede Griffiths in India. Realizing as he left Bede that he was near the Ramana Maharshi ashram, Laurence arranged an impromptu visit. On arrival, his hosts had suggested that he rest in the Old Hall while they took his bag to his room. It was the room where Ramana Maharshi had lived, meditated, and welcomed visitors from around the world each day and evening until his final illness.

Laurence had entered the room with no particular expectations; he was tired from the journey and glad to have a quiet moment to collect his thoughts. But, as he stepped into the empty room, he was startled and deeply moved to encounter a profound sense of Presence. The great teacher had died a half-century earlier, in 1950, on my birthday in fact, 14 April.

The photograph Laurence gave me was arresting. The revered mystic is peering into the eyes of the viewer, his attentive expression and slight smile evoking a sense of personal contact – no, more than that: radical presence, warmth, and understanding. His shoulders are bare, his engagement with the observer quietly riveting, his gaze conveying both questioning and understanding. It is abundantly clear that we are studying each other.

Placing the postcards in a hinged double frame, I sat them by my reclining chair-cum-bed, promising myself that someday I would read one of the biographies of this remarkable Indian contemplative. Trevor, who encounters the sacred through the great composers, had given me the Nazarene, while the Christian priest and monk had brought me the Hindu saint.

These new companions had found their way to my table as a result of the malignant perils at hand. Beneficence as a product of maleficence, as it were. I recalled Father Bede's recommendation that we honour each of the great wisdom traditions, going to depth in our own yet remaining open to the potential for new light being shed on mystery by each of the others. Bede's wisdom was echoed years later when Laurence observed:

> The connection between the historical Jesus and the Inner Christ
> is the most interesting and mysterious and exciting connection
> in my life, and to feel that I'm connected to that makes me feel
> connected to everything in this world. Through that connection,
> I can feel and love the truth in every religious tradition, and in
> individuals who manifest the essence of that tradition. And I think
> that means that to be a Christian, for me, is a process, not just
> an identity. It's a process; it's an evolution. But it does mean, that
> to be a Christian, there is no competition. Jesus did not compete
> with other religious leader, then why should Christians compete or
> pretend to be superior to anyone else? That would be un-Christian,
> unlike Jesus to do that.[2]

Jesus and Ramana Maharshi have been my daily chair-side companions, and so much more, since then, each shedding light on the mystery, grace, and reassurance exemplified by the other; each bringing with him the reminder of the words uttered by Cicely's patient so many decades ago – "I never would have thought that it would be safe to die here." In those words I find a memory of Mother's grit and grace. And once again a circle is complete.

KEEVIN AND AN IMPROBABLE CIRCLE OF FRIENDS

With my doctor's initial pronouncement prior to the esophagectomy, I recognized that the approaching surgery would confirm advanced cancer with a grim prognosis. With this in mind, I went immediately to my office in the Ross Pavilion and placed a phone call.

Keevin Robins, a Montreal businessman, is thirteen years younger than me. He had been a palliative-care volunteer since 1993. It was a Thursday afternoon. Realizing he would be on the PCU, I had him paged. Keevin listened to my news in silence. Then, following a brief pause, I asked if he would "please be there for Linda and Bethany should I not make it."

Our relationship had been warm yet not close, but, for reasons I would not have been able to explain, I felt this singularly unusual request was inevitable, if not natural and logical. There had been no searching fore-thought or discussion with Linda. It just seemed to be a loose end that I needed to deal with prior to the esophagectomy which, as it turned out, would take place within a day or two.

Remarkably, without hesitation, Keevin agreed. He later noted, "I spontaneously accepted, embracing the implied shift in our friendship. The trust and faith that had been expressed in that single request trans-formed our relationship into a deeper spiritual bond, a brotherhood."

I have always been struck by the synchronicity of the events that, through apparent chance, shape our lives. This was to be one of those occasions. A confluence of unrelated strangers were to be drawn into a support network of remarkable grace and depth. Who knew?

It had been a quarter-century since twenty-year-old Keevin quit uni-versity in September 1973 against parental advice and set out with Barry, his closest friend from childhood, on a world tour in search of a remedy for their deep-seated disenchantment with life. Keevin felt consumed by a post-1960s sense of angst and profound meaninglessness that he later would identify as Viktor Frankl's "existential anguish."

In due course, the two friends found themselves in Haridwar, India, a small town in the Himalayan foothills. There they met Sri Dilip Kumar Roy, known among his followers as Dadaji, one of India's great illumi-nates, a musician, poet, author, and mystic. While Barry continued on to Southeast Asia, and eventually home to Montreal, Keevin stayed behind at the Hindu ashram where Kumar Roy and his community lived.

Their disparate decisions would determine the course of their lives. As recounted earlier, Barry and I would meet for his retroperitoneal lymph-node dissection at the Royal Vic, an intervention that would not have been available in India; Keevin would discover, then embrace, the spiritual path that would henceforth guide his life.

Keevin was to remain a part of Dadaji's community in India as his student and attendant for six years until January 1980 when he became his personal caregiver during his guru's final illness. In March of that year, Keevin returned to Montreal to start an atypical new life as both a businessman and aspiring yogi and *sadhak*. In 1993 he applied to become a Royal Vic PCS volunteer in an effort to express his gratitude for Barry's surgery, and in time, over coffee, we became friends and PCS colleagues.

Through Keevin, I met his observant Jewish friend Michel, or, to be more specific, the Honourable Mr Justice M.J. Shore. Slight of frame and quick of mind, Michel has a natural twinkle in his eyes, the by-product of his intense focus on whatever is at hand. A surfeit of compassion and unwavering commitment to the Torah fuel his every thought. "May God bless you" colours each action, as does his ever-assessing analytical mind and his unquenchable passion for justice. To a discerning wisdom that is reminiscent of the prophets of old, Michel brings the enthusiasm of a newly minted believer.

So there they were, the Jew-cum-Hindu businessman and the intellectual Orthodox Jewish judge, united by the clarity of their awareness of the sacred, their creativity (Michel writes both prose and poetry), and their dedication to serving others. Their openness tended toward the universal. Nothing seemed more natural to them than escaping for a Hindu-Jewish retreat weekend of meditation at a rural Catholic monastery an hour or two from Montreal!

Thus, as Linda, Kappy, and Susan gathered in the family room during my esophagectomy on that March 2000 morning, Keevin and Michel, who had cancelled their commitments for that day, spent it in meditation close by. Indeed, thanks to Michel's ever-industrious caring, this group of dedicated supporters was not alone. Michel had recruited surprising, if not remarkable, further support.

As it happened, Michel's mother, Dr Lena Allen-Shore (a Polish-born philosopher, poet, writer, composer, and educator at Gratz College in Pennsylvania) had survived the Holocaust by masquerading as a Catholic and had vowed that, should she survive, she would devote her life to "building bridges" between faith traditions.

At the same time, a young pacifist Pole, Karol Wojtyla, was dodging Nazi entrapment and deciding to become a priest. Like Lena, he was an intellectual, possessed with both a strong faith and a love of literature, in particular the work of several Polish poets. In October 1978 the Catholic Church named Karol Wojtyla pope. Within days, Pope John

Paul II received a four-page handwritten letter in Polish from Lena, congratulating him, offering her continuing prayers, and sharing with him her passion for "building bridges" toward a healing of humanity.

A return letter thanked her warmly and their correspondence contin ued, the content enriched by their shared interests and personal goals, all of it expressed in their mother tongue. They finally met at the Vatican in 1996 and their close friendship continued with his invitation for her to join him for his historic visit to Jerusalem in 2000.[3]

Days before Lena was to join the pope's entourage for his pilgrimage to Israel, Michel spoke to his mother about my imminent surgery. She contacted the pontiff. He asked for the time the surgery would start on 10 March and requested that he be informed when the surgery had finished. Those involved would be in his prayers. Unknown to Linda, Kappy, Susan, and me, our support group had just increased to include Keevin, Michel, Lena, and His Holiness.

The brief encounter Pope John Paul II and I had shared on Queen Mary Road fifteen years earlier had long since faded from his mind, I am sure, but it remains in mine, enhanced by the sketch done that day and his interventions on my behalf a decade and a half later.

The surgery behind us, Keevin's presence was always available in times of need – a visit to the recovery room in the early post-operative hours; covering for Linda when she was called away from my bedside; and later, when I was home, the offer of twice-daily visits for meditation.

After a month of this daily meditation routine, Keevin suggested we include others who might like to join us. The meditation group that evolved swelled to more than twenty, though not more than five or six on any given day. I was intrigued by the diversity of our blossoming community. As time passed, Christians, Jews, Hindus, Muslims, Buddhists, and agnostics, as well as those with "no fixed allegiance," joined in. However, in due course, my persistent tendency to survive outwore the enthusiasm of most stalwarts and the numbers declined. A decade later (and beyond), the group gelled at three of us, twice daily on weekdays – Linda, our longtime friend Anita Mountjoy, and me. My persisting sense of frustration at remaining a meditation novice frequently brings to mind John Main's retort: "There is no such a thing as beginner or expert in meditation. There is just meditation!"

THE WAY OF PEACE

During the fall of 2000, two memorable milestones accompanied my return to health: in September, McGill's biennial Congress on Care of the

Terminally Ill (the 13th) featuring presentations by an outstanding international faculty of 177 colleagues; then, in October, "The Way of Peace" meeting in Belfast, Northern Ireland, convened by the Dalai Lama and Laurence, during which I offered a concurrent workshop for that event entitled "Lessons in Living from the Dying," a title chosen long before my diagnosis.

The closing plenary of the Belfast meeting would remain deeply etched in the memories of all present. "The Troubles," as our Irish hosts called them in a wonderfully Gaelic turn of phrase, had embroiled Northern Ireland in a bloody clash pitting the Unionist government and Ulster Protestants (inflamed by the fundamentalist preacher Ian Paisley) against Catholics, nationalists, and the paramilitary Irish Republican Army. Over the years the spiralling death toll had been augmented by intermittent bombings in England. From the mid-1960s until the 1998 Good Friday Agreement and beyond through 2001, this conflict resulted in more than 3,500 deaths.

As Trevor, cousin Joan Ormont, and I gathered in Belfast in October 2000, the killings were mostly a thing of the past, but they remained brutally fresh and raw in the collective psyche. Belfast was split in two, with the Catholics on one side of the road that ran through its heart and Protestants on the other.

The Dalai Lama was to be the speaker at the "Way of Peace" closing plenary and every seat in the large, airy auditorium was full. The platform facing us was empty as we arrived, save for an inverted v-shaped line of chairs which were soon to be filled by a line of young men and women who were discretely directed to one side or the other as the result of a quiet discussion with an organizer as each reached the stage. The Dalai Lama sat farthest from the audience, at the apex of the v. He appeared warmly attentive and relaxed.

I don't recall the details of His Holiness's opening remarks. I believe he may have commented on the complexity of the factors that shape our lives. Perhaps he spoke of his exile from Tibet and the troubles in *his* homeland. What I do recall is that his comments were delivered with the earnestness and energy that consistently fill his words with a sense of presence, depth, and meaning, a meaning that carries his audience with him as equal participants. On completing his remarks, he commented that he had invited his guests to tell us their stories.

The young people accompanying him on stage appeared to be in their late twenties or thirties. They were simply dressed, indistinguishable from those passing on the street – ordinary folk. There were five or six seated to his right, the same number on his left. Each had been born into a bloodstained world; from birth, each decision they made had been shaped in the shadow of the Troubles.

One after another, those seated on the Dalai Lama's right walked to the microphone, identified themselves, and told their story. Each had grown up in a Catholic family; each had experienced self, family, community, and every nuance of life filtered through a dark brooding presence of unpredictability and impending violence. A young lad had been wounded, his brother jailed; another had lost his father. A young woman spoke of her brother, killed by a British soldier's rubber bullet. Each quietly recounted a tale of suffering and then returned to his or her chair as the next came to the microphone. None of the speakers had previously met a member of "the enemy."

The Dalai Lama beckoned quietly to the Protestants on his left; they followed, one after another. Each was similarly scarred and none of them had ever known a person from the other side. As the last in line returned to his seat, a thick silence engulfed us. The stories we had heard were galvanizing, profoundly disturbing, but also, somehow, humbling, as the matter-of-fact absence of passion in each quiet narrative carried with it a stark contrast to the brutality of the events described.

What was most overwhelming for me was the eloquence of their words. Each young speaker told his or her tale in simple phrases that carried us into their world – a world of darkness rendered through simple but exquisite extemporaneous prose. I found it difficult to breathe. Brendan Behan, Samuel Beckett, Anne Enright, James Joyce, Oscar Wilde, W.B. Yeats, they were all present in spirit. We had been exposed to, then submerged in, a genetic pool of staggering richness and incredible depth. Elegance of Irish expression washed over us in waves, the product of countless back alleys, rain- soaked days, fireside chats, and endless nights of grief and loss that had progressively informed each speaker's understanding, and now ours.

Something powerful had transformed us. Each of us had become a player in this tragedy. The mirrored stories from right and left had been heard. Deeply. We found ourselves swallowed in an engulfing silence. And that included, most centrally, the Dalai Lama. His listening brought with it an immediacy that, through its evident depth, had taken each of us out of the formless, empty darkness into the incandescent light that dwells in the radical present.

And in that silence, all hurt and blame had given way to sadness, humility, and compassion, thus opening each of us to our own personal need for truth and reconciliation.

THE MAN WHO LEARNED TO FALL

Ten months had passed since my surgery. It was January 2001 when the postman delivered a package containing a brief letter and an accompanying book, *Learning to Fall: The Blessings of an Imperfect Life* by Philip Simmons. *Never heard of him.* I glanced at the letter. It was from the author. He was writing from Sandwich, New Hampshire. *Sandwich? Are you serious?* It was an invitation. It seems that, based on his book, Simmons had been invited to be a visiting lecturer at Harvard Medical School and he was planning to round out this commitment with a symposium titled "What Is Healing?" Would I agree to take part? *Strange. How did he get my name?* I turned to the book and glanced at the foreword. The opening paragraph is twelve lines long. As I reached the twelfth line I knew that I would happily walk to Boston on my knees simply to meet this man. He was a writer extraordinaire.

Philip Simmons was the quintessential man in motion – physically, intellectually, socially, and spiritually. He engaged life with enthusiasm. He was an English teacher and writer with a tenure-track position at a liberal-arts college in Lake Forest, Illinois; he was a naturalist and hiker (he had scaled all forty-nine of the New Hampshire peaks above 4,000 feet, having begun with Mount Washington at the age of six); as a singer, he was a Woody Guthrie aficionado and had made a number of quality recordings of songs by Guthrie and others; he was a proficient Alpine skier and a world-class storyteller, a gift that had helped him seduce his equally gifted wife, the sculptor and painter Kathryn Field; the son of a Jewish father and Catholic mother, he was an earnest student of his Judeo-Christian heritage as well as Eastern religious traditions and practices, commenting, "I'm grateful for insight wherever I find it, whether in modern poetry or physics or the Koran or the Old Testament or the sayings of the Christian Desert Fathers. Of all the sources of insight available to me, I turn to religion in particular because it is with religious language that human beings have most consistently, rigorously and powerfully explored the harrowing business of rescuing joy from heartbreak." He was also an accomplished orator, whether through lectures to students pursuing higher education or through readings of his written word (events he referred to as "performances") at Unitarian Universalist Church gatherings. His writing reveals a brilliant wordsmith, a discerning observer of the natural world, and a keen wit that could soften a hard insight by transforming it into an experience of shared hilarity and delight. Phil, Kathryn, and their children, Aaron and Amelia, did, indeed, have a home in Sandwich, New Hampshire – Center Sandwich, actually – a delightful town named in honour of John Montagu, 4th Earl of Sandwich, and nestled in the White Mountains on the shore of Squam Lake.

In 1993, at the age of thirty-five, Phil Simmons was informed that he had ALS and would likely be dead within three to five years. He and I met seven years following his diagnosis on Tuesday afternoon, 20 March, 2001, in the hallway adjacent to the Harvard auditorium. His four-hundred-pound motorized wheelchair came around the corner and bore down on me with sedate determination, his eyes sparkling over a neatly trimmed moustache and beard. He smiled broadly as we introduced ourselves; the warmth of his greeting was infectious.

Though the ravages of ALS had totally immobilized his wasting six-foot-plus body, he projected a sense of confidence and easy authority that left it clear who was in the driver's seat of both machine and symposium. As the session began we were joined by the third member of our panel, Rabbi Harold Kushner, author of the bestseller *When Bad Things Happen to Good People*.

The rabbi and I presented our respective thoughts on healing; Phil's reading drew on the foreword and first chapter of his book. An open discussion involving the audience followed.

I believe all present found nuggets to take home. But for me the impact was far greater than that. In Phil I had found a teacher who understood the inevitability of "falling" as an unavoidable consequence of human vulnerability and the path we share. Here was a man who had assessed and come to understand the implications of our recurrent fallings. For him, falling was not simply a problem to be solved but a mystery to be lived. Whatever the final outcome, he suggested, the challenge is to learn to accept the inherent limitations of our particular resources. There was respectful silence as he read: "We fall into humility, into compassion, into emptiness, into oneness with forces larger than ourselves, into oneness with others whom we realize are likewise falling. We fall, at last, into the presence of the sacred, into godliness, into mystery, into our better, diviner natures." Phil died 16 months later, on 27 July 2002; the message reached Linda, Bethany, and me early the next morning at a cottage on Lac Massawippi, Quebec. During the intervening months since the Sandwich symposium, Phil and I had become fast friends, bound by our sense of shared falling. It had been a rich journey together: my multiple visits to Sandwich, Phil's visit to Montreal to deliver a "performance" before an appreciative McGill Faculty of Medicine audience and to attend a Montreal Expos baseball game, all of us working with

Montreal filmmaker Garry Beitel as he crafted his lasting legacy to Phil, the award-winning documentary film *The Man Who Learned to Fall*. Phil was a great gift, a timely mentor, and an unforgettable confrère. He shone a bright light on the path that lies ahead for each of us.

"At one time or another, each of us confronts an experience so powerful, bewildering, joyous, or terrifying that all our efforts to see it as a problem are futile. Each of us is brought to the cliff's edge. At such moments we can either back away in bitterness or confusion, or leap forward into mystery. And what does mystery ask of us? Only that we be in its presence, that we fully, consciously, hand ourselves over. That is all, and that is everything."[4]

Phil's wisdom in recognizing *falling* as "an unavoidable consequence of human vulnerability and the path we share" was to be driven home with agonizing clarity over the ensuing years – and never more forcefully than following the death of Jean Vanier in May 2019. The founder, in 1964, of L'Arche, the international federation of communities for people with developmental disabilities that spanned thirty-seven countries, and then, in 1971, co-founder of Faith and Light, a network of families and friends of the disabled in over eighty countries, Jean had become my friend over the ensuing decades. We had kept in touch by letter – his small, tightly penned greetings always cherished – and then, in later years, by e-mail.

The news of Jean's death brought a heavy heart but it was to be a grief that was intensified and filled with unexpected turmoil when, in February 2020, a L'Arche investigation led to the report that Jean had sexually abused six women in Trosly-Breuil, France, between 1970 and 2005. My sense of loss gave way to depression, confusion, and despair. The suffering and disillusionment for all who suffered through this unexpected falling defies description. I had known Jean as an icon of faith, grace, and other-centred caring. He, like Marian Anderson, had for me embodied the spiritual quest personified. Then, as I looked back on words he had written, they took on new meaning:

There comes a moment when, with the help of a competent psychologist, we maybe have to look more closely at the powers of darkness hidden within us. No longer can we run away from them, but we must try to discover their origin and why they have such a hold over us. If we are to find healing and inner peace we have to face up to the real questions, to put names to them. We must not let ourselves be overcome by feelings of unworthiness that bring us into a terrifying, imaginary world ... The more we accept the truth in ourselves, the more we find the courage to acknowledge our mistakes and our responsibilities.[5]

A thoughtful 25 February 2020 letter from L'Arche Canada expressed our shared distress. My letter in response read:

Dear L'Arche colleague,
My path has been uniquely blessed by three *crossroad encounters* in meeting Marian Anderson, Jean Vanier and Kenny Jackson: the grace-filled contralto, the Spirit-filled teacher, and the terminally ill bank robber. They seemed a rather odd trinity of messengers concerning the transcendent/existential Reality that surrounds and embraces us all … Three disparate exemplars of the Nazarene's words; three incongruous signposts defining the human condition, that today I experience in the humbling admonition, "Let him that is without sin among you cast the first stone."

How easy it is for me, for us, to react to accounts of Jean's actions with hurt, defensiveness, disillusionment, judgment and anger, rather than compassion, humility and love! (*Father forgive me – to coin a phrase!*) During the hours since learning of Jean's reported actions I have been filled with anguish: for all involved; for the women; for L'Arche; for ourselves; but predominantly for Jean as I feel the suffering that this man of insight and grace must have experienced as he ran the gauntlet between his epic awareness of his Teacher's words and his abiding human nature … Curiously, as I began to identify my feelings in the wake of these revelations an unexpected voice from the past came to mind in the words, *Senator, you're no Jack Kennedy*. It was the retort made during the 1988 United States vice-presidential debate by Democratic vice-presidential candidate Senator Lloyd Bentsen to Republican Senator Dan Quayle in response to Quayle's mentioning the name of John F. Kennedy, the 35th President of the United States. Since then, the words *You're no Jack Kennedy* have become a personal reminder to not think too highly of myself, but also, to tread lightly when being judgmental of others. Now, in thinking about Jean, I realize that the dear friend that I knew to be a man of great spiritual depth and insight was also helplessly, hopelessly human, like the rest of us who share in this sacred, never trouble-free, journey along the challenging, stony and uncertain, if ever hopeful, migration from self to Self.

Robert Frost prophetically reminds us: *The woods are lovely, dark and deep, / But I have promises to keep, / And miles to go before*

I sleep, / And miles to go before I sleep. Sometimes the woods are darker and deeper than we expected or wish them to be. What a comfort it is that we are all in this together and that we can reach out to those who stumble, both to lend a hand and to steady our own, always uncertain, way home. Won't you join me in praying for Jean, for me, for each of us, as we set our path for today?

I give thanks for Jean, my cherished brother and fellow traveler as I recall the day my doorbell rang and on opening the door, there stood Jean with a slight smile on his face, saying, "Bal, I find myself in Montreal with nowhere to lay my head, will you take me in?" He entered and joined our party, such as it was. I felt deeply honored then, as I do today, to welcome this blessed soul into my life.

What a privilege to now feel part of the community loving, praying for, giving thanks for and celebrating Jean's life and his best intentions. May we, who have at times not measured up to the Nazarene's wise council, be forgiven, and, may L'Arche thrive in love! Agape, Bal

THE BOTTOM OF THE NINTH

I have always marvelled at three aspects of sport: athletic prowess, the frequency with which such events provide an apt metaphor for life, and the endless list of brilliant one-liners these contests generate – Yogi Berra's "It ain't over 'til it's over" or "The future ain't what it used to be." Some of these sports-generated zingers have particular relevance to palliative care: "It isn't the team with the best players that wins. It's the players with the best team that wins!" and "Winners are not teams who never fail, but teams who never quit." Then, there was the CBC hockey announcer who commented, "There is no such thing as an unassisted goal," which brings to mind Cicely's cogent observation, "What have I that I have not received?" And, finally, there is the baseball reference to "the bottom of the ninth," a phrase that has crept into the lingua franca to suggest "path certain; outcome uncertain"; "there is no going back"; "the stakes couldn't be higher"; "everything is on the line."

As the final decade of the century and millennium unfolded, I experienced a faint but persistent sense of the "bottom of the ninth" or at least something of its essence. My life journey gave way to the need for an emergency permanent tracheostomy in response to a sudden paralysis of my one remaining vocal cord, radiation therapy and chemotherapy for recurrent esophageal cancer in the lymph nodes of my neck, and, later, a third primary cancer, this time in the bladder. Yet I have been fortunate;

through it all I have been ever-renewed by abundant gifts – the love of ever-whistling Linda, the support of my children, the support of Keevin and other family members and close friends.

I retired in 2006, with the RVH PCS in good hands under thoughtful, grace-filled leadership. The Eric M. Flanders Chair in Palliative Medicine and the International Congresses were now being shaped by the always creative vision of colleague Bernard Lapointe. The McGill Programs in Whole Person Care and our annual public film series *Films That Transform* were now reaching new levels of excellence under the ever-Irish perceptiveness of Tom Hutchinson, who in 2011 published *Whole Person Care: A New Paradigm for the 21st Century* (Springer, 2011).

During these "bottom of the ninth" years, we lost two irreplaceable comrades in arms. One was Elisabeth; the other was Cicely.

EKR. On 23 June 2001 I spoke on "Quality of Life and the Total Pain-Healing Dialectic" at the opening plenary session of the American Academy of Hospice and Palliative Medicine meeting in Phoenix, Arizona. The large amphitheatre was full. Warm collegiality and focused attention were palpable. I felt deeply privileged to take part.

At some point during my presentation I noticed a figure hunched in a wheelchair parked off to my right, beyond the end of the front row. A watchful attendant hovered close by.

Following the lecture, on making my way toward the exit, I passed the wheelchair. I couldn't be certain whether the occupant was a man or woman but the attendant was discretely motioning to me as I moved toward them, directing me further into the shadows backstage. In the moments that followed, the swaddling wrap and coat were set aside and the figure straightened somewhat. I could see her clearly now. It was Elisabeth. My dear friend and mentor was seventy-five years old. Recent illness had been difficult but she had come a considerable distance to enable this opportunity to reconnect. I was profoundly grateful. It had been several years since we were last in contact. Now, here she was! Unbelievable! But "no," she quietly gestured, she would not go for coffee, or lunch, or a chat. She just wished to lend her support and say hello. She left with no one else realizing she had been present. It was the last time I would see her.

I believe we subsequently spoke by phone once or twice, but I can't be certain. She died three years later, on 24 August 2004, but has lived on in my thoughts as one of the most generous, compassionate, and trusting souls I have known. As an eloquent, often mesmerizing, communicator and shrewdly discerning listener, she had few equals. She was a global catalyst toward vanquishing the conspiracy of silence around death and dying; she was a cherished, faithful friend.

Cicely. Over the decades, Cicely and I kept in close contact through meetings in Montreal, London, and other international gatherings, as well as letters, phone calls, and e-mails, the latter accomplished in later years with the help of her indispensable assistant, Christine Kearney. In all these interactions Cicely radiated a powerful presence, her assertions ranging from edgy proclamations to a poet's brilliant encapsulation of the subtle essence of things. Exchanges with her were unfailingly informative, invigorating, and delightfully unpredictable, her mind having always been simultaneously set at both "detailed analysis required" and "fast forward."

Our correspondence during her last years conjures fond memories and speaks volumes about her as a groundbreaking global pioneer and generous friend. It was a privilege to read about her globetrotting lecture tours at age eighty-three as well as her news on assorted other matters such as funding, growth, and celebrations at St Christopher's: "The new wards enable us to offer single room accommodation to a greater number of patients. Our bed numbers have decreased as a ward closes, so Home Care, now fully staffed with 31 nurses, is busier than ever. There are currently 499 patients under Home Care. They all have access to our 24 hour on-call service, but with varying need for visits. Nearly half will stay at home to the end and this may mean many weeks of support. Those attending the Day Centre (around 20 a day) seem to have especially long and stable times, with some having remissions." On her evolving role: "I get used to being Founder/President at St Christopher's instead of Chairman and live much more on the sidelines of the Hospice." On her continuing enthusiastic participation in the International Work Group on Death, Dying and Bereavement: "[The meeting was] held in a castle in the Netherlands. We really worked hard in discussion groups for many hours. I joined the group discussing Transformations." And on her continuing exploration of the journey into depth: "I have just written a Guest Editorial for the European Journal of Palliative Care on keeping the balance of science and spirituality in our specialty. It is a continuing challenge, as it was from the beginning, but I remain optimistic that this is an area of life where we have something to say. The search for meaning is never more pressing, and seems to lead not necessarily to answers, but to an ability to live with the questions, finding the often anonymous Spirit of God present in them there. Many find unexpected peace."

Letters through 2004 shared details of her illness and loving care at St Christopher's. My 5 October 2004 e-mail gave her a full Montreal Congress report, including the news that it had attracted more than 1,400 participants from 39 countries.

In January 2005 Cicely wrote concerning an illness flair-up requiring the assistance of "Nigel Sykes, the St Christopher's team and the presence that is holding us all." She enclosed comments concerning the role of spirituality in hospice care that she had prepared for a worship service involving the archbishop of Canterbury, Rowan Williams.

Our resultant dialogue explored the challenge to faith posed by events such as the catastrophic 26 December 2004 Indian Ocean earthquake and tsunami that killed more than 230,000 from 14 countries, prompting the archbishop's remark that "the odd thing is that those who are most deeply involved – both as sufferers and as helpers – are so often the ones who spend least energy in raging over the lack of explanation." For her part, Cicely's discerning observations at countless bedsides led her to comment, "There is great strength in weakness accepted and perhaps it sums up much of what theology has to teach in a way more comprehensible than words."[6] Other correspondence during those years included the following.

3 March 2005: Dear Cicely, I hope you are weathering the storm, indeed, find yourself in a calm cove. I have just read once again your Foreword in Michael Mayne's book *Learning to Dance* that you so kindly sent me at Christmas 2001. It had been a restless night filled with unsettled thoughts and the stirring of ill-defined fears and doubts. How we do torture ourselves! And in the midst of all that I came across the words of Julian of Norwich that you clearly intended that I read tonight: "All this he showed me with great joy. See, I am God. See, I am in all things. See, I do all things. See, I never take my hands off my work, nor ever shall through all eternity. See, I lead all things to the end I have prepared for them." Thank you for that Cicely ... Lots of love this Easter and each day. Bal

1 April 2005, 11:29 A.M.: Dear Bal ... You may have heard that I am now a patient in St Christopher's and likely to remain so ... I am pleased to be here and to be cared for. Pain is being coped with and I am content. I am certainly not on my last legs yet! It is just that I really could not manage at home any longer ... Love to you and the family, Cicely.

4 April 2005, 4:17 P.M.: Dear Cicely, As you once said to me, "Oh Damn!" (or words to that effect. Said by you in response to news of medical challenges that *I* was facing at the time.) I am so glad that you have such a marvelous resource available for care – with all the competence and love that I know each of the St Christopher's

team members wishes to offer you. But I have no illusions that it is easy. Your prayer for humility and the response that you were given ("What have I that I have not received?") comes to mind with the marvelous twist that regarding St Christopher's it may well be stated, "What have you that you have not given?" In addition to all that comes your way in terms of physical care, please know that you are also held in the prayers of many. – with much, much love always, Bal

Saturday, 21 May 2005: 6:44 P.M.: Dear Cicely, The National Portrait Gallery painting is superb! It conveys an unmistakable sense of presence and gentleness in quiet strength. Catherine Goodman's powerful freedom of style breathes life into this wonderful legacy. Her brush and pallet knife work, modelling and use of colour are thrilling. I find the whole effect very moving. Cicely, your kind greeting written on the card will be cherished and will stay on my desk at home as a daily reminder of friendship and so much more. Let us have a virtual glass of Scotch together!! I toast you AND the grand portrait ... Bal

Friday, 17 June 2005, 12:17 P.M.: "Dear Bal, Just to make sure you are in the picture about Cicely. She would want you to know. She is with us on Nuffield Ward and will remain with us ... She has now perked up and is sitting in her chair ... David [David Oliviere, director of education and training, St Christopher's Hospice]

Tuesday, 21 June 2005, 7:24 P.M.: "Thank you David. We have been in touch in recent months/weeks and she has been in my thoughts daily. I am most concerned to have this update. Many, many years ago (summer of 1974 to be precise) when I was working on the wards at St Christopher's, I answered the phone and took the message for one of the patients, a Miss Vallor. Her friend, Miss Brown, had been her Sunday School teacher 60+ years earlier and was calling to say that she couldn't make it in to see her that day. She asked me to convey to Miss Vallor Isaiah 30:15. Later, at the bedside, Miss Vallor pointed out that the bit Miss Brown had undoubtedly wanted to pass on was the middle part – *in quietness and confidence shall be your strength!* Please tell Cicely that I now send that message to her and that with it comes all my love. Bal

Wednesday, 22 June 2005, 6:28 A.M.: Dear Bal, It is Cicely's birthday today, so your message is well timed. From a very sunny London. David

Thursday, 30 June 2005, 10:40 A.M.: Dear Bal, Cicely wanted me to thank you for the message you sent her via David Oliviere. She was so pleased to have it and sends her love, her prayers and her good wishes to you and the family ... She is not in pain, however, and as she says, is receiving the Palliative Care that she worked to promote and which every patient should expect ... I will keep you up to date with news. Christine [Christine Kearney, Cicely's personal assistant]

Thursday, 30 June 2005, 2:39 P.M.: Dear Christine and Cicely, Thank you so much for your letter. Monday I leave with Bethany and Linda for a cabin north of Montreal where there is access only by boat and no electricity. Shall be there for 3 weeks, then back in town. I am with you Cicely and so grateful for all we have shared. Much love, Bal

There is no road access around Bark Lake in the Laurentian Mountains and our secluded rented cottage was huddled on the northern shore of that pristine wilderness waterway, two and a half miles by boat from "civilization" (that is to say, the lone telephone at the small lakeside parking spot with its tiny store). The 18th of July was a lackadaisical Monday afternoon; I waited in the boat as Linda retrieved the messages recorded on our home telephone in Montreal. Her expression clouded. A message from St Christopher's seemed to suggest that Cicely had died. It was too late in the day to phone England.

We returned to our cabin in silence, the isolating throb of the outboard motor underscoring the bleak emptiness that echoed back to us from the surrounding vista of water and pines. No other boats were on the lake; the infrequent lakeside cottages hidden in the trees along the shore seemed abandoned. While the news was not surprising, the sharp reality of it stung with unexpected darkness and sense of void as we headed back to the cottage. I would phone St Christopher's early next morning.

Confirmation: Cicely had died Thursday-past, on 14 July 2005. The stunning immediacy and deafening silence that overtook that moment of realization reminded me of an insight of Cicely's in her book *Watch with Me*.

Many of us have had a fleeting experience of the still wholeness of some kind of Eternal Now – in love or vision. The world of nature is full of moments like that recently described to me by a friend when a sudden panorama of mountains in the snow was seen in a flash alongside a few snowflakes on a dark ski glove. We know how everything centres down into a point. We live with the paradox of immensity and focus, both holding the truth. Cannot the Beyond in the midst, the Prime Mover, the Ultimate Meaning, God Himself, come to such a point, the point of uttermost love? The greater the immensity, the finer, the more intense will be the focus.[7]

Cicely gone. Numb. I returned to the dock, untied the boat, and headed toward our cabin with a sense of emptiness and awe: that treasured germinal centre of inspiration no longer among us.

I had just gained the open strait between the mainland and a nearby island when, as on that day of trekking with Michael on the Burren in Ireland, I sensed that I was being watched. I scanned the shoreline.

Close by, on an abandoned raft, stood a great blue heron. It was stock-still, head held high but slightly at a tilt, long beak elevated; it was watching me intently. Its considerable magnificence measured at least five feet from the frayed canvas covering on which it stood to its penetrating "beady eye." It seemed to be holding me in a somehow familiar stare. It was a grand encounter to be sure! And from somewhere in that focused gaze, in the stillness of that moment, in the silence of that lake, I heard Cicely's voice, "The essence of it is found in scientific rigour and the friendship of the heart. Now just get on with it!" The circle seemed complete.

CROSSROADS

The edicts first heard in my childhood, so many decades ago, about the inevitability of responsibility, uncertainty, and loss, have led me to one final realization: *All endings may be viewed as a new beginning.*

When, as the last remaining member of my family of childhood, I face the multiple losses encountered with aging, I wonder how I may more effectively seek the path to an ever deepening experience of the immensity and focus that Cicely spoke of as she considered the Mystery that holds us in existence.

We have within us, it would seem, the potential for stillness and for an awareness of Self, Union, and Deep Centre, a place of inner peace, an awareness that cannot be reached through reasoning but instead is found in the Radical Present through letting go of ego and the compulsive thinking mind.

This insight has come down to us through the great teachers across the centuries. The fourth-century BCE Chinese sage, Lao Tzu, left us the *Tao Teh Ching*. It challenges us with a calls to embark on an inner path that celebrates our *Being* through effortless action that cannot be achieved by the discerning mind; a call to a leap-of-faith "descent" into compassion, humility, and forgiveness; a call to abandon our lust for power and wealth; a call to champion peace over violence; a call to move beyond knowledge as an end in itself while we open ourselves to silence and stillness.

Those ancient themes in the *Tao Teh Ching* have come to us again and again down the ages. They can be heard in the teachings of Jesus and, a millennium later, the legacy of St Francis of Assisi; and, eight centuries on from that, they are found in the writings of Joseph Campbell, who spoke to us about the "Hero Path." Campbell writes:

"We have not even to risk the adventure alone for the heroes of all time have gone before us. The labyrinth is thoroughly known ... we have only to follow the thread of the hero path. And where we had thought to find an abomination we shall find a God. And where we had thought to slay another we shall slay ourselves. Where we had thought to travel outwards we shall come to the center of our own existence. And where we had thought to be alone we shall be with all the world."[8]

Now I am eighty. Can it be? The path has been filled with both challenges and unmerited blessings. What can I conclude as my journey nears its end?

We shout questions at the Universe, and if we are listening, in the silence of our hearts, the Mystery that holds us in existence responds by whispering back, "You are not alone; I am with you always."

Healing connections, it would seem, exist as an integral part of the Unity that may surface when I trust enough to let go of me and mine; when I risk the journey from *self* to *Self* in the cloud of my unknowing.

The prevailing light, as we encounter our ten thousand crossroads, arises from one of two flames – self or Self. The former fosters fear and the need to defend, the need for fight or flight. The latter, healing and opening. It was always thus.

Which will it be at my next crossroad? And the next?

And what will be the cost – and to whom?

It matters.

Notes

CHAPTER ONE

1 "World War II Casualties by County," *World Population Review,* 2019, www. worldpopulationreview.com/countries/world-war-two-casualties-by-country/.

2 H.T.R. Mount, "Unpublished Memoir," 34.

3 J.M. Barrie, *Peter Pan and Wendy* (New York: Orchard Books, Scholastic Inc., 2004), 8.

4 Mount, "Unpublished Memoir," 35.

5 Was our Hudson a '45 or '46, or perhaps an earlier model – who knows? It didn't really matter since cars accumulated little mileage while the war was on and American Motors, preoccupied with building a fighting force, didn't come out with significant model changes until 1948.

6 Calgary oil baron C.C. Cross was born in Ottawa in 1895 and grew up in Toronto where he entered the brokerage business; he then moved to Regina to manage the company's western office. Following the stock market crash of 1929 and a move to Calgary (1936), he opened his own company specializing in oil stocks and bought the Buckhorn Ranch near Pincher Creek. When the federal government put a cap on speculative profits, Cross went into the oil industry and formed Globe Oil, the first independent oil firm to strike crude in the Leduc field (later becoming West Canada Oil). Cross was a major player in instituting many of the grand celebratory traditions of the Calgary Stampede (serving pancake breakfasts; popularizing western garb; organizing street square dances). He was a Stampede associate director in 1947; survived a plane crash in 1948; became chairman of the Calgary Horse Show; and served as honorary chief for two local Indian bands. He was also a ringleader behind the infamous train trip to Toronto to cheer Calgary on to the 1948 Grey Cup – an event that featured pancake breakfasts on the steps of Toronto's city hall, horses ridden into the elegant lobby of the Royal York Hotel, square dancing in the streets – thus permanently transforming the tone of Canada's annual

Grey Cup tradition. He and his family summered at Buckhorn Ranch for many years, including 1947.

7   Donna Munro, Personal communication, 12 July 2010.

8   Lois Hollingsworth, Personal communication, 4 December 2008.

9   M. Armstrong, Personal communication, 11 February 2011.

10   By the 1950s, services accounted for 51 per cent of London's economy; manufacturing, 41 per cent. Jobs were plentiful, and women were joining the workforce in record numbers. Roland Quinault, "Britain in 1950," *History Today*, 51, no. 4 (4 April 2001), www.historytoday.com/archive/britain-1950.

11   With the death of her father, King George VI, in February 1952, twenty-six-year-old Princess Elizabeth became head of the Commonwealth and queen regnant. That December, in her first Christmas broadcast, she pledged: "At my Coronation ... I shall dedicate myself anew to your service ... I want to ask you all, whatever your religion may be, to pray for me on that day – to pray that God may give me wisdom and strength to carry out the solemn promises I shall be making, and that I may faithfully serve Him, and you, all the days of my life."

12   An estimated three million people lined the parade route. The first coronation to be televised, the event also drew twenty-two million United Kingdom viewers and more than one million on the Continent.

13   Written by Handel in honour of the October 1727 Coronation of George II, "Zadok the Priest" has been sung at the coronations of all subsequent British monarchs. Rev. Dr Jocelyn Perkins, sacrist, Westminster Abbey, *The Queen*, 3 June 1953, 114.

14   Commissioned by King George III, it was completed for the extravagant sum of £8,000 in 1762, following two years of construction. Over the ensuing centuries it has undergone continual changes in design and costly upkeep.

15   This sense of magic, adventure, history, and tradition deepened over the following two weeks in England: Stonehenge; Plymouth; thatched-roofed "Hoops Inn" at Horns Cross, where the proprietors presented me with the gift of an eighteenth-century sword made in Paris by Liger of Rue Coquillière (which I enthusiastically christened Excalibur II); Lorna Doone country; Tintagel and the castle associated with the legends surrounding King Arthur; Bath; Stratford to attend the Shakespeare Memorial Theatre (Saturday, 13 June) for *Antony and Cleopatra*, and there to meet Charles Laughton, who signed my program, and Viscount Montgomery, who declined, saying, "My dear boy, if I did that I'd be ruined. I'd be signing autographs all night." Having seen *The Hunchback of Notre Dame*, but knowing nothing whatsoever of Field Marshal Rommel, the Desert Fox, the Afrika Korps, or El Alamein, I was thrilled beyond measure by the former but totally indifferent to the latter. Ah, the myopia of youth!

16 The Lyre's Club, founded in 1940 by Glebe Music Director Bob McGregor,
was a sixty-voice student choir committed to a broad repertoire. S.R. (Sam)
Berry, an accomplished performer on piano, sax, clarinet, trumpet, and trom-
bone, took over as director in 1950. The choir held thirty-five-minute noon-
time rehearsals on Mondays and Wednesdays; no academic time was allotted
to practices. In 1953 the Lyre's Club earned top rating in its class at the
Potsdam, New York, Music Festival and was praised as "one of the finest
choirs we have heard"; in 1954 it was invited to spend three days at a Syracuse
high school and in 1955 it again competed in the Potsdam Festival, earning
special praise for its rendition of Handel's "And the Glory of the Lord." During
the academic year, the choir performed in school concerts, special assemblies,
community and church concerts, and music competitions throughout the
Ottawa valley and beyond, including Toronto and Montreal. It also performed
an annual series of Christmas radio broadcasts on radio station CFRA. CBOT
television producer Pierre Normandin described the Lyre's Club as "one of the
finest choirs I've ever heard," this leading to a Lyre's Club telecast on 21
December 1955. The choir repertoire included: Handel's *Messiah* highlights
("And the Glory of the Lord," "There Were Shepherds Abiding in the Fields,"
"Glory to God," "He Shall Feed His Flock," and the "Hallelujah Chorus");
traditional Christmas carols; "Nightfall in Skye" (Hugh S. Robertson); "I
Beheld Her Beautiful as a Dove" (Healy Willan); "Country Style" (arr. H.
Simeone); "Ave Maria" (Schubert); "Nobody Knows the Trouble I've Seen"
(arr. Roy Ringwald); "Give Me Your Tired, Your Poor" (Irving Berlin); "There
Is a Balm in Gilead" (William L. Dawson); and, of course, the Lyre's Club
moving theme, Sir Arthur Sullivan's 1868 masterpiece, "The Long Day Closes."

17 My first concert as a Lyre featured "There Is a Balm in Gilead," Cynthia
Millman, soprano soloist; "Nobody Knows the Trouble I've Seen," John
Ambrose, baritone soloist; and three additional selections. That December,
each of our weekly Sunday afternoon radio broadcasts opened with a triumphant rendition of "Joy to the World," while the final 10 p.m. Christmas Eve
broadcast concluded with Schubert's "Ave Maria," Mozart's "Gloria in
Excelsis," Handel's "Hallelujah Chorus," and, finally, our beloved theme song.

18 It was the summer of 1956; Gord was seventeen and had to get to the airport
by bus since he didn't have a licence to drive a car. Gord's first experience of
flying was as a guest in Dad's Bellanca Cruisair in 1952. He was hooked.
Flying was to be his lifelong passion as he progressed from air cadet to Air
Canada where he had a distinguished career as captain, assigned to transatlantic flights. It was perhaps that same summer that Gord and I were in his bedroom when his Dad, the Norwegian-Canadian Arctic explorer Henry Larsen,
sauntered in and commented, grinning, "Well what are you two punks up to?"

When we protested his lack of respect, he continued, "Why I could pin the two of you down with one hand." We dove at him and in less than ten seconds found ourselves stacked one on top of the other like so much firewood under his burly right arm. With Henry Larsen as captain, the RCMP vessel the *St Roch* was the first to navigate the Northwest Passage from west to east (June 1940–October 1942), the first to sail the Passage both ways in a single season; and the first to circumnavigate North America.

19 Dad had known difficult times as a young man and had a strong sense of obligation in lending a hand to others in times of need, actions that also gave him much pleasure. For example, he did not charge ministers, missionaries, or those unable to pay for professional services. He also did not charge physicians, as a mark of courtesy. When Bruce MacDougall, a promising Chalmers member, decided to enter the ministry in spite of competing family demands for scarce resources, Dad supported him during his training. Similarly, when 38,000 Hungarians immigrated to Canada in the wake of their 1956 revolution, Dad and Mother were eager to respond to the call for help. Many were very highly trained, and my parents took in a young professional couple, supplying them with room, board, clothing, and useful contacts to get a new life started, and then welcomed them back to '37' following a January 1958 fire in their newly rented apartment. The day-to-day challenges, joys, and tensions associated with benevolence led to soul-searching discussions and fruitful family introspection regarding the motivation that lies behind helping others, the sources of gratification, and the importance of clear expectations on the part of all involved, issues that were omnipresent since our guests remained heavy smokers (in spite of Dad's asthma) and demonstrated a highly developed sense of entitlement coupled with understandable tinderbox irritability, the legacy of their disastrous multiple recent losses. All this resulted in steep learning curves all around.

20 The date of the dream is certain; it seems likely that my Sunday discussion outburst may have been a year or so later.

21 The Ottawa Auditorium opened in 1923 (demolished, 1967). It was the 7,500-seat arena at the corner of O'Connor and Argyle streets that was the home of the Ottawa Senators of the NHL (1923–34), winners of the 1927 Stanley Cup final in the building; and subsequently the Quebec Senior Hockey League (QSHL) Ottawa Senators (1934–54), the latter in the days of Legs Fraser, Butch Stahan, and Ottawa defenceman and dentist Bobby Copp. Other Auditorium events over the years included skating (the annual "Minto Follies"; Sonja Henie, competing in the North American Figure Skating Championships); boxing exhibitions (Jim Corbett, Jack Sharkey, Max Baer, Joe Louis, Joe Walcott, Rocky Marciano); basketball (Harlem Globetrotters); wrestling; track meets; tennis; concerts (Boston, Chicago, and Philadelphia

symphony orchestras); Gracie Fields; John McCormack; Ezio Pinza; Lily Pons; Frank Sinatra; John Philip Sousa; Red Army Chorus; Moscow Circus; Buddy Holly; Bob Dylan; Brenda Lee; Ray Charles; Fats Domino; the Everly Brothers; Paul Anka; the Rolling Stones. On 3 May 1947 the Percy Faith Orchestra and the Lyres Club performed for an audience of 10,000 at the opening of radio station CFRA. Having Legs Fraser deflect hockey pucks to me in the stands, attending the Red Army Chorus concert, and the CFRA opening (with brother Jim singing) were memorable highlights of my early childhood.

22 Presley's career had "started" with his July 1954 Sun recording of "That's All Right Mama." On arriving in Ottawa in April 1957, he commented that it was his first time in Canada (his Toronto concert had been the night before), adding that a year and a half earlier, when he had wanted to come, he was told that he wasn't well enough known to attract an audience. At the time of the two 3 April 1957 Ottawa concerts, he had just purchased his new Memphis home, Graceland, was living with his mother, and, he told reporters, neither smoked nor drank. While his "suggestive" pelvic gyrations were sufficiently controversial to lead to eight Notre Dame Convent students being expelled for attending the concert, he commented in an interview that he couldn't understand what the fuss was about; it was simply the only way he could sing the songs.

CHAPTER TWO

1 *Queen's Meds '63 Commemorative Book* (Toronto: Yearbook House 1963).
2 My 650cc BSA Golden Flash had been sold that spring for $250 and a 1952 Morris sedan purchased in the interest of safer Kingston-Ottawa travel over the coming years.
3 Of my daily "Inspector's Reports" for that summer, only one remains. Dated 2 August 1957, it records my report on that "sunny and hot" day: "*Contractor* (Grant); *Job Site* (Currell St, off Tweedsmur, Ottawa – *Materials Delivered* (one 6 x 6 single branch for lead, one 6" sleeve for lead, 100 lbs. pig lead); *General Comments* (opened approx. 159 feet of trench / laid fifty feet of pipe including one valve / one nozzle installed and one needs to be bored / joined with existing main on Tweedsmur / encountered sewer service for 239 Currell at exactly pipe level and called D.A.P. / workman lost half a finger when it was caught in the cable."
4 Ruth (whom everyone assumed would go on forever) astounded all by getting married at a mature age, several years after my graduation, leading her to wind down 164 Barrie and retire to nearby Adolphustown with her new husband for a deliriously happy, but all too brief, married life. Ruth was beyond special! Like Wilfred Grenfell, she believed in expressing her bedrock faith through

action rather than proselytizing. I am not certain what a saint is, but no matter how restrictive the definition, she was one! I loved Ruth. We all did. Ruth and I developed a particular bond; but then, I suspect each of her students felt that.

5 With such characters as "Rob Roy MacGregor" (the name shared with Dad's First World War buddy) and David Balfour (shared by me and my namesake, Dr Donald C. Balfour), how could I *not* identify with this stirring tale?

6 For example, James Richardson, twenty, died in the 1916 Battle of the Somme in France, having piped his regiment on to victory. Unprotected, he strode up and down outside a barbed-wire barrier, playing his pipes with the greatest coolness. The impact was instantaneous. Inspired by his splendid example, the company rushed the wire with such fury and determination that the obstacle was overcome and the enemy position captured. Richardson served with the 16th Battalion of the Canadian Expeditionary Force (Canadian Scottish), which had regiments from Victoria, Vancouver, Winnipeg, and Hamilton. He died later that same day after putting his pipes down to attend to a wounded comrade. He is the only Canadian piper ever awarded the Victoria Cross, Canada's highest medal for military gallantry. "Legendary WWI Bagpipes Makes Long Journey Home," CBC *News*, 8 November 2006, www.cbc.ca/news/canada/british-columbia/story/2006/11/08/bagpipes-victoris.html.

7 "Oil Thigh" refers to the hallowed Queen's tradition of erupting in song while joining a low-kicking can-can dance line at moments of pride and joy, usually during sporting events and other informal occasions. The celebratory song "Queen's College Colours" was written in 1898 and built on the rousing 1891 Gaelic chorus, "Oil thigh na Banrighinn a Banrighinn gu brath *(repeat x 3)* Cha-gheill! *(repeat X 3),*" sung to the tune of the Battle Hymn of the Republic. The oft-repeated first verse proclaims: "Queen's College colours we are wearing once again, / Soiled as they are by the battle and the rain, / Yet another victory to wipe away the stain! / So boys go in and win!" (the last line was changed in 1985 to "So, *Gaels* go in and win" to include Queen's women athletes). The beloved Gaelic chorus translates as "The college of the wife of the king forever" (x 3) + "no surrender" (x 3). "Oil Thigh," *Queen's University Encyclopedia*, 2019, www.queensu.ca/encyclopedia/o/oil-thigh.

8 I first met Harley Smyth at Glashan in grade 7; we parted company for high school and then reunited in Meds '63. He arrived at Queen's with the decided advantages of ability and energy, displayed, among other places, on stage and radio as a tenor in a quartet of some fame. As class president, he put his efficiency to early use, resulting in a flood of moralistic class debates. His subsequent activities would eventually include acting, playing the organ, choirmaster, athlete (intramural football, hockey, volleyball), a summer African Christian Mission stint, impersonator, reading authors in the original Latin, Rhodes scholar, husband, father, and neurosurgeon.

9   Born in Holland, Hans completed upper-school examinations in English while
    working as a carpenter's assistant prior to assuming his place as 'Meds 63
    moralist, workhorse, water-polo competitor, and soccer player prior to a career
    in pathology and pediatrics in Timmins, Ontario.

10 In that, his rotating internship year, Jim was on call and thus slept in the hospi-
    tal every other night and weekend, unable to get home at all. The nights *off*
    that Betty refers to in her letter are the 50 per cent of the nights when he is *off-
    duty* but still does not get home until eight to ten o'clock and yet is expected to
    be back on duty by seven the next morning.

11 The Reverend Laverty served as Queen's chaplain from 1947 to 1983. Character-
    ized by his effortlessly low-key deportment, "the Padre," as he was universally
    known, had a legendary memory for names and relationships that engendered
    a sense of community across the campus and beyond during the terms of six
    principals. Confidential counsellor, trusted friend, and adviser to countless stu-
    dents, he was respected as a man of faith and boundless generosity. I received
    his thoughtful advice and support on a number of occasions while at Queen's,
    although I had never consulted him and we had only a passing acquaintance.
    He was a man of integrity and tireless commitment. He died in April 2011.

12 Claude T. Bissell (1916–2000), educated at the University of Toronto and
    Cornell, was a Second World War veteran. He joined the University of
    Toronto's English Department and was dean in residence at University College
    (1946), later serving as the university's vice-president prior to becoming presi-
    dent of Carleton University (1956). He was president of the University of
    Toronto from 1958 until 1971. His writings include a two-volume biography
    of Vincent Massey and his memoir of his University of Toronto years. "Claude
    Bissell," *Wikipedia*, 2019, www.en.wikipedia.org/wiki/Claude_Bissell.

13 John V. Basmajian (1921–2008) served in the Royal Canadian Army Medical
    Corps in the Second World War, later obtaining his MD at the University of
    Toronto in 1945. He joined that university's faculty, was promoted to full
    professor of anatomy in 1956, and then was recruited to Queen's as department
    head (1957–69). I always found it puzzling that Dr Basmajian would
    disparage both me and the general practitioner's role in the course of such a brief
    exchange. It was a half-century later that I learned that I was not the only one to
    receive a foreboding prediction during those interviews. Classmate Bob Vaughan,
    a Belleville native, was informed that recent students from Belleville had a high
    fail or dropout rate, while Dave Skene, our all-star Golden Gaels linebacker, was
    told that athletes frequently did badly, or at least failed to live up to their poten-
    tial. "Bas" was giving us a pep talk: he was goading us on! He had a "nose-to-
    the-grindstone" message to get across, and he cared enough to express it!

14 In a letter home written 4 October 1959, I comment, "Faye may drop out of
    Meds so that we can get married sooner than now seems feasible. This has

been her idea & I have not even encouraged it for I now like the idea of her in
Meds if that is what she wants. She would still get her BA of course."

15 Yousuf Karsh, *Portraits of Greatness* (Toronto: University of Toronto Press
1960), 16.

16 An inner-ear condition characterized by vertigo and dizziness.

17 The senior fellow's name has been changed but *all* other details of this account
of my first foray into liaison psychiatry are as they unfolded.

18 There were some objections to including "beat Edmonton," but the guys were
playing for my hometown team. The wording stayed!

19 Two copies of the telegram were made: the one for Stew, Lou, and Gary; and
the copy that lies in front of me more than a half-century after the fact. As I
unroll the whole thirty-plus feet, reading the names, I am surprised at the number that are familiar. I see a cloud of faces. We all remain twenty-ish, filled with
enthusiasm and bright-eyed.

20 Ron Stewart (known to us all as "Stew") was an icon of our student years at
Queen's. While playing for the Gaels (1953–57) he was on two Yates Cup
championship teams (1955, 1956) and was voted the team's MVP three times
and the league MVP for the 1957 season. Though diminutive at 5'7", he went
on to play thirteen years with the Ottawa Rough Riders (1958–70) and was
named an Eastern Conference all-star in 1960, 1961, and 1964. He played on
four Grey Cup teams, winning in three (1960, 1968, 1969) and losing in 1966.
On 10 October 1960 Stewart set a CFL record for yards rushing in one game
(287 yards for an amazing 17.9 yds per carry) while scoring four touchdowns
(with runs of 37, 51, 51, and 59 yds) against the Montreal Alouettes. As the
game ended, his accomplishment was acknowledged with a standing ovation
by the 22,000 Montreal fans. He was named the CFL's Most Outstanding
Canadian and winner of the Lionel Conacher Award as Canada's top male
athlete that year. He was inducted into the Queen's, Ottawa, CFL, and
Canadian Sports halls of fame. I did a portrait of Stewart and sent it to him on
behalf of Meds '63. The Queen's Alma Mater Society's executive expressed
warm appreciation for the telegram project and the favourable publicity
accorded Queen's as a result.

21 131–133 King Street East, a Georgian-style limestone double house by architect William Coverdale, was erected in 1842–43 for Noble Palmer, founder of
the *Kingston Spectator* newspaper. Half of the building was occupied by Sir
Charles Metcalfe, governor general of Canada (1843–45), while his predeces-
sor, Sir Charles Bagot, lay dying in the vice-regal residence, Alwington House,
Kingston. "Government House 1832," Ontario Plaques, www.ontarioplaques.
com/Plaques/Plaque_Frontenac26.html.

22 I had thrilled to *Tigrero*, Sasha Siemel's gripping 1953 autobiographical
account of becoming the only white man to earn the title of "Tigrero," that is,

one who hunts livestock-killing jaguars in Brazil's Matto Grosso, armed only with a seven-foot spear. I was astonished to learn he was passing through Kingston. Faye and I attended his lecture, then spoke to him afterwards and invited him to our home. A wonderful chat ensued and he assured us that the chance to talk with new friends, rather than returning alone to his motel, was a joy. The joy, in fact, was mine. Born in 1890, Sasha Siemel was seventy-two when we spent that evening together.

23 R. Wesley Boston went on to train in pediatrics at Harvard and then returned to Queen's, pediatrics, with a special interest in neonatology and, subsequently, palliative care.

24 John Ruedy went on to develop the first academic Division of Clinical Pharmacology in Canada. He has been a leading catalyst and architect in Canadian medical research, teaching, and program development and served as dean of the Faculty of Medicine at Dalhousie University (1993–99).

25 Dr Bingham joined the Queen's Faculty of Medicine in 1945 as professor of surgery. Educated in England and Switzerland, he served in the Royal Navy (1923–27) and won the King's Prize Sword as the best cadet in his class. His medical training was at the University of Edinburgh (1928–34), while his post-graduate training as house surgeon was at the Royal Infirmary, Edinburgh, and later the British Postgraduate Medical School, London; he became a fellow of the Royal College (Edinburgh) in 1936. He served as a surgeon in the British Army as major (1939–42) and then as lieutenant-colonel (1942–45), participating in the North African Campaign (1941–42). *Queen's Alumni Review* (Kingston, 1945), 193–4.

26 Queen's Meds '53 cousin Don Connor was once asked, "Did Bingham give your class the *whole* surgery course from beginning to end, as he did ours?" The response was immediate. "Yes, he sure did, every morning beginning at 8:00 A.M. for the whole year."

27 I have only met two individuals who consistently avoided the first-person-singular pronoun, Marian Anderson and DLCB. In her case, this was based on her clearly articulated recognition that anything she ever did, thought, or held to be true largely depended on others. As for DLCB, the affectation appeared to result from the conclusion that *one* summed up himself quite nicely, and did so in an appropriate, vaguely deferring, British sort of way.

28 Catriona Bingham, who referred to her husband as "the Great One," was an ardent Roman Catholic and a formidable being in her own right. In her last years she was chief of her hereditary clan.

29 The committee chair, anesthetist Stu Vandewater, would later describe the underlying concerns: "Through the late 1950's and early '60's there was a creeping deterioration in clinical education and research in general as the faculty continued to be dominated by many of the 'old guard' and their

pre-Second World War methods, with emphasis on private practice and less on clinical teaching of medical students, house-staff and research. The Queen's teaching hospitals were essentially community hospitals that failed, or refused, to recognize the enormous growth in specialty medicine, the changing public demands in health care and necessary integration of the various health professions arising from wartime stunting and introduction of universal hospital insurance. Kingston was no longer competing with Toronto or Montreal or even non-university affiliated centres such as Hamilton or Ottawa, with the increasing demands for quality post MD intern and resident training to meet licensing and Royal College requirements.

"With the input of a trio of consultants (Drs H. Agnew, R. Janes, and W. Macleod), corrective measures included: 400 of the 600 beds were designated clinical-teaching units reserved for attending staff; patient fees were pooled into a fund for academic expenses; attending staff were deemed "Geographic Full Time" and assigned salaries and ceilings; a central billing and collecting agency was established; patient care was to be provided by teams (students, interns, residents, staff); private staff offices were closed; ambulatory specialty clinics organized by department were established; clinical research was promoted. S.L. Vandewater, Personal communication; "November 22, 1962: Future of Queen's Medical School: Resuscitate or Bury It? A Memoir" (9 November 2007).

30 The impact of these changes is indicated by the data reflecting house-staff appointments for the year 2007–08: 339 positions (all filled); first-year residents [R1] (interns), 94, 23 of them Queen's grads of a class of 100, 52 from other Canadian schools, 19 international graduates; R2, 109; R3, 58; R4, 44; R5, 36; R6, 3; R7, 1.

31 As honorary president of our class, Dr Bingham was in good company. The other Meds '63 honorary presidents during our years at Queen's were: Pre-Med I, Malcolm Perry; Pre-Med II, Elof Axel Carlson; Med I, Rae Laurenson; Med II, J.D. Hatcher; Med IV, John A. Milliken.

32 Dr Balfour received recognition from the Mayo Clinic as well as from numerous national and international organizations. He became director of the Department of Surgery in 1937, and he held honorary fellowship in the royal colleges of surgeons of England, Edinburgh, and Australasia. He was one of the founders of the World Medical Organization and a charter member of the World Health Organization and of the Central Surgical Association.

33 Queen's Meds '63: Dick Barry, Charlie Bateman, George Biro, Ken "Brad" Bradley, Don "Chads" Chadsey, Merv Connery, Earl Covert, Jim Coyle, Helen Currie, Cliff Derry, Sid Dinsdale, Morty Dolman, George Drew, Peter Dunlop, Mike Eisenstat, Ken Embree, Jim Farr, Dick Flindall, Clarke Forbes, Bill Forrest, George Gerula, Bob Hall, "Herbie" Hayes, Mary Horsey, Roger

Hughes, Bill James, Gary Johnson, Dick Kennedy, "Rich" Kidd, Aube Kurtz, Joe McClure, Hugh McGuire, John McKinney, Bill Mabee, "King" Mahon, "Al" Mark, "Art" Moody, Bal Mount, Gord Paprica, Sheila Paprica, Tanya Pietak, Terry "Tort" Porter, Don "Ding" Pringle, "Andy" Simone, Dave "Skener" Skene, Harley Smyth, Micky Sole, David "Sneaker" Sutton, John Taylor, Bob "Vaughaner" Vaughan, "Hans" Verbeek, "Penny" Walsh, Alayne "Steve" White, Garry Willard, and the elusive George Crabb.

CHAPTER THREE

1 The Royal Victoria Hospital was opened in 1893, the legacy of two Scottish immigrants, Sir Donald Alexander Smith, Lord Strathcona (1820–1914), and George Stephen, Lord Mount Stephen (1829–1921). The same Lord Strathcona was the foundational benefactor of Sir Wilfred Grenfell and namesake for the early Grenfell fleet (*Strathcona I* and *Strathcona II*). The Royal Vic's three proud baronial-style wings would acquire new additions as the years passed: in 1905, the Hershey Pavilion nurses' residence; in the 1920s, the Women's and the Ross Memorial pavilions; in the early 1950s, the Medical and Surgical pavilions; and in 1993 the Centennial Pavilion housing emergency, birthing, and ICU facilities. In 1920 this impressive 687 Pine Avenue landmark overlooking downtown Montreal from the slopes of Mount Royal became a research institute of the Faculty of Medicine of McGill University, and in 1929 Dr Wilder Penfield established the Montreal Neurological Institute adjacent to it and connected to the main buildings by a third-floor walkway somewhat resembling Venice's Bridge of Sighs as it crossed over the north end of University Street.

2 Rachelle had married McGill grad Dr Michael Laplante in December 1962. Mike was thus a year my senior when he entered urology training and would become a lifelong mentor and friend.

3 Dr Kenneth Joseph Chisholm MacKinnon (1921–2007): As a graduate of St Francis Xavier University and Dalhousie Medical School, Kenneth MacKinnon practised medicine with his father in Antigonish and with his father-in-law, Dr Lloyd Meech, in North Sydney, Nova Scotia, prior to moving to Montreal in 1945 for post-graduate medical training at McGill. He was appointed to the staff of the Royal Victoria Hospital and McGill in 1953. On 28 May 1958 he joined vascular surgeon Joe Luke and internist John Dossetor in carrying out the first successful organ transplant in the British Commonwealth, a kidney transplant between teenage identical twins following seizure-induced acute renal failure in one of the girls. MacKinnon was named RVH urologist-in-chief in 1959, chairman of the Medical Board (1965–69), and subsequently director of professional services. He served as president of both the Canadian Urological Association and the Canadian Academy of Urological

Surgeons. During their Montreal years, Ken and his wife, Ann Frances Meech, raised their nine children, and in 1979 Ken and Ann moved to Nairobi, Kenya, where he was the executive director of the Aga Khan Hospital. Returning to Nova Scotia in 1982, he became chief of staff at the Halifax Infirmary and adjunct professor of urology, Dalhousie University. In 1986 he founded the Palliative Care Service at the Halifax Infirmary and remained its director until semi-retirement in 1991. From 1991 to 1994, he acted as palliative-care consultant in Antigonish and helped to establish palliative-care services across Nova Scotia. In 1995 he was named the first honorary patron of the Nova Scotia Hospice Palliative Care Association. Among his many honours, Dr MacKinnon was awarded a doctor of laws by both Dahousie and St Francis Xavier universities and received the Canadian Urological Association Achievement Award. A man of deep faith, humility, compassion, and intellectual curiosity, Ken MacKinnon was a thoughtful leader in medical education and administration; he was an influential architect in the development of academic urology at McGill and beyond, both nationally and internationally. He was to play a critical role in the development of the Royal Victoria Hospital Palliative Care Service. Ken MacKinnon influenced the lives of countless people. He was a mentor and healer of remarkable stature, a man among men.

4 Following internship and assistant-resident training in medicine at the Royal Vic (1963–65), Martin Raff was a resident in neurology at the Massachusetts General Hospital in Boston (1965–68). He did post-doctoral training in immunology with Avrion Mitchison at the National Institute for Medical Research in Mill Hill, London (1968–71), after which he moved to University College, London. He was president of the British Society of Cell Biology (1991–95). The recipient of numerous international awards for his research, he continues to serve on various scientific advisory boards in Europe and America. He is a co-author of two widely used cell-biology textbooks: *Molecular Biology of the Cell* and *Essential Cell Biology*.

5 The Ugandan letters from Dad repeatedly commented on the unbecoming sense of superiority he perceived in his British acquaintances. A holdover, it seemed, from colonial times, it was an attitude that British friends had acknowledged during our 1953 coronation visit to the United Kingdom. Time and again, the Englishman at home and abroad felt himself to be a member of the "superior race" and lacked any sense of the "brotherhood of all races." While many of Mother and Dad's colleagues in Uganda clearly felt they were there to "serve" according to their Christian faith, those whom they were "serving" were considered to be fit only for roles of service. This did not sit well with Dad. Though he repeatedly expressed regret at mentioning it and had great affection for their British hosts, who had shown them the warmest hospitality and friendship, it bothered him greatly.

6 In the typesetting of the page, Wordsworth's word "past" has been reproduced as "cast," suggesting the volitional aspect of this tragic event. A Freudian slip (?) with sad historic accuracy.

7 And with the world, Faye and I watched the television drama unfold all weekend as the accused killer was apprehended and then himself killed before our eyes. On Monday, 25 November, the president was buried in a sailor's grave at Arlington National Cemetery.

8 Born in Hungary, Peter immigrated to Canada in 1956 and was a 1963 Ottawa University medical graduate. Following post-graduate training, he would practise dermatology in Toronto, making annual volunteer visits to village hospitals in India over a twenty-seven-year span and working at the Toronto Street Health Clinic for the homeless.

9 Their caring provided me with an important lesson regarding the significance of our attachments. Messages from my Queen's mentors offered a particular lift: D.L.C. Bingham (a phone call, "MOUNT, how are you doing? ... Get on with it!"); Peter Morrin (a plant); OB/GYN professor Edwin Robertson (an inscribed book, *Runes of the North*). All were, and remain a half-century later, powerful reminders of the healing power of expressed caring.

10 American physician and founder of MEDICO, Thomas Anthony Dooley III (1927–61) had written three books concerning his work in Asia before dying with a malignant melanoma at the age of thirty-four. On my graduation from Queen's, I received a gift volume of his writings from my brother-in-law and his wife. Ironically, it bore the inscription "To Bal with our love, Hoping you'll find fulfillment as he did, Jane & Ted."

11 *Faust* was also the first opera performed when the Met opened on 22 October 1883. The Met moved to its vibrant new home on Broadway at Lincoln Square in April 1966.

12 Betty Mae Swerdfager Mount (25 May 1934–7 February 1964). Her death was a catastrophe that deeply wounded each of us. Jim wrote the eulogy for her 14 February memorial service at Dominion-Chalmers United Church. Following a reading of Proverbs 31: 10–31, Jim summed up our loss:
   "Across the constellation representing the spectrum of human personality and ability flashes the occasional individual who sends forth a spray of warmth, energy and support, bathing all those about. Such a person was Betty. Her rushing, full life touched many, and each of us treasures his own memories.
   "Her face shone with open, honest generosity and interest. Her graceful hands were rarely still and equally at home in the tumult of the Liszt Funérailles or the turning of a hem. She loved the mystic beauty of things Scottish and the wildly rhythmic music of Eastern Europe. She frequently played the Khachaturian 'Toccata' but equally enjoyed a quaint, lacy blouse.

Her winning, gracious social approach as hostess or guest spread ease about the room. A sparkle in her eye betrayed her sense of humor, while soft, loving warmth could overflow about those she loved.

"The silver medals, prizes and cups of high school, her Associateship in the Toronto Conservatory of Music at 16 years, and the seven scholarships at Queen's University represent an intellectual endowment and capacity for work graciously bestowed by a bountiful Lord through her parents. Her ability, honesty and warmth led to her election to the office of Head Girl at Lisgar and to the Levana Executive at Queen's. The same qualities led to the request that she deliver what proved to be a memorable valedictory address for her graduating class in high school.

"Her abilities could have been channeled in any direction. She chose, however, to give freely of herself to the Swerdfager home, her friends, whether longtime or acquaintances of moments, and to Jim, Heather Lynn and Howie. Never was this endowment used to wound another or to elevate herself; the days were too short, there was too much to do. There were so many projects underway ... books to read, hours to practice, then later, too many coats, dresses and meals to make, too many letters to write, too many acts of thoughtfulness to carry out. She chose to live for others and was successful. She gave us David Bruce on February 7.

"Her passing at 29 must have an immediately obvious positive facet. To interpret the responses she elicited from each of us, to understand what we received on dipping into the pool of her love, we must understand the needs in ourselves which she so willingly relieved. Only through understanding ourselves can we return in kind, love for love. The inwardly blind man may trample his benefactor. We can open our eyes only with effort, continual effort in the scrutiny of the source of each emotion and act. Only then can the Betty in our environment be rewarded with our true love.

"We have been replenished from the fullness of her spirit and can still return love to the Betty about us."

13 Dr John H. Duff was a University of Toronto medical graduate (1957) with post-graduate training in surgery at McGill (1961–66); FRCSC (1965); RVH co-director of the Accident Service and associate professor (1966–72); Markle Scholar in Academic Medicine (1968–73). In 1972 he was appointed chief of surgery at Victoria Hospital, London, and professor of surgery at the University of Western Ontario. He served as Department of Surgery chair, University of Western Ontario, and chief of surgery at the University Hospital (1984–97). From residency days on, John was recognized as a surgeon's surgeon, a man of rare stature.

14 Frank D. Selke, Jr was a noted Montreal Canadiens NHL executive (1951–65). HIs father, Frank J. Selke, was the general manager of the team during this period.

15 Hector "Toe" Blake (1912–95) did it all: player on the 1932 Sudbury Memorial
Cup champions; player on 1935 Stanley Cup-winning Montreal Maroons;
player on the Montreal Canadiens (1935–47); left wing on the "Punch Line"
with Rocket Richard and Elmer Lach (1943–47); Habs' captain (1940–48);
NHL MVP and scoring champion (1938–39). As captain, hc lcd thc Habs to
two Stanley Cups (1944 and 1946). He was the Habs' head coach (1955–68),
winning the Stanley Cup eight times (1956–60, 1965, 1966, 1968) – one of
the greatest players and head coaches in hockey history.

16 In addition to the Stanley Cup, there was a second trophy awarded that evening. The Conn Smythe Trophy was presented for the first time, for the playoff's
MVP. That landmark "first" was awarded to Jean Béliveau, who had eight
goals and eight assists in thirteen playoff games.

17 Lloyd D. MacLean was chairman of the McGill Department of Surgery
(1968–73 and 1987–88). He was the Edward W. Archibald Professor of
Surgery at McGill (1987–93) and surgeon-in-chief at the Royal Victoria
Hospital (1962–88). His wide-ranging research interests included septic shock,
peritonitis, the relation of host defences to trauma and disease, the surgical
treatment of obesity, and the emerging field of organ transplantation.

18 D. Ackman, H. Khonsari, B.M. Mount, P. Rege, and J.B. Dossetor,
"Arteriovenous Fistulae for Haemodialysis: Advantages with Cadaver Renal
Transplantation," Proceedings of the Fourth Conference of the European
Dialysis and Transplant Association, Paris, June 1967.

CHAPTER FOUR

1 "Pierre Elliot Trudeau," Dictionary of Canadian Biography, vol. 22,
www.biographia.ca.

2 The "Quiet Revolution" refers to the 1960s period of rapid liberalization and
nationalization in Quebec that was made possible by the defeat in 1960 of the
Union Nationale (in power since 1944) under Maurice Duplessis. Policy changes introduced by Jean Lesage's victorious Quebec Liberal Party included the
nationalization of education and health care (previously heavily influenced by
the Catholic Church); an attack on political patronage; the revision of the elec-
toral map to better represent urban areas; increased state support of provincial
economic, social, and cultural growth, in particular the nationalization of
private electricity companies in 1962 to form Hydro-Québec, the creation,
in 1965, of the Caisse de Dépot et Placement du Québec to administer the
Quebec pension plan, and subsequent nationalizations – SIDBEC (iron and
steel); SOQUEM (mining); REXFOR (forestry); and SOQUIP (petroleum). René
Durocher, "The Quiet Revolution," Canadian Encyclopedia, 30 July 2013,
www.thecanadianencyclopedia.ca/en/article/quiet-revolution.

3   The flag of Quebec (adopted in 1948) consists of a blue base with a white
    cross through the centre, dividing the flag into quarters. In each quarter there
    is a white fleur-de-lys (also spelled fleur-de-lis), a symbol of purity representing
    the Virgin Mary. Whitney Smith, "Flag of Quebec," *Encyclopedia Britannica*,
    2019, www.britannica.com/topic/flag-of-Quebec.

4   During the riot, 292 were arrested; 123 were injured (including 43 police);
    12 patrol cars were burned or damaged; 6 horses were injured. The violence of
    the police was roundly criticized by French commentators. Journalist Marc
    Laurendeau, commenting on the fires and mayhem, called them "understand-
    able," noting, "When people are provoked they react." "PM Trudeau won't let
    them rain on his parade," CBC Archives, 24 June 1968. www.cbc.ca/archives/
    entry/pm-trudeau-wont-let-em-rain-on-his-parade.

5   Haynes Johnson, "1968 Democratic Convention: The Bosses Strike Back,"
    Smithsonian Magazine August 2008, www.smithsonianmag.com/history/
    1968-democratic-convention-931079/.

CHAPTER FIVE

1   Memorial Sloan Kettering Cancer Center occupied the New York City block
    bounded by 67th and 68th streets, from York to First avenues. It comprised
    James Ewing Hospital (fronting on York) and the Sloan-Kettering Institute,
    Memorial Hospital, and the Tower Outpatient Building (fronting on York
    Avenue). The Norman Winston House residence faced this conglomerate from
    across 67th Street at York Avenue.

2   In Jungian psychology the ego (self) is the centre of consciousness whereas
    the Self is the centre of the total personality, which includes consciousness, the
    unconscious, and the ego; the Self is both the whole and the centre.

3   Sources regarding Dr Whitmore include: personal observations and inter-
    actions; "A Tribute to Willet F. Whitmore, Jr., the Willet F. Whitmore Tribute
    Evening, Memorial Hospital Alumni Society Memorial Sloan-Kettering Cancer
    Center New York City," 10 November 1983; *New York Times* obituary, 9 May
    1995; James E. Montie and Joseph A. Smith, Jr, "Whitmoreisms: Memorable
    Quotes from Willet F. Whitmore, Jr., MD," *Urology*, 63 (2004): 207–9.

4   Ted Beattie offered his assessment of Whit at the 10 November 1983 tribute
    held at his retirement: "James Ewing made Memorial Hospital famous with his
    concept of anatomical cancers treated by aggressive 'compleat oncologists.'
    Whit typifies, par excellence, this concept ... For a professional lifetime, Whit
    has delivered the best-known cancer care. He has educated a distinguished
    group of cancer oncologists. His research and development have made possible
    enormous strides in the successful treatment of the most serious urologic can-
    cers. Whit has done this without apparent effort and with an aequanimitas and

kindliness that places him in the Oncologic Hall of Fame. As the Founding Father of urologic oncology, he is without peer."

5 Bob Donohue, Personal communication.

6 To work with Whit was to admire him. Flinty Ann "Poppy" Joachim, his long-time administrative assistant, quipped, "[He] was my boss for 32 years and the very best. But it took me all 32 to train him to his high peak of executive excellence. His tenderness and compassion led all his patients to love him" ("Tribute," 10 November 1983).

7 Among Bing's many accomplishments while at the Met, one stands out. It was his insistence that led to the Met's artist roster being racially integrated when, at his invitation, Marian Anderson became the first African American to sing a leading role in the house, as the fortune teller Ulrica in Verdi's *Un Ballo in Maschera* on 7 January 1955. The cast included Richard Tucker (Riccardo), Leonard Warren (Renato), and Zinka Milanov (Amelia). The sold-out hall, including Eleanor Roosevelt, Margaret Truman, and the Duchess of Windsor, gave her a tumultuous welcome, as did the *New York Times*: "There was no moment in which Miss Anderson's interpretation was commonplace or repetitive in effect. In Ulrica's one-half act, by her native sensibility, intelligence, and vocal art, Miss Anderson stamped herself in the memory and the lasting esteem of those who listened." Other African Americans soon followed, starting with Robert McFerrin and, in due course, such beloved divas as Leontyne Price and Jessye Norman. James Bennett, "The Complicated History of Marian Anderson's Met Debut," WQXR, 27 February 2017, www.wqxr.org/story/complicated-history-marian-andersons-met-debut/.

8 Dad and I later had the pleasure of hearing L.M. sing a leading role at the Met and I am humbled to report that the marvellous voice was as thrilling on stage as it had been in the recovery room.

9 As a result, when Whit was invited to give a lecture tour in Australia, he accepted more commitments than usual, knowing the films could be used in many of the sessions. With plans completed, he asked his departmental research assistant and Jill of all trades, Ann-Marie Sundra, to send the too-heavy-to-carry films to his contact person in Sydney so they would be there when his flight arrived. The phone call from Australia was brief and perhaps the only time the team could recall Whit losing his cool. "Where are the films?!" Ann-Marie had sent them by sea; they arrived six months after Whit returned home, exhausted by his countless arduous make-up lectures. Ann-Marie survived.

10 Launched by a Saturn V rocket from Kennedy Space Center on 16 July, Apollo 11 was the fifth manned mission of NASA's Apollo program. The *Apollo* spacecraft had three parts: a Command Module, with a cabin for the three astronauts, the only part that returned to Earth; a Service Module, which supplied the

Command Module with propulsion, electrical power, oxygen, and water; and a Lunar Module, for landing on the Moon. After being sent toward the Moon by the Saturn V's upper stage, the astronauts separated the spacecraft from it and travelled for three days until they entered into lunar orbit. Armstrong and Aldrin then moved into the Lunar Module and landed in the Sea of Tranquility at 3:17 P.M. EST, 20 July 1969, stating, "The Eagle has landed. Tranquility base here." They stayed approximately 21.5 hours on the lunar surface, 2.5 hours in extra-vehicular activity. Armstrong became the first to step onto the lunar surface, remarking, "That's one small step for man, one giant leap for mankind." The live TV coverage of the event was broadcast worldwide. After lifting off in the upper part of the Lunar Module and rejoining Collins in the Command Module, they returned to Earth, landing in the Pacific Ocean on 24 July.

11 The public did not learn how close Apollo 11 had come to disaster until decades later. We were not told about the tenuous computer capacity of Mission Control, the presence of apparent UFOs flying alongside Apollo 11 when 200,000 miles from earth, the unexpected "z particles" penetrating their small ship, the perilously thin skin of the lunar module, the dismal 3/6 success rate of its single-ascent engine on pre-flight testing, the crashing of the onboard computers as lunar landing was imminent, the treacherous off-course flight path and lack of fuel with only fifteen seconds of fuel remaining at touchdown on the Moon, the broken circuit that was crucial for lift-off from the Moon and its seat-of-the-pants repair by Aldrin (who jammed his pen into the broken connection), and the danger of the angle of re-entry as they hit the Earth's atmosphere (too steep meant burning up; too shallow meant bouncing back into space). Sarah Loff, "Apollo 11, Mission Overview," 15 May 2019, www.nasa.gov/mission_pages/apollo/missions/apollo11.html.

12 The full identity of the strain in question is 129/Sv-CPS1^J. B. Mount and J.C. Stevens, "The Early Natural History of Murine Germinal Testicular Tumors," *Journal of Urology*, 105 (1971): 812–16.

13 Our two published papers were B. Mount, L.C. Stevens, and W.F. Whitmore, Jr, "The Effect of Chemotherapy on Testicular Germinal Tumors in Mice, Cancer," *Journal of Urology*, 26, no. 3 (September 1970), and Mount and Stevens, "The Early Natural History of Murine Germinal Testicular Tumors."

14 An editorial titled "A Stem Cell Legacy: Leroy Stevens" in *The Scientist* read: "When *Science* voted stem cell research its 1999 'Breakthrough of the Year,' the congratulatory article traced the field's origin to the 1981 successful culture of mouse embryonic stem cells. But the roots of exploring these multipotential cells go back considerably further to a little-mentioned researcher who worked with mice at the Jackson Laboratory in Bar Harbor Maine." The editorial went on to detail the work of Leroy Stevens and Don Varnum in identifying cells from early 129 embryos that could support differentiation. Stevens called them

"pluripotent embryonic stem cells." The editorial concludes, "Leroy Stevens is truly the unsung hero of stem cell research." Ricki Lewis, "A Stem Cell Legacy: Leroy Stevens," *The Scientist* (6 March 2000), www.the-scientist.com/news/a-stem-cell-legacy-leroy-stevens-56114.

15 Paul Simon and Art Garfunkel would subsequently be responsible for countless memorable hours throughout my life. They still are! Where in heaven's name had I been? My "What or who is Simon and Garfunkel" query *still* wakens me at 2 A.M.! As life's ironies would have it, I finally spent an evening in the Vivian Beaumont Theater forth-three years later. Following a memorable performance of *War Horse*, we stopped for a cup of coffee at the local Starbucks and, as we entered, Simon and Garfunkel's "The Boxer" was playing. Sweet retribution! A sense of time standing still.

16 Marc Laurendeau, "Front de libération du Québec," *Canadian Encyclopedia* (11 August 2013), www.thecanadianencyclopedia.ca/en/article/front-de-liberation-du-quebec.

17 "The October Crisis: Civil Liberties Suspended," CBC Archives, 2019, www.cbc.ca/archives/categories/politics/civil-unrest/the-october-crisis-civil-liberties-suspended/flq-backgrounder.html.

CHAPTER SIX

1 We would learn only much later that Laurin's change in position resulted from pressure by Lévesque. Remarkably, Lévesque later added to Laurin's humiliation by pronouncing in the *Journal de Montréal* on 30 October that calling in the army had been the *right* thing to do. Lésveque later changed sides once again, claiming that Trudeau had overreacted. D. Poliquin, *Réne Lévesque* (Quebec: Boréal 2009).

2 Sequence of events as documented by Bernard Amyot, past president of the Canadian Bar Association, *Montreal Gazette*, 5 October 2010.

3 "Love Itself," Leonard Cohen, in *Ten New Songs*, 2001, Sony Music Entertainment.

4 Carl Jung, *The Self*, www.carl-jung.net/self.html.

5 The left-cerebral hemisphere analyzes over time, the right synthesizes over space. The former is analytical, verbal, logical; the latter, spatial, intuitive, and imaginative, and may feature leaps of insight. A cognitive shift toward increased right-brain perception can be learned. B. Edwards, *Drawing on the Right Side of the Brain* (Los Angeles: J.P. Tarcher 1979). Bede Griffiths, *Return to the Centre* Collins (Fount Paperbacks: William Collins and Company 1984), 81.

6 For a fuller discussion, see Sarvepalli Radhakrishnan, *Indian Philosophy* (London: George Allen and Unwin 1927), vols. 1 and 2.

7 Georges-Philéas Vanier (1888–1967) was appointed nineteenth governor general of Canada (1959–67) by Queen Elizabeth II on the recommendation of Prime Minister John Diefenbaker. As a soldier in the First and Second World Wars, he reached the rank of major-general. Of their children, Thérèse became a doctor; Bernard, an artist; Byngsie (Father Benedict), a monk at the Cistercian monastery in Oka, Que.; and Jean, founder of L'Arche. In the 1999 *Maclean's* list of the 100 most influential Canadians of all time, Georges Vanier ranked number one. S.J. Jacques Monet, "Georges Vanier," *Canadian Encyclopedia*, 15 January 2008, www.thecanadianencyclopedia.ca/en/article/georges-phileas-vanier.

8 Officially named the Institute of Experimental and Clinical Oncology, Academy of Medical Sciences of the Soviet Union.

9 Harry Grabstald had been Whit's colleague and long-standing "student" for years. While he lacked the unique Whitmore surgical finesse, his results were equal to those of the boss; his slightly acid sense of humour was delightful; and our correspondence, as the years passed, was a continuing volley of rejoinders that kept me on my toes. I cherished his friendship.

10 The official record of the series notes: "This was more than just a sporting event, because for Canadians hockey is more than just a sport. It's our national game, a part of our culture, our history, our national identity. Hockey is the one thing about which we have always been able to say, 'We are the best.' The Soviets have their writers, their musicians, their scientists. Our heroes, with names like Morenz, Clancy, Conacher, Chabot, Schriner, Duran, Bauer, Bentley, Richard, Howe, and Beliveau, have been hockey players. Not that there haven't been other men in other fields just as worthy, but the hockey player with his speed, his grace, his strength, his physical bearing has touched something that runs strong and deep in the Canadian consciousness. If the Soviets lost this series, they would lose no more than that, a hockey series. But for Canadians, haunted by the knowledge that the world doubted our superiority at the game we called our own, there was more at stake. To lose this series, would be to lose face." John Macfarlane, *Twenty-Seven Days in Septembe: The Official Hockey Canada History of the 1972 Canada/U.S.S.R. Series* (Hockey Canada/Prosport Productions 1973), 4–5.

CHAPTER SEVEN

1 This account is compiled from the following: indelible memory; personal diary; CBC television coverage; *Time Magazine*, 9 October 1972; John Macfarlane, *Twenty-Seven Days in September: The Official Hockey Canada History of the 1972 Canada/U.S.S.R. Series* (Hockey Canada/Prosport Productions 1973); Gilles Terroux, *Face-off of the Century: The New Era*

(Toronto: Collier-Macmillan Canada 1972); Patrick White, "The Story of the Summit Series, as It's Never Been Told Before," *Globe and Mail*, 15 September 2012, www.theglobeandmail.com/sports/hockey/the-story-of-the-summit-series-as-its-never-been-told-before/article4546471/?page=all.

2 Yevgeni Yevtushenko made an important contribution to promoting progress, openness, human rights, and freedoms in the Soviet Union. "Yevgeni Yevtushenko," *Poetry Foundation*, 2019, www.poetryfoundation.org/poets/yevgeny-yevtushenko.

3 In August 1968 Soviet tanks invaded Czechoslovakia to crush the liberal policies introduced by the newly elected first secretary of the Czechoslovak Communist Party, Alexander Dubček. While a campaign of civil resistance to the occupation persisted, the momentum for change had been lost. In April 1969 Dubček was replaced. In the 1970s the dissident movement in Czechoslovakia re-emerged under the leadership of Václav Havel, among others. Yevtushenko, like Solzhenitsyn, chose to raise his liberal views from within the system.

CHAPTER EIGHT

1 Darrell David Munro (1919–2012) joined the staff of the Royal Victoria and Royal Edward Laurentian Chest hospitals in 1952. He was chief surgeon at the Royal Edward from 1964 to 1984 and principal thoracic surgeon at the RVH where he was also coordinator of planning and development in the late 1960s. A pioneer in thoracic surgery, he focused on pulmonary tuberculosis at the Royal Edward and on lung cancer at the Vic. He pioneered the use of the fiberoptic flexible bronchoscope and the stapling devices used to secure transected bronchi; he was an early crusader against smoking as a probable cause of lung cancer, launching the first hospital-based anti-smoking program in Canada in 1954; and, in 1965, he was leader of the team carrying out Canada's first lung transplant. His colleagues noted, "He was open in the sense of being non-secretive, popular, convivial and frank; he expressed himself clearly, had energy, charisma and was fun to be with. He was good with his hands as surgeon, fly-fisherman, wood-worker and landscape gardener." Though our contact was intermittent, and on this occasion brief, he influenced my life as few others did. "The Square Knot" (summer 2012), 26, *Square Knot Newsletter*, McGill Archives, https://www.mcgill.ca/squareknot/archives.

2 Members were: Anne Morgan, administrative director of RVH Medical Services; Jenny MacDonald, clinical coordinator in the Department of Surgery; and four physicians –MacKinnon, Mount, Munro, and Shibata (Surgical Oncology).

3 Medical representation included Arvanitakis (Psychiatry), Baxter (Otolaryngology), Bromage (Anesthesia), Hacker (Dermatology), Kendall (Medicine), Latour (Gynacology), MacKinnon and myself (Urology), Cantlie (Medical Oncology), Robb (Neurology), Roy (Medicine, Veterans' Hospital), Shapiro (Medicine), Shibata (Surgery). Presentations were made by myself as chairman; Nursing Coordinator MacDonald; Chaplain McDowell; Williams, social service; Morgan, administration; Cantlie, Oncology; and Arvanitakis, Psychiatry.

4 B. Mount, A. Jones, and A. Patterson, "Attitudes toward Death and Dying in a Teaching Hospital," *Urology*, 4, no. 6 (1974): 741–47.

5 B. Mount, "Christian and Agnostic Attitudes toward Death," *Ontario Medical Review*, January 1970, 11.

6 Material dealing with St Christopher's Hospice and Dame Cicely Saunders is based on personal discussions and correspondence over three decades with Dame Cicely and her colleagues, as well as the following: Shirley Du Boulay, *Cicely Saunders: The Founder of the Modern Hospice Movement* (London: Hodder and Stoughton 1984); Shirley Du Boulay and Marianne Rankin, *Cicely Saunders: The Founder of the Modern Hospice Movement* (London, SPCK 2007); Cicely Saunders, *Cicely Saunders: Selected Writings, 1958–2004* (Oxford: Oxford University Press 2016); David Clark, *Cicely Saunders: Founder of the Hospice Movement. Selected Letters 1959–1999* (Oxford: Oxford University Press 2002); Cicely Saunders, *The Management of Terminal Malignant Disease*, 2nd ed. (London: Edward Arnold 1984); Cicely Saunders, D.H. Summers, and N. Teller, *Hospice: The Living Idea* (London: Edward Arnold 1981); Cicely Saunders, *St Christopher's in Celebration: Twenty-One Years at Britain's First Modern Hospice* (London: Hodder and Stoughton 1988); Cicely Saunders, *Hospice and Palliative Care: An Interdisciplinary Approach* (London: Edward Arnold 1990); Cicely Saunders, *Watch with Me: Inspirations for a Life in Hospice Care* (Sheffield, UK: Mortal Press 2003); Cicely Saunders, *Beyond All Pain: A Companion for the Suffering and Bereaved* (London: SPCK 2008); Cicely Saunders, *Beyond the Horizon: A Search for Meaning in Suffering* (London: Darton, Longman and Todd 1990); Drian Gallery, *Marian Bohusz* (London: Ranelagh Press 1977); D. Clark et al., *A Bit of Heaven for the Few? An Oral History of the Hospice Movement in the United Kingdom* (Lancaster, UK: Observatory Publications 2005); Mary Baines, "Dr. Mary Baines Reflects on the Pioneering Days of Palliative Care," *European Journal of Palliative Care*, 18, no. 5 (2011): 223–7.

7 I received Shirley Du Boulay's biography from Cicely when it was published in 1984 and read it immediately. Subsequently, Cicely and I discussed it and the relevant crossroad experiences in both our lives on numerous occasions. In this

summary of Cicely's life I have attempted to include only material that I have direct knowledge of through the above interactions. To accurately report specific dates and locations, however, I have referred to details cited in the Du Boulay and Du Boulay/Rankin biographies. I have endeavored to use only those details and quotes that reflect statements that I have heard either verbatim or in essence from the persons quoted. I enthusiastically refer the reader to the aforementioned superb biographies.

8 Saunders, *Beyond the Horizon*, 2.

9 John Hinton received medical training at King's College Hospital and psychiatric training at the Maudsley. He was professor of psychiatry at the Middlesex Hospital from 1966 to 1983. *Dying* reported his study of the needs of the dying in the United Kingdom. John Hinton, *Dying* (London: Penguin Books 1972), 159.

CHAPTER NINE

1 Terry Neville, *The Royal Vic: The Story of Montreal's Royal Victoria Hospital, 1894–1994* (Montreal and Kingston: McGill-Queen's University Press 1994), 197–9.

2 Instead of meeting with our Core Group, Elisabeth agreed to give a one-and-a-half-hour seminar to more than three hundred colleagues representing a broad cross-section of the hospital and university family. The impact of this "spontaneous" session on the credibility of our PCS proposal appeared to be considerable.

3 Balfour Mount, "Letter to Elisabeth: Dedicated to Carol," in *Death: The Final Stage of Growth*, ed. Elisabeth Kubler-Ross (New Jersey: Prentice Hall 1975), 127–33.

4 Professor Florence Wald, dean of the Yale School of Nursing from 1959 to 1966, is considered the "mother of the American hospice movement." She developed Hospice New Haven after having been inspired by a 1963 lecture given at Yale by Cicely.

5 William Smith, *Dictionary of Greek and Roman Antiquities* (London, 1890), 851–3; C.T. Onions, *The Oxford Dictionary of English Etymology* (London: Oxford University Press 1966), 643.

6 The Brompton Chest Hospital, London, dates from the 1840s. Pain management using a strong analgesic solution bearing its name ("the Brompton mixture"), given by mouth at regular intervals, was practised at St Luke's Hospice and introduced by Dr Saunders at St Christopher's.

7 Cicely Saunders, *The Management of Terminal Illness* (London: Hospital Medicine Publications 1967), 1–29. The doses reported here are "morphine equivalente" doses; Cicely was using diamorphine (heroin) in those early years.

Later, Twycross found that, when given by mouth, morphine and diamorphine are interchangeable with the dose adjustment used here.

8 The doctor's unjustified fear of tolerance and addiction leads to ordering doses to be given "as required," which dictates that the patient must again experience pain before having the next dose. Tolerance and addiction are *very* rare if the drug is given regularly in doses carefully adjusted to prevent the pain consistently.

9 Neville, *The Royal Vic*, 171–5.

10 The PCS Core Group included: Drs Mount, Ajemian, Peter Geggie; PCS administrator Dottie Wilson; Dietetics, Kay Watson; Psychology, Drs Ronald Melzack, Stephanie Dudek, Margaret Kiely; Nursing, Lois Hollingsworth, Jennie MacDonald, Anita Mountjoy; Physical and Occupational Therapy, Ann Morrison; Social Services, Dr Jean-Pierre Duplantie, Jean Cameron; Clergy, Mel McDowell; RVH administration, Bes, Anne Morgan, Ken MacKinnon.

CHAPTER TEN

1 Mary Baines et al., *Lancet*, 2 (1985): 990–3.

CHAPTER ELEVEN

1 PCS planning team: MDs: B. Mount, I. Ajemian, K. Arvanitakis, P. Geggie, P. Mansell, D. Popkin, H. Shibata; Registered nurses: N.C. Macauley, L. Hollingsworth, J. MacDonald, A. Mountjoy, D. More; Administration: D. Wilson, J. MacPhail; Psychology: S. Dudek, M. Kiely, R. Melzack; Dieticians: K. Watson; Physical and Occupational Therapy: A. Morrison, J. Kinghorn; Social work: J.-P. Duplantie, J. Cameron; Pastoral: M. McDowell, L. Temple-Hill; Philosohy: C. Allen; RVH administration: L. Besel, A. Morgan; Photography: P. Byszewski; Library: S. Jack.

2 Evaluation Committee: B. Mount, I. Ajemian, R. Melzack, S. Dudek, M. Kiely, J. Hoey, D. Arvanotakis, D. Wilson.

3 *OMEGA: Journal of Death and Dying*: "Aims & Scope." "This Journal brings insight into terminal illness; the process of dying, bereavement, mourning, funeral customs, suicide. Fresh, lucid, responsible contributions from know-ledgeable professionals in universities, hospitals, clinics, old age homes, suicide prevention centers, funeral directors and others concerned with thanatology and the impact of death on individuals and the human community ... Drawing significant contributions from the fields of psychology, sociology, medicine, anthropology, law, education, history and literature, *OMEGA* has emerged as the most advanced and internationally recognized forum on the subject of death and dying. It serves as a reliable guide for clinicians, social workers, and

health professionals who must deal with problems in crisis management, e.g., terminal illness, fatal accidents, catastrophe, suicide and bereavement." OMEGA: *Journal of Death and Dying, Sage Journals*, journals.sagepub.com/home/ome.

4 IWG I, 1974 participants (a partial list): Claus Bahnson, Jean Quint Benoliel, Sandra Bertman, Ned Cassem, Frederick Coleman, Clarence Collins, Herman Feifel, Loma Feigenberg, John Fryer, Robert Fulton, Doris Howell, Richard Kalish, Bob Kastenbaum, Bunny Kastenbaum, Mel Krant, Joan Kron, Elisabeth Kübler-Ross, Bill Kutscher, Sylvia Lack, William Lamers, Dan Leviton, Robert Lifton, Jack Lynch, Balfour Mount, Roy Nichols, Russell Noyes, Colin Murray Parkes, Vanderlyn Pine, Cicely Saunders, Edwin Schneidman, Michael Simpson, Kenneth Spilman, Florence Wald, Henry Wald, Bill Worden, Mary Vachon, Laurens White.

5 Details of the full legacy of John Fryer's complex personality would not be known for two decades. No one in the room knew the impact on his field that he had already left in his wake. John Ercel Fryer was born in Kentucky in 1938. He attended medical school at Vanderbilt University and completed medical-residency training at the Ohio State Hospital. His psychiatry residency program at the University of Pennsylvania was, however, aborted when it was discovered that he was gay, leading him to complete his psychiatry training at Norristown State Hospital in Philadelphia.

That would not be the only time he was fired based on sexual orientation. It was, after all, the early 1970s and the American Psychiatric Association (APA), in its *Diagnostic and Statistical Manual of Mental Disorders* (DSM), clearly defined homosexuality as a "mental disorder": i.e., a disease. In 1972, as a result of earlier protests, gay-rights advocates Barbara Gittings and Dr Franklin E. Kameny were invited to organize a presentation at the APA annual meeting in Dallas to educate members about homosexuality. Initial plans called for Gittings and Kameny to form a panel along with two "straight" psychiatrists but Gittings felt that a panelist was needed who was both a psychiatrist *and* gay. They invited thirty-four-year-old John Fryer, who was a staff psychiatrist at Temple University but did not yet have tenure. He agreed to participate on condition that his identity remain secret and his voice distorted during the presentation. Wearing an oversized tuxedo, mask, and wig, he joined the panel as "Dr Henry Anonymous" and started his presentation with the words, "I am a homosexual. I am a psychiatrist." The audience found the presentation "electrifying"; it was the first time a gay psychiatrist had spoken about his sexual orientation in public. Fryer's presentation played a crucial role in the subsequent APA decisions both to remove homosexuality from its list of mental disorders and to urge that "homosexuals be given all protections now guaranteed other citizens." The members ratified those decisions in April 1974, seven months before our Columbia meeting.

Thus, when we met in Columbia, Fryer had already been the protagonist of one of the most important moments in the history of the American gay-rights movement. He went on to play an active role in several organizations, including the International Work Group on Death, Dying and Bereavement; the Philadelphia Aids Task Force; Physicians in Transition; Temple's Family Life Center; and the Institute of Religion and Science. For more than three decades, John Fryer was also organist and choirmaster at St Peter's Episcopal Church in Germantown, Philadelphia. He retired as a full professor of psychiatry and family and community medicine in 2000 after teaching for more than thirty years. He spent a sabbatical year at St Christopher's Hospice at the invitation of Dr Saunders. He died as a result of sarcoidosis in 2003. The identity of the man behind the mask during the historic 1972 APA meeting was not revealed until 1994. Dudley Clendinen, "John Fryer, 65, Psychiatrist Who Said He Was Gay in 1972, Dies," *New York Times*, 5 March 2003, www.nytimes. com/2003/03/05/us/dr-john-fryer-65-psychiatrist-who-said-in-1972-he-was-gay.html.

6 Elaine Woo, "Herman Feifel, 87; Pioneer in Study of Death," *Los Angeles Times*, www.articles.latimes.com/2003/jan/24/local/me-feifel24. See also *Mortality: Promoting the Interdisciplinary Study of Death and Dying*, 17, no. 1 (Taylor and Francis, 2012); William Dicke, "Edwin Shneidman, Authority on Suicide, Dies at 91," *New York Times*, www.nytimes.com/2009/05/21/us/21shneidman.html?_r=0.

7 Education: stenographer, Shaw's Business School; honours sociology, University of Toronto; non-directive counselling in industry, Institute of Industrial Relations, Toronto; rapid reading, Harvard; French, McGill. Employment: Clinical/research secretary and hospital administration, Massachusetts General Hospital, Harvard; creating standard- practice instructions, purchasing, budget management, liaison (internal/external) for RCA Victor Canada; consultant to client firms regarding systems analysis for Riddell, Stead, Graham and Hutchinson, Chartered Accountants; small-business management (all aspects) for Dayrand and the AudioShop, Montreal.

8 Twelve sessions (Fridays at 2–4 p.m., repeated at 5:30–7:30 p.m.) were provided for thirty-nine volunteers. Topics: 1) Introduction: RVH study, St Christopher's as a model, the team approach; 2) North American attitudes toward death and dying; 3) Psychological reactions of dying persons; 4) Hazards and challenges in caregiving; 5) Guidelines for interacting with dying persons; 6) Viewpoint: the dying patient and family; 7) Viewpoint: the helping professions; 8) Presentation by Volunteer Bureau, Princess Margaret Hospital, Toronto; 9) Religious needs of the dying patient; 10) Psychological reactions of dying persons; 11) "How Could I Not Be Among You?" (film); 12) Funeral arrangements, wills, Do Not Resuscitate (DNR) orders, legal issues.

9 Cicely Saunders, *Watch with Me: Inspiration for a Life in Hospice Care* (Sheffield, UK: Mortal Press 2003), 24.

10 J. Aitken, "Fond Farewell: Compassion and Honesty for the Dying," *Weekend Magazine*, 25, no. 25 (21 June 1975): 4.

11 In the interval since palliative-care plans started to gel in September 1973, I had made fifty-four presentations – most of them local, but also in Toronto, London (Ontario), Calgary, the United Kingdom, the USSR, and Plattsburgh, NY, and had authored twelve publications. A busy time.

12 "Magoo," or Donald Bruce MacGowan, was the PCU "night orderly." He was an eclectic man, his interests spanning old René Claire films, American jazz, philosophy, and religion; his heroes were Woody Allen, Thomas Merton, and René Lévesque. One night when, as a student in France, he was driving drunk in Paris, he killed an eleven-year-old boy and was charged with manslaughter and fined. He turned to nursing as a "way of life," expiation, and a path toward meaning. Magoo was a team favourite; his sardonic edginess gave voice to our waxing and waning discomfort in our dance with death. His ongoing contrived charades served as an effective veil for his questing spirit, as we would learn a little later.

13 Of the admissions, six were readmissions, twenty-five were direct admissions to the PCU, and twenty-two were transfers from other hospital wards; twenty-four were male; seven remained on PCU at the completion of the four months; and forty were discharged (twenty-nine died, nine went home, one was transferred off-service, and one went to a nursing home). The PCU length of stay: range of 1–82 days, average 16.7 days. Home Care (1 nurse): 86 visits to 13 patients.

14 Mild, moderate, and severe pain, vomiting, anorexia, nausea, dyspnea, cough, anxiety, and mental distress, confusion, depression, insomnia, constipation, fungating growths, urinary frequency, and the need for catheterization.

15 RVH PCS team, 1975: PCU nurses: Anne Dubrofsky and Sue Britton (heads), Mary Carol Case, Joan Armstrong, Glynis Williams, Leslie Vincent, Nancy Stevenson, Diane Harnden, Bobbe LaughtonChristel Mueller, Jackie Podasky, Mabel Dufresne, Sadie Kaplan, Dorothy More, Sharon Randall; Certified nursing assistants: Barbara Carter, Denis McLaughlin; Nursing assistants: Pat Gladwish, Ross Anderson; Nursing aide: Dorothy Jacobs; Nursing orderly: Don MacGown; Physicians: Ina Ajemian (director, Clinical Care), John Scott, Akos Beszterczey, Balfour Mount (PCS director); Administrative director: Dottie Wilson; Secretary: Rollande Poulin; Unit co-ordinator: Lynn Filiatrault; Domiciliary care: Head nurse, Cathy Macaulay; Registered nurses: Aileen MacDonald, Shirley Elliottl; Social worker: Anne Chant; Physiotherapist: Sharon Manson; Chaplains: Mel McDowell, Lionel Temple-Hill; Secretary: Joanne McPhail; Research: Ron Melzack, John Hoey, Margaret Keily,

Stephanie Dudek, Miriam Gillett; Volunteers: Director Kathleen Markey,
Evelyn Allan, Christine Allen, Jane Allen, Blanche Baxter, Sophia Bey, Olga
Biollo, Jean Cameron, Don Carver, Pat Cogan, Dorothy Danacker, Jean
Davidson, Gilles Deslauriers, Gwendoline Desmier, Sybil Etmekdgian, Anne
Faller, Rolande Faubert, Francine Freeman, Georgina Gajewski, Janet Gill,
Miriam Gillitt, Patricia Gladwish, Pierre-Yvan Graftieaux, Gloria Graham,
Betty Gratias, Naomi Guttman, Judy Gutwillig, Gael Harrison, Michele Horny,
Judi Hymovitch, Mary Kennedy, Judy Kinghorn, Elizabeth Langenbach, Gail
MacLauchlan, Barry Martin, Heather McFarland, Betty McLeod, Anne Marie
McTurner, Stella Mikosz, Dorothy More, Lorna Morse, Mary Muir, Brian
Murphy, Frances Murphy, Bob Ozoris, Agnes Perkins, Betty Pickard, Pierrette
Prevost, Dorothy Ranger, Gill Reilly, Donna Robertson, David Roche, Alicia de
Roussy, Nora de Saint Romain, Margo Savard, Fred Sawyer, Vivian Saykaly,
Diana Scott, Diana Severs, Conchita Street, Adeline Swabey, Charles Taylor,
Wanda Teas, Hilda Temple-Hill, Maggie Torrey, Kathleen Wakeham, Betty
Whiting, Darris Wiles, Isabelle Wright.

16 Balfour Mount, Ina Ajemian, John Scott, Akos Beszterczey, Dottie Wilson,
Miriam Gillitt, Ann Hampson, Sue Britton, Cathy Macaulay, Pierrette
Lambert, Lynn Filiatrault, Kitty Markey, Christine Allan, Jean Cameron,
Sharon Manson, Mel McDowell, Lionel Temple-Hill, Sheila O'Neill, Al Lyall,
Ron Melzack.

17 The RVH *Manual on Palliative/Hospice Care: A Resource Book*, I. Ajemian and
B. Mount, eds. (Salem, NH: Ayer Company 1982), became an internationally
used resource book for program development.

18 Balfour Mount, "Death: A Part of Life?" CRUX: *A Quarterly Journal of
Christian Thought and Opinion*, 1, no. 3 (1973–74); B.M. Mount, A. Jones,
and A. Patterson, "Death and Dying: Attitudes in a Teaching Hospital," *Journal
of Urology*, 4, no. 6. (1974): 741–7; D.A.E. Shephard, "Terminal Care:
Towards an Ideal," *CMAJ*, 115 (1976): 97–8; B.M. Mount, "The Problem of
Caring for the Dying in a General Hospital: The Palliative Care Unit as a
Possible Solution," *CMAJ*, 115 (1976): 119–21; B.M. Mount, I. Ajemian, and
J.F. Scott, "Use of the Brompton Mixture in Treating the Chronic Pain of
Malignant Disease," *CMAJ*, 115 (1976): 122–4; R. Melzack, J.G. Ofiesh, and
B.M. Mount, "The Brompton Mixture: Effect on Pain in Cancer Patients,"
CMAJ, 115 (1976): 125–9; J. Garner, "Palliative Care: It's the Quality of Life
Remaining That Matters," *CMAJ*, 115 (1976): 179–80; R.W. Buckingham,
S.A. Lack, B.M. Mount, and L.D. MacLean, "Editorial," *CMAJ*, 115 (1976):
1211–15; W.B. Murray and R.W. Buckingham, "Implications of Participant
Observation in Medical Studies," *CMAJ*, 115 (1976): 1187–90; D.A.E.
Shephard, "Principles and Practice of Palliative Care: Conference Report,"
CMAJ, 116 (1977): 522–6; M.A. Simpson, "Living with the Dying" (letter),

CMAJ, 117 (17 December 1977): 14; B. Mount, "Living with the Dying" (response), *CMAJ*, 117 (17 December 1977): 14–5; C. Saunders, "Living with the Dying" (letter), *CMAJ*, 117 (17 December 1977): 15.

19 D. Rosenhan, "On Being Sane in Insane Places," *Science*, 179 (1973): 250–8. Rosenhan's study should be seen in the context of the challenges to institutional norms that were the hallmark of the 1960s, in this case, the challenge to contemporary psychiatry that was voiced by R.D. Lang and many others. An earlier participant- observation study occurred when Caucasian Texan journalist John Howard Griffin posed as a black man in the southern United States, later publishing an account of the experience in his 1961 book *Black Like Me*. Qualitative-research techniques that evolved during the subsequent decades would eventually provide new strategies for examining phenomena that are poorly captured by quantitative research.

20 The peer reviewed journal *Science* is universally held in the highest regard. David L. Rosenhan obtained his PhD in psychology at Columbia University and was a recognized expert in psychology and the law. He was a fellow of the American Association for the Advancement of Science and a visiting fellow at Oxford University. He joined the Stanford Law School faculty in 1970, having previously been a member of the faculties of Swarthmore College, Princeton University, and Haverford College. He was also a research psychologist and lecturer at the University of Pennsylvania. Ann. E. Kazak, "David Rosenhan," *APA PsychNet*, 2019, www.psycnet.apa.org/record/2013-31242-003.

21 Alan Lyall, Mary Vachon, and Joy Rogers, representing the Clarke Institute Community Resources Services. *RVH Manual*, 498–509.

22 High-stress levels were anticipated given the pioneering nature of the program; the high ambient-stress levels generally associated with death; the "high expectations of doing a superlative job"; the recognition that "the eyes of the world were upon us"; the use of a non-hierarchical team approach in the context of a traditional, hierarchical teaching hospital; and the understanding that death presents threats to intra-psychic defences for all.

23 This meant that each of the following items was experienced by over 50 per cent of the nursing staff: restless, disturbed nights; losing sleep on account of worry; decreased energy levels; feeling constant strain; "taking things hard"; feeling nervous. In addition, each of the following were experienced by at least 25 per cent of the nursing staff: shaky hands, eating excessively, stomach upset, constipation, weight gain of more than five pounds in the past month, butterflies in the stomach, rapid heart rate.

24 The Clarke authors noted: "The director was such a key and charismatic figure in bringing this unit into being, and had somehow managed to devote an enormous amount of time to it, so that he seemed ever present and ever available at this early stage and this ill prepared some staff for the reality that he would

have to draw back to pursue other duties in the near future. This set the stage for the inevitable disillusionment experienced by all followers of charismatic leaders."

25　Jean, a British social worker, was a research assistant with orthopedic surgeon Richard Cruess (later dean of medicine, McGill) on immigrating to Canada, and then joined the PCS planning group in 1973. She provided bereavement support by telephone to countless grieving family members as a long-time member of the bereavement follow-up program and developed the Jean Cameron Fund for the purchase of otherwise unavailable patient amenities.

26　Interviews were carried out at the anniversary + 2 weeks (54 weeks) following the death. "Key persons" (KP) were relatives or friends who had been "closest" to the patient. The relationship of the "key persons" to the deceased was matched so that the PCU and comparison group each included eight widows, five widowers, four daughters, two parents, one sister.

27　Buckingham, who at the time was paid through Health, Education, and Welfare funds, was on leave without pay while preparing the study.

28　RVH PCS team, December 1976: MDs (1 director, 1 clinical director, 1 staff MD, 1/5 psychiatrist); PCU (nursing: 1 head nurse, 5 staff RNs, 7 RNs-part time, 2 nursing assistants, 1 aide, 1 orderly); 1 unit coordinator; Home Care: (1 head RN, 3 staff RNs); Consult: 1 RN; support staff: 6 MDs of various specialties, 1 social worker, 1/2 physiotherapist, 1 dietician, chaplains; Research and administration: 1 administrator, 1 research assistant (part-time), 1 secretary; Volunteers: 1 director, 5 committee chairs, 48 staff.

29　PCU admissions: 332 (171 male); by transfer from another ward (158), by direct admission to PCU (174); department admitted from: Medical (65), Surgery (122), OB/GYN (5), Neurology (11), Oncology (99), Other (3), Readmit (27). PCU median length of stay, 9.85 days. PCU discharges: 325 (171 male); discharge to home (32), died (285), transfer off-service (7), transfer to nursing home (1). PCU admissions with cancer diagnosis: lung 56, colon 50, breast 44, female reproductive 27, stomach 18, head and neck 18, pancreas 17, kidney and bladder 13, prostate 11, lymphatic 10, others 41. Home Care admissions: 194 (94 male); from PCU (10), Medical (17), Surgery (32), OB/GYN (2), Neurology (2), Oncology (102), other (10); readmit (19). Home Care discharges: 176 (88 male); discharged to PCU (103), RVH (34), died at home (21), nursing home or other hospital (10), other (8). Home Care cost-savings estimate: a three-month detailed analysis by the RVH Department of Nursing estimated that 50 per cent of patient days on Home Care would otherwise have been days spent in hospital. Home Care visits, total: 2,372; nature of visits: primary nursing care, 1,757; hospital follow-up, 252; assessment, 180; bereavement, 75; crisis, 69; consultation, 39. Home Care patients with cancer diagnosis: lung 37, breast 34, colon 29, female reproductive 12, pancreas 11, stomach 7, kidney and bladder 7, head and neck 5, others 33. Home Care evaluation: All patients and their KPs completed a fifteen-question multiple-choice questionnaire on 1 May 1976 (or between their fourth and fifth visits if new patients) and KPs were interviewed two weeks following discharge. An overwhelming majority of respondents claimed a high degree of satisfaction. It was interesting to note that retrospective KP satisfaction levels were higher than on their first response. The only consistent negative response was to the question concerning pain control. While that may be due to the progressive nature of the patient's disease with its inevitable deterioration, it is a reminder of the need for further excellence (Final Report, 493–501). Consultations by PCS MDs, 490. Consult outcome (Tr = "Transfer to"): Tr PCU, 149; Tr Home Care, 72; Tr PCU + Home Care, 34; Off-service follow-up 110; Tr home/nursing home, 19; no follow-up needed, 49; died off-service, 57.

30 The gold was won by Jacek Wszola of Poland; Stones got the bronze.

31 Director's Comments, RVH PCS *Newsletter*, 2 (December 1976).

32 University of Chicago Billings Hospital, Department of Psychiatry.

33 On each day, registrants sat at the same table during the morning and afternoon sessions. The table-discussion leaders had received detailed instructions prior to the conference and met daily during the meeting to review progress. "Your role is not that of teacher but of catalyst, stimulator, host (in terms of putting people at ease and facilitating introductions) and general 'animateur' for the table.".

34 Dr John D. (Jack) Morgan, professor of philosophy, King's College, University of Western Ontario, Personal communication. These points were intended in my remarks from the floor but undoubtedly were much less clearly stated prior to my subsequent, most helpful, discussion with Jack.

35 Bill 101 made French the official language of government and of the courts in the province of Quebec, as well as the language of the workplace, of instruction, of communication, of commerce, and of business. Education in French became compulsory for immigrants, even those from other Canadian provinces, unless a "reciprocal agreement" existed between Quebec and that province (the so-called Quebec clause). Michael Behiels and R. Hudon, "La langue française," *Canadian Encyclopedia*, 31 July 2013, www.thecanadianencyclopedia.com/articles/bill-101.

36 Donnella H. Meadows, Dennis L. Meadows, Jorgen Randers, and William W. Behrens III, *The Limits to Growth* (New York: Universe Books 1972).

CHAPTER TWELVE

1 Pierrette had arrived at my office unannounced in the middle of a busy wall-to-wall press of patients. "Says she needs to speak to you for a minute or two,"

the secretary explained, adding, "doesn't speak much English." She was all too aware of my many failed French courses and their stunted, stumbling results. The next patient was asked to wait; Pierrette blew into the room. We had perhaps a dozen or so words of shared vocabulary between us, but that was sufficient. Here was a leadership person in the francophone nursing community – a very animated leadership person! Having never heard of Elisabeth or Cicely, she had, on her own, come to a detailed understanding of the needs of the dying, their families, and their caregivers. It was then that she heard of the Vic PCS. She couldn't believe it. She couldn't believe it and came right over. I called Bes and filled her in. Always ready to capitalize on a good bet, Pierrette was offered a job on the spot. "Travailler avec les Anglais? Mon Dieu!" After a day or two of pondering, she acquiesced. I noted with more than a little humility and anglophone awe that here was the Quebec version of EKR and Dame Cicely – unknown internationally because she was a Québécoise! Had she been anywhere else in North America, she would have been a household name. Pierrette joined the team days later.

2 With slight clarifications in wording being introduced as time passed, this document became the working paper for the RVH *Manual on Palliative/ Hospice Care*, edited by I. Ajemian and myself (Salem, NH: Ayer 1980).

3 The candid disclosures included in this account of Chip and his family were agreed to by Chip and his mother, Janet, who also graciously permitted the inclusion of his story in my lectures and publications over the years.

4 Canadian Army brigadier-general, Second World War; Liberal MP (Westmount) in governments of Pearson and Trudeau and then chairman of National Capital Commission; officer of the Order of Canada.

5 Gregory L. Fricchione, *Compassion and Healing in Medicine and Society: On the Nature and Use of Attachment Solutions to Separation Challenges* (Baltimore, MD: Johns Hopkins University Press 2011).

6 T.S. Eliot, "Four Quartets, Little Gidding."

7 RVH PCS Executive Committee: W. Edward Bembridge, Marcel Cazavan, Janet Drury, Tom Markey, Richard P. Sargent, Mrs B David Tessler. Advisory Board: Dr Gregory Baum, Michel Bélanger, André Charron, Frank B. Common, Jr, Chipman Drury, Leonard Ellen, Dr John Evans, Maureen Forrester, Dr Sam Freedman, Sidney Maislin, W. Earle McLaughlin, Paul Paré, Dr Cicely Saunders, Gilles Vigneault.

8 PCU; Emergency Holding Unit; Plastic Surgery; Ophthalmology and Otolaryngology; "Tabah Surgery," including four oncology beds; offices for two plastic surgeons; Surgical ICU; an endoscopy unit; and, finally, further expansion of the PCU into freed-up Surgical ICU space.

9 Later, I was interested to receive a letter of thanks from a colleague in the Department of Medicine at Tulane University School of Medicine who had

been present at that Roswell Park Rounds. She had been writing a master's
program assignment at Roswell Park on new concepts in end-of-life care. Her
own earlier troubling experiences when her husband had died, coupled with
the attitudes she encountered while writing the paper ("I again ran into skeptics, people who felt that the terminally ill need no special attention!") had
prompted her letter of thanks. President Richard Nixon had embarked on
"The War on Cancer" with the signing of the National Cancer Act of 1971;
Roswell Park and Dr Murphy were major players in the battle. One assumes
that Dr Murphy felt he could not afford to leave any doubt where he and his
institute stood regarding cancer-treatment goals.

10 *Universities: Canada*: Queen's (x4); Western (x2); Sherbrooke; McMaster;
Toronto; Ottawa; Mount Allison; Alberta. *United States*: Temple; Rochester;
Chicago; Wisconsin; Miami (x2); UCSF; Cornell; Oral Roberts; Georgetown;
Columbia.
Hospitals: Canada: Ottawa General; Montreal Children's, Montreal
General; Jewish General (Montreal); Chest Hospital (Montreal); Riverside
(Ottawa); Cornerbrook General (Newfoundland); St Michael's (Toronto);
Cowansville General (Quebec); Hôtel-Dieu (Quebec City); Halifax Infirmary.
United States: Roswell Park (Buffalo); Church Home and Hospital
(Baltimore); Strong Memorial Hospital (Rochester); Burlington General (VT);
Cedars Sinai (Los Angeles); Wausaw General (WI); New York Hospital
(New York City); Sidney Farber Cancer Center (Boston); University
Nebraska Medical Center; Albert Einstein Medical Center (New York City).
International: Charing Cross (London, England); Hôtel-Dieu (Paris); Royal
Prince Alfred (Sydney, Australia); Radiumhammet, Karolinska Sjukhuset
(Stockholm, Sweden); King Edward VII Memorial (Hamilton, Bermuda).
Meetings: Canada: Royal College of Physicians and Surgeons of Canada;
Oncology Nurses of Montreal; World Congress of Family Physicians;
International Home Care Workshop; International Seminars on Care of the
Terminally Ill (1976, 1978, 1980); Quebec Urologists Asssociation; Academy
of Medicine (Ottawa); Ontario Medical Association; International Seminar
on Stress, Cancer and Death; NCI (Canada) Oncology Workshop; Canadian
Society Hospital Pharmacists Annual Meeting; Ontario Hospital Association;
Research Methodologies Seminar; Family MD Refresher Courses (x5). *United
States*: Northeast Section AUA; Massachusetts Public Health Association
(Boston); International Work Group on Death Dying and Bereavement;
2nd World Congress on Pain; Forum for Death Education and Counselling
(Washington); National Hospice Organization Annual Meeting, Problems in
General Practice; American Cancer Society National Conference on Urological
Cancer; Nebraska Medical Society Annual Meeting; Canadian-American
Hospital Association Health Management Conference; American College

Physicians Annual Meeting. *International*: International Association for
Enterostomal Therapy; International Association for Suicide Prevention;
International Association for Study of Pain; International Seminar on Terminal
Care (Milan, Italy). *Other*: Inst. J. Paoli I. Calmattes (Marseille, France);
St Christopher's Hospice (London, England); Center Laennec (Paris); Osler
Society (McGill); London District Health Council (Ontario); Carl Kouba
Hospice (WI); Comprehensive Cancer Center (Miami); Lethbridge
Rehabilitation Center (Montreal); Hospice of Santa Barbara (CA); NCI
(Bethesda, MD); Hospice of Los Angeles; Rand Corporation (Los Angeles);
Cross Cancer Institute (Edmonton); Center for Bioethics (Montreal);
Palliative Care Work Group (Toronto).

11 Robert A. Johnson, *Balancing Heaven and Earth: A Memoir of Visions,
Dreams and Realizations* (New York: HarperCollins 1998), 64–5.

12 Ajemian and Mount, eds., *The R.V.H. Manual on Palliative/Hospice Care*,
489–97.

13 Jacques was honoured with membership in the Order of Quebec (1998) and
Order of Canada (2005). On 18 April 2005, at the age of fifty-seven, he and
his wife, Francyne Blackburn, were killed in a catastrophic head-on collision
with a bus on the Champlain Bridge as he headed to Quebec City to deliver a
lecture, leaving behind a grieving community. Elisabeth Wassermann, "Beyond
on Call: Quadriplegic Tragedy Shapes a Giving Life," *National Review of
Medicine*, 15 (30 August 2004), www.nationalreviewofmedicine.com/
issue/2004_08_30/beyond_on-call_15.html.

14 The term "music therapist" refers to a specially trained individual whose
intervention is based on a thorough knowledge of all facets of music
(historical, theoretical, practical), the behavioural sciences, treatment and
educational models, and accepted therapeutic approaches.

15 S. Munro and B. Mount, "Music Therapy in Palliative Care," *CMAJ*, 119,
no. 9 (1978): 3–8; Susan Porchet-Munro, *Music Therapy in Palliative/Hospice
Care* (St Louis, MO: Magnamusic-Baton 1984).

16 Balfour Mount, "The Advance Retreat: An Experiment in Organizational
Development on the RVH PCS," *RVH Manual*, 510–19.

17 D.B. Jones, *The Best Butler in the Business: Tom Daly of the National Film
Board of Canada* (Toronto: University of Toronto Press 1996), 132–7;
Thomas de Hartmann, *Our Life with Mr. Gurdjieff* (New York: Cooper
Square Publishers 1964). With customary insight, Tom had long recognized
the need for greater consciousness on our journey through life. He was, however, always respectful of the boundaries of others and I was at that time perhaps too often reticent in discussing inner-life topics. My propensity to cut
short such discussions would lead to a cherished memento of our friendship,

the gift of a 1964 edition copy of de Hartmann's *Our Life with Mr. Gurdjieff*, with the inscription, "To Bal, with love, Tom. November 22, 1991."

18 The other NFB film-crew members would join her on the PCU during the final pre-filming days.

19 Jones, *The Best Butler in the Business*, 211–14.

20 *Last Days of Living* awards include: HEMA Film Festival, Best of Show (April 1981); Chicago International Film Festival, Gold Plaque (November 1980); and San Francisco International Film Festival, Honorable Mention, 1980.

21 The 1978 Second Seminar Program, 2 November: "Care of the Dying" (Cicely Saunders); "The Case for Active Treatment" (Irwin Krakoff); "Communicating Diagnosis & Prognosis with Patient & Family" (Eric Cassell); "Evaluating Terminal Care" (Robert Kastenbaum); "How the Health Professional Deals with Stress" (Merville Vincent); "Stress & the RVH PCS" (Jacques Voyer); "Music Therapy for the Terminally Ill" (Susan Munro). 3 November: "Pain Physiology Update" (Ronald Melzack); "Assessing Pain" (Ramon Evans); "Pain Management" (Balfour Mount); "Specific Problems of Patients with Non-Malignant Disease at St Christopher's Hospice" (Cicely Saunders); "Management of Gastrointestinal Symptoms" (Sylvia Lack); "Control of Other Symptoms" (Ina Ajemian); "Spiritual Concerns: Their Relevance" (John Scott); "Spiritual Cross-Cultural Considerations" (Robert Fulton); "Spiritual Counseling" (Brenda Halton); "Interest Groups regarding the RVH PCS Experience" (Home Care; Consult Team; Social Work; Volunteers); "Palliative Care Nursing and the Dying Child" (Barrie de Veber). 4 November: "Normal and Abnormal Grief" (Merville Vincent); "Bereavement Follow-Up Programs" (Colin Murray Parkes); "Grief & Loss: Cross-Cultural Considerations" (Robert Fulton); "Dying Children & Their Families" (William Lamers); "Children, When Parents Die" (Morris Wessell).

22 Frankl and his wife and parents were deported to the Nazi Theresienstadt Ghetto in September 1942. His father died there. On 19 October 1944 Frankl and his wife were transported to Auschwitz where his mother and brother died; his wife was later transferred to Bergen-Belsen where she died. On 25 October 1944 Dr Frankl was moved to Kaufering, a concentration camp affiliated with Dachau. There he worked as a slave labourer for five months. In March 1945 he was moved to Türkeim (also affiliated with Dachau) where he worked as a physician until he was liberated by the Americans on 27 April 1945. In 1947 Frankl married his second wife, Eleonore Katharina Schwindt, a practising Catholic. "Viktor Frankl," *Good Therapy*, 2019, www.goodtherapy. org/famous-psychologists/viktor-frankl.html.

23 Viktor E. Frankl, *Man's Search for Meaning* (New York: Washington Square Press 1984), 55–6.

24 Ibid., 54–8.
25 Ibid., 86.
26 Research Methodologies, 5 October: "Research Needs in Hospice Care: Separating Assumptions from Facts" (Cicely Saunders); "Clinical Trials, Methodologic Considerations: Pointers & Pitfalls" (John Kreeft); "Content Analysis & Other Non-Double Blind Methodologies" (Lesley Degner); "Pain Research: Approaches to the Problem of Measuring the Unmeasurable" (Ron Melzack); "Pall Care: Epidemiological Considerations" (Walter Spitzer); "Bereavement Research: Predictive & Outcome Measures & Other Variables I Have Known" (Colin M. Parkes); "The Omega Project: A Decade of Research Observations at the Mass. Gen'l Hosp." (Bill Worden); "Evaluating Educational Programs for the Hospice Team" (Michael Simpson).

   Third International Seminar, 6 October: "Children & Death: Things I've Learned Along the Way" (Ida Martinson); "Life-Death Decision Making in Health Care" (Lesley Degner); "The Symptom Control Team in a General Hospital: Impact on an Institution" (Pierrette Lambert); "A Daycare Centre for the Terminally Ill" (Eric Wilkes); "The RVH Bereavement Follow-Up Program: Development & Evaluation" (Margaret Kiely and Ann Hampson); "A Widow-Widow Self-Help Program" (Mary Vachon and Joy Rogers); "Group Intervention Bereavement" (Gary Davis); "The Last Days of Living" (Balfour Mount and Malca Gillson). 7 October: "Understanding Pain: A Physiological Update" (Ronald Melzack); "Updating the Assessment & Treatment of Chronic Pain" (Sylvia Lack); "But What Else Can We Do? The Nurses' Role in Terminal Care" (Margo McCaffery); "Practical Pointers in the Control of Other Symptoms" (Cicely Saunders, Tom Leicht, Ina Ajemian); "The Problem Patient" (Cicely Saunders); "Enterostomal Therapy" (Rosemary Watt); "Music Therapy" (Susan Munro); a choice of fourteen evening workshops on aspects of palliative care. 8 October: "Staff Stress As We Have Experienced It: Etiology, Diagnosis, Prevention" (Jacques Voyer); "My Experience with Staff Stress among Those Caring for the Terminally Ill" (Sam Klagsbrun); "Staff Stress: New Staff & the Pall. Care Culture" (Lorine Besel); "Staff Selection" (Balfour Mount); "The Meaning of Suffering for the Terminally Ill" (Viktor Frankl); "Bridging the Gulf of Meaning" (Christine Allen).
27 Royal Vic PCS, Medical Students' Society; Faculty of Religious Studies; Faculty of Medicine, Department of Psychiatry; Department of History of Medicine; Department of Neurology and Neurosurgery; Montreal Clinical Research Institute; Arts and Science Undergraduate Society; McGill Debating Union.
28 Dr Christine Allen, later Sr Mary Prudence Allen, a volunteer on our PCS team, spoke after Dr Frankl on "Bridging the Gulf of Meaning." She addressed the issue of forming a bond between caregiver and care recipient through four

strategies: the discovery of common ground; the exploration of differences; the mutual release of energies; and the creation of new life. Her superb analysis was published in the RVH *Manual*, 231–42.

29 Composer (nine symphonies; *Das Lied von der Erde*) and conductor (Vienna Opera), Gustav Mahler was for many symbolic of the unsettled, questing, doubting, guilt-ridden angst of the second half of the twentieth century. A Jew turned Catholic, he was preoccupied with questions of meaning. His music expresses with riveting clarity the unrest that has stirred countless souls then and since. After working on his Second Symphony for eight years, Mahler attended the February 1894 funeral of conductor Hans von Bulow and was overwhelmed by Klopstock's ode "Resurrection" that was part of that service. He wrote, "This struck me like lightning! Everything was revealed clear and plain to my soul in a flash." His *Resurrection Symphony* was soon completed and Mahler himself conducted its premiere in Berlin on 13 December 1895.

CHAPTER THIRTEEN

1 Elizabeth Lesse, *Broken Open: How Difficult Times Can Help Us Grow* (New York: Villard Books 2005). The words quoted here are the opening lines of the Introduction to this highly recommended, insightful guide to navigating life's lee shores, by the co-founder of the OMEGA Institute.

2 Squirrelled away with Marian and Joan's letters and the condolence letters and telegram from the Grenfell Mission at St Anthony that all too soon would follow was Maude's last Valentine Day's card to Harry. It read: "Sweetheart, to me you've always been the very sweetest part of all the precious hopes and dreams I have within my heart / You've brought the deepest happiness that I have ever known, Sweetheart, that's why my love belongs to you – and you alone." The card was signed with the code initials that they never explained – *Your S.S.E.* – and bore the telltale remnants of the scotch tape that had kept it prominently displayed close at hand during the final years of Harry's life.

3 Later published as B. Mount, *Sightings in the Valley of the Shadow: Reflections on Dying* (Downers Grove, IL: InterVarsity Press 1983).

4 Ibid., 107, and, to follow, 113 and 114.

5 Diane K. Osbon, *Reflections on the Art of Living: A Joseph Campbell Companion* (New York: Harper Collins 1995), 23–5.

6 Neil initiated the Cross Cancer Institute Palliative Care Program on his return to Edmonton during the summer of 1981. In 1984 he recruited Eduardo Bruera – a notable landmark in the international growth of the field. In 1994 Neil returned to Montreal to join the McGill palliative-care team.

7 John Wilson McConnell (1877–1963), the youngest of seven children born to
  Irish immigrants, had been a major benefactor of Quebec institutions since the
  early years of the twentieth century: McGill University and its teaching
  hospitals, the YMCA, churches (both Catholic and Protestant), the Salvation
  Army and Old Brewery Mission, the Victorian Order of Nurses, and the
  Montreal Symphony Orchestra, as well as youth initiatives, mission projects,
  and needy individuals, including a promising young Montreal contralto,
  Maureen Forrester, whose musical training he enabled. During the First and
  Second World Wars, McConnell was a tireless organizer, fundraiser, and instrumental figure behind a number of successful war efforts. The philanthropic
  foundation bearing his name was founded in 1937 and, with his death in
  1963, was renamed the J.W. McConnell Family Foundation.
  See www.mcconnellfoundation.ca/en/about.

8 Montreal's "Golden Square Mile" (bounded by Atwater Avenue to the west,
  Bleury Street and Avenue du Parc to the east, the slopes of Mount Royal to the
  north, and La Gauchetière to the south) found its genesis in the industrializa-
  tion, population explosion, flourishing commerce, and "age of unbridled capitalism" that swept Montreal during the period 1850–1930, when the wealthy
  "established families" of "polite" society were joined by the swelling ranks of
  the nouveau riche, resulting in an increasing polarization between the rich and
  the poor. The crowded inner city, with its disease, vermin, noise, and fumes,
  was said to be "almost uninhabitable." In addition to magnificent homes, the
  newly settled tree-lined neighbourhood for the influential and affluent boasted
  new churches, convents, schools, and parks. At its peak (c. 1900),
  three-quarters of Canada's millionaires lived in the Golden Square Mile;
  indeed, fully 70 per cent of the entire country's wealth was in the hands of its
  residents. A core group of influential French Canadian families had been joined
  in the area by a mixed, but predominantly Scottish, population. Between 1850
  and 1930, the Golden Square Mile's inhabitants were 60 per cent Scots, 13
  per cent English, 10 per cent French Canadian, 8 per cent American, 4 per cent
  Irish, and 5 per cent Other (Germans, Jews, Italians, Belgians, etc.). François
  Rémillard and Brian Merrett, *Mansions of the Golden Square Mile, Montreal
  1850–1930* (Montreal: Meridian Press 1987).

9 Neil McKenty, *In the Stillness Dancing: The Journey of John Main* (London:
  Darton, Longman and Todd 1986); Paul T. Harris, *John Main by Those Who
  Knew Him* (Ottawa: Novalis 1991). I also rely on personal communications
  from Father Laurence Freeman and Polly and Mark Schofield for details
  regarding the life of John Main and the early years of the meditation
  community he founded.

10 As John Main was developing his centre for "Christian meditation," the
   Trappist monk and priest Thomas Keating and his colleagues at St Joseph's

Abbey in Spencer, Massachusetts, were teaching a similar approach under the name "centering prayer."

CHAPTER FOURTEEN

1 McGill's Fourth International Congress, 4–6 October 1982. Plenary sessions: "Chronic Pain with Advanced Cancer: Diagnostic Approaches" (Kathleen Foley), and "Comments" (Cicely Saunders); "Children Facing Death" (Elisabeth Kübler Ross); "Psychogeriatrics: Understanding the Elderly Patient" (Sir Ferguson Anderson); "Medical Management of Malignant Bowel Obstruction" (Mary Baines); "Nursing Care of the Terminally Ill: Selected Issues" (Mary Ann Comartin); "Teaching Health Care Professionals about Terminal Care" (Derek Doyle); "Screening of Films of Merit: When Jewish Patients and Families Confront Death" (Lea Baider); "Care of the Dying in Bombay" (Luis de Souza); "Diagnostic Variables in Pastoral Care" (Paul W. Pruyser); "Pastoral Care of the Terminally Ill" (Phyllis Smyth); "Euthanasia and Assisted Suicide" (pro: Derek Humphrey; con: Cicely Saunders; legal aspects: Edward Keyserlingk); "The Family Facing Death & Bereavement" (Peter Lynch); "The Montreal Bereavement Study" (Margaret Kiely); "Volunteers in Hospice" (Kitty Markey); "Suicide & Its Impact on Survivors" (Edwin Schneidman); "Death the Inner Journey" (John Main); "Suffering as Teacher" (Jean Cameron); "Serving Others" (Thérèse Vanier). Workshops: "Problems in Starting a Hospice" (Dottie Wilson); "Hospice Administration" (John Hackley); "Home Care" (Sue Britton); "Social Worker Role" (Peter Lynch); "Pastoral Care" (Phyllis Smyth); "Children and Death" (Michael Whitehead); "Fund Raising" (David English); "Symptom Control in a General Hospital" (John Scott); "Bereavement" (Mary Vachon); "Volunteers" (Kitty Markey); "Nursing Issues" (Mary Ann Comartin); "Training the Team" (Derek Doyle); "Physicians in Terminal Care" (Dan Hadlock); "Hospice in a Small Community Hospital" (Wilma O'Connell); "Physical & Occupational Therapy" (Francis Howard); "Death Education" (Jack Morgan).

2 The participants included: Bob Fulton, Herman Feifel, Ida Martinsen, Jeanne Quint Benoloil, Inge Corless, Bob Kastenbaum, Myra Bluebond-Langner, John Hinton, Mort White, Mary Vachon, Thelma Bates, Bill Lamers, Lea Baider, Michael Levy, John Fryer, Ina Ajemian, and John Scott.

3 Philip Simmons, *Learning to Fall: The Blessings of an Imperfect Life* (Sandwich, NH: 2000), 13.

4 Vickie's family, the Sixts, were Linda's closest friends; their son was her godson. They had been posted to Hong Kong for two years.

5 28 January 1985: Steve Herbert, RVH executive director, offered welcoming comments; I gave an historical overview; Sue Britton spoke on "The Nature of

Whole Person Care"; and our guest speaker, Dr Dorothy Ley, executive director of the Palliative Care Foundation, addressed "Palliative Care: The Canadian Reality."

6 PCS alumni, January 1985. Nurses: Joan Armstrong, Pat Bartle, Saidie Caplin, Barbara Carter, Mary Carol Case, Barbara Chatterley, Mary Ann Comartin, Ann Dubrovsky, Mabel Dufresne, Elizabeth Emond, Carmen Felisi, Elma Foster, Pat Gladwish, Diane Harder, Dorothy Jacobs, Audrey Kost, Pierrette Lambert, Cathy Macaulay, Pam Manzo-Paz, Denis McLaughlin, Dorothy More, Crystal Mueller, Marjorie Northrup, Ann O'Callaghan, Lorraine Peters, Mary Ann Piette, Jackie Podasky, Sharon Randall, Ursula Rau, Valerie Richards, Dorothy Scofield, Lydia De Simone, Nancy Stevenson, Babs Swami, Janet Taylor, Annette Thibodeau, Rosemary Valenti, Barbara Vessie, Glynis Williams. Physicians: Akos Beszterczey, Warren Bell, Charlie Hackett, Michael Kay, Sharon Mintz, Heather Pushie, John Scott, Janet Christie Seely. Volunteer director: Kitty Markey. Social service: Anne Chant. Music therapy: Susan Munro, Eugene Bereza. Physiotherapy: Sharon Manson, Delia Doutrie; Danielle Poulin. Pastoral care: Sister Brenda Halton, Arlen Bonner, Dale Cuff, Ian Smith. Bereavement coordinator: Ann Hampson. Education coordinators: Jocelyn Tanguay, Susan Dermit. Secretaries: Diane Legault, Maria Pantano, Lorraine Pilon, Rollande Poulin, Ginette Robert, Susan Smyth.

7 Father John had spoken of his dream of oblates living in community in a centrally located high-rise with a mix of private and shared spaces for singles, families, young and old, noting that the facility might be located in the downtown core, not far from the priory.

CHAPTER FIFTEEN

1 Christopher Hibbert, ed., *James Boswell: The Life of Johnson* (Penguin ed., 1979), 231.

2 T. Pyszczynski, S. Solomon, and J. Greenberg: *In the Wake of 9/11: The Psychology of Terror* (Washington, DC: American Psychological Association 2003).

3 John Denver, "Forest Lawn"; The Beatles, "A Day in The Life"; Sting, "Russians"; Paul Simon, "The Boy in the Bubble"; Metallica, "Enter Sandman"; Pink Floyd, "The Wall."

4 Dave Williams, "A Moment in Time," *CMAJ*, 180, no. 13 (2009): 1335.

CHAPTER SIXTEEN

1 Fifth International Congress on Terminal Care, 1–3 October 1984. Plenary sessions: "Hospice in America: The Reality" (Barbara McCann); "Our Greatest Challenges in Palliative Care" (Balfour Mount); "Clinical Pharmacology,

Quality Assurance and Hospice" (Marcus Reidenberg); "The Interdisciplinary Team in the Management of Selected Symptoms" (Mary Baines); "The United States National Hospice Study: A Further Report" (David Greer); "The Meaning of Life Index: A New Outcome Measure in Terminal Care" (Stephanie Shenker and Walter Spitzer); "Non-Verbal Communication: Non-Pharmacologic Support" (Susan Munro); "Sexuality and the Dying Patient" (David Wellisch); "AIDS: Current Concepts" (Daniel William); "The Interdisciplinary Team in the Management of Selected Patients, Part II" (Mary Baines); "Power, Politics and Woman's Work: Nursing in a Changing World" (Jeanne Quint-Benoliel); "Pastoral Care: A Non-Confessional Approach" (Phyllis Smyth); "Stress in Hospice: What Are the Facts?" (Mary Vachon); "Bereavement Counseling" (William Warden); "The Nature of Suffering and the Goals of Medicine" (Eric Cassell); "The Nature of Suffering and the Goals of Hospice" (Thomas West).

Workshops: "Hospice Administration: USA Perspective" (Lynne Côté?); "Home Care" (Sue Britton and Donna Blake); "Social Work" (Peter Lynch); "Pastoral Care" (Phyllis Smyth); "Children & Death" (Dennis O'Connor); "Symptom Control Team in a Hospital" (Marcel Boisvert); "Volunteers" (Mary Coughlan); "Nursing Issues" (Jeanne Belair, Leslie Vincent, and Rhoda Hoffman); "Physicians in Terminal Care" (Dan Hadlock); "Problems for the Rural Hospice" (Sarah Thompson, Judy Lund, and Marjorie Hickey); "Death Education" (Charles Corr).

2 Mother Teresa (1910–97), born Agnes Bojaxhiu in Skopje, Macedonia, experienced a religious calling at age twelve, joined Loreto Sisters of Dublin at eighteen, taught in India for seventeen years (speaking English, Bengali, and Hindi), and then, in 1946, had a further calling to work with the poorest of the poor in Calcutta. She founded the Missionaries of Charity in 1950, establishing a home for the dying, a school, a leper colony, an orphanage, a nursing home, a family clinic, and a series of mobile health clinics. She was awarded the Nobel Peace Prize in 1979 and was canonized in 2016. At her death in 1997, there were 4,000 Sisters of Charity, thousands of lay volunteers, and 610 foundations on all seven continents.

3 Speaking commitments, 1981–85. *Universities: Canada*: Queen's (x5); Dalhousie; McMaster; Calgary; Saskatchewan (at Regina and Saskatoon); Ottawa. *United States*: Penn. State; UCLA; State University of New York (Buffalo). *International*: Bergen (Norway).

Hospitals: Canada: Jewish General (Montreal) (x4); Chest (Montreal); Montreal General Hospital (x2); Queen Elizabeth (Montreal); St Vincent de Paul (Brockville); Elizabeth Bruyère Centre (Ottawa); Homewood Sanitorium (Guelph); St Paul (Saskatoon); Ottawa Civic. *United States*: Memorial (Sarasota, FL); Bon Secours (Grosse Pte, MI); Veterans' Administration Med.

Center (Shreveport, LA); Merch Hospital Oncology Center (Pittsburgh, PA); Grand View (Sillarsville, PA); Cleveland Clinic (x2); Long Island Jewish; Harbor UCLA Medical Center (Tarrence, CA). *International*: Haukeland (Trondheim, Norway); Red Cross (Oslo, Norway).

Meetings: *Canada*: College of Family Physicians of Canada Annual Meeting; Quebec Medical Secretaries Annual Meeting; Women's College Hospital Medical Staff Annual Meeting; BC Medical Association Annual Meeting; 6th World Congress of International College of Psychosomatic Medicine; Royal College of Physicians and Dentists; La Fondation québécoise du Cancer; Anglican Synod of Bishops; Royal College of Physicians and Surgeons of Canada; International Congresses on Care of the Terminally Ill (l982, 1984); Newfoundland/Labrador Hospital Association; Canadian Cancer Society; Ontario Medical Student Symposium; Palliative Care Work Group (Ontario); Society of GYN/OB Oncologists; Canadian National Conference on Palliative Care; King's College Conference on Children and Death; Quebec Cancer Foundation Annual Meeting. *United States*: New England Cancer Society Annual Meeting; Northeast Canadian-American Health Council; Genesee Region Home Care Association; Vermont Medical Association; American Society of Consultant Pharmacists Annual Meeting; NHO Annual Meeting; New York Cancer Society Annual Meeting; Catholic Health Association of the United States Annual Meeting; Ontario Psychiatrists Association; *American Journal of Hospice Care* National Conference; Richmond Academy of Medicine (VA); Annual Cancer Symposia for Nurses and Physicians (San Diego, CA); Connecticut Hospice (New Haven); Florida State Hospice Association meeting. *International*: IWG (Rosenon, Sweden); 9th International Seminar of Life Planning Center (Tokyo, Japan); seminars (Kyoto and Osaka, Japan); Seminar on Palliative Medicine (Sydney, Australia); Norwegian National Conference on Palliative Care (Loen, Norway); International Conference on Terminal Care (London); Australian National Meeting on Hospice Care (Adelaide); International Symposium on Human Value (London); St Christopher's Hospice (London).

4 I remained director of Palliative Care McGill, a network of programs in McGill-affiliated hospitals, the biennial McGill International Congresses, and the Montreal Children's Hospital needs-assessment study. I would also continue as an RVH PCS physician.

5 Kollwitz found haunting beauty in the plight of the anguished and downtrodden. Her deepening empathy through life would be hard-earned. Peter, the youngest of her two sons, was killed in the First World War; her beloved grandson of the same name, in the Second. She became the voice of the imprisoned, the starving, the helpless, the raped, and the dying. She was evacuated from her long-time Berlin home in 1943 shortly before it was bombed (with the loss of

many of her drawings, prints, and documents). She died just before the end of the war. Naomi Blumberg, "Kathe Kollowitz: German Artist," *Encyclopedia Britannica*, 2019, www.britannica.com/biography/Kathe-Kollwitz.

6 Ruth Leger Sivard, *World Military and Social Expenditure*, vol. 16, 1996, 7.

7 Bernard Grun, *The Timetables of History*, 3rd rev. ed. (New York: Simon and Schuster 1991), 613.

8 Leonard Cohen, Sony Music Entertainment, 1992.

9 The committee of twenty-six included nine nurses, five pediatricians, four parents, two child-life specialists, two social workers, one administrator, one ethicist, one psychologist, and one palliative-care physician. One of the nurses, Linda McHarg, a McGill PhD candidate, played an invaluable liaison and leadership role. Seven areas of inquiry were initiated: 1) Demographics (age and diagnosis) for five years of MCH deaths; 2) Key Person semi-structured interviews of MCH staff concerning existing resources, problems, and suggestions; 3) Staff and parent survey (multiple-choice questionnaire) relating to children dying during 1984–85; 4) Case studies (selected problems in terminal care); 5) Physical-resource assessment, all wards; 6) Review of previous MCH studies in target areas; 7) Study of trial bereavement-support program (offering pre-death, at death, and post-death support) – PhD project, L. McHarg.

10 Bob Geldof, *Is That It?* (London: Penguin Books 1986), 20–1.

11 Sixth International Congress on Care of the Terminally Ill, 27 September-1 October 1986. The remaining plenary sessions included one on "Hospice an International Response": Tibet (Queen medical student Bob Clendenning); New Zealand (Richard Turnbull); Norway (John Mauritzen); Italy (Georgio Di Mola). The vulnerability of life in our global village was suggested once again when a planned participant from Gdansk, Poland, Father Eugeniusz Dutkiewicz, was unable to be with us because of his arrest and impending trial as a member of the Polish Solidarity Union. Other plenary sessions addressed "The Deepening Shade: The Psychological Aspects of Life-Threatening Illness" (Harvard psychologist Barbara Sourkes); "Life Transitions & the Human Response to Change" (Colin Murray Parkes of St Christopher's Hospice, the Royal London Hospital Medical College, and the Tavistock Institute of Human Relations); "Ethical Considerations in Life/Death Decisions" (Edmond Pellegrino, American ethicist, medical historian, philosopher, and pioneer in teaching humanities as part of the medical-school curriculum); "The Thanatology Movement: Yesterday's Successes & Today's Challenges" (Herman Feifel, the American psychologist whose publication *The Meaning of Death* in 1959 broke the taboo on discussions of death and dying and established it as a legitimate field for scholarly and scientific study). Feifel also participated with Edmund Pellegrino and Phyllis Smyth in a lively exchange on "The Overlap between Humanism, Spirituality, Religion & Philosophy."

Delegates participated in workshops covering a wide range of clinical and research issues, the faculty including: Robert Twycross, Declan Walsh, Robert Buckman, Ben Crul, Gerry Wiviott, Judith Vogel, Jean Cameron, Lorine Besel, Joyce Clifford, Norman Paul, Jean-Paul and Rejeanne Blais, Therese Rando, Jacques Voyer, Marcel Boisvert, Michael Simpson, June Penney, Lesley Degner, Eduardo Bruera, Martin Levitt, Harvey Schipper, Gordon Lang, Barry De Veber, Paul Henteleff, Elizabeth Latimer, Frank Brescia, Jeanne Belair, Irene Corbett, Linda Edgar, Lynda Kabbash, Claire Lavirne-Pley, H. Rapin, D.R. Longo, R.D. Narkiewicz, Anne Rooney, Susan Warner, A.M. Wald, Betty Ferrell, Rosemary Fry, J.M. Hall, Linda Kristjanson, Karen Wright, N.R. Stearns, Ulla Qvarnstrom, L. Platt, L. Scruby, S. Dubik-Unruh, C. Wares, Roger Branch, Monroe Wright, Maurice Lamm, Clyde Nabe, Robert Jenks, S. Brissettee, Lucie Fréchette, Sarie Mai, Claudia Ospovat.

12 Based on Dr Eitinger's work, the World Health Organization reversed the long-standing assumption that a chronic psychiatric disorder indicated premorbid vulnerability, devising in 1992 a new category, "enduring personality change after catastrophic experience," and thus laying the foundations for the concept of post-traumatic stress disorder. In 1980 Eitinger and colleague Lars Weisath documented the "Stochkolm Syndrome." Tessa Chelouche, "Leo Eitinger MD: Tribute to a Holocaust Survivor, Humane Physician and Friend of Mankind," *IMAJ*, 16 (April 2014): 208–11.

13 Elie Wiesel was sixteen years old in January 1945 when his right foot began to swell with frostbite. Continuing ability to work in the labour camp depended on immediate surgery. Dr Eitinger examined him, arranged for the surgery to take place the next day, and reassured Wiesel, "Don't be afraid. Everything will be alright." Years later, in his book *Night*, Wiesel wrote: "At ten o'clock in the morning they took me into the operating room. 'My doctor' was there. I took comfort from this. I felt that nothing serious could happen to me while he was there. There was balm in every word he spoke and every glance he gave held a message of hope." Elie Wiesel, *The Night Trilogy: Night, Dawn, The Accident* (New York: Hill and Wang 2000). Also, Eddy Polak, personal discussion, 2014.

14 "Current World Population," *Worldometers: Real-time World Statistics*, www.worldometers.info/world-population/.

15 "World Population by Year," *Worldometers: Real-time World Statistics*, www.worldometers.info/world-population/world-population-by-year/.

16 David Biello, "Human Population Reaches 7 Billion: How Did This Happen and Can It Go On?" *Scientific American*, 28 October 2011, www.scientificamerican.com/article/human-population-reaches-seven-billion/.

17 "Global Climate Change: Vital Signs of the Planet," National Aeronautics and Space Administration, 2019, www.climate.nasa.gov/evidence/.

18 W.R.L. Anderegg, "Expert Credibility in Climate Change," *Proceedings of the National Academy of Sciences*, 107, no. 27 (21 June 2010): 12107–09; DOI: 10.1073/pnas.1003187107.

19 James A. Folley, "Seven Nations Contributed to 60 Percent of Global Warming: Study," *Nature World News*, 16 January 2014, www.natureworldnews.com/articles/5664/20140116/seven-nations-contributed-60-percent-global-warming-study.htm.

20 John Upton, "Super Euros: Top 10 Climate-Change-Fighting Countries Are All in Europe," *Grist*, 20 November 2013, www.grist.org/news/the-top-10-climate-change-fighting-countries-are-all-in-europe/.

21 "The Stock Market: Bulls, Bears, Booms, and Busts," CBC Archives, www.cbc.ca/archives/categories/economy-business/stock-market/the-stock-market-bulls-bears-booms-and-busts/1987-black-monday-hits-worlds-stock-markets.html.

22 Grun, *The Timetables of History*, 618, 620.

23 RVH Annual Report, 1981.

24 Terry Neville, *The Royal Vic. 1894–1994* (Montreal and Kingston: McGill Queen's University Press 1994), 199–201.

25 Dr L.J. de Souza noted the opening of palliative-care ashrams in Bombay and Goa; Mrs C. Couvreur, president of Continuing Care in Brussels, reported news of a new home-care program and plans for a PCU; Professor Eric Wilkes, at the pioneering St Luke's Nursing Home, Sheffield, UK, stated that a working party was planned to explore the possible development of new hospices for children; our 1986–87 trainee Harri Helle, in Helsinki, sent word of developing palliative-care programs in Finland; and from Dr Maurice Abivan at l'Hôpital International de l'Université de Paris, there was word of their newly opened PCU. Dr Douglas MacAdam, head, Department of Community Practice, University of Western Australia, wrote to inform us of the opening of the "Cottage Hospice," a new, purpose-built, twenty-five-bed facility, and word arrived from M.E. Kingsley in Seoul Korea about the work of their Hospice Committee at the one-thousand-bed Severance Hospital and Cancer Treatment Centre of Yonsei University and their plans for a palliative home-care program. Mun Wan Chan-Ho, a lecturer in clinical psychology at the Chinese University of Hong Kong, visited us to discuss her planned QOL research, and there was a report from Dr S.L. Erel in Toledo, Ohio, about a new World Health Organization project in Cancer Pain Relief for the Toledo region. Closer to home, Professor Neil MacDonald in Edmonton indicated that plans were afoot for a PCU to complement the existing palliative consultation and home-care programs at the University of Alberta hospitals, while colleagues at Calgary's Rockyview General Hospital wrote to inform us of their expanding palliative-care program.

26 The gifts were donated or purchased with the money raised through a volunteer fundraising project. Examples of items on the gift cart: stuffed toys,

candles, handkerchiefs, scarves, window bird feeders, toiletries, candy, picture frames, ornaments, novelty items, and games. The stockings were filled with such items as lip balm, assorted herbal teas, moisturizing lotion, home-made jellies, candy, Christmas ornaments, and so on.

27 Our first paper was "Quality of Life in Terminal Illness: Defining and Measuring Subjective Well-Being in the Dying," *Journal of Palliative Care*, 8, no. 3 (1992): 40–5. Then came, with John Scott, "Status of Cancer Pain and Palliative Care in Canada," *Journal of Pain & Symptom Management*, 8, no. 6 (1993): 395–8; "Phototherapy in the Treatment of Depression in the Terminally Ill," *Journal of Pain & Symptom Management*, 9, no. 8 (1994): 534–6; and, as a product of our synergistic discussions with Neil MacDonald and Eduardo Bruera, "Ethical Issues in Palliative Care Research Revisited," *Palliative Medicine*, 9 (1995): 79–80.

28 S.R. Cohen, B.M. Mount, M.G. Strobel, and F. Bui, "The McGill Quality of Life Questionnaire: A Measure of Quality of Life Appropriate for People with Advanced Disease. A Preliminary Study of Validity and Acceptability," *Palliative Medicine*, 9 (1995): 207–19; B.M. Mount and S.R. Cohen, "Quality of Life in Terminal Cancer Patients" (presented as keynote address at the 1995 Hospice Congress in Taipei, Taiwan, 29 July 1995), *Journal of the Hospice Foundation of Taiwan* (in Mandarin), 18 (1995): 8–16; B.M. Mount, "Quality of Life in Terminal Care Patients," *Journal of the Hospice Foundation of the Republic of China*, 18 (September 1995): 9–16; B.M. Mount and S.R. Cohen, "Quality of Life in the Face of Life-Threatening Illness: What Should We Be Measuring?: *Current Oncology*, 2, no. 3 (September 1995): 121–5; S.R. Cohen, S.A. Hassan, B.J. Lapointe, and B.M. Mount, "Quality of Life in HIV Disease as Measured by the McGill Quality of Life Questionnaire," AIDS, 10 (1996): 1421–7; S.R. Cohen, B.M. Mount, and N. MacDonald, "Defining Quality of Life," editorial in *European Journal of Cancer*, 32A, 5 (1996): 753–4; S.R. Cohen, B.M. Mount, J. Tomas, and L. Mount, "Existential Well-Being Is an Important Determinant of Quality of Life: Evidence from the McGill Quality of Life Questionnaire, *Cancer*, 77, no. 3 (1996): 576; B.M. Mount and S.R. Cohen, "Quality of Life in Patients with Life-Threatening Illness in Death and the Quest for Meaning," in Stephen Strack and Herman Feifel, eds., *Death and the Quest for Meaning: Essays in Honor of Herman Feifel* (New Jersey: Jason Aronson 1997), 137–52; S.R. Cohen et al., "Validity of the McGill Quality of Life Questionnaire in the Palliative Care Setting: A Multi-Center Canadian Study Demonstrating the Importance of the Existential Domain," *Palliative Medicine*, 11 (1997): 3–20; S.R. Cohen et al., "Well-Being at the End of Life: Part 1, A Research Agenda for Psychosocial and Spiritual Aspects of Care from the Patient's Perspective; Part 2, A Research Agenda for

the Delivery of Care from the Patient's Perspective," *Cancer Prevention & Control*, 11 (1997).

29 Adaptation to illness may entail a "response shift," that is, a change in the individual's empiric QOL score resulting from: 1) changes in the person's internal standards of measurement (scale recalibration in psychometric terms); 2) changes in values (the perceived importance of domains determining QOL); or 3) a redefinition of QOL (reconceptualization). M.A.G. Sprangers and C.E. Schwartz, "Integrating Response Shift into Health-Related QOL Research: A Theoretical Model," *Society of Science and Medicine*, 48 (1999); 1507–15.

30 J.E. Bower et al., "Cognitive Processing, Discovery of Meaning, CD4 Decline and AIDS-Related Mortality among HIV-Seropositive Men," *Journal of Consultative Clinical Psychology*, 66, no. 6 (1998): 979–86.

31 Balfour Mount, P.H. Boston, and S.R. Cohen, "Healing Connections: On Moving from Suffering to a Sense of Well-Being," *Journal of Pain and Symptom Management*, 33 (2007): 372–88. Twenty-five candidates met the selection criteria; of these, four declined to sign the consent form and eight were unable to complete more than one ninety-minute interview owing to death, progressive weakness, or increasing priority of other issues. The remaining thirteen subjects participated in at least three interviews. (Total number of interviews, fifty-four.) Subject accrual continued until additional data failed to lead to further development of the suggested properties in the target categories. Three (more, as required) semi-structured interviews, designed according to accepted qualitative techniques, were conducted with each participant in order to explore the "inner-life" experiences prior to and during illness. Interview Guideline Topics included: the meaning of "spirituality" and "inner life" for the patient; the influence of these domains in shaping the experience of illness; evolution of QOL over the illness; perception of pain and suffering; patient response to caregiver initiatives; communication issues; the meaning and purpose of life; illness beliefs and cultural issues; ethical issues; the quality and meaning of family and caregiver relationships; and sense of personal health. Pre-study trials suggested that synergistic value was achieved by joint interviewing (Boston and Mount), with one alternately being assigned to record field-note observations. Independent thematic analysis of the transcribed interviews was followed by a detailed iterative discussion according to Moustakas's reflective process of data analysis. Major emerging themes across cases were determined according to accepted qualitative strategies.

32 G.L. Fricchione, *Compassion and Healing in Medicine and Society: On the Nature and Use of Attachment Solutions to Separation Challenge* (Baltimore, MD: Johns Hopkins University Press 2011).

33 P.H. Boston and B.M. Mount, "The Caregiver's Perspective on Existential and Spiritual Distress in Palliative Care," *Journal of Pain and Symptom Management*, 32 (2006): 13–26.

CHAPTER SEVENTEEN

1 Joe Romm, "World's Scientists Warn: We Have 'High Confidence' 'in the 'Irreversible Impacts' of Climate Inaction," *Think Progress*, 2 November 2014, www.thinkprogress.org/climate/2014/11/02/3587485/climate-panel-final-plea/. Physicist and climate expert J. Romm, holder of a PhD from MIT, is a senior fellow at the Center for American Progress and is the founding editor of *Climate Progress*. In 1997 he was acting assistant secretary of the U.S. Department of Energy, responsible for energy efficiency and renewable energy, where he oversaw $1 billion in R&D and demonstration and deployment of low-carbon technology. His books include *Hell & High Water*, *Straight Up*, and *Language Intelligence*. He was chief science adviser for the 2014 Emmy Award-winning documentary series *Years of Living Dangerously*.

2 "Climate Change 2014 Synthesis Report Summary for Policymakers," *Intergovernmental Panel on Climate Change*, www.ipcc.ch/pdf/assessment-report/ar5/syr/AR5_SYR_FINAL_SPM.pdf.

3 Kevin van Paassen, "Canada Dead Last in Ranking for Environmental Protection," *Globe and Mail*, 31 August 2010, www.theglobeandmail.com/news/world/canada-ead-last-in-oecd-ranking-for-environmental-protection/article15484134/.

4 Personal communication. Among his many accomplishments, Dr Doyle led the negotiating team which saw palliative medicine become a medical specialty in Great Britain; he co-founded the Association for Palliative Medicine of Great Britain and was its first president; he was first chairman of the Committee for Professional Education in Palliative Care for Europe; he was co-editor and contributor to the *Oxford Textbook of Palliative Medicine*; he co-founded and was first editor-in-chief of the journal *Palliative Medicine* and has served on eight editorial boards of palliative-care journals worldwide.

5 The Task Force included: Drs I. Cummings-Ajemian, F. Burge, L. Dionne, M. Downing, N. MacDonald, B. Mount, J. Poulson, J. Scott, M. Scott; and legal adviser Neil Roberts. The potential for the College of Family Medicine and the Royal College to jointly promote palliative medicine through a two-year training program subsequent to certification by either college was considered by both colleges and it was suggested that the Quebec College might be a third licensing body. The document "Palliative Medicine: Toward Recognition as a Discipline in Canada" was presented to the relevant directors of both the Royal College and the College of Family Physicians at a joint meeting

in May 1994. A senior Royal College spokesman called the document "the strongest application for discipline recognition that the Royal College has received in a decade."

6 Neil MacDonald, Personal communication.

7 "OMA Palliative Care: Backgrounder," OMA's *End of Life Care Strategy*, April 2014, www.oma.org/Resources/Documents/PalliativeCare.pdf.

8 Dr Shigeaki Hinohara was born in 1911. He was a cardiologist and is said to have authored 150 books and numerous medical articles. At age 101, he remained professionally active as an author and educator, as the head of five foundations and president of St Luke's International Hospital, Tokyo, and as patron of the Asia Pacific Hospice Palliative Care Network.

9 M. Kearney and B. Mount, "Spiritual Care of the Dying Patient," in *Handbook of Psychiatry in Palliative Medicine*, Harvey M. Chochinov and William Breittbart, eds. (New York: Oxford University Press 2000), 357–73.

10 At successive Congresses I invited Michael to present a stream of rich, informative seminars and master classes: "Suffering and the Human Spirit," "Image Work in Pain Management," "Using Imagery in Patient Care and Teaching," "Who Am I Who Cares?" (a master class with Nurse-Tutor Anne Hayes, Dublin), "Western Traditions of Spirituality and Healing in Health Care" (examining the ancient foundations of Western medicine, both Hippocratic and Asklepian, on the Greek island of Kos, the birthplace of Hippocrates), "Working with Dreams in Palliative Care," "Suffering, Healing & the Limits of Medicine: A Dialogue with Dan Callahan, the Hastings Center New York, and Michael Kearney," and "Teaching Holistic Care in a Clinical Setting."

11 Kearney and Mount, "Spiritual Care of the Dying Patient."

12 Notes for "Reflections v: 'I & Thou,'" International Congress, 28 September 2000; Parker Palmer, *Let Your Life Speak* (San Francisco: Jossey-Bass 2000).

13 Terror Management Theory linking death anxiety and the need for self-esteem is based on the research of Ernest Becker (see the Pulitzer Prize-winning *The Denial of Death*, 1973) and of S. Solomon, J. Greenberg, and T. Pyszczynski (*The Worm at the Core: On the Role of Death in Life*, 2015).

14 Palliative Care McGill was created by me with the support of Dean Cruess in July 1991 as a means of developing an interactive palliative-care system in McGill-affiliated hospitals; as well, two hospitals acquired "McGill-affiliated" status for palliative care only – Mt. Sinai and Notre Dame de la Merci – thus fostering development of shared standards of clinical care and enhanced capability for research and teaching. In November 1994 the nine hospitals involved were Royal Victoria Hospital, Montreal General Hospital, Jewish General Hospital, Mt Sinai Hospital, Notre Dame de la Merci, St Mary's Hospital, Queen Elizabeth Hospital, Montreal Children's Hospital, and

Douglas Hospital. They provided a total daily census of 66 PCU beds, 70–102 consult patients, and 148–93 home-care patients.

15 Those copied on the letter were Drs Sylvia Cruess, Henry Shibata, Richard Cruess (dean), Gordon Crelinsten, and Claude Forget, chairman of the board, RVH.

16 On 17 November I received a copy of a letter written by the head nurse of an RVH surgical ward. It was addressed to the Nursing Council (responsible for the quality of nursing care). In it she documented the unrelieved pain that one of their patients had suffered as a result of the bed closures. Having pointed out that in the past such a patient would be rated *high priority* for PCU transfer within twenty-four hours, she noted that with the bed closures the patient remained on the surgical ward for days. The head nurse closed with this observation: "Despite our best efforts in using the expertise of PCS consultants, we were unsuccessful at bringing her pain under control. The one other option for Mrs T. would be to insert an epidural catheter with an ongoing infusion drip of anesthesia by this route. That would require a specialized infusion pump, inservice education as well as the support of the anesthetist who works with PCU. This was a familiar procedure for the PCU staff. The PCU is extremely responsive, but they are restrained by resources. I felt it important to bring this case to your attention to illustrate how monetary decisions can impact on quality of care." During this same period, the administrative fusion of the RVH and the Montreal General occurred and plans were established to close three Montreal hospitals serving the anglophone community since the nineteenth century: the Queen Elizabeth (1894), the Reddy Memorial (1870), and the Catherine Booth (1890).

17 While she was not given to public pronouncements, Kappy's quiet determination brings to mind the unrelenting effectiveness of a heat-seeking missile. Once convinced, she plans. With plans in place, she makes it happen. In 1972 Kappy had organized and led the first Women's Mission to Israel. In 1974 she was elected president of Women's Division, United Israel Appeal of Canada; in 1973/74 she was chairman of Women's Division, Combined Jewish Appeal and National Missions. In 1982 she organized the vernissage of the Precious Legacy Exhibition at the Montreal Museum of Fine Arts for the Jewish Community Foundation. She also had acted as chairman of the Israel Cancer Research Fund and its fundraising gala. Among the many rewards Kappy would receive from a grateful nation were: the Governor General of Canada's Meritorious Service Award (2003), a McGill University Honorary Doctorate of Laws (2009), the Queen Elizabeth II Diamond Jubilee Medal (2013), and the Order of Canada (2015).

18 Indeed, as the years passed, the ripple effects of the Eric M. Flanders Chair continued to extend in a manner that was astounding: enhanced community trust and support; increased administrative motivation for the continued

existence of Palliative Care McGill and our related teaching and research activities; support for creation of the McGill Programs in Integrated Whole Person Care; support for the two-year part-time visiting professorship of Dr Michael Kearney to study concepts related to healing in the undergraduate and graduate medical setting, resulting in recommended curriculum changes in McGill undergraduate medical training; support for recruiting Dr Tom Hutchinson to develop the Centre for Integrative Medicine at McGill; the establishment of a remarkable list of annual public-education lecture series at McGill (including "Mini-Med," "Mini-Science," "Mini-Law," "Mini-Music," "Mini-Biz," "Mini Ed-Psych," "Mini-Enviro," and "Mini-Pharma"); Kappy's election to McGill Board of Governors; the creation of an extended community through the hosting of countless guests in all settings, from annual formal banquets to more intimate affairs in Kappy's home.

19 Neil completed medical studies at McGill and then post-graduate training at the Royal Vic and Memorial Sloan Kettering Cancer Center prior to returning to McGill where he founded the Royal Vic Oncology Day Centre and served as a Faculty of Medicine associate dean. In 1971 he was named director of Edmonton's Cross Cancer Institute, later becoming director of the Division of Oncology, University of Alberta, and executive director of the Provincial Cancer Hospitals Board. He served as medical oncology chief examiner for the Royal College (1987–90), president of the Canadian Oncology Society, chairman of the Service to Patients Committee of the Canadian Cancer Society, and chairman and secretary-treasurer of the Finance Committee of the American Society of Clinical Oncology. Following a sabbatic year in palliative medicine at McGill (1980–81), he was named professor of palliative medicine and was recipient of the first Canadian Chair in Palliative Medicine in Canada (1987). Subsequently, he coordinated development of the undergraduate medical Canadian Palliative Care Curriculum and was co-editor of the highly acclaimed *Oxford Textbook of Palliative Medicine*. In 1994 Neil was chairman of the newly formed Canadian Society of Palliative Care Physicians, which worked toward Royal College acceptance of palliative medicine as a recognized discipline. In 1990–91 he worked as medical officer in the Cancer/Palliative Care Unit at the World Health Organization's Geneva office. His research interests have included: ethical issues in clinical trials and in palliative care, the role of chronic inflammation in cancer syndromes, the cancer cachexia syndrome, and cancer-patient selection for early palliative support.

20 Participants at the 16 June 1995 meeting were: Principal Shapiro, Dean Abe Fuks, Kappy Flanders, Richard Pound, David Bourke, Gerard Douville, Charles McDougall, Richard Cruess, Sylvia Cruess, Brian Leyland-Jones, David Goltzman, Mona Kravitz, Henry Shibata, Larry Stein, Gordon Crelinsten, Jean Morin, and Joy Shannon.

CHAPTER EIGHTEEN

1 The reflections of John Shelby Spong on God as metaphor are included here with his kind permission (2009).

2 P.W. Martin notes that by "Deep Centre" he means the germinal higher part of the person, the element of our being that is conterminous and continuous with "the More," an aspect of our personhood that has been recognized and variously named in all wisdom traditions. P.W. Martin, *Experiment in Depth: A Study of the Work of Jung, Eliot and Toynbee* (Boston: Routledge and Kegan Paul 1955), 132–5.

3 W.H. Vanstone, *The Stature of Waiting* (Harrisburg, PA: Morehouse Publishing 1982) 79–87.

4 Florence spent the final year of her life on the PCU. One day early in her admission, a young McGill medical student and Keevin Robbins, a volunteer with several years' experience, found themselves at her bedside struggling to understand Florence's evident anguish. It was during our pre-alphabet-board days and her futile gestures became increasingly frantic as she repeatedly, silently, struggled to make them understand. Finally, a shot in the dark. Did she want the window open a little? "Yes!!" her contorted face silently shouted in reply as she sank back into her pillow. They hastily complied, and then Keevin and the student departed, totally exhausted. Once in the hall they spontaneously turned to each other, hugged each other tightly, and burst into tears, telling evidence of the daunting level at which they had set their expectations in their effort to provide whole-person care. The medical student, Krista Lawlor, would in due course join our team to become a peerless and universally loved physician, teacher, and mentor for us all, while Keevin became my fellow traveller in exploring issues contemplative and my weekly meditation partner.

5 Bede Griffiths: *The Golden String* (1954), *Return to the Centre* (1976), *The Marriage of East and West* (1982), *A New Vision of Reality* (1990), *The Universal Christ: Daily Readings with Bede Griffiths* (1990), *A New Creation in Christ* (1992).

6 S. Du Boulay, *Beyond the Darkness: A Biography of Bede Griffiths* (London: Rider 1998).

7 Our New Harmony, Indiana, gathering got off to a bumpy start for Laurence, Bede, and the core group of organizers. Our distinguished guest, now eighty-four, had flowing white hair and beard, a saffron robe, high-pitched Oxford accent, and twinkling, effervescent eyes. To the locals he undoubtedly suggested nothing quite so much as a Cecil B. DeMille casting reject. We had descended on a town whose character and name, New Harmony, appeared to constitute an oxymoron as the burly Good Old Boy burghers greeted us by flexing their all-too-evident prejudices while repeatedly demanding to know who Bede and

Laurence were and what it was that they were about that might upset *their* New Harmony. Laurence found his customary patience and compassion on edge as concern for the well-being of our speaker became a consideration. Our hosts were suspicious. We were planning to do what? Discuss the challenges of siting still? While doing nothing? And saying nothing? It seemed to them that this group needed watching. And that they did, although generally at a distance. Nevertheless, the final service in the community chapel featured the muffled thunder of a half-ton pickup and an additional car or two which pulled up at the door in mid-proceedings to disgorge their brawny occupants, who entered our cloistered meeting to form a threatening row along the rear wall, arms folded across their chests, as they scrutinized the peculiar celebrant at the front. In turn, I found it important to join their line as a precautionary gesture. Ah, the joy of exploring New Harmony.

8 By 2015, the World Community for Christian Meditation had grown to nearly 3,000 meditation groups meeting weekly in more than 100 countries, 63 of them having national coordinators.

9 Ernest Becker, *The Denial of Death* (New York: Macmillan 1973).

10 Irvin D. Yalom, *Existential Psychotherapy* (New York: Basic Books 1980).

11 For a comprehensive summary of Terror Management Theory, see T. Pyszczynski, S. Solomon, and J. Greenberg, *In the Wake of 9/11: The Psychology of Terror* (Washington, DC: American Psychological Association 2003), and the 2006 prize-winning documentary film *Flight from Death: The Quest For Immortality.*

12 "Liepzig Gewandhaus Orchestra," *Wikipedia*, www.en.wikipedia.org/wiki/Leipzig_Gewandhaus_Orchestra. The Gewandhausorchester was founded in 1743 and inaugurated its new home, the Gewandhaus, in 1781. The storied history of the orchestra includes its 1789 concert with Mozart, the premiere of Beethoven's 5th Piano Concerto (1811), and the first complete cycle of Beethoven's symphonies (1825–26). Medelssohn became its conductor in 1835. His *Scottish Symphony* and Violin Concerto in E were both premiered there, as were symphonies by Schubert and Schumann. Other premieres, conducted by the composer, included Richard Wagner's *Meistersinger Prelude* and Johannes Brahms's Violin Concerto. In 1884 the orchestra moved to its new concert hall, where they hosted, among others, conducting their own works, Johannes Brahms, Peter Tchaikovsky, Edvard Grieg, and Richard Strauss. Anton Bruckner gave an organ recital in the hall. Following various temporary post-Second World War homes, the New Gewandhaus opened in 1981, the only dedicated concert hall to be built in the former Communist East Germany. The orchestra also performs in the Leipzig Opera and in St Thomas's Church, offering an unparalleled symphonic, operatic, and sacred repertoire. (Notes by Claudius Bohm.)

13 Eric J. Cassell, "The Nature of Suffering and the Goals of Medicine," *New England Journal of Medicine*, 306 (1982): 639–45.

14 H. Schipper, "Guidelines and Caveats for Quality of Life Measurement in Clinical Practice and Research," *Oncology*, 5, no. 5 (1990): 51–7.

15 S.R. Cohen and B.M. Mount, "Quality of Life in Terminal Illness: Defining and Measuring Subjective Well-Being in the Dying," *Journal of Palliative Care*, 8, no. 3 (1992): 40–5; S.R. Cohen, B.M. Mount, M.G. Strobel, and F. Bui, "The McGill Quality of Life Questionnaire: A Measure of Quality of Life Appropriate for People with Advanced Disease. A Preliminary Study of Validity and Acceptability," *Palliative Medicine*, 9 (1995): 207–19; S.R. Cohen, S.A. Hassan, B.J. Lapointe, and B.M. Mount, "Quality of Life in HIV Disease as Measured by the McGill Quality of Life Questionnaire," *AIDS*, 10 (1996) 1421–7; S.R. Cohen, B.M. Mount, J. Tomas, and L. Mount, "Existential Well-Being Is an Important Determinant of Quality of Life: Evidence from the McGill Quality of Life Questionnaire," *Cancer*, 77, no. 3 (1996): 576.

16 In the Dalai Lama's 1994 John Main Seminar, he presented, from a Buddhist perspective, his reflections concerning various tenets of Christianity: loving your enemy, the Sermon on the Mount, the Beatitudes, equanimity, the Kingdom of God, the transfiguration, faith, and the resurrection. These talks were published as *The Good Heart* (Boston: Wisdom Publications 1996).

17 Born in 1935, Tenzin Gyatso was enthroned in Lhasa in 1940 as the fourteenth Dalai Lama. He assumed full political powers over Tibet in 1950 at the age of fifteen as the Chinese People's Liberation Army invaded the country. His desire to see Tibet function as an autonomous region within the People's Republic of China was rejected by China and during the Tibetan uprising of 1959 he escaped to India. He was awarded the Nobel Peace Prize in 1989 in recognition of his service to humanity, his advocacy on behalf of the people of Tibet, his global teaching of Tibetan Buddhism, and his lifelong interest in the link between modern science and Buddhism. In addition, he has been a tireless advocate for the environment, non-violence, interfaith dialogue, physics, astronomy, women's rights, and reproductive health. He is a rare gift to humanity as a champion of peace, dialogue, and community, and as an explorer of human potential in the face of suffering.

18 *The Four Noble Truths:* 1) the inevitability of suffering in life; 2) the source of suffering is ego-generated desires and reactions; 3) our capacity to be free from attachment to desire; 4) the way to end suffering that is the eightfold path. *The Eightfold Path:* 1) Right Viewpoint – to view things negatively so that results are better than expected; 2) Right Values – commitment to mental and ethical growth in moderation; 3) Right Speech – to speak in a non-hurtful, not exaggerated, truthful way; 4) Right Actions – wholesome actions, avoiding harm;

5) Right Livelihood – taking a job that does not harm self or others, directly or indirectly; 6) Right Effort – working to improve; 7) Right Mindfulness – ability to see with clarity things as they are; 8) Right Meditation – state of enlightenment and loss of ego.

19 Jack Kevorkian (1928–2011) was an American pathologist and euthanasia activist.

20 R. Brownrigg, *Who's Who in the New Testament* (London: Weidenfeld and Nicolson 1971), 254.

21 A. Humphreys and A. Tilbury, *Israel & the Palestinian Territories: Lonely Planet Travel Survival Kit* (London: Lonely Planet Publications 1996), 177.

22 The Russian Church of the Ascension; Mosque of the Ascension; Church of the Paternoster; Tombs of the Prophets; Dominus Flevit Chapel; Church of St Mary Magdalene; Church of All Nations; and Tomb of the Virgin.

23 Historical references to Jesus outside the books of the New Testament are scarce but sufficient to support his historicity. They include: two references by the historian Josephus (Christopher Price, "Did Josephus Refer to Jesus? A Thorough Review of the Testimonium Flavianum," *Bede's Library*, www.bede. org.uk/Josephus.htm); a letter of Pliny the Younger when he was governor of Bithynia; an allusion to his work by the historian Tacitus; references to him in the Talmud that depict him as a rabbi, list his disciples, refer to his execution, and condemn him for "practising sorcery and leading Israel astray." Brownrigg, *Who's Who in the New Testament*, 155.

24 Stanislao Loffreda, *Recovering Capharnaumi* (Jerusalem: Franciscan Printing Press 1993).

25 Ibid., 51.

26 These lines from the *Tao Te Ching*, chapter 42, as translated by Stephen Mitchell, come to mind as I recall St Colman's cave. Appropriately, this inspired and highly recommended text was a gift from my long-time mentor, Michael Kearney. Stephen Mitchell, *Tao Te Ching, A New English Version* (New York: Harper and Row 1988).

CHAPTER NINETEEN

1 Cicely Saunders, *Beyond the Horizon: A Search for Meaning in Suffering* (London: Darton, Longman and Todd 1990), 2.

CHAPTER TWENTY

1 Philip Simmons, *Learning to Fall: The Blessings of an Imperfect Life* (Center Sandwich, NH: Home Farm Books 2000), Foreword.

2 Laurence Freeman, Personal communication.

3 The pope later invited her to Assisi in 2002. A year later, in 2003, he hosted
   Lena and her family (including Michel and his children) at a birthday party he
   held for her at the Vatican. During this glorious event she presented to him her
   book tracing their shared dreams, *Building Bridges: Pope John Paul II and the
   Horizon of Life*. In his warm response, he thanked her "for seeing deep into
   my thoughts and understanding the intentions guiding my actions." The
   correspondence and visits continued until his death in 2005 when Lena was
   honoured to have a private viewing at her friend's coffin and to be seated with
   the papal household during the service that followed.
4 All Philip Simmons quotes are from his *Learning to Fall*.
5 Jean Vanier, *Seeing beyond Depression* (Mahwah, NJ: Paulist Press 2001).
6 Cicely Saunders, *Watch with Me: Inspiration for a Life in Hospice Care*
   (Sheffield, UK: Mortal Press 2003), 15.
7 Cicely Saunder, "Faith," in ibid., 16–17.
8 Joseph Campbell, *The Power of Myth* (New York: Doubleday 1988), 123.

Index